Handbook of
Pediatric Dentistry

FIFTH EDITION

Handbook of Pediatric Dentistry

Edited by

ANGUS C. CAMERON, BDS (Hons), MDSC, FDSRCS (Eng), MRACDS (Paed), FRACDS, FICD, FADI
Specialist in Private Practice
Paediatric Dentistry
Sydney
Visiting Associate Professor
University of Newcastle (AUS)
Charles Sturt University (NSW) and the University of Leeds (UK)
NSW
Australia

RICHARD P. WIDMER, BDSc (Hons), MDSc (Melb), FRACDS, FICD
Head, Department of Dentistry
Sydney Children's Hospital Network
Westmead Sydney
Clinical Associate Professor
Paediatric Dentistry
The University of Sydney
Senior Consultant
Paediatric Dentistry
Westmead Hospital
NSW
Australia

For additional online content visit ExpertConsult.com

ELSEVIER

ELSEVIER

HANDBOOK OF PEDIATRIC DENTISTRY, FIFTH EDITION

First edition 1997
Second edition 2003
Third edition 2008
Fourth edition 2013

Notices

Practitioners and researchers must always rely on their own experience and knowledge in evaluating and using any information, methods, compounds or experiments described herein. Because of rapid advances in the medical sciences, in particular, independent verification of diagnoses and drug dosages should be made. To the fullest extent of the law, no responsibility is assumed by Elsevier, authors, editors, or contributors for any injury and/or damage to persons or property as a matter of products liability, negligence or otherwise, or from any use or operation of any methods, products, instructions, or ideas contained in the material herein.

ISBN: 978-0-7020-7985-6

Printed in India
Last digit is the print number: 9   8   7   6   5   4   3   2   1

Content Strategist: Alexandra Mortimer
Content Development Specialist: Veronika Watkins
Project Manager: Umarani Natarajan
Publishing Services Manager: Shereen Jameel
Design: Patrick Ferguson
Illustration Manager: Narayanan Ramakrishnan

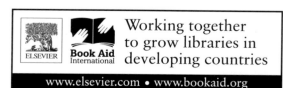

CONTENTS

APPENDICES

I find it a great honour to write a foreword for this fifth edition of the *Handbook of Paediatric Dentistry* which is edited by Angus C. Cameron and Richard P. Widmer. I have had the pleasure of interacting with these fine paediatric dentists over the past four decades. Through organized dentistry and academia our collaborations have been intertwined, efforts always focused on improving the oral health of infants, children, adolescents and children with special healthcare needs.

I have always been impressed with the *Handbook of Paediatric Dentistry* which Angus and Richard have so thoroughly put together. Many of the cases presented in the handbook were patients seen at Westmead Hospital, where both Angus and Richard were faculty members for a number of years. I came to appreciate not only the patient experience provided at Westmead but also the vast amount of clinical information that has been made available to dentists throughout the world to help them provide the best possible care for their patients.

In these trying times of the coronavirus, infecting adults and children, paediatric dentistry has had to face challenges. The need for personal protective equipment, which was difficult to obtain at the onset of the pandemic, emphasizes that oral healthcare is a medical necessity, and providing oral healthcare with the utmost safety for patients and the dental team has been at the forefront of our recent endeavours when offering optimal oral care to the children we see. This pandemic will bring paediatric dentistry to the highest level of research and patient care, always focused on what is best for children.

I extend my thanks to all dentists who treat children, to Angus and Richard for this new edition of the handbook published in six languages and to the reader who will respect the Handbook for what it is intended for: optimal oral health for children.

Respectfully,
Kevin J. Donly, DDS, MS
Immediate Past-President
American Academy of Pediatric Dentistry

Professor and Chair
Department of Developmental Dentistry
UT Health San Antonio

PREFACE

Well, here we are, almost a decade on from the last edition and 24 years from our first.

Our first edition grew from our undergraduate student notes in a way we could not have anticipated, and to have expanded internationally was fanciful, but here we are, a popular contemporary handbook now translated into eight languages.

We all expect change, but the reality of the pace and extent of change is always a surprise. Take the concepts in cariology, for example, with the extensive inputs from biochemistry, microbiology, genetics and public health! These extensive changes flow onto all aspects of paediatric restorative oral health care from what the clinician can offer, what our families can expect and what the community expects. However, it is the much broader concept of the paediatric oral physician that has become our overall focus, and it is this focus that we hope comes through even more strongly in this fifth edition.

For the clinician, it is striving to practice with a mindset that is tempered and improved by lifelong learning and practice that brings with it the immense, spiritual satisfaction of helping others. For the child patient who has a "good" experience of dentistry, there is an everlasting positive memory that hopefully brings about a desire for maintaining their oral health as they become adults.

As far as the community is concerned, it is now recognised, more than ever, that oral health is part of total health and cannot be ignored. Recent declarations from several important institutions have reinforced the previous impetus from the US Surgeon General and the United Nations (UN) and provide a new impetus for this integration to be actively promoted by dental clinicians. To recap:

In 2000, the final summary from the US Surgeon General's Report on Oral Health in America stated, 'You cannot have health without oral health.' This report received wide international acceptance and drove the UN to eventually pass an important resolution in 2011.

This UN resolution on Prevention and Control of Non-Communicable Diseases recognized, for the first time ever, that oral diseases are public health problems worldwide.

The World Health Organization resolution of 2016 further supports this by stressing that children are a priority group for prevention. Oral health assessment needs to be part of all routine community activities, such as immunisation, dietary advice, well-baby checks, infant record keeping and so on.

More recently, *The Lancet* (2019) published an editorial and two influential articles on oral health, as well as five further short comments in response to these articles.

In addition, the American Academy of Pediatrics made a strong policy statement (October 2020): Maintaining and Improving the Oral Health of Young Children; and the Australian government (2019) published Clinical Guidelines on Pregnancy Care 2019 which stressed the importance of inculcating oral health during pregnancy.

However, the extent of the global oral health disaster cannot be underestimated. Untreated caries in children is associated with impaired quality of life including pain, feeding problems, disturbed sleep and absence from school. Furthermore, severe caries early in life may affect the child's growth and development, especially when left untreated.

Dental decay is the most common chronic childhood disease of children 5 to 17 years, on a par with cardiovascular disease, asthma and diabetes. Dental decay is five times more common than asthma and seven times more common than hay fever, affecting over 600 million preschool children worldwide.

Untreated dental caries in permanent teeth is the most prevalent disease (35% for all ages combined) across all medical conditions assessed in the Global Burden of Disease Study with at least 2.4 billion individuals affected (Marcenes et al., 2015).

In addition, oral diseases are the fourth most expensive human disease to treat. Current annual European Union spending of €79 billion is predicted to reach €93 billion by 2020, with 5% to 10% of public health expenditure relating to oral health. Globally, there is an increase in the burden of oral disease especially in countries with emerging economies.

What is our role in addressing these inequalities in our communities? Paediatric dental clinicians need to be integral in this drive to raise awareness of the problems to which poor oral health leads. There needs to be a greater involvement with our local "health community" and regular communication with all our other health colleagues, health bureaucrats and government organisations. This contact may be in the form of a "care plan" for a patient, sent to their general medical practitioners, or outlining concerns about a government programme to bureaucrats. Whatever the activity, it will help raise awareness of paediatric dental health. We need to act as paediatric oral physicians. This embraces the aspiration of total patient care, a model expressing the broad scope of child development and oral health.

This handbook, our 5th edition, will provide the interested clinician with the information, evidence and support to provide up to date, safe, contemporary paediatric oral health care—from chairside to the community—and help to address the huge challenges in paediatric oral health not only in your local setting but in all countries and have children's oral health at the forefront of our children's total health.

We are extremely grateful to all the members of the Australasian Academy of Paediatric Dentistry and our international colleagues for their support in the publication of this book.

Angus C. Cameron and *Richard P. Widmer*
Westmead, Sydney, Australia
May 2021

The editor(s) would like to acknowledge and offer grateful thanks for the input of all previous editions' contributors, without whom this new edition would not have been possible.

Paul Abbott, BDSc (WA), MDS (Adel), FRACDS (Endo)
Winthrop Professor of Clinical Dentistry
UWA Dental School/Oral Health Centre of Western Australia (OHCWA)
The University of Western Australia
Australia

Eduardo A. Alcaino, BDS (Hons), MDSc, FRACDS, MRACDS
Grad. Dip. Clin. Dent (Sedation)
Specialist Paediatric Dentist
Specialist Clinical Associate
University of Sydney
Visiting Specialist Westmead Centre for Oral Health
Principal
Sydney Paediatric Dentistry P/L

Johan KM Aps, DDS, MSc Paed Dent, MSc DMFR, PhD
Oral Health Care
Artevelde University of Applied Sciences
Gent
Belgium

Mariana Pinheiro Araujo, PhD, BDS
NHS Education for Scotland
Dental Clinical Effectiveness
Dundee Dental Education Centre – DDEC, Small's Wynd
Dundee
UK

Wendy Bellis, BDS, MSc (Paed Dent)
Specialist Paediatric Dentist and Honorary Clinical Senior Teaching Fellow
The Eastman Dental Institute
University College London
UK

Angus C. Cameron, BDS (Hons), MDSC, FDSRCS (Eng), MRACDS (Paed), FRACDS, FICD, FADI
Specialist in Private Practice
Paediatric Dentistry
Sydney
Australia;
Visiting Associate Professor at the University of Newcastle
Charles Sturt University (NSW) and the University of Leeds (UK)
NSW
Australia

Yasmi O. Crystal, DMD, MSc
Clinical Professor
Pediatric Dentistry
New York University, College of Dentistry
New York
USA

Marcio da Fonseca, DDS, MS
Professor and Head
Pediatric Dentistry
University of Illinois at Chicago
Illinois
USA

Julia Dando, BDS (Wales), MMedSci (Sheffield), FDSRCS (Edin), MOrthRCS (Eng), MRACDS (Orth)
Orthodontist
Cleft and Craniofacial Services
The Childrens Hospital at Westmead
NSW
Australia

Stephen Fayle
Consultant and Honorary Senior Clinical
    Lecturer in Paediatric Dentistry
School of Dentistry
University of Leeds;
Consultant
Leeds Dental Institute
Leeds
UK

John Featherstone, PhD, MSc
Professor of Preventive and Restorative
    Dental Sciences at the University of
    California
San Francisco (UCSF) and Dean of the
    School of Dentistry
California
USA

Anastasia Georgoiu, BDS, MDSc, MRACDS (Oral Med), FRACDS, FICD, FOMAA
Oral Medicine
Macquarie Oral & Maxillofacial Specialists
Sydney
NSW
Australia

Mike Harrison, BDS, MScD, FDS RCS, MPhil
Consultant in Paediatric Dentistry
Department of Paediatric Dentistry
Guy's and St Thomas' Hospitals
London
UK

Andrew A.C. Heggie, MBBS, MDSc, BDSc, FRACDS (OMS), FFDRSC (I), FRCS (Ed)
Professor
Oral and Maxillofacial Surgery Unit,
    Department of Plastic and Maxillofacial
    Surgery
Royal Children's Hospital of Melbourne
Parkville
Victoria
Australia

Nicola Innes, PhD, BDS, BMSc, BSc, MFDS, MFGDP
Professor
Child Dental and Oral Health
University of Dundee
Dundee
Fife
UK

Evelina Kratunova, BDS, MDS, DChDent, FFD
Clinical Associate Professor
Department of Pediatric Dentistry
College of Dentistry, University of Illinois
    Chicago
Illinois
USA

James Lucas AM, BSc, BDSc, MDSc, FRACDS, FICD
Paediatric Dentist Principal
Lucas Dental Care
Paediatric Dental Specialist
Clinical Associate Professor
University of Melbourne
Parkville
Victoria
Australia

Erin Mahoney, BDS (Otago), MDSc (Syd), PhD (Syd), FRACDS
Specialist Paediatric Dentist
Hutt Valley District Health Board
Clinical Senior Lecturer
University of Otago
New Zealand

Cheryl B. McNeil, PhD
Professor
Psychology
West Virginia University
Morgantown
West Virginia
USA

Daniel W. McNeil, PhD
Eberly Distinguished Professor
Departments of Psychology, and Dental
    Practice & Rural Health
West Virginia University
Morgantown
West Virginia
USA

Benjamin Moran, MBBS, BMedSci (Hons), MMedStats, FANZCA, FCICM
Specialist Anaesthetist
Dept of Anaesthesia and Pain Medicine
Gosford Hospital
NSW
Australia

Neeta Prabhu, BDS (Bombay), MDS (Mangalore), MPhil (Newcastle upon Tyne), MRACDS (Paed), FRACDS FICD
Staff Specialist
Head of Discipline, Paediatric Dentistry,
    Sydney School of Dentistry, Faculty of
    Medicine and Health
Staff Specialist, Paediatric Dentistry,
    Westmead Centre for Oral Health, Western
    Sydney Local Health District
NSW
Australia

Mark Robertson, BDS, MSc, MFDSRCS (Ed)
Clinical Lecturer in Paediatric Dentistry
School of Dentistry
University of Dundee
UK

Clement Seeballuck, BA, BDentSc, MFDS RCS (Ed)
Clinical Lecturer
Paediatric Dentistry
Dundee Dental School, University of Dundee
UK

Marc Semper
Endodontist
Bremen
Germany

Sarah Starr, MHealthScEduc, BAppSc (Speech Pathology)
Director, Speech Pathologist
Speech Pathology
Speech Pathology Services
Burwood
NSW
Australia

Richard Steffen, Dr. WBA KZM SSO
Clinic for Paediatric Oral Health
UZB University Center for Dental Medicine
Basel
Switzerland

Svante Twetman, Odont Dr
Professor
Odontology
University of Copenhagen
Copenhagen
Denmark

Richard P. Widmer, BDSc (Hons), MDSc (Melb), FRACDS, FICD
Head, Department of Dentistry, Sydney
    Children's Hospital Network
Westmead
Clinical Associate Professor, Paediatric
    Dentistry
The University of Sydney
Senior Consultant, Paediatric Dentistry
Westmead Hospital
NSW
Australia

The editors are extremely grateful for the support of all those involved in the teaching of paediatric dentistry throughout Australia and New Zealand and the members of the Australasian Academy of Paediatric Dentistry. The international list of contributors reflects the depth of experience in paediatric oral health care that has been gathered to complete our fifth edition.

We would especially like to thank the staff of Westmead Hospital and the Children's Hospital at Westmead, particularly Mr Paul De Sensi, Chief Medical Photographer, and Mr John Yeats, Medical Photographer. We would also like to give special thanks to the many registrars who have worked in our departments for their support.

Our families and close friends must not go unmentioned for their quiet support and encouragement; and finally, we would like to thank our child patients, the responsibility of whose care we are entrusted with. They give us wonder as we watch them grow, the joy in our daily work and the motivation for our endeavours.

CONTRIBUTORS TO PREVIOUS EDITIONS

The Editors would like to acknowledge the great support and contributions made to the earlier editions by the following people, who made this book possible:

Michael J. Aldred
BDS (Wales) PhD (Wales) GradCertEd (QUT) FDS RCS (Eng) FRCPath (UK) FFOP (RCPA)

Sherene Alexander
BDS (**Mangalore**) MDS (**Mangalore**) MRACDS (**Paed**) FRACDS FICD

Anthony Blinkhorn
OBE

Louise Brearley Messer
AM BDSc LDS MDSc (**Melb**) PhD (**Minn**)

Roland Bryant
MDS (**Syd**) PhD FRACDS

Santo Cardaci
BDSc Hons (**WA**) MDSc (**Adel**) FRACDS

Peter J.M. Crawford
BDS, MScD, FDSRCS (**Edin**), FDSRCS (**Eng**), FRCPCH

Michael G. Cooper
MB BS FANZCA FFPMANZCA

Peter J. Cooper
BSc MB ChB MRCP (**UK**)

Bernadette Drummond
BDS (**Otago**) PhD FRACDS

Rebecca Eggers
BDS (**Syd**) MDSc (**Syd**) FRACDS

John Fricker
BDS MDSc (**Syd**) Grad Dip Adult Ed FRACDS

Peter Gregory
BDSc MDSc (**WA**) FRACDS

Roger K. Hall
OAM MDSc (**Melb**) FRACDS FICD

Kerrod B. Hallett
BDSc (**Hons**) MDSc (**Qld**) FRACDS

Linda Hayes-Cameron
BPsyc (**Hons**) (**UNE**) MPsyc (**Macq**) BHeathSc (**Nursing**)

Fiona Heard
BDSc (**Melb**) LDS MDSc (**Syd**) FRACDS

Justine Hemmings
B App Sc (**Speech Path**)

Sally Hibbert
BDS MPhil (**Liverpool**) FDS (**Paed Dent**) RCS

David Isaacs
MB BChir MD MRCP FRACP

Tissa Jayasekera
MDSc (**Melb**) MDS (**Syd**) FRACDS

Timothy Johnston
BDSc (**WA**) MDSc (**Melb**) FRACDS FADI

Allison Kakakios
MB BS (**Hons**) FRACP

Om P. Kharbanda
BDS (**Lucknow**) MDS (**Lucknow**) MOthRCS (**Edin**) MMEd (Dundee)

Nicky Kilpatrick
BDS (**Birm**) PhD (**Newcastle**) FDSRCPS FRACDS (**Paed**)

Nigel M. King
BDS Hons (**Lond**) MSc Hons (**Lond**) PhD (**Hong Kong**) LDSRCS (**Eng**) FDSRCS (**Edin**) FDSRCS (**Eng**) MRACDS (**Paed Dent**) FHKAM (**Dent Surg**) FCDSHK (**Paed Dent**)

Linda Kingston
B App Sci (**Speech Path**)

Peter King
MDS (**Syd**)

Judy Kirk
MB BS (**Syd**) FRACP

Sandy Lopacki
MA (**Speech Path**) (**Northwestern**)
CCC-ASHA

James Lucas
MDSc (**Melb**) MS (**LaTrobe**) FRACDS
LDS

Simrit Malhi
BDS (**Hons**) (**Punjab**) MDS (**PGIMER**)
MRACDS (**Paed**) FDSRCS (**Eng**)

Jane McDonald
MB BS (**NSW**) FANZCA

David J. Manton
BDSc MDSc PhD FRACDS FICD

Kareen Mekertichian
BDS (**Hons**) MDSc FRACDS FPFA FICD

Craig Munns
MBBS PhD FRACP

Stephen O'Flaherty
MB ChB FRACP FAFRM

Christopher Olsen
MDSc (**Melb**) FRACDS

Sarah Raphael
BDS (**Adel**) MDSc (**Syd**) FRACDS

Tony Sandler
BDS (**Witw**) HD Dent (**Witw**)

Mark Schifter
BDS MDSc (**Syd**) MSND RCS (**Edin**)
MOM RCS (**Edin**) FFD RCSI (**Oral Med**)
FRACDS (**Oral Med**) FICD

Sarah Starr
B AppSci (**Speech Path**), M Health Sci (**Ed**),
CPSP

Neil Street
MB BS (**NSW**) MAppSci (**UTS**) FANZCA

Sarah Raphael
BDS (**Adel**) MDSc (**Syd**) FRACDS

Julie Reid
BAppSci (Speech Pathol) (**La Trobe**)
GradDip (Gerontol) (**Syd**) PhD

W. Kim Seow
BDS (**Adel**) MDSc (**Qld**) DDSc PhD
FRACDS

Margarita Silva
CD (**Mexico**) MS (**Minn**)

Joe Verco
BDS (**Adel**) LDS (**Vic**) BSc Dent (**Hons**)
MDS FAAPD

Meredith Wilson
MBBS, FRACP, MBioeth

John Winters
BDSc MDSc (UWA) FICD

Peter Wong
BDS (**Hons**) MDSc (**Syd**) FRACDS

CHAPTER 1

The philosophy of paediatric dentistry: What is paediatric dentistry?

Richard P. Widmer ■ Angus C. Cameron

What is paediatric dentistry?

Paediatric dentistry is a specialty based not on a particular skill set, but rather encompassing all dentistry's technical skills against a philosophical background of understanding child development in health and disease. This latest edition of the handbook emphasizes again the broader picture in treating children (Appendix J). A dental visit is no longer just a dental visit; it should be regarded as a 'health visit'. We are part of the team of health professionals who contribute to the well-being of children, both in an individual context and at the wider community level. Children often slip through childhood to adolescence seemingly in the blink of an eye, and family life is more pressured and demanding. Commonly, children spend more time on social media than

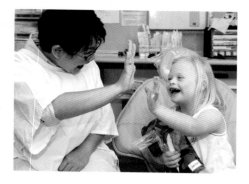

Figure 1.1 The dental visit should be a positive experience. Children with special needs may present different challenges in their care; however, their involvement and joy are the greatest reward.

interacting directly with family and friends, and more than ever, the major influences on their lives come from outside the family.

The pattern of childhood illness has changed, and, with it, clinical practice. Children presenting for treatment may have survived cancer, may have a well-managed chronic disease or may have significant behavioural and learning disorders (Figure 1.1). There are increasing, sometimes unrealistic, expectations among parents/carers that the care of their children should be easily and readily accessible and pain-free and result in flawless aesthetics.

Caries and dental disease should be seen as reflective of the family's social condition, and the dental team should be part of the community.

Your [patients] don't have to become your friends, but they are part of your social context and that gives them a unique status in your life. Treat them with respect and take them seriously and your practice will become to feel part of the neighbourhood, part of the community.
(HUGH MACKAY, PSYCHOLOGIST, SOCIAL RESEARCHER AND NOVELIST)

In the evolving dynamics of dental practice, we feel that it is important to change, philosophically, the traditional 'adversarial nature' of the dental experience. It is well recognized that for too many, the dental experience has been traumatic. This has resulted in a significant proportion of the adult population accessing dental care only episodically, for the relief of pain. Thus, it is vital to see a community, and consumer, perspective in the provision of paediatric dental services. The successful practice of paediatric dentistry is not merely the completion of any operative procedure but also ensuring a positive dental outcome for the future oral health behaviour of that individual and family. To this end, an understanding of child development – physical, cognitive and psychosocial – is paramount. The clinician must be comfortable and skilled in talking to children, and interpersonal skills are essential.

Patient assessment: history

A clinical history should be taken in a logical and systematic way for each patient and should be updated regularly. Thorough history-taking is a skill. It may be time consuming and requires practice. However, it is an opportunity to get to know the child and family. Furthermore, the history facilitates the diagnosis of many conditions, even before the clinical examination. There are often specific questions pertinent to a child's medical history that will be relevant to their management, thus it is desirable that parents be present. The understanding of medical conditions that can compromise treatment is essential, and this will be expanded on in later chapters. Be aware that the parent(s) or carer(s) may be unaware of the full medical and/or social history of the child. This may be the case in those children who are adopted or are the offspring of differing social arrangements.

Clinicians need to be empathetic and flexible with their history-taking that may require a private discussion with the carers.

The purpose of the examination is not merely to check for caries or periodontal disease, as paediatric dentistry encompasses all areas of growth and development. Having the opportunity to see the child regularly, the dentist can often be the first to recognize significant diseases and anomalies.

CURRENT COMPLAINTS

The history of any current problems should be carefully documented.

- Assessment of pain
  Nature and type (e.g., acute, chronic, aching, sharp, dull)
  Onset and duration
  Exacerbating factors (e.g., biting, cold or heat)
  Relieving factors (e.g., relief with analgesics)

Remember that dental pain in children is usually episodic, and the first presentation of the child as a patient to your practice may be because of pain. A wakeful night with a child in pain that is not relieved by analgesics is a huge incentive for a parent to seek care. However, this may give rise to unrealistic expectations on the part of the carer as to the ability of the clinician to resolve the cause of the pain at the initial appointment, especially if the child has multiple carious teeth. From a specialist perspective, once a referral has been made, the child is frequently in no discomfort at all having had to wait a period of time before attending the specialist appointment.

- Parental concerns

DENTAL HISTORY

- Previous treatment; how the child has coped with other forms of treatment.
- Eruption times and dental development.
- What preventive treatment has been undertaken previously.
- Methods of behaviour management used previously.

MEDICAL HISTORY

For the majority of children, taking a medical history will be uncomplicated. These following questions will cover most major issues for fit and well children:

- Has your child had any serious illnesses?
- Have they been admitted to hospital or had any operations?
- Are they taking any medications?
- Have they any allergies?

If the answer to all of these is 'No', then it is safe to assume that the child is generally fit and well, and it is not necessary to ask about each body-system.

Notwithstanding this, when required, a more thorough medical history is needed, and this should be undertaken in a systematic fashion, covering all system areas of the body. The major areas include:

- Cardiovascular system (e.g., cardiac lesions, blood pressure, rheumatic fever).
- Central nervous system (e.g., seizures, cognitive delay).
- Endocrine system (e.g., diabetes).
- Gastrointestinal tract (e.g., GORD, coeliacs).
- Respiratory tract (e.g., asthma, bronchitis, upper respiratory tract infections).
- Bleeding tendencies (including family history of bleeding problems).

- Urogenital system (renal disease, ureteric reflux).
- Allergies – note the type of reaction
- Past operations or hospital admissions.
- Current treatment and medications.
- Specialists involved in the care of the child

It is always preferable to communicate with the specialist physician responsible for the care of the child; however, the child's general medical practitioner should also be informed if any major treatment is undertaken.

PREGNANCY (OBSTETRIC) HISTORY

It is important to keep in mind that asking about obstetric history maybe triggering for some parents/carers, as they may not be expecting such questioning at a dental consultation. Introduce the topic in general terms and be prepared to leave the topic to a later stage if it is obviously a sensitive topic.

- Gestational age (full term is considered to between 38 and 42 weeks).
- Birth weight.
- APGAR (appearance, pulse, grimace, activity, and respiration) scores.
- Delivery: natural birth, assisted delivery, Caesarean section – elective (planned) or emergency
- Antenatal and perinatal problems, especially during delivery.
- Prematurity and management in a special care or neonatal intensive care unit.
- Feeding: breast/bottle, duration and transition to solids.

Obstetric history is an essential part in the taking of a paediatric history. As will be discussed in later chapters, the formation of both primary and permanent teeth provides a record of past disease experience. The ameloblast is exquisitely sensitive to changes in oxygen saturation and temperature. Consequently, those teeth that are calcifying at delivery, namely the second primary molars and the first permanent molars, are often affected by foetal distress or perinatal infection for example. Children who are born severely preterm may demonstrate anomalies in their primary dentition.

GROWTH AND DEVELOPMENT

In many countries, an infant record book is issued to parents to record postnatal growth and development, childhood illness and visits to health providers. Areas of questioning should include:
- Developmental milestones and motor skills
- Height and weight over time (see Appendix L)

Single growth measurements are not as important as growth velocity
- Speech and language development (see Chapter 15).
- Socialization.

CURRENT MEDICAL TREATMENT

- Medications, including complementary medications.
- Current treatment and care.
- Immunizations.

FAMILY AND SOCIAL HISTORY

- Family history of serious illness or inherited conditions.
- Siblings.

- Family pedigree tree (see Appendix N).
- Schooling, performance in class, social issues.
- Speech and language problems.
- Pets/hobbies or other interests.

This last area is useful in beginning to establish a common interest and a rapport with the child and the parent. When asking questions and collecting information, it is important to use lay terminology. For example, the distinction between rheumatic fever and rheumatism may often be not be understood, and more specific questioning may be required. Furthermore, questions regarding family and social history must be neither offensive nor intrusive. An explanation of the need for this information is helpful and appropriate. It is important to recognize the changing patterns of family units, and the carer accompanying the child may not always have a full knowledge of the past medical history.

Examination

EXTRAORAL EXAMINATION

The extraoral examination should be one of general appraisal of the child's well-being. The clinician should observe the child's gait on entering the surgery and the general interaction with the parents or peers in the surgery. A regular assessment of height and weight is useful, and dentists should routinely measure both height and weight and plot these measurements on a growth chart (see Appendix L).

A general physical examination should be conducted. In some circumstances, this may require examination of the chest, abdomen and extremities. Although this is often not common practice in a general dental surgery setting, there may be situations where this is required (e.g., checking for other injuries after trauma, assessing manifestations of syndromes or medical conditions). Speech and language are also assessed at this stage (see Chapter 15).

The following should be assessed:
- Facial symmetry, dimensions and the basic orthodontic facial types.
- Eyes, including appearance of the globe, sclera, pupils and conjunctiva.
- Movements of the globe that may indicate squints or palsy.
- Skin colour and appearance.
- Temporomandibular joints.
- Cervical, submandibular and occipital lymph nodes.

INTRAORAL EXAMINATION (Figure 1.2)

- Soft tissues.

  Soft tissue examination should include the oropharynx, tonsils, soft palate and uvula. It is important to identify upper airway obstruction early. Snoring and sleep apnoea affect up to 5% of children and may lead to issues with growth and development, cognition, behaviour and school performance (Figure 1.3).

  Abnormalities or lesions should be documented and photographed (see Chapter 10).
- Oral hygiene and periodontal status.

  Gingivitis is common in children, but periodontitis is rare and often associated with systemic disease. An oral hygiene assessment is an introduction to all aspects of preventive oral healthcare. As a grading system, the CPITN (Community Periodontal Index of Treatment Needs) is the most convenient to use.
- Quantity and quality of saliva.
- Dental hard tissues.

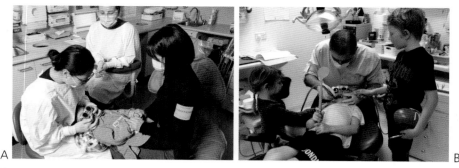

Figure 1.2 (A) One of the most convenient ways in which to examine very young children is in the knee-to-knee position with the child's head in the dentist's lap. The child can see the parent, who gently restrains the arms. This gives an excellent view of the upper teeth and jaws, in a similar position to normal operating in a dental chair. (B) Involving children in their dental care.

Dental charting is the standard procedure that should be thorough and detail the current state of the dentition and the plan for future treatment. It is our way of systematically documenting pathology (caries), anomalies and tooth substance loss and provides a record of past treatment.

Occlusion and orthodontic relations

The child should be assessed for skeletal and dental problems and abnormalities of functions of the stomatognathic system. Clinical assessment is performed in all the three dimensions of space, that is, vertical, anteroposterior and transverse (Figure 1.4).

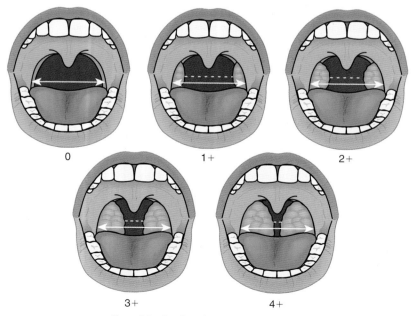

Figure 1.3 Grading of tonsillar enlargement.

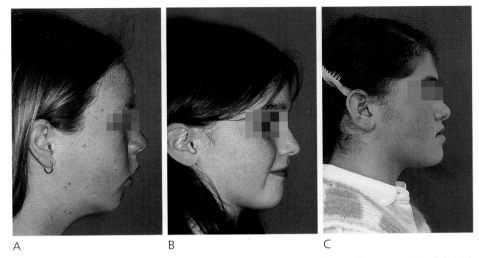

A   B   C

Figure 1.4 Evaluation of facial profile. (A) Child with retrognathic chin and convex face suggestive of skeletal: class II pattern. (B) Class I pattern. (C) Prominent chin with concave profile, suggestive of class III skeletal pattern.

Skeletal classification; this describes the anteroposterior relationship between the maxilla and mandible relative to the cranial base:

- Skeletal class I: the maxilla and mandible are in an orthognathic relationship.
- Skeletal class II: the mandible appears small relative to the maxilla (retrognathic). This could be because of a small mandible, a large maxilla or a combination of both.
- Skeletal class III: the mandible appears larger than the maxilla (prognathic). This could be attributed to a large mandible, a small maxilla or a combination of both.

DENTAL RELATIONSHIPS

Dental relationships are recorded with the teeth in occlusion. Angle's classification of malocclusion is based on the relationship of the upper and lower first permanent molars.

MOLAR RELATIONSHIP (Figure 1.5)

- Class I implies an anteroposterior relationship with the mesio-buccal cusp of the upper first permanent molar occluding between the mesial and distal cusps of the lower first permanent molar.
- Class II molar relationship implies distoocclusion of the lower first permanent molar with the upper first permanent molar and is a reflection of a retrognathic skeletal pattern with increased over jet.
- Class III molar relationship implies a mesially positioned lower first permanent molar and is a reflection of a prognathic mandible and anterior cross-bite.

INCISOR RELATIONSHIP (Figure 1.6)

- Class II division 1 (proclined upper incisors).
- Class II division 2 (retroclined upper incisors).

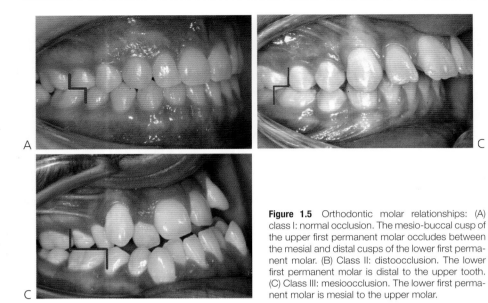

Figure 1.5 Orthodontic molar relationships: (A) class I: normal occlusion. The mesio-buccal cusp of the upper first permanent molar occludes between the mesial and distal cusps of the lower first permanent molar. (B) Class II: distoocclusion. The lower first permanent molar is distal to the upper tooth. (C) Class III: mesioocclusion. The lower first permanent molar is mesial to the upper molar.

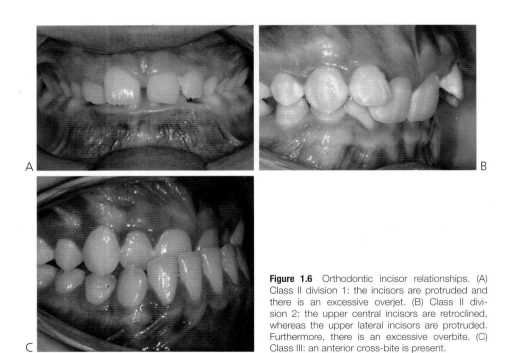

Figure 1.6 Orthodontic incisor relationships. (A) Class II division 1: the incisors are protruded and there is an excessive overjet. (B) Class II division 2: the upper central incisors are retroclined, whereas the upper lateral incisors are protruded. Furthermore, there is an excessive overbite. (C) Class III: an anterior cross-bite is present.

- Class III cross-bite of the anterior segment or negative over jet.
  Vertical assessment includes normal or abnormal vertical overlap of the incisors, that is, normal, deep or open bite.
  Transverse assessment should include any cross-bite or scissors-bite of the buccal segments of the dental arches.

Special examinations

RADIOGRAPHY AND OTHER IMAGING

The guidelines for prescribing radiographs in dental practice are presented in Appendix I. The overriding principle in taking radiographs of children must be to minimize exposure to ionizing radiation consistent with the provision of the most appropriate treatment. Radiographs are essential for accurate diagnosis. If, however, the information gained from such an investigation does not influence treatment decisions, both the timing and the need for the radiograph should be questioned. Paediatric radiology is discussed in Appendix I.

PULP SENSIBILITY TESTING

- Thermal (i.e., carbon dioxide pencil).
- Electrical stimulation.
- Percussion.
- Mobility.
- Transillumination.

BLOOD INVESTIGATIONS (see Appendix A)

- Full blood count with differential white cell count.
- Clinical chemistry.

MICROBIOLOGICAL INVESTIGATIONS

- Culture of microorganisms and antibiotic sensitivity.
- Cytology.
- Serology.
- Direct and indirect immunofluorescence.

ANATOMICAL PATHOLOGY

- Histological examination of biopsy specimens.
- Hard-tissue sectioning (e.g., diagnosis of enamel anomalies; see Figure 9.26).
- Scanning and transmission electron microscopy (e.g., hair from children with ectodermal dysplasia; see Figure 9.2B).

PHOTOGRAPHY

Extraoral and intraoral photography provides an invaluable record of growing children. It is important as a legal document in cases of abuse or trauma, or as an aid in the diagnosis of anomalies or syndromes. Consent will need to be obtained for photography.

DIAGNOSTIC CASTS

Casts are essential in orthodontic or complex restorative treatment planning, and for general record keeping.

CARIES ACTIVITY TESTS (see Chapter 4)

Although these are not definitive for individuals, they may be useful as an indicator of caries risk. Furthermore, identification of defects in salivation in children with medical conditions may point to significant caries susceptibility. Such tests include assessment of:

- Diet history.
- Salivary flow rates.
- Salivary buffering capacity.
- *Streptococcus mutans* and *Lactobacillus* colony counts.

Steps in diagnosis

Differential diagnosis: This is a list of all the possible diagnoses that, with further investigation and examination, is refined to the provisional diagnosis.

Provisional diagnosis: This should be formulated for every patient. Whether the child has early childhood caries, simple periodontal disease such as gingivitis or any other pathology or functional issue, it is important to make an assessment of the current conditions that are present. This will influence the ordering of special examinations and the final diagnosis and treatment planning.

Definitive diagnosis: The final diagnosis determines the final treatment plan.

Assessment of disease risk (see Chapter 4)

All children should have an 'assessment of disease risk' before the final treatment plan is determined. This is particularly important in the planning of preventive care for children with caries. This assessment should be based on:

- Past disease experience.
- Current dental status.
- Family history and carer status.
- Diet considerations.
- Oral hygiene.
- Concomitant medical conditions.
- Future expectations of disease activity.

Social factors, including recent migration, language barriers and ethnic and cultural diversities, can impact access to dental care and will therefore influence caries risk.

LOW RISK OF DISEASE

- No caries present.
- Favourable family history (appropriate diet, dentally healthy siblings, motivated parents and caregivers).
- Good oral hygiene.
- Access to community water fluoridation.

MODERATE RISK

- One or two new lesions per year.

HIGH RISK OR FUTURE HIGH RISK

- Three or more new lesions per year.
- Orthodontic treatment.
- Chronic illness or hospitalization.
- Medically compromised children.
- Social risk factors.

TREATMENT PLAN

1. Emergency care and relief of pain.
2. Preventive care.
3. Surgical treatment.
4. Restorative treatment.
5. Orthodontic treatment.
6. Extensive restorative or further surgical management.
7. Recall and review.

Clinical conduct

INFECTION CONTROL

It is now considered that 'universal precautions' are the expected standard of care in current paediatric dental practice. The principles of universal precautions are:

- Prevention of contamination by strictly limiting and clearly identifying a 'zone of contamination'.
- The need for elimination of contamination should be minimal if this zone of contamination is observed.

Universal precautions regard every patient as being potentially infectious. Although it is possible to identify some patients who are known to be infectious, there are many others who have an unknown infectious state. It is impossible to totally eliminate infection; thus, observing universal precautions is a sensible approach to minimizing the risk of cross-infection.

All children must be protected with safety glasses, and clinicians must also wear protective clothing, eyewear, masks and gloves when treating patients.

RECORDING OF CLINICAL NOTES

Care must be taken when recording clinical information. Notes are legal documents and must be legible. Clinical notes should be succinct. The treatment plan should be reassessed at each session so that at each subsequent appointment, the clinician knows what work is planned. Furthermore, at the completion of the treatment for the day, a note should be made regarding the work to be done at the next visit.

CONSENT FOR TREATMENT (see Chapter 3)

There is often little provision in a dental file for a signed consent for dental treatment. The consent for a dentist to carry out treatment, be it cleaning of teeth or surgical extraction, is implied when the parent or guardian and child attend the surgery. It is incumbent on the practitioner, however, to provide all the necessary information and detail in such a way as to enable 'informed consent'. This includes explaining the treatment using appropriate language to facilitate a complete understanding of proposed treatment plans.

It is important to record that the treatment plan has been discussed and that consent has been given for treatment. This consent would cover the period required to complete the work outlined. If there is any significant alteration to the original treatment plan (e.g., an extraction that was not previously anticipated), then consent should be obtained again from the parent or guardian and recorded in the file.

Generally, when undertaking clinical work on a child patient, it is good practice to advise the parent or guardian briefly at the commencement of the appointment what is proposed for that appointment. Also, it is helpful to give the parent or guardian and child some idea of the treatment anticipated for the next appointment. This is especially relevant if a more invasive procedure such as the use of local anaesthesia or removal of teeth is contemplated.

SPECIAL NOTES REGARDING ORAL HEALTHCARE FOR CHILDREN IN THE HOSPITAL SETTING

The care of children in hospitals provides many challenges: from the acute presentations in the emergency department to the care of children requiring long-term hospitalization who are seriously ill. Most specialist training programmes will involve some rotation through a children's hospital, and it is the complex day-to-day activity within these institutions where many of the theories and practicalities of your specialist work in paediatric dentistry are put into practice.

As will be discussed in later chapters, children can require oral healthcare and advice from birth. Developmental anomalies of orofacial structures are many and varied, with all tissues being potentially involved. With over 700 syndromes expressing an orofacial manifestation, liaisons with departments such as genetics, ear, nose and throat (ENT/otorhinolaryngology), paediatric surgery, immunology, oncology and many others are essential in providing important diagnostic input and, later, treatment for children.

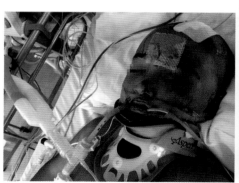
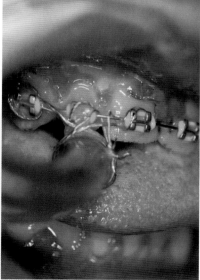

A   B

Figure 1.7 Management of a severely burnt, intubated child in the paediatric intensive care unit. Taping of the endotracheal tube to the corner of the mouth may result in ulceration, scarring and stricture. Placement of passive orthodontic appliances allows the tube to be wired to the teeth and stabilizes the position of the tube in the mouth.

Most university training in dentistry centres around the individual practitioner undertaking the responsibility for a patient's care. In the hospital setting, care must be interdisciplinary (rather than multidisciplinary), where multiple specialists are participating together in the overall care of the child.

It is crucial to build networks with the hospital for the beneficial integration into medical, surgical and allied health departments. Paediatric dentists are unique in the hospital setting, as they are (oral) physicians as well as (oral) surgeons. However, too frequently, the 'dental department' and the 'teeth' are considered separately from the rest of the body. The involvement of the paediatric dental team and the inculcation of appropriate oral health advice into a cardiac or haematology clinic, for example, have so many positive benefits for the journey of a child through their hospital visit. This might include providing dental restorative care concurrently with a child undergoing an ENT procedure under one general anaesthesia session rather than two. Communication, consultation and cooperative relationships with medical and paramedical colleagues are essential to facilitate the best outcome for each child.

It is also essential that the paediatric dentist has sound knowledge, flexibility and ingenuity to solve complex management issues that might never previously have been encountered or published. This might include the construction of an appliance to prevent self-mutilation (see Figure 13.6) or wiring an endotracheal tube in the paediatric intensive care unit (PICU) to the teeth to prevent dislodgement of the tube and lip commissure scarring (Figure 1.7). The incredibly varied nature of the special needs and comorbidities that a clinician is confronted with in a children's hospital makes every clinic and every day a stimulating experience.

CHAPTER 2

Child development, relationships and behaviour management

Richard P. Widmer ■ Daniel W. McNeil ■ Cheryl B. McNeil

Promoting positive behaviour among children, adolescents and their caregivers in the dental surgery

This section is a practical guide for specific modes of interacting in the dental environment which can help produce positive and adherent behaviours in child and adolescent patients, as well as their parents and other caregivers (e.g., grandparents). These guidelines are based on principles and research findings from behavioural dentistry as well as behavioural, developmental, child and paediatric psychology.

It is probably true for most of us that the meaning of our lives is centred on our personal relationships. These are the source of our sense of personal identity; they are the source of our emotional security or insecurity that might define us; they are the source of our greatest joys, of our deepest comforts, but, of course, they are also the source of our most bitter disappointments. However, without personal relationships life for most of us would be meaningless. We might dream of escape to the proverbial 'Desert Island', but we wouldn't want to stay there for more than an hour or two or possibly a week, because we would soon realize that the lifeblood of our lives is in our relationships. That is where we get all the rich material for coping with life (Hugh MacKay, ABC radio, 26 March 2010). So at home and at work, we need to nurture our relationships constantly. In dentistry, this is particularly relevant because we are working intimately, not only with those we are caring for but also with their carers and indeed the entire dental team. We spend a great deal of our waking hours at work, which we want to enjoy as much as possible, and so our relationships become crucial and can be used to positively affect the behaviour of the child in the dental environment.

Much has been written about management of problem behaviour among children receiving oral healthcare, with a focus on the use of various techniques. This guide, however, emphasizes specific, simple methods that can be used with children and adolescents to enhance their comfort and cooperation. The general idea is to use finesse instead of trying to achieve absolute behavioural control. Because a sense of lack of control is one of the major components of anxiety and fear (along with a lack of predictability), using methods that are encouraging rather than demanding can go a long way in promoting comfort in the dental environment.

Dentists, dental hygienists and dental therapists are integral members of the healthcare team for children and adolescents and must have an awareness of practical methods of behaviour management that are based on knowledge of psychological principles and stages of growth and development. The adage that 'children are not small adults' promotes the idea of special knowledge and behaviours that are important in caring for younger dental patients. Oral health professionals must have a knowledge base in child and adolescent medicine, as well as in social, emotional and cultural factors affecting the health and behaviour of this age group.

It is imperative that dental appointments in infancy, childhood and adolescence are positive, as research clearly shows that early experiences have strong effects on whether dental advice and treatment are sought in adulthood. Having a rapport with the parents/caregivers (e.g., grandparents) is essential because they typically are the most influential people in the child's life.

Child behaviour and development

Working with children is, of course, different from working with adults; therefore, it is essential to be familiar with age-appropriate skills and functioning, and development. Infants, children and adolescents are undergoing progressive changes in cognitive, receptive and expressive language; fine and gross motor ability; and social/emotional development. Each child is unique and may develop at varying rates relative to their same-aged peers; for example, one child may present with strong motor skills but less well-developed language, whereas this may be the opposite for another same-age peer.

DEVELOPMENTAL MILESTONES AND ISSUES

There are two essential needs that remain constant from birth to adulthood: the desire to feel important and having an emotional connection with others. Oral health professionals who are aware of their patient's age-appropriate development and needs can use that information to develop a rapport with the child and have appropriate expectations of the behaviour of that particular child in the dental setting.

With international guidelines suggesting dental visits by age 1 year or at the emergence of the first tooth, it is essential that oral healthcare providers be prepared for these earliest dental visits, and to work with their carers, as the interactions are 'triadic' ones that involve not only the child and the provider(s) but the carer as well.

GENERAL DEVELOPMENTAL MILESTONES AND CHILD BEHAVIOUR

Age 3 to 4 months

- In their first 3 to 4 months, babies become extremely interested in their world of people, places and objects.

Age 6 to 8 months

- By 6 to 8 months, infants are discovering new ways to share and express their curiosity, joy, frustration and fear within their world. Babies can shift their attention while keeping in mind the object on which they were focusing. They can look at a teddy bear and be delighted by it, then turn to look at the parents to share those feelings.
- By 8 months, babies are beginning to crawl and discover their surroundings, learning to distinguish differences in their world and people.
- Mobility sets the stage for the first significant appearance of fear. Stranger awareness begins at this time.
- Understanding of spoken words and nonverbal communication (receptive language) develops at a much greater rate than expressive language.
- The infant learns to 'social reference', where he/she shows interest in an object or person and then turns to the parents for emotional feedback. The infant can read the parent's/caregiver's facial expression, tone of voice and words to understand the concept of a particular danger or safety.

Dental implications

- Advice regarding tooth eruption, initial oral hygiene measures and teething.

It is generally accepted that teething has the potential to cause local irritation; however, there is no accepted evidence connecting the systemic symptoms, such as diarrhoea, flushed cheeks and fever, to teething. It is important to seek medical advice if an infant has persistent febrile illness.

Age 9 to 12 months

- By 9 months, two-way conversations about feelings are now possible. Infants become aware of the possibility of others sharing their thoughts and feelings. Understanding and labelling the infant's feelings and experiences can help with relationship building, acceptance and trust.
- Object constancy or permanence is developing in which infants begin to realize that objects and people still exist even when out of sight (e.g., repeatedly throwing the spoon off the high chair and it magically reappearing).
- Separation anxiety is a consequence of this stage and may continue in varying degrees until 18 months.

Dental implications

Children's behaviour is a function of their learning and development, and so it is reasonable to expect that their behaviour in the dental environment will also vary.

- The child has limited ability to understand dental procedures. Nonetheless, with sensitivity to the child's normal emotional development and play expectations, even without cooperation, an oral examination and some treatment can often be accomplished without sedation.
- Good rapport with the parents is required, as the dentist can educate the parent on the importance of sending positive and appropriate feedback to the infant/child about the dental experience.

Age 1 to 3 years (toddler years: egocentric)

- Infants begin to develop a sense of self and explore their autonomy. They may become noncompliant for the first time, as they practise asserting themselves, trying to establish themselves as independent and avoiding situations that make them feel out of control and with a limited sense of self.
- Language develops and 'No' becomes a favourite in their repertoire of words.

- Sharing and cooperative play are meaningless at this stage because the 'toddler rules of ownership' outweigh all concepts, such as: If I see it, it's mine. If it's yours and I want it, it's mine. If it's mine, it's mine and mine only!

Dental implications
- In the dental room, the clinician may identify an object of particular ownership, such as a doll or another toy, and praise the child for taking good care of it rather than trying to remove it.
- Giving toddlers lots of little choices (a choice of two at any time) will assist in enhancing their sense of self and importance, resulting in greater cooperation.
- Preferences for 'boy' and 'girl' objects is common at this age: many toddler boys show interest in cars, trains, the colour blue and other boys, whereas many toddler girls show interest in dolls, fairy dresses, the colour pink and other young girls, for example. Play remains solitary, however, and is 'parallel play' to their peers.
- The ability to communicate varies according to the level of vocabulary development, which is expected to be limited. Thus, the difficulty in communication puts the child in a 'precooperative' stage.
- These children are too young to be reached by words alone, and shyness may mean that the child must be allowed to handle and touch objects to understand their meaning.
- Children of this age typically should be accompanied by a parent or other carer.

Age 3 years

- By this age, children are less egocentric and like to please adults.
- They have very active imaginations and like stories; back-and-forth communication is possible, and children at this age typically have the capacity for some reasoning.
- In times of stress, they will turn to a parent and not accept a stranger's explanation. Typically, these children feel more secure if a parent is allowed to remain with them until they have become familiar with the dental professionals. Then a positive approach can be adopted.

Dental implications
- Liberal use of praise for adherence to requests in the surgery is indicated, given the child's desire to please adults.
- Telling stories during the course of treatment may help to capture the child's attention and to distract him/her from any unpleasant aspects of care being provided.

Age 4 to 5 years (early childhood years)

- By this age, children are exploring new environments and relationships in their world. They prefer one-on-one friendships, as more than one is difficult to manage. Once at school, however, they have to learn to sit quietly in groups and pay attention. Further development of social skills and regulation of emotions is occurring while mixing with their peers.
- These children listen with interest and respond well to verbal directions. They have lively minds and may be great talkers who are prone to exaggeration. In addition, they will participate well in small social groups.
- Four-year-old children are extremely creative, as fantasy and imaginary play allows them to work through confounding problems, emotions and the stressors of daily life. Therefore, pretend play can open the door to a young child's thoughts and worries and provide the dentist with valuable information. Showing great interest, listening and reflecting back to the child what they just said or taking on the role of another toy in conversation with them will encourage them to explore further.

Dental implications

- At this age, these children can be cooperative patients, but some may be defiant and try to impose their views and opinions. They are familiar with and respond well to 'thank you' and 'please'.
- Promotion of autonomy and the development of self-esteem by allowing decision-making and choices in their treatment and encouraging them to take responsibility for tasks such as manoeuvring the dental chair is important.
- Children at this age typically are still fearful about leaving their parents/carers in the waiting room, so they should be accompanied by the parent/carer to the operatory. Nevertheless, there is less fear of new experiences than earlier in life. They take pride in their possessions, and comments about clothing can be effectively used to establish communication and develop a rapport. By this age, children usually have relinquished comfort objects such as thumbs and 'security blankets'.
- Use of 'labelled praises' and 'direct commands' has been found to be important in promoting child and carer comfort, and reducing anxiety and fear, in this age group and in earlier years as well. A labelled praise is a specific praise that lets the child know the exact behaviour that the dental provider appreciates. Labelled praise frequently results in an increase in the frequency of the behaviour that is praised. As an example, the labelled praise of 'Lucas, you are doing such a good job being still in the chair, just like a statue' will often result in the child sitting still more often during the appointment. A direct command is a clear and specific instruction that is told to the child rather than asked of the child. Children are more likely to follow a direct command than an instruction presented in an unclear or questioning manner. For example, the direct command of 'Keep your hands close to your side, Claire' will typically result in better adherence than a questioning instruction such as 'Would you like to keep your hands close to your side, Claire?' After a direct command is given, it is important to give the child a labelled praise for following the direction ('Good job putting your hands by your side') to increase the probability of future compliance to instructions during the appointment.

Age 6 to 8 years

- By 6 years, children are established at school and are moving away from the security of the family.
- They are increasingly independent of parents and will play without their parents being in close proximity.
- For some children, this transition into greater independence may cause considerable anxiety and distress, with outbursts of screaming, temper tantrums and even striking parents. Furthermore, some will exhibit marked increase in fear responses.

Dental implications

- This age may be an ideal time to help the child and parent/caregiver move from the parent/caregiver being in the surgery to the child being able to go back alone from the waiting room to the surgery.
- The increased tendency towards fearfulness prompts special care in working with children at this age, accepting that new fear(s) may develop, even if the child has been a prior patient who earlier was comfortable in the dental setting.

Age 8 to 12 years (the middle or 'tweener' years)

- At this age, children are part of larger social groups and are strongly influenced by them. They notice who is accepted and who is excluded from groups. With this comes the growing concern of embarrassment, which they will avoid at all costs. Although parents might wish

for them to become leaders, they appropriately become followers because this is perceived as healthier and safer.
- As a consequence, children learn to hide their feelings and thoughts at this time and adopt a 'cool' attitude.
- Intellect becomes more important as they develop cognitively and begin to reason. The preteenager becomes concerned with what is moral and just and becomes more literal (e.g., a parent asks: 'Pick up your clothes'. The child picks them up and places them back down stating, 'You didn't tell me where to put them!').

Dental implications
- Be cautious to not embarrass the child through criticism of his/her self-care (e.g., tooth-brushing).
- Be patient in not expecting the child to freely share information without considerable rapport-building.
- Given the developing capacity to reason, children in this age range may respond well to explanations about the need to engage in toothbrushing and flossing on their own, without parental prompting.

Adolescence
- The adolescent is faced with solving major questions such as: Who am I? Who am I becoming? Whom should I be? With such tasks in mind, it is understandable that teenagers are often perceived as self-absorbed, excluding themselves from family and, to some degree, their peers. Many interactions with the teenager tend to result in a narcissistic view of any situation.
- Adolescents are on a journey of self-discovery and, not unlike the toddler, are looking for greater autonomy, such as experimenting with new identities, realities and self-concepts, all of which are healthy. Experimentation and use of tobacco and other substances are common.
- Adolescents typically believe they are invulnerable, and that they will not encounter adverse results from their actions. They do not expect, for example, that negative health outcomes will result from tobacco use, as 'other people' get addicted and only 'old people' have health problems.
- Appearance becomes increasingly important during the teenage years.
- Teenagers often feel that their experiences are unique, so listening with an open mind, providing independence as would be done with an adult and supporting them in reaching their goals (within safety limits) will earn trust and cooperation.
- Greater rapport is gained when the dentist adopts a nonjudgemental, nonpreaching and respectful approach towards the teenager.

Dental implications
- Treating the teenager as his/her own person, independent from the parent/caregiver, typically will be well received.
- Taking some time to talk about nondental topics in an 'adult' way may be a good way to develop rapport.
- Emphasizing the importance of self-dental care to maintain their smile may be a way to 'reach' adolescents in terms of preventive behaviours.

UNDERSTANDING CHILD TEMPERAMENT

There has been a long-standing debate in the literature on child development about the degree to which a child's development is influenced by 'nature' versus 'nurture'. Studies suggest that children do indeed enter the world with a characteristic temperament or personality that stays with them, to some degree, for the rest of their life. Thomas and Chess (1977) suggested that there are three basic temperaments that influence later personality. Approximately 65% of infants can fit into one of these three categories. The remainder have a mixture of traits.

Easy temperament

These children have a positive mood, have regular bodily functions, are adaptable and flexible and have a positive approach to change or new situations.

Difficult temperament

These children are more irritable and intense. They have irregular body functions and take some time to develop feed, play, sleep patterns and routines. They have difficulty with new situations and adapting to change and tend to withdraw in social settings.

Slow-to-warm-up temperament

These children have a shy disposition and a low activity level. Initially, they are slower to adapt to new situations, but once they are comfortable with their environment, they begin to engage.

Dental implications of child temperament

Dentists working with children must use different approaches and techniques, depending on the personality type of the child. Whereas an easy-temperament child may be flexible enough to handle a quick change in plan, a slow-to-warm-up child may need to be given a longer time to adjust. Difficult children respond best to a dentist who provides a great deal of structure in a sensitive but confident manner. The slow-to-warm-up child is best served by dental personnel who are calm, patient and encouraging (without being demanding).

Use of verbal and nonverbal communication to promote positive behaviour in children

The following principles are some of the important considerations in positive communication with children and their families.

- Show respect for the child and his/her feelings and interests.
- Show interest in the child as an individual. Find out his/her preferred name (e.g., nickname if any) and use it frequently in speaking with the child (and caregiver).
- Share 'free information' as much as the child/caregiver seems to want and to be able to handle.
- Give well-stated instructions (e.g., 'Please open your mouth now', instead of questions, such as, 'Would you like to open your mouth now?'). Tell the child kindly what he/she needs to do, not what they should not do.
- Communicate at the child's level, both physically (Figure 2.1) and cognitively/emotionally.

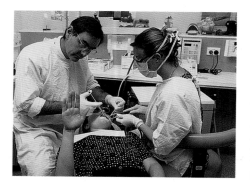

Figure 2.1 Giving children control in the dental surgery. It is essential to listen to your patient. A prearranged signal of a hand raised tells the clinician that the procedure is uncomfortable. This gives the child some control over what is happening without interfering with the procedure. The provider can even ask the child to 'practise' using the hand signal once, to demonstrate that this procedure will in fact work. Thereafter, however, the provider can praise the child for remaining calm and not having to raise their hand.

- Focus on the positive aspects of a child's (and parent's) behaviours. In most situations, ignore negative behaviours.
- Avoid stereotyping and making assumptions about children (e.g., that boys are interested only in sports; that young girls are interested in dolls).
- Show ethnic, cultural and gender sensitivity.

Physical structuring and timing during the dental visit

SETTING THE STAGE FOR POSITIVE BEHAVIOUR

In addition to communications from the dentist and dental staff, many aspects of the dental situation can be arranged in such a way that it promotes positive reactions in infants, children and adolescents. McNeil and Hembree-Kigin (2010) describe PRIDE (praise, reflection, inquire, describe, enthusiasm) skills, modified here for relevance to the dental situation, which is a conceptualization that can help prompt members of the dental team to structure their behaviour with children and teenagers. This approach is not to discourage spontaneity with youngsters, which can be so important in working positively with 'kids', but may provide a way for adults to think about including skills as part of their repertoire with children. In fact, the final point of the PRIDE skills is enthusiasm, which speaks of communicating joy, spontaneous fun and action to youth.

PRAISE, REFLECTION, INQUIRE, DESCRIBE, ENTHUSIASM

- Praise: These 'social reinforcers' can be either 'labelled' or 'unlabelled'. Labelled praises (e.g., 'That's a great job keeping your mouth open, Medika!') typically are more effective at managing behaviour than unlabelled praises (e.g., 'Well done, Danny!').
- Reflection: Such phrases are a demonstration of the dentist listening to the child and can involve a simple repeating of some of the child's words, perhaps with embellishment.
- Inquire: These questions involve asking a child for information, or otherwise prompting him/her to reply ('I'm wondering how you feel about coming to see me today.'). Open-ended questions typically produce more information and promote a more positive interview atmosphere, relative to closed-ended questions that can be answered with a Yes or No or a simple fact. Question-asking typically is greatly overused by adults with children and should instead be used judiciously.
- Describe: These statements focus on the child's behaviour, and portraying the child's actions, typically in a positive light (e.g., 'Now you're keeping your mouth open and letting your feet and legs be still'.).
- Enthusiasm: There is a time for animation and play on the part of the dentist and dental team and a time for more reserved professionalism. Particularly with younger children in a dental environment, enthusiasm on the part of the dentist and team is often needed to combat the negative images of dental care portrayed in the media, by peers and sometimes by parents and other caregivers.

Use of these PRIDE skills will be well received by children and youth and can help make the dental appointment reinforcing and enjoyable. PRIDE skills, however, should not be used in some automaton fashion, but rather flexibly and in concert with the dental professional's own personality and the procedures at hand. Not only are these interpersonal communication skills essential, but the physical and structural aspects of the dental appointment are also crucial.

PRACTICAL GUIDELINES FOR PHYSICAL AND SOCIAL ASPECTS OF THE DENTAL SURGERY

- Everyone in the surgery (dentist, auxiliary, parent) should transmit positive, comforting expectations to the patient.

- Use stimulating visual distracters in the surgery (child- and adolescent-oriented posters).
- Have age-appropriate materials (safe toys, magazines) in the waiting room. Include materials for parents.
- Have toys available for younger children as distracters or tangible rewards.
- Greet the child in the waiting room without a mask and not wearing surgical garb. Use the child's preferred name. Smile at the child! Depending on the child's height and your height, you may wish to squat in greeting him/her, to be at eye level.
- Try to decrease wait time both in the waiting room and in the operatory, as longer wait times have been shown to be related to more disruptive behaviour during the appointment.
- Pace procedures during the appointment, based on how the patient is coping, so that they are neither rushed nor bored. Periodically ask how he/she is coping with the appointment, sometimes using closed-ended (e.g., 'Are you doing OK?') and sometimes open-ended questions.
- Inform and discuss with parent/caregiver before the appointment and at the end.
- Include children, and especially adolescents, in the decision-making and practicalities of treatment.
- Provide information in advance about the procedures to be performed at the next appointment so that the child and parent/caregiver are prepared.
- Allowing a child a visit to the 'treasure chest' to get a tangible reward at the end of an appointment, finding some positive behaviour to reinforce (even if much of the child's behaviour was challenging), can leave a child with positive memories of the dental experience.
- Structuring what is remembered about a dental appointment has been shown to be an important issue in how children perceive dental care. The oral health professional may wish to provide a short summary statement after the 'treasure chest' visit, emphasizing certain (positive) parts of the dental visit (e.g., 'Rickie, today you came in bravely and sat in the chair and kept your mouth open for a long time, even when you got a bit tired. Well done for keeping still for so long! Now, what was the best part of your visit today?').

Presence or absence of family members in the surgery

- It is appropriate that a parent be present in the surgery to support their children during treatment, particularly in their younger years. Parents/caregivers can be coached by dental professionals regarding how to be most helpful during a visit.
- If a parent is unable or unwilling to provide appropriate support, then it may be more desirable for them to wait outside the surgery. Note that parental access to their children should never be denied.
- When there are other siblings, who enjoy or readily cope with dental treatment, it often is helpful to use them as a model.

Transmission of emotion to the child or adolescent

- Children acquire some of their parents' fear and anxiety about the dental treatment both in the dental environment and in the long term.
- Emotion is transferred from parents, siblings, dentist and auxiliaries to the child, whose emotional state also impacts all of those persons. Dental staff who are calm and confident and use humour will promote positive experiences for their patients.

Physical proximity and touching

- Initially, work from the front, at eye level.
- Be aware of the child's physical distance, that is, the 'intimate zone'. This zone is approximately 45 cm but varies in different cultures. By necessity, the dentist must 'invade' this space, but frequent stopping between procedures allows the child some time for coping.

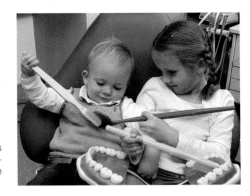

Figure 2.2 Involving children in their treatment. It is important for children to feel that the dental environment is nonthreatening and safe and can be a place for enjoyment.

- Touching the child can be used in nonprivate bodily regions, such as the lower arms and shoulders, to encourage, soothe or reward. The oral health professional should be attuned to the child's reaction to such touching, however, and whether it is well received. There are wide cultural variations in the appropriateness of such touching, both in terms of the child's background as well as that of the oral health professional.

Timing

- It is best to introduce new procedures at an appropriate rate to avoid either rushing or boring the patient.
- Conducting less invasive procedures first will usually be more tolerable for the patient.

Stimulating and distracting objects and situations (Figure 2.2)

- Be aware of popular culture. In some settings, it is possible to have different areas of the surgery orientated to particular patient age ranges.
- One area might include puppets and pictures of colourful cartoon characters for children up to 8 years.
- For older children, have wall posters of pop groups.
- Adolescents, like adults, are best treated in a modern, friendly environment.
- In some settings, popular electronic games and videos are appropriate.
- Fish tanks provide interesting stimulation for children of all ages, as well as adults.

Surgical clothing and instruments

- Never greet a child while wearing a face mask and gloves.
- Explain the need for protective clothing. With younger children, you can make putting on the mask and other gear a fun task that you describe to the child as you are doing it.
- Familiarize children with appropriate instruments and use child-friendly terms to describe the equipment to young children (e.g., Mr. Squirty, tooth counter).

Greetings in the waiting room

- It is ideal, particularly in initial meetings, for the dentist/hygienist/therapist to greet the child and parent/carer in the waiting area.
- An interview room or nonsurgical environment is useful for new patients (Figures 2.3–2.5).

Involving and communicating with parents

It is helpful for the dentist and other members of the oral healthcare team to have a positive relationship with both children and their parents. Keep parents well informed. While asking personal information, always remember to involve the child in the discussion when appropriate. Be

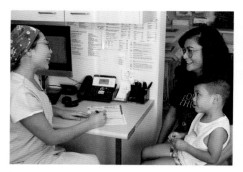

Figure 2.3 At the first visit, it is often good to see the child and parent away from the surgery. It provides an opportunity to talk with the child and establish rapport.

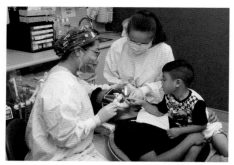

Figure 2.4 Introducing a child to the dental environment; part of the familiarization.

prepared to separate the child from the parent to discuss more sensitive issues if necessary. The chairside assistant can be asked to occupy the child during this discussion.

Talking with children and adolescents

Children, like adults, typically respond best if they are treated as individuals, somehow special to the provider. Consequently, using the child's name to refer to him/her, and repeating it in conversation periodically during the dental appointment, is helpful in producing a positive environment and in capturing and maintaining the child's attention. It usually helpful for the dentist and members of the dental team to speak with (not at) the child at the child's level, both physically and psychologically. Dental jargon typically is best avoided with most patients, but particularly with children. Table 2.1 suggests terminology that might be used with younger patients. Of course, use of these terms should be at a developmentally appropriate level for the child. Some mid- and older adolescents, for example, may actually respond well to learning dental jargon because it gives them a sense of being cognitively advanced.

Special arrangements for first-time dental visits

Certain steps are appropriate for an initial visit. In general, the pace of a first appointment is much slower.

- Use preappointment letters giving information about the visit that also includes photographs of the rooms and what might be expected of the child and parent.
- Use an interview room for the initial contact.

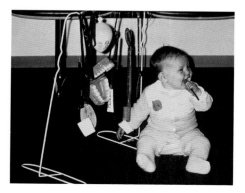

Figure 2.5 A dental mobile: every child should have one!

TABLE 2.1 ■ Dental terminology and lay language equivalents for use with children (age levels are approximate and should be based on the cognitive level)

Dental terminology	Lay language
Ages 1–5	
Air syringe	Wind blower
Water syringe	Water pistol
High evacuation suction	Vacuum cleaner
Saliva ejector	Straw
Radiograph	Picture of your tooth
Prophylaxis	Electric toothbrush
Explorer	Tooth counter
Rubber dam	Raincoat for your tooth
Local anaesthesia	Putting the tooth to sleep
High-speed handpiece	Tooth whistle
Low-speed handpiece	Tooth tickler
Extraction	Wiggle your tooth
Stainless steel crown	Helmet for your tooth
Ages 6–10	
Anaesthetize	Numb
Extract	Take out or wiggle
Caries, carious lesion	Hole
Pain	Tickle or pressure
Drill	Electric motor
Dental surgery	Treatment room

The emphasis is on educating the child, promoting comfort and allowing the visit to be exciting and fun. Relatively simple and less invasive procedures are preferred. Introducing the child to the office, staff and equipment and pointing out posters and other materials of interest in the treatment room can be helpful.

Behavioural methods for reducing fear and pain sensitivity

Table 2.2 gives eight methods that can be used across a variety of situations with children and adolescents of all ages. The particular uses depend on the patient's developmental age and personality, as well as on a variety of other factors such as the quality and depth of the dentist's relationship with the child or adolescent.

Intervening with children and adolescents who are agitated, fearful or uncooperative

The dental clinic or office is novel and unlike most situations children encounter. Typically, youth go for dental care once or twice per year, which does not allow them to readily become accustomed

TABLE 2.2 ■ **Behavioural methods for reducing anxiety**

Tell–show–do	Informing, then demonstrating, and finally performing part of a procedure
Playful humour	Using fun labels and suggesting use of imagination
Distraction	Ignoring and then directing attention away from a behaviour, thought or feeling to something else
Positive reinforcement	Tangible or social reward in response to a desired behaviour
Modelling	Providing an example or demonstration about how to perform a behaviour
Shaping	Successive approximations to a desired behaviour
Fading	Providing external means to promote positive behaviour and then gradually removing the external control
Systematic desensitization	Reducing anxiety by first presenting an object or situation that evokes little fear, then progressively introducing stimuli that are more fear-provoking

to this unique environment with its own sights, sounds and smells that can arouse fear and other distress. Children and adolescents can become 'dysregulated' emotionally and behaviourally during dental treatment because of fear, boredom and frustrating demands (e.g., keeping one's mouth open for long periods). Interventions are age dependent, but some possibilities follow here.

- Redirection often is helpful, in the form of distraction or focus on a nondental topic. Questions are typically not a good idea, as they place a demand on the child/adolescent, but remarking about something else may be helpful (e.g., a cartoon program that is playing on an overhead video monitor).
- For toddlers, the CARES protocol (Girard et al. 2017) may be helpful, taking a break from the ongoing dental treatment, with the dental providers moving away from the child but still in the room and involving the parent/caregiver in the following steps. (The CARES acronym is reflected in the bolded letters below.)
  - '**C**ome in calm and close' (parent is physically next to child, perhaps sitting on the side of the dental chair, or placing the child on their lap, without being smothering/suffocating)
  - '**A**ssist child' (parent asks provider to move light out of child's eyes for a bit)
  - '**R**eassure child' ('It's OK. Mommy is here.')
  - '**E**motional validation' ('I know it's scary having all these people look into your mouth, but they really want to help make your teeth all better.')
  - '**S**oft and **S**oothing' (parent cuddles child for a moment and coos)
- For older children and adolescents, asking them to breathe slightly deeply and rhythmically with the dental provider also may allow for more regulated breathing and distraction, counting as they do so, in and out.

Integrating behavioural and pharmacotherapeutic approaches

The behavioural principles and methods described earlier are used routinely, many in virtually every encounter with a youngster in a dental setting. When medications are needed for pain and/or anxiety control, or for sedation, sensitive behavioural approaches on the part of the oral health professional are particularly important. Using medication alongside behavioural approaches may be the most effective way to deal with many clinical scenarios. In fact, behavioural approaches can and should be used to prepare phobia patients, for example, before and after pharmacotherapy, as described by Milgrom and Heaton (2007).

Referring for possible mental health evaluation and care

WHEN TO REFER

It is a role of the dental professional to refer a child or family when there seem to be significant emotional or psychological issues. Even when such problems do not interfere with dental treatment, it is the dentist's role, as a member of the healthcare team, to identify possible psychopathologies and to refer for proper care. A sensitive conversation with the parents/caregivers regarding your concern for the child is essential before making the referral.

COMMON REASONS FOR REFERRING A CHILD OR ADOLESCENT FOR MENTAL HEALTH CONCERNS

- Evidence of abuse or neglect (e.g., bruises, broken teeth, cigarette burns, inappropriate clothing for weather, severe hygiene problems, untreated breaks or sprains).
- Extremes of behaviour, anxiety or emotion (e.g., attention deficit hyperactivity disorder, dental phobia).
- Neurological signs or symptoms (e.g., possible seizure activity, tics).
- Severe developmental or cognitive delay (e.g., possible learning disabilities, motor problems, possible autism spectrum disorder, feeding problems).
- Extremely poor parenting (e.g., sole use of excessive physical restraint and punishment).

REFERRAL SPECIALTIES

Referrals for mental health concerns should be made to psychologists, psychiatrists or social workers. In a hospital setting, it is possible to refer to one of the available departmental services. In a dentist's private surgery, referrals can be made to professionals in private practice, community agencies or hospitals. The following guidelines are suggested when selecting a specialty for referral.

Psychologists

Refer in the case of abuse or neglect, extremes of behaviour, developmental or cognitive delay or extremely poor parenting. When there is a need for sophisticated cognitive, personality, neuropsychological and/or behavioural assessment, referral to a psychologist is best, as standardized psychometric tests can be used. Psychologists also can provide individual child/adolescent, parent/child and/or family therapy to address problems in the child/adolescent and family system.

Psychiatrists

Refer when there are neurological signs or symptoms. When psychoactive medications may be needed, such as when a child demonstrates signs of psychosis, referral to a psychiatrist is most appropriate, similar to cases in which there are complicating medical factors.

Social workers

Refer for social problems, abuse or neglect. Referral to social workers is appropriate when there are existing social problems in the family that require mobilization of community resources. Social workers know about and help patients use available services in the community.

HOW TO REFER

It is acknowledged that suggesting mental healthcare to parents can be an anxiety-provoking task for the dentist. Nevertheless, it is essential that such referrals are made, because the dentist is in a unique role as a healthcare provider. If referrals are not made in a timely fashion, then a condition can progress and worsen.

- Speak to the parents/caregivers in a private setting, informing them of the signs or symptoms that are the cause for concern, without blaming or ascribing responsibility. When the parents understand the problems and your concern, referral to a specific professional or service can be made. It is often helpful to emphasize it is for the well-being of the child and the necessity to address the problem for their proper development.
- Ensure that the parents and the child or adolescent are aware of the referral and know the specialty of the referral. (It is not appropriate merely to describe the referral as 'to a doctor who will help your child').
- Refer first to only one of the mental health specialties. If additional referral is necessary, it can be arranged by the first referral source. In making the referral, one can ask for feedback from the mental health professional after the appointment. If there is behavioural disruption in the surgery, the mental health professional may have recommendations for management once the child or family has been evaluated.
- Mental health concerns are considered private by many individuals. Given this desire for privacy, releases to exchange relevant information, signed by a parent or guardian and the child if of an age to understand it, are required. Such a form can be signed in the dental surgery and sent to the mental health professional, along with a request for feedback.

Acknowledgements

The contributions of DWM and CBM are supported by the US National Institutes of Health/ National Institute of Dental and Craniofacial Research (R21 DE026540).

Further reading

Girard, E., Wallace, N.M., Morgan, S., et al., 2018. Parent–child interaction therapy with toddlers: improving attachment and emotion regulation. New York: Springer.

McNeil, C.B., Hembree-Kigin, T.L., 2010. Parent–child interaction therapy, second ed. New York: Springer.

McNeil, C.B., Hembree-Kigin, T., Eyberg, S.M., 1996. Short-term play therapy for disruptive children. King of Prussia, PA: Center for Applied Psychology.

McNeil, C.B., Quetsch, L.B., Anderson, C. (Eds.), 2019. Handbook of parent-child interaction therapy for children on the autism spectrum. New York: Springer.

McNeil, D.W., Randall, C.L., Cohen, L.L., et al., 2019. Transmission of dental fear from parent to adolescent in an Appalachian sample in the USA. International Journal of Paediatric Dentistry 29, 720–727.

McNeil, D.W., 2020 March. Can it be fun?: best behavioral practices in dental care for preschoolers. Symposium conducted at the meeting of the International Association for Dental Research [abstract]. Journal of Dental Research 99, A-0259 and A-0260.

Milgrom, P., Heaton, L.J., 2007. Enhancing sedation treatment for the long term: pre-treatment behavioural exposure. SAAD Digest 23, 29–34.

Thomas, A., Chess, S., 1977. Temperament and development. Oxford: Brunner/Mazel.

CHAPTER 3

Pharmacological behaviour management

Eduardo A. Alcaino ■ Benjamin Moran

Pain management for children

The proper treatment of pain in children is often inadequate and involves misconceptions that:

- Children experience less pain than adults.
- Neonates do not feel or remember pain.
- Pain is character-building for children.
- Opioids are addictive and too dangerous in terms of respiratory distress.
- Children cannot localize or describe their pain.

DEVELOPMENT OF PAIN PATHWAYS

Even premature neonates have the physiological pathways and mediators to feel pain. The statement that infants and children do not experience pain, either partially or completely, is not physiologically valid.

VARIATION OF PAIN RESPONSES IN CHILDREN

Pain is a bio-psycho-social entity which can affect the individual response of each child to a painful stimulus. A history directed at each of these domains may guide how pain is assessed and managed. For example:

- Previous procedures may increase current stress and current analgesic requirements
- Age and developmental level
- Social situation
- Psychological development or disorders
- Medical conditions

Methods for paediatric pain assessment

- Observer-based techniques which are useful in preverbal children, that is, scales that measure blood pressure, crying, movement, agitation and verbal expression/body language.
- Self-reporting of pain is valid in children over 4–5 years of age. For instance, the use of visual analogue scales such as Baker-Wong Faces.
- Children with severe developmental delay can be extremely difficult to assess regarding pain, even by their regular carers. Unusual changes in behaviour from normal may represent an expression of pain.
- Observation of nonverbal cues and behaviour is important. A quiet, withdrawn child may be in severe pain. Simple measures are there to measure pain in children of all ages.

NONPHARMACOLOGICAL PAIN MANAGEMENT

- Nonpharmacological analgesia should be attempted in all patients where pain is an expected outcome.
- It should involve the child and the parent (if possible).
- Attempt to have an environment that reduces fear and anxiety, as this may decrease pain perception.
- Techniques include diversion/distraction (videos, magic, games, storytelling), deep breathing, music, comforting touch (usually the parent).

ANALGESIA BEFORE PROCEDURES (PREEMPTIVE ANALGESIA)

- Giving adequate analgesia before a procedure will result in less overall analgesia being required.
- Consideration should be given to ensure adequate systemic and/or local analgesia before the commencement of a procedure. Appropriate time for absorption and effect should be allowed.
- A stronger analgesic may be required for the procedure with regular simple analgesics for the postoperative period.

Routes of administration

- Oral analgesia is the preferred route of administration in children. Absorption for most analgesics is generally rapid (within 30 min).
- Attention to formulation suitable to the individual child can help greatly with compliance, that is, liquid versus tablets in younger children, pleasant taste.
- The rectal route of administration can be valuable in a child not tolerating oral fluids. Absorption may vary, as medications absorbed in the lower part of the rectum avoid first-pass metabolism, where the upper part of the rectum does not. Doses and time to peak levels may

vary compared with oral preparations and are usually much longer. Peak levels after rectal paracetamol may take 90 to 120 min. Adequate explanation should be given and consent should be obtained for the rectal administration of a drug. This route is not used in an immunocompromised child because of the risk of infection or fissure formation.

- Parenteral paracetamol and parecoxib (cyclo-oxygenase 2 [COX-2] nonsteroidal antiinflammatory drug [NSAID]) are now available.
- Intranasal or sublingual administration of opioids have been described as an alternative to injection, which avoids first-pass metabolism by the liver.
- Repeated intramuscular injection should be avoided in children. They will often tolerate pain rather than have a painful injection. A subcutaneous cannula, inserted after using topical local anaesthetic cream (EMLA), can be used if repeated parenteral opioid analgesia is applied.
- In obese children, the dosage given should be based on ideal body weight, which can be estimated as the 50th centile on an appropriate weight-for-age percentile chart.

ANALGESICS

See Table 3.1.

Paracetamol

- Dosage 20 mg/kg orally, then 15 mg/kg every 4 hours.
- 30 mg/kg rectally as a single dose.
- Maximum 24-hour dosage of 90 mg/kg (or 4 g) for 2 days, then 60 mg/kg per day by any route of administration.
- Ensure adequate hydration.
- Useful as a preemptive analgesic.
- No effect on bleeding.

TABLE 3.1 ■ **Analgesic agents for children**

Drug	Oral dose	IMI, SCI, IVI dose	Notes
Paracetamol	20 mg/kg initially, then 15 mg/kg every 4 hours		Maximum 90 mg/kg/day (up to 4 g) for 2 days, then 60 mg/kg/day
Ibuprofen	10 mg/kg every 6 hours		Maximum 40 mg/kg/day up to 2 g/day
Celecoxib	2–4 mg/kg every 12 hours		Maximum duration 5 days
Naproxen	5 mg/kg every 12 hours		Maximum 10–20 mg/kg/day up to 1 g/day
Diclofenac	1 mg/kg every 8 hours 1 mg/kg every 12 hours (rectally)		Maximum 3 mg/kg/day up to 150 mg/day
Morphine	0.2–0.3 mg/kg every 4 h	0.1–0.15 mg/kg every 3 hours	
Tramadol	1–1.5 mg/kg every 6 hours	1 mg/kg every 6 hours	Maximum 6 mg/kg/day up to 400 mg/day

IMI, Intramuscular injection; *IVI*, intravenous injection; *SCI*, subcutaneous injection.

- Intravenous (IV) paracetamol is available (10 mg/mL). The same dose is used and administered over 15 min.
- Take care with dosages, as many different strengths and preparations are available.

Nonsteroidal antiinflammatory drugs

- Effective alone after oral and dental procedures.
- May be used in conjunction with paracetamol.
- Have an opioid-sparing effect.
- Increased bleeding time because of inhibition of platelet aggregation.
- Useful analgesic once haemostasis has been achieved.
- Best given if tolerating food and drink.
- Can be used in infants over 6 months of age.

Relative contraindications for the use of nonsteroidal antiinflammatory drugs in children

- Bleeding or coagulopathies.
- Renal disease.
- Haematological malignancies, in children who may have or develop thrombocytopenia.
- Severe asthma, especially if the child is sensitive to aspirin or is steroid dependent or has coexisting nasal polyps.

Aspirin

- Rarely used in children for mild pain because of the risk of Reye syndrome.
- However, aspirin is commonly used in the management of juvenile rheumatoid arthritis.

Ibuprofen

- Commonly used in children for mild pain with less gastrointestinal side effects compared with aspirin.
- Should be avoided in patients with renal impairment.

Cyclo-oxygenase 2 inhibitors

- Include celecoxib and parecoxib (parenteral preparation).
- No effect on platelet function or gastrointestinal side effects (compared with aspirin or ibuprofen).
- Useful analgesic adjunct for moderate to severe pain.

Codeine

- There is now consensus that codeine should not be generally given to children and not used in children under 12 years of age.
- Repeated administration causes constipation.
- Main action is attributed to metabolism to morphine (approximately 15%).
- 10% of patients of European descent and up to 30% of Hong Kong Chinese patients cannot metabolize codeine and find it an ineffective analgesic.
- IV use may cause profound hypotension.

Oxycodone

- Good oral bioavailability.
- No pharmacological differences in metabolism.
- Available as a liquid.
- Useful alternative to codeine.

- Useful analgesic when combined with simple analgesia.
- May cause nausea and vomiting.

Morphine

- About 30% oral bioavailability as morphine sulphate.
- May cause nausea and constipation similar to all opioids.
- There is a low risk of addiction for supervised analgesic use in children.

Tramadol

- May be used for moderate pain in children over 12 years of age.
- A weak μ-opioid agonist and has two other analgesic mechanisms (increasing neuronal synaptic 5-hydroxytryptamine and inhibition of noradrenaline uptake).
- 70% oral bioavailability.
- No effect on clotting.
- Avoid use in children with seizure disorders and those taking tricyclic or selective serotonin reuptake inhibitor (SSRI) antidepressants.

CLINICAL HINT: SCENARIO

A compliant 8-year-old boy is having several teeth extracted under local infiltration and inhalation sedation with nitrous oxide. Consider:
- Preoperatively: paracetamol 20 mg/kg orally, 30 min preoperative.
- Postoperatively: ibuprofen 10 mg/kg and paracetamol 15 mg/kg every 6 hours or 30 min before bedtime that night.

DISCHARGE CRITERIA

Many drugs that are used for combination sedation and analgesia in children have a long half-life of several hours. Discharge criteria should be used to assess that the child is well enough before discharge from a free-standing facility. Criteria should include:

- Self-maintenance of airway.
- Easily rousable and able to converse.
- No ataxia, that is, can walk properly.
- Tolerating oral fluids.
- Discharge in the care of a responsible adult with appropriate information about after-hours contact if a problem arises.

Local anaesthesia

The use of local anaesthesia (LA) in paediatric dentistry varies significantly between countries, and there are also individual preferences. Every clinician must be proficient at administering painless LA. Although it is the mainstay of our pain control for operative treatment, it also represents one of the greatest fears in our patients. Use of many of the nonpharmacological techniques described in the previous chapter may enable the dentist to deliver an injection without the child being aware. There are few patients, old or young, who are not genuinely afraid of injections, and there are obvious disadvantages in the physical size of the dental cartridge syringe.

TECHNIQUES AND TIPS

- It makes little sense to hold the syringe in front of a young child to see. Although it is essential not to lie to the child, distractions such as having the dentist or dental assistant talk, use visual aids such as TV monitors or movie goggles or use of the low-velocity suction are useful.

- The use of topical anaesthetics is essential to create the optimal experience for the child. A multitude of agents are available with different flavours and properties; however, topical creams such as EMLA® (a eutectic mixture of two local anaesthetics: lignocaine and prilocaine) penetrate deeper through the mucosa. Despite several studies on the use of EMLA in dentistry, the manufacturers do not list its use on mucous membranes.
- The most common needles used in paediatric dentistry are 30G needles (short, 25 mm, and ultra-short, 11 mm) for infiltration and 27G long needles (38 mm) for block injections in older children.
- The use of block injections has decreased over time, and many paediatric dentists no longer use this technique in young children
- Electronic devices for slow injection techniques are also widely used and may replace more conventional techniques. Other distraction and vibrating devices may also be useful (Figure 3.1).
- The use of infiltration versus block injections in the mandible is subject of some debate, and clinicians differ in their choice of technique. The approach of the needle to the mandibular foramen differs in younger children, as the angle of the mandible is more obtuse and a

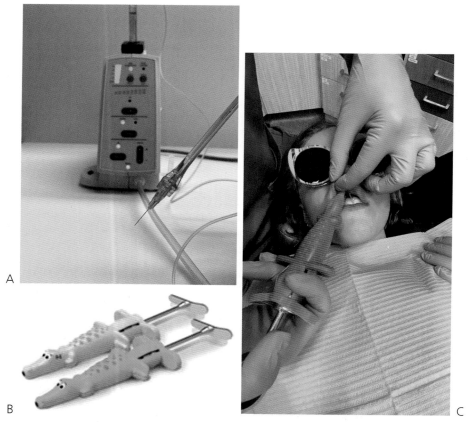

Figure 3.1   (A) An example of an electronic local anaesthetic injection device. (B, C) Many devices (autoclavable) are available to hide and distract from the relatively large dental cartridge syringe. It is preferable not to show the needle to the child.

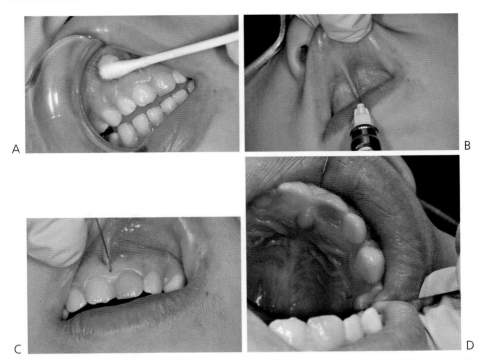

Figure 3.2 Techniques for administering palatal anaesthesia. (A) Use topical anaesthetic and leave adequate time to work. (B) Good retraction of the upper lip, injecting slowly and high into the labial sulcus. (C) Inject from the already anaesthetized labial side, through the interdental papilla. (D) Note the blanching of the palatal mucosa indicating spread of the anaesthetic solution.

shorter needle (25 mm) may be sufficient. However, even with the best technique, a mandibular block injection may still be extremely uncomfortable for children.

- Infiltration injections supplemented with intraperiodontal injection are useful in extraction cases (Figure 3.2A).
- Palatal anaesthesia is best achieved by slowly infiltrating through the inter-dental papilla after adequate labial or buccal anaesthesia to minimize discomfort to the child (Figure 3.3).
- Intraosseous dental anaesthesia may be useful in obtaining profound anaesthesia without the complications or regional (block) injections. A wider-bore needle (25G short) may be used in children, as their bone is much less dense than in adults. Care must be taken not to damage unerupted teeth or adjacent structures (Figure 3.2B).

NEED FOR LOCAL ANAESTHESIA UNDER SEDATION AND GENERAL ANAESTHESIA

Some form of pain control is required when invasive procedures are performed under any form of sedation (including inhalation sedation, oral sedation, or intravenous sedation). However, the need for local anaesthetic under general anaesthesia (GA) is controversial. There are no clear guidelines in the Australasia, United States of America (USA), United Kingdom (UK) or other countries as to the use of LA under GA. It is well recognized that a patient's vital signs may change in response to painful stimuli (e.g., extraction), depending on the depth of anaesthesia.

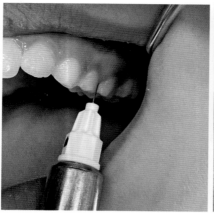
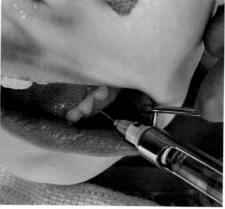

A   B

Figure 3.3 (A) Technique for intraperiodontal injection. An ultra-short needle is inserted parallel to the long axis of the tooth into the periodontal ligament following normal buccal or labial infiltration. Inject slowly under pressure. Only a small amount of solution is required. (B) Intra-osseous technique. After a small buccal infiltration, penetrate the bone with a larger-bore short needle into the bone, avoiding sensitive adjacent structures.

Good communication with your anaesthetist regarding the delivery of intravenous analgesia in a timely fashion (a minute or so before the painful stimuli or extractions) is important for proper patient care. LA is not routinely used for extractions of primary teeth under GA. Studies have observed that the child's postoperative recovery is usually independent of the procedure performed, and preschool children waking after having a general anaesthetic can be more distressed by the sensation of numbness in the mouth. However, the use of LA is recommended for dentoalveolar surgery or the removal of permanent teeth, especially first permanent molars. Another issue in the use of LA is the risk of damage to the lips and/or the tongue during emergence from the general anaesthetic. This is of particular concern in the care of those children with special needs who may not understand the sensation of numbness.

CLINICAL HINTS: LOCAL ANAESTHESIA

Successful local anaesthesia depends on:
- Communication with the child and parent.
- Routine use of topical anaesthesia, and leaving adequate time for it to act.
- Slow injection of warm solution.
- Avoiding direct palatal injections.
- Adequate anaesthesia for procedure being performed.

The 'coldness' of 'ice blocks' (popsicles, ice lollies) may help children cope with the numbness sensation postoperatively.

COMPLICATIONS WITH LOCAL ANAESTHESIA

The most significant complication encountered is overdosage. Consequently, maximum doses (Table 3.2) need to be calculated according to weight and preferably written in the notes if more than just a short procedure is being performed. This clinical complication is highlighted in a paper that reviewed significant negative outcomes (death or neurological damage) in children resulting from local anaesthetic overdose (Goodson & Moore, 1983) or in combination with sedation (Chicka, 2012).

TABLE 3.2 ■ **Maximum dosages for local anaesthetic solutions**

Anaesthetic agent	Maximum dose
2% Lidocaine with 1 : 100 000 adrenaline	7 mg/kg
4% Prilocaine with felypressin	9 mg/kg
0.5% Bupivacaine with 1 : 200 000 adrenaline	2 mg/kg
4% Articaine with adrenaline 1 : 100 000 (approximately 1.5 cartridge of 2.2 mL in 20 kg child)	7 mg/kg

Calculation of maximum local anaesthetic dosage:
2% lidocaine = 20 mg/mL
2.2 mL/carpule = 44 mg/carpule
A 20 kg child (~5 years old) can tolerate a maximum dose of 2% lidocaine with vasoconstrictor of:
7 mg/kg × 20 kg = 140 mg equivalent of 3 carpules (6.6 mL)

Other complications include:

- Biting of the lower lip (most common) or tongue postoperatively.
- Failure to adequately anaesthetize the area.
- Intravascular injection (inferior alveolar nerve blocks or infiltration in the posterior maxillae, directly into the pterygoid venous plexus).
- Facial nerve paralysis by injecting too far posteriorly into the parotid gland.
- Although rare, allergic reactions to local anaesthetics and needle breakage can occur.

Consequently, adequate postoperative instructions to both children and parents are necessary to minimize these complications. As noted earlier, inadequate local anaesthetic technique (inexperienced operator, fast delivery of solution and inadequate behaviour management) for initial procedures in young children may diminish the effect of adequate analgesia in subsequent procedures (Weisman et al., 1998).

The use of 4% articaine with adrenaline has gained popularity over the last two decades. However, its safety and effectiveness in children under the age of 4 years have not been established.

Sedation in paediatric dentistry

The decision to sedate a child requires careful consideration by an experienced team. The choice of a particular technique, sedative agent and route of delivery should be made at a prior consultation appointment to determine the suitability of the child (and their parents) to a specific technique. Dentists who practice sedation must comply with sedation guidelines and legislation in their local country and undergo ongoing training in sedation as well as advanced resuscitation skills.

Procedural sedation and/or analgesia imply that the patient is in a state of drug-induced tolerance of uncomfortable or painful diagnostic or interventional medical, dental or surgical procedures. Lack of memory of distressing events and/or analgesia may be desired outcomes, but lack of response to painful stimulation is not assured.

There are different levels of sedation, including minimal, moderate or deep sedation, and GA.

MINIMAL SEDATION

Minimal sedation (old terminology, 'anxiolysis') is a drug-induced state during which patients respond normally to verbal commands. Although cognitive function and coordination may be impaired, ventilatory and cardiovascular functions are unaffected. Children who have received minimal sedation generally will not require more than observation and intermittent assessment of their level of sedation. Some children will become moderately sedated despite the intended level of minimal sedation; should this occur, then the guidelines for moderate sedation apply.

MODERATE SEDATION

Moderate sedation (old terminology, 'conscious sedation' or 'sedation/analgesia') is a drug-induced depression of consciousness during which patients respond purposefully to verbal commands or after light tactile stimulation. No interventions are required to maintain a patent airway, and spontaneous ventilation is adequate. Cardiovascular function is usually maintained. The loss of consciousness should be unlikely, and this is a particularly important aspect of the definition of moderate sedation; drugs and techniques used should carry a margin of safety wide enough to render unintended loss of consciousness unlikely.

DEEP SEDATION

Deep sedation is characterized by depression of consciousness that can readily progress to the point where consciousness is lost and patients respond only to painful stimulation. It is associated with loss of the ability to maintain a patent airway, inadequate spontaneous ventilation and/or impaired cardiovascular function, and has similar risks to GA, requiring an equivalent level of care.

The use of any form of sedation in children presents added challenges to the clinician. During sedation, a child's response is more unpredictable than that of adults. Their proportionally smaller bodies are less tolerant to sedative agents and they may be easily over-sedated and, subsequently, anaesthetized. Anatomical differences in the paediatric airways include:

- The vocal cords positioned higher and more anterior.
- The smallest portion of the paediatric airway is at the level of the subglottis (below cords) at the level of the cricoid ring.
- Children have a relatively larger tongue and epiglottis.
- Possible presence of large tonsillar/adenoid mass (Figure 3.4).
- Larger head to body size ratio in children.
- The mandible is less developed and retrognathic in younger children and infants.
- Children have smaller lung capacity and higher metabolic rate, resulting in a smaller oxygen reserve. Hence children desaturate faster than adults.

Presedation patient assessment

The preoperative assessment is among the most important factors when choosing a particular form of sedation. This assessment must include:

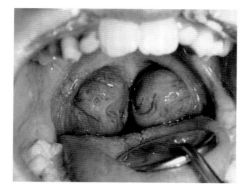

Figure 3.4 Large tonsils cause a significant risk of airway obstruction.

TABLE 3.3 ■ Resting vital signs in children

Age	Heart rate (beats/min)	Blood pressure (mmHg)	Respiratory rate (breaths/min)
Neonate	120–170	75–85/45	45–60
2–4 years	110–130	90/50	40
4–6 years	100	100/60	30
10 years	90	110/60	25
15 years	80	120/65	12

- A thorough medical and dental history (including birth and neonatal history, current medications taken, previous hospitalizations and past operations).
- Patient medical status (see American Society of Anesthesiologists [ASA] classification, below). Caution must be taken with children under 5 years of age.
- Patient's weight and vital signs.
- History of recent respiratory illness or current infections.
- Airway assessment to determine suitability for sedation or GA.
- Fasting requirements and the ability of the carer to comply with instructions.
- Proposed procedures being performed.

The clinician should be aware that children have resting vital signs that differ according to their age (Table 3.3).

Use of immobilization devices (protective stabilization)

Immobilization devices, such as papoose boards, must be applied in such a way as to avoid airway obstruction or chest restriction. The child's head position and respiratory excursions should be checked frequently to ensure airway patency. If a papoose board is used, a hand or foot should be kept exposed, and the child should never be left unattended. Monitoring devices must be used at a level consistent with the level of sedation achieved.

Patient monitoring

The use of monitoring devices such as pulse oximetry is desirable for minimal sedation and mandatory for moderate and deep sedation. Although not currently mandated during relative analgesia in dentistry, it is suggested that pulse oximetry should be used in all instances when a child is sedated. Sedation is a continuum, and any dentist who sedates children must be capable of recognizing a deeper level of sedation than intended and be able to rescue the patient from this unintended level of sedation (Cote & Wilson, 2016).

Regulations vary in each country, and cultural aspects and socio-economic factors will also influence which particular approach to sedation is chosen. Parental attitudes will also determine the appropriateness of a particular sedation technique or the need for restraint.

Pharmacological agents may be administered in a number of ways, but the more common routes of delivery include:

- Inhalational sedation.
- Enteral route: oral or nasal or rectal sedation.
- Parenteral or IV sedation.
- GA.

INHALATION SEDATION (RELATIVE ANALGESIA/NITROUS OXIDE SEDATION)

Nitrous oxide (N_2O) has been used for over 150 years; however, its mechanism of action is not fully understood. Its analgesic effect is opioid in nature and its anxiolytic effect resembles a benzodiazepine effect. Nitrous oxide is a weak inhalational anaesthetic agent, which is extremely useful in relieving anxiety. The use of N_2O offers the clinician a safe and relatively easy technique to use as an adjunct to clinical care. It can provide a gentle introduction to operative dentistry for the very anxious patient, or an ongoing aid for those who need assistance to accept routine operative dental care. It is effective for children who are anxious but generally cooperative. An uncooperative child will often not allow a mask or nasal hood to be placed over the nose. It also requires a child of sufficient maturity, age or understanding to help during the dental procedure. Can the child breathe through the nose? A good tip is to do a 'sniff test'; that is, if the child can breathe through the nose with the mouth closed, then this often means this patient is probably a good candidate for N_2O.

Advantages

- Very safe and relatively easy technique when only light sedation is required.
- Rapid induction and easily reversible with short recovery time.
- Can be titrated to required level.

Contraindications

The only specific contraindication to N_2O in children is a blocked nose. The following conditions may significantly affect the efficacy of this technique and are best avoided:
- Children with severe psychiatric disorders.
- Cystic fibrosis.
- Chronic upper airway obstruction (i.e., large adenoids).
- Communication problems.
- Unwilling patients.
- Pregnancy.
- Acute respiratory tract infections.
- Malignant hyperthermia (MH) is not a contraindication to the use of N_2O.

Precautions in the use of nitrous oxide

Nausea and vomiting may be a problem in some children; this is usually minimized with the routine use of rubber dam during restorative dentistry (Figure 3.5A). Nausea is often brought about by fluctuating concentrations of N_2O caused by alternating mouth and nose breathing.

ADMINISTRATION OF INHALATION SEDATION

For the safe and effective use of inhalation sedation, it is necessary to have an understanding of the different stages of analgesia and anaesthesia, the various delivery systems and nitrous circuits. This requires training in its administration and the careful monitoring of children. Most countries have specific courses for accreditation in the use of N_2O sedation.
- Dental N_2O delivery machines must have the capacity to deliver 100% oxygen, and a minimum of 30% oxygen.
- Before commencing sedation with N_2O, always carefully inspect the apparatus and circuit for any leaks. If the reservoir bag does not inflate, examine for a tear.
- A range of nasal masks is available with different colours and smells, that is useful in making the child feel more comfortable.

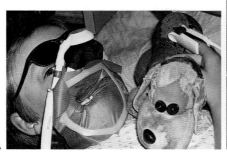
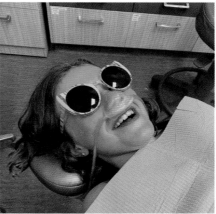

A B

Figure 3.5 (A) The use of nitrous oxide with rubber dam. Placement of dam minimizes mouth breathing and children are usually more settled. Note the pulse oximeter on the finger. Although the use of pulse oximetry is not mandatory, it measures oxygen saturation and heart rate, which provides added safety. A disadvantage of the shape of the nasal mask is that it may make placement of protective glasses difficult. (B) A low-profile nasal mask that is often better tolerated in some children.

- The acceptance of a disposable nasal mask is usually the biggest hurdle clinically, and it may be useful to lend a mask to the child before their treatment visit so they can practice and familiarize themselves with it.

Procedures

- Recline the dental chair and place the mask on the child's nose so that it fits properly. Once in place, check that the mask sits comfortably on the child's face in close proximity to the skin, and secure the mask so that it covers the nostrils completely and does not move unnecessarily during the procedure.
- Determine the amount of gas (volume per minute) required for the child. Variable-flow N_2O machines are preferred for use in children.
- Start the procedure with 100% oxygen with active scavenging. Monitor the reservoir bag as the child breathes; it should move at the same rate as the child's breathing with each inspiration and expiration.
- Constant monitoring is critical, and the use of pulse oximetry is advised. Assess the child's eyes, general responses and level of consciousness throughout the procedure.
- Induction techniques include titration (most common) or by rapid induction for more experienced operators. Appropriate training and experience are necessary. When using a titration technique, the N_2O is titrated in 10% intervals.

Effects of nitrous oxide sedation

Children are very open to suggestion. Their thoughts and behaviours can be guided by the dentist, especially under N_2O sedation. Describe (suggest) the sensations that the child will feel:

- Anxiolysis and analgesia.
- Initial 'heaviness' or sinking into the chair.
- Tingling and numbness of the extremities.
- A warm sensation and a feeling of 'lightness' or floating off the chair with increasing depth of analgesia.
- Time compression (a 30-minute visit may feel more like 10 minutes to the child)

Determining levels of nitrous oxide sedation

- Most children will sedate well between 30% and 40% level of nitrous oxide (30:70 to 40:60 levels of $N_2O:O_2$).
- Once LA has been administered successfully, the N_2O should be lowered to 30% or below and maintained at this level. Repeatedly adjusting the levels can be quite disconcerting, and so changes should be kept to a minimum.
- Once the procedure is complete, or near completion, the concentration of gas should be lowered, so that the child is maintained on 100% oxygen. This displaces nitrous oxide from the child's body and decreases the amount of exhaled gas into the operatory room. Diffusion hypoxia is a concern with N_2O under general anaesthesia, not a concern with dental N_2O machines which deliver a minimum of 30% oxygen concentration.
- The level at which a patient will be comfortable under N_2O will be different for every child. Excessive amounts of N_2O may put the child into the excitement stage of anaesthesia (Guedel stage II) and may induce vomiting, a feeling of fear or excessive movement.
- In certain countries (in Europe, for example), nitrous oxide is supplied as a premixed gas of 50% N_2O and O_2 and so levels cannot be varied.

Give clear written postoperative instructions to the parent. In most cases children will go home after N_2O sedation, but some children will attend school that same day. Keeping children under supervision is recommended and taking precautions is important.

CLINICAL HINTS: NITROUS OXIDE SEDATION

- Can the child breathe through the nose? (Crying, upper respiratory tract infection and obstructions can all make nose breathing difficult.)
- During treatment, ensure the child is breathing through the nose and not the mouth.
- Most children will be adequately sedated between 30:70 and 40:60 levels of $N_2O:O_2$.
- Rubber dam is desirable with restorative procedures and minimizes mouth breathing (Figure 3.5).
- Excessive body movement may be a sign of over-sedation.

Ideal patient:

- American Society of Anesthesiologists I or II
- A cooperative 5-year-old or older (larger nose allows better use of nasal hood).
- A child able to follow commands (e.g., nose breathing).
- A 30- to 45-minute treatment time.

Adverse events during sedation

Sedation is a continuum. Any technique which depresses the central nervous system (CNS) may result in a deeper sedation state than intended, and consequently, clinicians who sedate children require a much higher level of skill with a particular technique, the relevant training and experience, and proper accreditation with the relevant regulating authority.

Sedation of children for diagnostic and therapeutic procedures remains an area of rapid change in medicine and one of considerable controversy. Studies (Cote et al., 2000) have identified several features associated with adverse sedation-related events and poor outcomes, including:

- Adverse events occur more frequently in a nonhospital-based facility (private practice settings).
- Inadequate resuscitation was often associated with a nonhospital-based setting.
- Inadequate preoperative assessment.
- Inadequate and inconsistent physiological monitoring.
- Adverse events often associated with drug overdoses or the use of multiple agents, especially when three or more drugs were used.

- Lack of an independent observer.
- Errors in medication.
- Inadequate recovery procedures.

Considerations for paediatric sedation in the dental setting

- Proper accreditation in your country of practice and following established guidelines for monitoring children during sedation are essential.
- The same level of care should apply to hospital-based and nonhospital-based facilities (Figure 3.6).
- Pulse oximetry should be mandatory whenever a child is sedated, irrespective of the route of drug administration or the dosage.
- Monitoring devices such as oximeters, blood pressure and heart rate monitors, end-tidal CO_2 monitors or others will depend on the level of sedation administered.
- Age- and size-appropriate equipment and medications for resuscitation should be immediately available in a designated 'crash cart', regardless of the location where the child is sedated.
- All healthcare providers who sedate children, regardless of practice venue, should have advanced airway management skills, resuscitation skills and ongoing training.
- Practitioners must carefully weigh the risks and the benefits of sedating children beyond the safety net of a hospital or hospital-like environment.
- Practitioners must understand that the absence of skilled backup personnel could pose significant risks in the event of a medical emergency (Cote et al., 2000; Cote & Wilson, 2016; Cravero & Blike, 2006).

The use of N_2O sedation of children has already been discussed earlier. Other forms of sedation used across the world will be discussed briefly. These include oral/nasal sedation, rectal sedation and IV sedation. Techniques such as intra-nasal sedation or intra-muscular sedation are not commonly used in dentistry.

Oral sedation. Oral sedation is the most popular route used by paediatric dentists because of the ease of administration for most children. There are a number of agents used for this technique, including:

- Benzodiazepines (e.g., midazolam).
- Hydroxyzine.
- Promethazine.
- Ketamine.
- Clonidine.
- Dexmedetomidine.

Midazolam has increased in popularity in the last two decades because of its safety and short-acting nature, allowing a quick recovery and discharge of the patient. Oral dosage varies

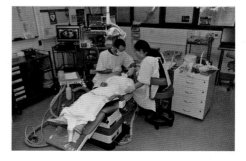

Figure 3.6 An intravenous (conscious) sedation clinic has a similar setup to a normal operating room environment with monitoring and resuscitation equipment.

from 0.3 to 0.7 mg/kg; however, a maximum ceiling dose (e.g., 10 mg) is usually determined for the older age groups. There are a number of studies that report on the use of oral midazolam as a successful technique for children with the following selection criteria:

- Children of ages 24 months to 6 to 8 years (depending on individual characteristics, e.g., body weight).
- ASA 1 or 2.
- Short or simple procedures (<30 min).
- Parents who are 'fit' for the technique; that is, they are able to care adequately for the child after the procedure.

Although this drug may be used successfully in the older age groups, it may be more difficult to deal or move children of a larger size, once sedated. Children over 6 years may become disinhibited, and there is a higher frequency of paradoxical reactions in this age group. In addition, obese children may present added airway complications and issues with pharmacokinetics of the drug. Appropriate fasting for elective procedures is preferable.

The main disadvantage of the oral route is that the drugs given cannot be titrated accurately. As most drugs undergo hepatic metabolism, only a fraction of the original dose is active. This makes titration difficult and unreliable, unlike other techniques such as N_2O and IV sedation. Equally, an overdose cannot be easily reversed. Oral sedation requires enough cooperation of the child to be able to take the medication orally. A child may also spit out the medication. Never re-dose, as it is impossible to accurately determine how much of the drug was ingested.

In the precooperative age group, a knee-to-knee position offers good access for the delivery of oral medications. This technique is also used to treat young children, as it allows good control of the patient, easy restraint by the parent/carer and good vision into the mouth by the clinician.

CLINICAL HINTS: ORAL SEDATION

- Weigh the child at both the consultation and treatment visit (to minimize dosage errors).
- The dentist should administer the drug which is checked by a second person for accuracy of dose.
- Record time when drug was administered and dosage.
- Onset of effect is usually 20 to 30 minutes.
- Administer local anaesthetic.
- Use of rubber dam is recommended.
- Recover child to preoperative state (that is, awake, alert and responsive).

Rectal sedation. Although used routinely in Scandinavia and other European countries, the use of this form of sedation is less common in Australia, Asia, UK and the USA. It is, however, an excellent route for drug administration and provides a more reliable and controllable absorption than the oral route.

Intranasal sedation. This implies delivery of medication directly to the nasal mucosa by spray or drops. The most common drugs used include midazolam, ketamine and sufentanyl (a synthetic opioid analgesic). This route has a shorter onset of action when compared with oral drugs. There are some adverse reactions, such as burning of the nasal mucosa, stinging sensation, bitter taste and the unpleasant squirting of a drug into the nose. There are also cases of oxygen desaturations; therefore, experienced sedationists and staff are required for the safe use of this technique. Its mechanism of action is not fully understood (either absorbed directly into the blood stream or directly into the CNS), and this is not a common technique used in paediatric dentistry.

Intravenous sedation. This technique requires a highly trained team, including an experienced and appropriately qualified sedationist (medical or dental practitioner) or a specialist anaesthetist and medical nurses experienced in sedation and recovery, but also a proceduralist dentist familiar with the effects of sedation in clinical dentistry. Appropriate monitoring, adequate facilities and recovery options are mandatory for the safe delivery of IV drugs. The relevant regulating body in each country dictates these guidelines.

IV sedation has the advantage of the procedure being controllable and may be readily reversible, but as most children are frightened of needles, the placement of a cannula on the dorsum of the hand or anticubital fossa is often distressing, especially in anxious children. Although different drug combinations may be used under IV, in Australia, a combination of midazolam and an opioid analgesic (e.g., fentanyl or alfentanyl) is often used. These drugs are readily reversible by flumazenil and naloxone, respectively.

Patients with the following criteria are suitable for intravenous sedation

- Child patients 8 years of age or older.
- ASA 1 or 2. Must have a degree of cooperation to allow injection and have adequate venous access.
- Must have a cooperative parent/carer to look after the patient.

Some children may not be suitable for IV sedation. Some 'red flags' include:

- Children with significant respiratory disease such as cystic fibrosis, poorly controlled asthma or sleep apnoea.
- Obese children (where resuscitation procedures may be difficult and the airway more unpredictable).
- Dysphagia, liquid diet or thickened fluids, history of aspiration pneumonia.
- Poorly controlled epilepsy or reflux.
- Parents who may not provide adequate care to the child postoperatively.

Suitable procedures for intravenous sedation

- Ideally, procedures that require approximately 30–45 min duration.
- Primary teeth extractions, premolar extractions or up to two permanent molars.
- One to two quadrants of restorative dentistry.
- Short surgical procedures with good access to surgical area.

Procedures usually not suitable for intravenous sedation

- Three to four quadrants of dentistry (unless minor restorative).
- Extractions of permanent molars in each quadrant (invasive procedure and bleeding from all four quadrants make airway management more difficult).

CLINICAL HINTS: INTRAVENOUS SEDATION

- The technique is highly dependent on the sedationist, the dentist performing the clinical work and clinical support staff with experience working under intravenous (IV) sedation.
- Elevate the chin to minimize/avoid airway obstruction.
- Body movement may be present and may interfere with treatment.
- Watch breathing pattern, coughing or signs of obstruction.

IV sedation is usually performed in a hospital environment or in dental surgeries that have been duly accredited for the use of these more advanced sedation techniques.

Sedation protocols are strictly defined in many countries by regulations and guidelines. A comprehensive document (PS9) applies to several medical and dental colleges in Australia and New Zealand (PS9, 2014), as well as similar guidelines in other countries.

General anaesthesia

The use of GA for dental treatment has increased globally. This is because of increased awareness and acceptance by parents and the increase in availability, safety and an understanding that it is the most appropriate way in which to manage young children requiring extensive dental treatment. Additionally, restorative dental care for the child with special needs often necessitates GA. Dental GA is also in line with the management of most other invasive medical procedures that are performed under anaesthesia around the world.

Mortality rates from anaesthesia have decreased around the world. In Australia, in 2005, deaths attributed to anaesthesia in all age groups were estimated to be 1:53,000. The mortality rate for children, although unable to be accurately quantified, was much lower than this, and is estimated to be 1:150,000. The mortality risk for dental GA would be expected to be lower than this, as it is elective surgery that has a lower risk profile than other major operations.

SAFETY OF ANAESTHETIC AND SEDATIVE DRUGS IN CHILDREN

In 2016, the US Food Drug Administration (FDA) issued a safety announcement, stating that anaesthetic and sedation drugs could affect the neurocognitive development in young children, that is, being neurotoxic to the developing human brain (https://www.fda.gov/media/101937/download). At present, there is no worldwide consensus, and more information may be obtained at https://smarttots.org.

There are important ongoing prospective studies at the time of editing of this chapter. The GAS (general anesthesia spinal) Study is an international, randomized controlled trial being conducted at 28 hospitals in 7 countries. This study found that children who had undergone either general anaesthesia or regional anaesthesia in a surgical procedure lasting less than 1 hour showed no difference in cognitive development at the 2-year time point. Five-year results await (McCann, 2019). The Pediatric Anesthesia Neurodevelopment Assessment (PANDA) study used a sibling-matched cohort design to test the hypothesis that a single exposure to general anaesthesia in healthy children younger than 3 years was associated with, at ages 8 to 15 years, an increased risk of impaired global cognitive function (IQ) as the primary outcome and abnormal domain-specific neurocognitive functions and behaviour as secondary outcomes (Sun, 2016). The PANDA study, along with the preliminary GAS trial findings, provides some clinical evidence that a single, relatively brief early exposure to general anaesthesia in generally healthy children is unlikely to cause clinically detectable deficits in global cognitive function or serious behaviour disorders.

CLINICAL HINT: RISK VERSUS BENEFIT

Although most children will cope with dentistry in a normal setting, many may benefit from delivery of extensive dentistry in one session under general anaesthesia (GA). The decision to arrange a general anaesthetic should not be taken lightly, and benefits of providing treatment must always outweigh the risks of providing GA. Economic variables (public health access and private health insurance), cultural factors and access to anaesthetic facilities may also influence the use of GA. When deciding to place the child under general anaesthesia, the clinician must assess the whole situation.

What is the dental condition?

- Is there gross dental caries or dentoalveolar trauma?
- Does the child have a facial swelling?

- Is the child in pain?
- Is it reasonable for the child to cope with the anticipated treatment?

Is the treatment absolutely necessary?

- Could the patient be managed more conservatively?
- Has the child undergone a period of familiarization?
- Has there been a history of emotional trauma associated with the dental environment?

Certain clinical situations indicate automatically the need for GA:

- Multiple carious and abscessed teeth in multiple quadrants in very young children.
- Severe facial cellulitis.
- Facial or complex dental trauma.
- Children with medical conditions (e.g., cerebral palsy, autism spectrum disorder, attention deficit hyperactivity disorder) where treatment in the dental chair is unsafe for the child and staff.

Treatment planning under GA requires experience and careful consideration to avoid treatment failures or repeat GAs. Consequently, GA treatment in paediatric dentistry ideally should only be carried out by dentists with the appropriate postgraduate qualifications. In other words, the skill is in the treatment planning, not doing the fillings or extractions.

CONSENT FOR TREATMENT

In many countries, consent is dependent on the age of the child. For descriptive purposes, only the age of consent has been described as it applies in Australia.

Consent for children younger than 14 years of age

In children under 14 years of age, a specific 'Consent form' is required. The parent or guardian must sign the form and a dentist must witness the signature.

Consent for children 14 to 16 years of age

Children aged 14 to 16 years must give their own consent for the treatment to be performed. Although a 'responsible informed child' can give this consent, the parent or guardian should also give consent and sign the form. The dentist should explain the procedure and witness the signatures.

Although there is no authoritative statement in statute law regarding consent for children younger than 16 years, common law (Australasia and the UK) dictates that:

> …*as a matter of law the parents' right to determine whether or not their minor child below the age of 16 will have medical treatment terminates if and when their child achieves a sufficient understanding to enable him to understand fully what is proposed.*
> (GILLICK V WEST NORFOLK AREA HEALTH AUTHORITY [1986] AC 112, UK)

Consent over 16 years

A patient 16 years and over must consent for their own treatment.

EMERGENCY TREATMENT

In emergency situations, dental treatment may be performed without the consent of the child or parent or guardian if, in the opinion of the practitioner, the treatment is necessary and a matter of urgency to save the child's life, or to prevent serious damage to the child's health (Section 20B of the Children [Care and Protection] Act [1987] NSW, Australia). Fortunately, there are few situations where this will occur in the dental environment, although situations do arise for those working in hospital settings. The overriding point is to 'do no harm'.

It is important that, when possible, 'informed consent' be obtained. The clinician must carefully explain all the procedures planned using lay language as appropriate. All potential risks need to be mentioned, discussed and documented. Alternative therapies and the likely outcomes of each therapy also need to be discussed. When completing the sections on standard forms on the nature of the operation, be specific, do not use abbreviations and include all the procedures planned. Where appropriate, use simple terminology to describe the operation, such as 'extractions of baby teeth', 'fillings of teeth and extraction if needed', 'removal of extra tooth', etc.

PREANAESTHETIC ASSESSMENT FOR GENERAL ANAESTHESIA

A medical history and examination by the anaesthetist are required before the procedure. If a patient has complex medical problems, a preoperative anaesthetic assessment may be required as a separate consultation before the day of surgery.

The anaesthetist will particularly want to be aware of:

Past anaesthetic history:

- Any previous general anaesthetics.
- Any adverse events (e.g., emergence delirium, postoperative nausea and vomiting, problems with induction such as being held down, difficult intubation).

Past medical history

- Behavioural issues (e.g., autism, developmental delay, extreme anxiety and needle phobia).
- Syndromes and pansystemic disease (e.g., Down syndrome, velocardiofacial syndrome).
- Cardiac disease, heart murmurs, previous surgery for congenital defects.
- Respiratory disease (e.g., asthma).
- Airway problems (e.g., history of croup, cleft palate, micrognathia, previous tracheostomy, known history of intubation difficulties, sleep apnoea).
- Neurological disease (e.g., epilepsy, previous brain injuries, cerebral palsy).
- Endocrine and metabolic disorders (e.g., diabetes, genetic metabolic disorders).
- Gastrointestinal problems (e.g., reflux, difficulty swallowing or feeding).
- Haematological (e.g., haemophilia, thrombocytopenia, haemoglobinopathies).
- Neuromuscular disorders (e.g., muscular dystrophy).
- Allergies must be noted, including latex, food or medication allergies.

Medications must be documented. Most medications should be continued until the time of anaesthesia unless there is a clear reason to withhold (e.g., with anticoagulants or insulin). Consultation with the original prescriber should be made before warfarin or aspirin is ceased to make an assessment of the risk or benefit of ceasing these drugs. Management of diabetic patients will require consultation with the patient's endocrinologist.

Upper respiratory tract infection

If a child has had an upper respiratory tract infection within the previous 2 weeks, they are at an increased risk of laryngospasm and bronchospasm (if a lower respiratory tract infection was present). If the child presents with an upper respiratory tract infection on the day of surgery and is systemically unwell, it may be appropriate to delay elective anaesthesia for 2 to 3 weeks. This decision can be balanced against economic and social issues and patient factors such as the child's age, urgency of treatment, severity of the infection and any other medical problems the child may have. Ultimately, the decision to cancel or proceed is up to the anaesthetist.

Fasting

Current consensus guidelines regarding paediatric fasting times are as follows:
Child aged older than 6 months
- 6 hours from solids.
- 4 hours from formula or breast milk.
- 1 hours from clear fluids.

Infants under 6 months
- 6 hours from solids and milk.
- 4 hours from formula.
- 3 hours from breast milk.
- 1 hour from clear fluids.

Keeping fasting instructions close to these guidelines will cause the least distress for the patient. Unfortunately, difficulties with organizational factors often result in longer fasting times.

There is no evidence that oral medications taken during the time of fasting increases the risk of aspiration during anaesthesia.

OPERATING THEATRE ENVIRONMENT

There is often a misconception that everything that happens in an operating room is sterile, and unless staff are familiar with dental procedures, the experience for many children and parents can be overly bureaucratic. Although clinicians must follow the protocols of the individual institution under which they operate, it is essential that auxiliary staff appreciate the anxiety that our patients feel and why they are having their treatment performed under GA. To reduce the child's fear and anxiety, strategies should be used to help them to cope with the operating theatre environment. For example:
- Minimizing the waiting time before the procedure by staggering admission times.
- Leaving children in their own clothes. It is not necessary to change into theatre attire for routine restorative procedures.
- Allowing a parent to stay with the child during induction of anaesthesia.
- Using inhalational/gas inductions as opposed to IV inductions in young children.
- Allowing a parent into the recovery area to be with the child as soon as they are awake and stable.
- Reassuring parents at all stages about what to expect.

Premedication (Table 3.4)

Some children may require oral premedication before anaesthesia. Suggested medications include midazolam, clonidine or ketamine.

Induction

Having an environment that minimizes anxiety and fear is essential to a successful induction. This requires cooperation and trust between the dentist, anaesthetist, dental staff, nursing staff and theatre staff. Anxiety is minimized by allowing a parent to be with the child during induction. Anaesthesia induction may be IV or gaseous. Sevoflurane with N_2O and O_2 can be given for a gaseous induction. It is not too unpleasant and, with skill, can be used with little distress to the patient. The use of topical local anaesthetic cream before insertion of a cannula into a vein alleviates some of the pain of obtaining IV access. Some extremely uncooperative children may require induction with intramuscular ketamine 2 to 3 mg/kg. These are usually older children with autism or developmentally delay.

TABLE 3.4 ■ **Premedication for general anaesthesia**

Drug	Route	Dose	Onset	Side effects
Midazolam	Oral/Buccal	0.3–0.5 mg/kg	20–30 min	Disinhibition and hyperactivity is not uncommon, both immediately and postoperatively. Causes amnesia.
	Intranasal	0.2 mg/kg	10–15 min	Can sting.
Clonidine	Oral	4 µg/kg	45–60 min	Sedation, bradycardia, no amnesic effects.
	Intranasal	2 µg/kg	30–60 min	
Ketamine	Oral	5–10 mg/kg	10–20 min	Can cause increased salivation, bronchospasm, tachycardia, psychomimetic effects (dissociative state).
	Intranasal	3–5 mg/kg	10–15 min	
	Intramuscular	3–5 mg/kg	3–5 min	

Sharing the airway (Figure 3.7)

- The anaesthetist and dentist must share the airway, so teamwork, and mutual understanding and respect of each other's needs, is necessary.
- Nasotracheal intubation with a nasal RAE (Ring-Adair-Elwyn) tube provides good access for the dentist and a secure airway for the anaesthetist. A throat pack is usually used, and it is essential to ensure the removal of a throat pack at the end of the case. Direct visual laryngeal inspection by the anaesthetist is preferred.
- The throat pack should not be so bulky that the tongue is forced anteriorly, limiting the access to the mouth for the dentist. In young children, reduce the size of an adult-sized pack to one-third (ribbon gauze of about 30 cm moistened with saline).
- An oral laryngeal mask airway (LMA) or endotracheal tube provides a satisfactory airway for the anaesthetist, but may or may not give the dentist the access they require because it encroaches on the work area. However, this is a useful technique for less extensive dental work, such as extractions of primary anterior teeth after trauma or when a nasal tube is contraindicated. If an LMA is used, a flexible one is most appropriate, but it is a less secure airway than an endotracheal tube.
- A face-mask-only technique by the anaesthetist may be used for simple extractions. The mask is removed for a short time while the extraction is performed. However, the airway must be protected. This can be done by placing a gauze swab behind the teeth being extracted. This technique should be discussed with and performed under the discretion of the anaesthetist.
- During anaesthesia, it is important to protect the eyes from injury by taping them shut. Avoid padding to the eyes, as this can result in inadvertent globe pressure and cardiac arrhythmias.
- Before waking the patient, all foreign material such as rolls, gauze and throat packs must be removed and accounted for.

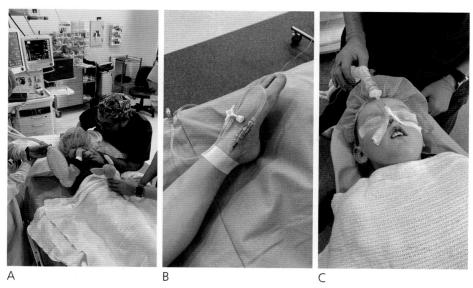

A   B   C

Figure 3.7 Management under general anaesthesia: sharing the airway. (A) Anaesthetic induction is a stressful time for parent and child and should be performed as atraumatically as possible. This relies on empathy and understanding and a close working relationship with your anaesthetist. (B). Children will often get quite distressed in recovery, being aware of the intravenous line. Siting of the cannula in the foot using the long saphenous vein, rather than in the back of the hand or the antecubital fossa, gives excellent IV access, and the child is unaware of the line when they awaken. (C) Intubation with a nasal Ring-Adair-Elwyn tube. This endotracheal tube gives excellent access to the oral cavity, and tubing is out of the way of the operator but is safely secured, avoiding extubation. Note the taping of the eyes without packs to avoid compression of the orbit.

Analgesia

Intraoperative analgesia should be given as appropriate. The use of IV opioids may be required. A short-acting opioid, such as fentanyl, may be a preferred opioid, as pain is not commonly experienced postoperatively. It has the added benefit of being less emetogenic as the other opioids (such as morphine and oxycodone). As mentioned earlier, local anaesthetics may be used, but often the feeling of numbness around the mouth causes even more distress than the discomfort of the procedure. Intraoperative parecoxib, a selective COX-2 NSAID, can be administered at a dose of 1 mg/kg. Paracetamol 15 mg/kg every 4 hours may also be used.

Emergence

Ideally, parents should be able to come into the recovery area once the child is awake and in a stable condition. Distress on waking is not uncommon and can be attributed to emergence delirium. This condition may be caused by the choice of anaesthetic drugs, lack of local anaesthesia, the child may be upset by the unfamiliar environment, an unpleasant taste in the mouth or because their mouth feels different because of missing teeth or new crowns. Intraoperative administration of clonidine 0.3 to 0.5 μg/kg IVI or proprofol 0.5 to 1 mg/kg at the end of the case can mitigate against emergence delirium.

CLINICAL HINTS: TREATMENT UNDER GENERAL ANAESTHETIC

1. Preoperative assessment, written consent and information provided to parents at the consultation visit.
2. Dental treatment planning. This is an important part to reduce repeat procedures under sedation.
3. Parent contacted 24 hours prior by dentist and hospital staff confirming fasting instructions and admission protocols.
4. On day of general anaesthetic (GA)/surgery
   a. Assessment by anaesthetist: confirms fitness of child for procedure (e.g., upper respiratory tract infection, illnesses).
   b. Assessment by dentist and treatment plan discussion with parent(s). In many cases one parent will attend the consultation and the other parent presents on the day of treatment. An important step regarding informed consent.
   c. Check that all dental equipment is operational before commencing GA.
5. Induction. Protocol differs in each hospital, but often the induction is with a parent present (current trends in paediatric GA).
6. Radiographs and photos. In cases of dental caries and extractions, intra-oral radiographs are 'mandatory'. The absence of x-rays during dental GA may be considered negligent in some countries. Preoperative photos are strongly recommended to record the preoperative status.
7. Use of rubber dam is strongly recommended in restorative cases (further protection to the airway).
8. The use of local anaesthesia (LA) is not constant in all cases and highly dependent on the operator's choice/experience. Some dentists will only use LA for extractions of permanent teeth and surgical procedures.
9. Review your initial treatment plan, account for all extracted teeth and disposable materials.
10. Dentist to discuss postoperative outcome with parents on the day of GA.
11. Arrange a post-GA follow-up appointment.

CATEGORIES OF ANAESTHETIC RISK

American Society of Anesthesiologists

- Class 1: Healthy patient.
- Class 2: Mild to moderate systemic disease without significant limitations.
- Class 3: Severe systemic disturbance without limitations.
- Class 4: Life-threatening systemic disorder.
- Class 5: Moribund patient not expected to survive more than 24 hours.
- Class E: Emergency patient.

Suitability for day-stay anaesthesia

Most children who are ASA 1 or 2 will be suitable for day-stay anaesthesia (Figure 3.8). However, children with more severe systemic disease may need preoperative and overnight hospital care to ensure that they are maintaining their airway, tolerating oral food and fluids, that any pain is satisfactorily managed and that there is no ongoing bleeding.

Ward instructions

Postoperative instructions and consultation notes in the medical file must be clear and legible. It is important for nursing staff to understand what procedures have been performed and by whom. They should also know whom to contact if complications arise.

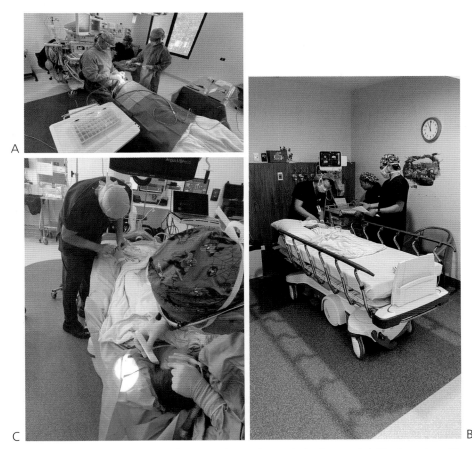

Figure 3.8 (A) Treatment under general anaesthesia must be conducted in a comfortable atmosphere. There must be cooperation between the anaesthetist and the operating dental surgeon, both of whom need access to the oral cavity and the airway. Nasal intubation is invaluable. Note the anaesthetic machine in close proximity but out of the way of the operating surgeon, and the dental assistant also has all the required equipment close at hand. Protocols in individual institutions will vary, however, and it is not usually necessary to scrub for restorative procedures, as these are considered to be 'nonsterile'. (B) A day-stay recovery ward with one-to-one nursing care after general anaesthesia. Normal day-stay recovery is 1 to 2 hours after the operation. Most children recover quickly and, once fully recovered, are better at home than waiting for extended periods in the hospital setting. (C) Consider other medical and social needs of a child undergoing anaesthesia. A routine dental operation might be an opportunity for blood tests to be performed. In this case, a child with severe autism is having his finger and toenails cut and his hair trimmed, commonplace events that might have been impossible when he was awake.

Further reading

Analgesic Expert Group, 2007. Therapeutic guidelines: analgesic version 5. Therapeutic Guidelines Ltd. Melbourne.

Australian and New Zealand College of Anaesthetists and Faculty of Pain Medicine, 2010. The paediatric patient. In: NHMRC acute pain management: scientific evidence, third ed. Australian and New Zealand College of Anaesthetists and Faculty of Pain Medicine. Online. Available www.anzca.edu.au /publications/acutepain.htm.

Herschell, A.D., Calzada, E., Eyberg, S.M., et al., 2003. Clinical issues with parent–child interaction therapy. Cognitive and Behavioral Practice 9, 16–27.

Lamacraft, G., Cooper, M.G., Cavalletto, B.P., 1997. Subcutaneous cannulae for morphine boluses in children: assessment of a technique. Journal of Pain Symptoms and Management 13, 43–49.

NSW Health, 2006. Paracetamol use, 2006. PD2006_004. Available: www.health.nsw.gov.au/policies /pd/2006/PD2006_004.html.

Royal Australasian College of Physicians, 2005. Paediatrics and Child Health Division. Guideline statement: management of procedure related pain in children and adolescents. Available: www.health.nsw.gov.au /policies/pd/2006/PD2006_004.html.

The Therapeutic Goods Administration (TGA), Australian Government Department of Health, 2015. Codeine use in children and ultra-rapid metabolisers. Pharmacovigilance and Special Access Branch Safety Review. Available: https://www.tga.gov.au/alert/safety-review-codeine-use-children-and-ultra -rapid-metabolisers.

Use of Local Anesthesia for Pediatric Dental Patients. Latest Revision 2020:318–323. https://www.aapd.org /globalassets/media/policies_guidelines/bp_localanesthesia.pdf.

Weisman, S.J., Berstein, B., Schechter, N.L., 1998. Consequences of inadequate analgesia during painful procedures in children. Archives of Pediatrics and Adolescent Medicine 152, 147–149.

Sedation

Adewale, L., Morton N., Blayney, M., 2016. Guidelines for the management of children referred for dental extractions under general anaesthesia. Available: http://dentalanaesthesia.org.uk/wp-content/uploads /2016/08/full_guidelines_dopd_ga-1.pdf.

Aldecoa, C., Bettelli, G., Bilotta, F., et al., 2017. European Society of Anaesthesiology evidence-based and consensus-based guideline on postoperative delirium. European Journal of Anaesthesiology 34, 192–214.

Chicka, M.C., Dembo, J.B., Mathu-Muju, K.R., 2012. Adverse events during pediatric dental anesthesia and sedation: a review of closed malpractice insurance claims. Pediatric Dentistry 34, 231–238.

Cote, C.J., Notterman, D.A., Karl, H.W., et al., 2000. Adverse sedation events in pediatrics. A critical incident analysis of contributing factors. Pediatrics 105, 805–814.

Cote, C.J., Notterman, D.A., Karl, H.W., et al., 2000. Adverse sedation events in pediatrics: Analysis of medications used for Sedation. Pediatrics 106, 633–644.

Cote, C.J., Wilson, S., 2016. Guidelines for monitoring and management of pediatric patients during and after sedation for diagnostic and therapeutic procedures. Update 2016. Pediatrics 138, e1–e31.

Cravero, J.P., Blike, G.T., 2006. Review of pediatric sedation. Anesthesia and Analgesia 99, 1355–1364.

Goodson, J.M., Moore, P.A., 1983. Life-threatening reactions after pedodontic sedation: an assessment of narcotic, local anesthetic, and antiemetic drug interaction. Journal of the American Dental Association 107, 239–245.

Guidelines on sedation and/or analgesia for diagnostic and interventional medical, dental or surgical procedures 2014. Available: https://www.anzca.edu.au/documents/ps09-2014-guidelines-on-sedation-and -or-analgesia.

Houpt, M., 2002. Project USAP, 2000—use of sedative agents by pediatric dentists: a 15-year follow up survey. Pediatric Dentistry 24, 289–294.

Kupietzky, A., Houpt, M.I., 1993. Midazolam: a review of its use for conscious sedation of children. Pediatric Dentistry 15, 237–241.

Lee, H.H., Milgrom, P., Starks, H., et al., 2013. Trends in death associated with pediatric dental sedation and general anesthesia. Paediatrics Anaesthesia 23, 741–746.

Lee, J.Y., Vann, W.F., Roberts, M.W., 2000. A cost analysis of treating pediatric dental patients using general anesthesia versus conscious sedation. Pediatric Dentistry 22, 27–32.

McCann, M.E., de Graaff, J.C., Dorris, L., et al., 2019. Neurodevelopmental outcome at 5 years of age after general anaesthesia or awake-regional anaesthesia in infancy (GAS): an international, multicentre, randomised, controlled equivalence trial. Lancet 393, 664–677.

NICE clinical guideline 112. Developed by the National Clinical Guideline Centre. Sedation in children and young people. Sedation for diagnostic and therapeutic procedures in children and young people. Issue date: December 2010. Available: https://www.nice.org.uk/guidance/CG112.

Primosch, R.E., Buzzi, I.M., Jerrell, G., 1999. Effect of nitrous oxide-oxygen inhalation with scavenging on behavioral and physiological parameters during routine pediatric dental treatment. Pediatric Dentistry 21, 417–420.

Royal College of Dental Surgeons of Ontario, Canada, 2009. Guidelines: use of sedation and general anaesthesia in dental practice. Available: http://www.rcdso.org/sedationAnaesthesia_pdf/Guidelines _sedation_06_09.pdf.

Society for the Advancement of Anaesthesia in Dentistry, 2009. Standardised evaluation of conscious sedation practice for dentistry in the UK. Available http://www.saad.org.uk/files/documents/Standardised%20 Evaluation%20of%20Conscious%20Sedation%20Practice%20for%20Dentistry%20in%20the%20UK. pdf.

Sun, L.S., Li, G., Miller, T.L., et al., 2016. Association between a single general anesthesia exposure before age 36 months and neurocognitive outcomes in later childhood. JAMA 315, 2312–2320.

Townsend, J.A., Hagan, J.L., Smiley, M., 2014. Use of local anesthesia during dental rehabilitation with general anesthesia: a survey of dentist anesthesiologists. Anesthesia Progress 61, 11–17.

Wilson, S., Houpt, M., 2016. Project USAP 2010: use of sedative agents in pediatric dentistry—a 25-year follow-up survey. Pediatric Dentistry 38, 127–133.

Yagiela, J.A., Cote, C.J., Notterman, D.A., et al., 2001. Adverse sedation events in pediatrics. Pediatrics 107, 1494.

Dental caries

Svante Twetman

Introduction

Dental caries is a biofilm-mediated, sugar-driven, multifactorial disease that results in a phasic de- and remineralization of the dental hard tissues (Pitts et al., 2017). The complex interplay among biological, genetic, social and behavioural factors classifies caries as a noncommunicable disease (NCD), sharing risk factors with other NCDs, such as overweight and diabetes (Figure 4.1). Untreated dental caries in permanent teeth is the most prevalent disease (35% for all ages combined) across all medical conditions assessed in the Global Burden of Disease Study, with at least 2.4 billion individuals affected (Marcenes et al., 2013). In addition, dental caries is the most common chronic childhood disease, affecting over 600 million preschool children worldwide. Untreated caries in children is associated with impaired quality of life including pain, feeding problems, disturbed sleep and absence from school. Furthermore, severe caries early in life may affect the child's growth and development, especially when left untreated. This makes children a priority group for prevention (World Health Organization [WHO], 2017). This chapter deals with the microbial events involved in dental caries and the key factors that influence the carious process. It will also cover caries detection, risk assessment and the preventive principles with special reference to early childhood caries (ECC).

Oral biofilm

The oral microbiome is the ecological community of commensal, symbiotic and pathogenic microorganisms of the mouth, their genetic information and their environment in which they interact (Kilian et al., 2016). In the oral cavity, most bacteria are located on the tongue and the oral

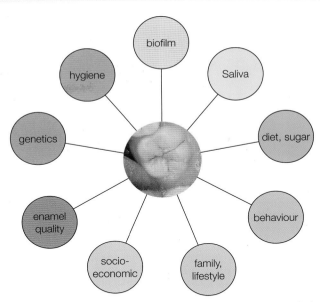

Figure 4.1 Examples of factors that influence the caries process. Some can be controlled and/or modified by parents and dental professionals whereas others are more or less fixed.

mucosa while approximately 20% constitute the dental biofilm (dental plaque). The composition of the oral biofilm is unique for each individual and is formed during the first 1000 days of life according the 'first come, first served' principle. Modifying factors are genetics, order of exposure, timing, diet and the location (ecological niche). The mode of delivery and other perinatal factors have a strong impact on the early microbiome; for example, vaginal birth and breastfeeding are associated with a health-associated salivary microbiome and reduced risk for caries (Boustedt et al., 2018). The 'early' colonizers (3–6 months) belong to the genera *Streptococcus*, *Veillonella* and *Lactobacillus* spp. (Dzidic et al., 2018). In connection with tooth eruption, the 'constant' colonizers appear (*Gemella*, *Granulicatella*, *Haemophilus*, *Rothia*) whereas the 'late' colonizers, such as *Actinomyces*, *Porphyromonas*, *Abitrophia* and *Neisseria*, are detectable after the first year of life. The established dental biofilm is typically arranged with hedgehog filaments and corncob structures, as illustrated in Figure 4.2.

The current understanding is that the oral microbiota does not play a passive role but actively contributes to the maintenance of health. The dental biofilm is dynamic and contains a large number of different types of bacteria with various properties and functions; a rich, diverse and balanced biofilm in symbiosis with the host is associated with health and acts as a fluoride reservoir and a protective barrier to erosion. A persisting environmental low-pH stress (<5.0) may, however, induce a dysbiotic shift in the oral/dental biofilm with an overgrowth of acidogenic and acid-tolerating commensal species (Figure 4.3). The organic acids formed by these abundant acid-producing bacteria create a net mineral loss at the tooth surface, and the first clinical signs of demineralization can be visually detected within 2 months after a significant biofilm shift. A typical example of such acid-tolerating strains is the mutans streptococci family. Elevated levels of *Streptococcus mutans* and *Streptococcus sobrinus* are strongly associated with the initiation of dental caries, in particular early in life and in high-caries populations with poor oral hygiene and limited access to care. They are, however, not 'classical pathogens', because many children harbour the bacteria without developing caries (Marsh, 2018). Mutans streptococci can be transmitted vertically from the parents and horizontally from other caregivers, but this is 'normal' and causes no harm

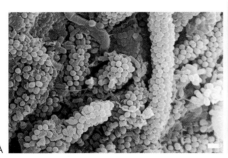
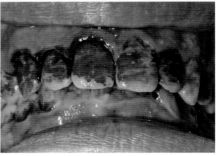

A   B

Figure 4.2 (A) Scanning electron micrograph of dental plaque (×4555 magnification). This image shows the typical 'corncob' arrangement of streptococci held by an extracellular polysaccharide matrix on a web of central filamentous microorganisms. (Courtesy Institute of Dental Research, SEM Unit, Westmead). (B) Disclosing plaque is an important part of teaching children about oral hygiene and educating parents. (Courtesy Dr Andrew McNaught.)

as long as the biofilms remain in an unstressed and symbiotic state. Thus, measures to avoid early acquisition of caries-associated bacteria are not a cost-effective caries-preventive strategy. The individual biofilm composition, stress tolerance and resilience are important to keep in mind; the classical but infamous 'Vipeholm study' showed that some persons could consume large amounts of sugars without having any caries lesions. Recent research suggests that individuals with a 'saccharolytic' ecotype of their salivary microbiome seem most vulnerable for caries development (Zaura et al., 2017).

The most common drivers of biofilm dysbiosis among children are excessive sugar intake, irregular mechanical tooth cleaning and impaired saliva functions. Biofilm eradication is neither possible nor desirable. Therefore, the sustainable way to deal with the causes of caries should focus on measures to ecologically modulate and control the oral biofilm to maintain a stable symbiosis (primary prevention) or to restore a caries-associated microbiome (secondary prevention). Population-based and/or personalized approaches are useful for these purposes and the main strategies for children are daily fluoride exposure, dietary sugar reduction and regular oral hygiene (Twetman, 2018).

The caries process

The caries process is not a continuous cumulative loss of tooth minerals but a dynamic process characterized by alternating periods of demineralization and remineralization. When there is a

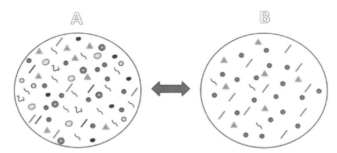

Figure 4.3 Principal drawing of the ecological low-pH shift from a dynamic and diverse health-associated symbiotic oral biofilm (A) to a dysbiotic state (B) with reduced diversity and abundance of acid-tolerating caries-associated species. The process can go both ways; by dealing with the drivers of dysbiosis, a symbiotic biofilm may be re-established.

net loss of minerals over time, a lesion will develop and progress whereas a net gain results in repair.

    A. Enamel demineralization is a chemical process involving the dissolution of hydroxyapatite. The biofilm-produced organic acids (lactic acid and acetic acid) diffuse through the biofilm and into the enamel pores between the rods where they dissociate and decrease the pH of the fluid surrounding the enamel crystals. Once dissociated, the protons dissolve the hydroxyapatite crystal surface:

$$Ca_{10}(PO_4)_6(OH)_2 + 10H^+ \rightarrow 10Ca_2 + 6H(PO_4)^{3-} + 2H_2O$$

    Depending on the degree of saturation of the specific apatite and the inter-rod fluid, calcium (Ca^{2+}) and phosphate (PO_4^{3-}) ion concentration increases. The buffering of these ions at the enamel surface leads to the development of a subsurface lesion with a hypermineralized surface layer. The whitish optical changes of an early lesion occur because of the increased pore spaces between the thinned rods. A continuation of mineral net loss will eventually undermine the support opening a physical cavity. This surface breakdown may take from months to years, depending on the intensity and frequency of the caries-related factors as elaborated later.

    B. Enamel remineralization occurs as a natural repair process where biofilm/salivary calcium and phosphate ions are deposited into crystal voids of the demineralized tooth structure, resulting in net mineral gain. The presence of free fluoride ions in the oral environment can drive the incorporation of the Ca^{2+} and PO_4^{3-} ions into the crystal lattice, forming a fluoroapatite mineral that is significantly more resistant to a subsequent acid challenge.

Factors influencing the caries process

Host factors. The hereditary components of dental caries were clinically evitable already in the dawn of modern dentistry. The recent advances in genetics and genomics have significantly increased the molecular understanding of the disease (Divaris, 2019), but there is still a long road to the translation of these findings into daily practice. Up to date, the quality of the tooth structures and the saliva flow rate and composition are the major host factors that should be considered. Poor hypomineralized enamel is associated with increased prevalence and incidence of dental caries, especially in the primary dentition (Figure 4.4). Saliva plays a critical role in the caries process, as it provides a stabilized supersaturated solution of calcium and phosphate ions as well as fluoride ions from extrinsic sources. The major constituent is water (~99.5%), providing acid clearance and mechanical cleaning. In addition, saliva contains a wide

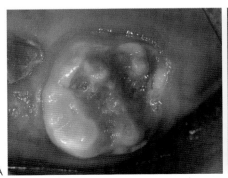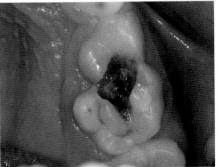

A   B

Figure 4.4 (A) Hypomineralized and/or hypoplastic teeth are predisposed to caries, particularly if the enamel deficiencies are plaque retentive. If the enamel is completely absent and dentin is exposed, these teeth can deteriorate rapidly. (B) Interproximal lesions that are cavitated and unable to be thoroughly cleaned do not arrest.

range of inorganic (salts, electrolytes) and organic (mucins, glycoproteins, enzymes, immuno-globulins) components with antibacterial, antifungal and antiviral activity that contributes to maintaining a symbiotic oral biofilm. Chewing-stimulated saliva has increased buffer capacity and elevated calcium and phosphate concentrations, which aid in reducing demineralization and assist remineralization as mentioned previously. Consequently, impaired saliva functions can significantly increase the caries risk. The saliva secretion rate increases with age, and it is uncommon that healthy children have compromised saliva functions. During sleep, how-ever, the flow rate is low and insufficient to buffer nocturnal feeding. Radiation therapy and prescribed antidepressive drugs are xerogenic and may jeopardize oral health, particularly in teenagers. The chewing of pH-neutral sugar-free gums increases the salivary flow and may be recommended for children and adolescents with objective or subjective signs of dry mouth.

Substrate. Fermentable carbohydrates are metabolized to acids by the oral biofilm via the glycolytic pathway. Sucrose is the 'arch criminal', but the oral bacteria can use all fermentable carbohy-drates, including cooked starches. Sucrose is digested into its components glucose and fructose, and the availability of glucose is the main of source of lactate, subsequently excreted from the bacterial cells as lactic acid. Traditionally, dentists have focused on the frequency of sugar con-sumption, but both the amount and frequency of sugar intake are important determinants for caries and overweight. The overall consumption of sugar has increased over the past 50 years in most Western countries, especially related to an increasing consumption of fast food and carbon-ated beverages. To reduce caries and overweight, the WHO has issued strong recommendations to reduce the intake of free sugars among children and adults to less than 10% of total energy intake (Moynihan et al., 2018). They further suggest nations to reduce, over time, the intake of free sugars to below 5%. Free sugars are those added to food and beverages and sugars naturally present in honey, syrups, fruit juices and fruit juice concentrates.

Sociobehavioural factors. Dental caries prevalence differs between countries and across regions; a low caries prevalence is commonly observed in developing countries, whereas the prevalence is higher in the industrialized and western countries. There is, however, a strong socio-economic gradient in caries in the latter societies; children from families with lower socio-economic status have, on average, three times more decayed teeth than those with a higher socio-economic background (Peres et al., 2019). In addition, children belonging to ethnic minorities often pres-ent an elevated caries risk. These disparities are partially explained by health beliefs, locus of control and self-efficacy, as these factors exert an influence on parents' knowledge as well as their attitudes and practices, including dietary and hygiene practices undertaken with their children. Such oral health-related behaviour includes tooth cleaning and feeding practices and use of preventive services. Several initiatives over the years have been designed to reduce the caries inequality gaps, but there is no 'one-size-fits-all' approach. Common success factors are that the programmes contain a component of fluoride, are adopted to the local culture and use the local day-care/school system as an integrated arena for oral health promotion.

Caries detection

Caries detection aims to find present lesions and assess their severity, activity and risk of progres-sion. The best clinical practice for this process is visual and tactile inspection. The teeth must be dry and clean to enable detection of the very early lesions. Sharp dental probes have little diag-nostic benefit, so it is advisable to use a blunt or ball-ended probe to check surface integrity and to avoid damage to demineralized enamel. Bitewing radiographs should be exposed on individual indications when the proximal surfaces cannot be inspected, or when existing lesions are moni-tored over time. The development of commercial caries detection systems, such as DIAGNOdent, Canary and Soprolife, increases not only the number of correctly detected early lesions but also the number of false-positive tests (over-detection). Thus, these methods should not be used alone but may be a valuable adjunct to the traditional methods. For research purposes, quantitative light

TABLE 4.1 ■ **Clinical evaluation of lesion activity according to the International Caries Detection and Assessment System**

	Signs of a likely active lesion	**Signs of a likely inactive lesion**
Colour	Enamel surface whitish/yellowish	Enamel surface whitish, brownish or black
Texture	Opaque with loss of luster, feels rough on gentle probing across the surface	Shiny and feels hard and smooth on gentle probing across the surface
Location	Lesion in the entrance of fissures, near the gingival margin or below or above the contact point (proximal surfaces)	Lesion is typically located at some distance from the gingival margin
Dentin	Soft or leathery on gentle probing	Shiny and hard on gentle probing

fluorescence (QLF) can quantify very small changes in mineral content, and this technology is useful in monitoring the impact of preventive measures on the caries process.

The caries process is a continuum and the severity of lesions must be scored on tooth level. Unfortunately, the commonly used DMFT/dmft (decayed/missing/filled teeth) score (WHO) has limitations because it counts caries only when there is a cavitation into the dentin and the subsequent treatment decisions are mostly restorative. For example, the caries prevalence in 15-year-olds is 21% when dentin caries is scored compared with 52% when also the early lesions are included. Therefore, a caries scoring system that allows detailed staging of lesions and activity assessment is best clinical practice. One example is the International Caries Detection and Assessment System (ICDAS) that has gained popularity among both clinicians and epidemiological researchers in recent years (Ekstrand et al., 2018). The original ICDAS has seven scores, but for clinical practice, lesions are graded as sound (ICDAS 0), early (ICDAS 1–2), moderate (ICDAS 3–4) or extensive (ICDAS 5–6). In addition, the colour, texture and location of each lesion are evaluated as 'likely active' or 'likely inactive', which is important information for the subsequent disease management (Table 4.1). ICDAS has been validated in a large number of clinical trials and generally shows a good overall performance (see Figure 4.5).

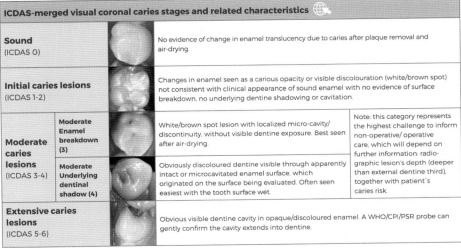

Figure 4.5 ICDAS-merged visual coronal caries stages and related characteristics.
Note: Non-carious surfaces with developmental defects of enamel (including fluorosis), erosive tooth wear, and extrinsic/intrinsic stains are considered as sound for caries.

> **BOX 4.1 ■ Examples of risk factors and protective factors associated with caries in children**
>
> Social/medical/behavioural risk factors for caries
> - Parent/family/caregiver has life-time of poverty, low health literacy, habitual smokers
> - High intake (amount/frequency) of free sugars from meals, snacks or beverages
> - Bottle or nonspill cup containing natural or added sugar used frequently or at bedtime
> - Breastfeeding beyond 12 months, especially if frequent/nocturnal
> - Mother/primary caregiver has active dental caries
> - Child has special healthcare needs and or disabilities
>
> Clinical risk factors for caries
> - Early noncavitated lesions or enamel defects
> - Visible cavities or fillings or missing teeth because of caries
> - Visible dental biofilm (plaque) on teeth
>
> Caries protective factors
> - Fluoridated drinking water or other community fluoride vehicles
> - Teeth brushed twice daily with fluoridated toothpaste
> - Topical fluoride from health professional
> - Access to a dental home/regular dental care
>
> (Modified from Tinanoff, N., Baez, R.J., Diaz Guillory, C., et al., 2019. Early childhood caries epidemiology, aetiology, risk assessment, societal burden, management, education, and policy: global perspective. International Journal of Paediatric Dentistry 29, 238–248; Martignon, S., Pitts, N.B., Goffin, G., et al., 2019. CariesCare practice guide: consensus on evidence into practice. British Dental Journal 227, 353–362.)

Caries risk assessment

Caries risk assessment is the clinical process of establishing the probability of an individual patient to develop carious lesions over a certain period of time and/or the likelihood that there will be a change in size or activity of lesions already present (Twetman, 2016). The risk assessment is a key element for personalized care plan, clinical decision-making and patient motivation. Informed parents and children that understand key factors about the disease and their own role are more likely to take action and modify their behaviour (Martignon et al., 2019). The caries risk is assessed by collecting and compiling data from the family and patients' social, medical and dental history with a comprehensive clinical examination. The balance between protective and pathological factors will ultimately determine the level of caries risk, and three categories are commonly used: low, moderate and high risk. There is consensus that 'low risk' means absence of disease (risk) factors and presence of protective factors, but there are no accepted definitions on the moderate- and high-risk categories. Examples of aspects to be addressed in the risk assessment process are shown in Box 4.1.

Because the risk assessment ideally should precede the disease, it is appropriate to carry out a comprehensive caries risk assessment at the child's first dental visit. Current research indicates that around 50% of all children change their risk category over time, for better or for worse, so the current caries risk should be re-evaluated periodically (Figure 4.6). Particular 'risk ages' to be considered are those linked to tooth eruption when a large number of susceptible tooth surfaces are exposed: 1 to 3 years, 5 to 6 years and 12 to 15 years. It is reported that most dentists perform caries risk assessment in children but they do so in an informal, subjective and nonstandardized way. The 'educated guess' is commonly based on the patient's past caries experience and the therapist's 'gut feeling'. There is evidence to suggest that multiple factor models combining clinical and various background factors are more accurate than the use of single predictors, in particular among preschool children (Mejàre et al., 2014). Thus the use of a structured age-adopted checklist

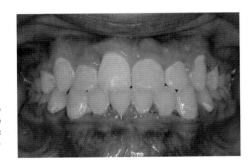

Figure 4.6 Note that risk can change. A child who was previously free of caries has developed 'white spot lesions' during treatment with fixed orthodontic appliances. The onset of brackets induced a dysbiotic shift in the adjacent biofilm.

or computer software is considered best clinical practice because it enhances objectivity, consistency and documentation and adds structure/routines to the clinical work. Examples of such validated caries risk assessment tools for children are CAMBRA (Featherstone & Chaffee, 2018) and Cariogram (Bratthall & Hänsel Petersson, 2005) that can be downloaded and used free of charge. When the individual risk level has been determined and communicated, a preventive care plan should be tailored to meet the need of the child. A suggested framework to a risk-based caries management is shown in Table 4.2.

Preventing dental caries

During the recent decades, systematic reviews of literature have examined the evidence for the common caries-preventive methods, and Table 4.3 shows a summary of the certainty of the evidence. A high certainty means that a true effect is supported by extensive high-quality research with a minimal risk of bias. A low, or very low, certainty does not rule out the possibility that the intervention is useful but its effectiveness has not been demonstrated in multiple randomized controlled trials with low risk of bias.

FLUORIDES

Fluoride is the cornerstone in the dental caries prevention, and research has shown that fluoride is most effective when a low level of fluoride is constantly maintained in the oral cavity (O'Mullane et al., 2016). The principal mode of action of all fluoridated modalities (community-based, self- and professionally applied) is the topical effect at the enamel surface. Therefore, presence of fluoride in the biofilm and the microenvironment around the teeth around the clock is crucial. Low concentrations of fluoride, such as after toothpaste use, inhibit demineralization and promote remineralization of the tooth surface. As mentioned earlier, the incorporation of fluoride (as fluoroapatite) into the enamel decreases its solubility and increases its resistance to caries. Likewise, the presence of supersaturated calcium and phosphate in an amorphous form (casein phosphopeptide-amorphous calcium phosphate [CPP-ACP]) in adjunct to fluoride may boost and enhance enamel remineralization. Higher concentrations of fluoride (after professional varnish or gel applications) increase amount of CaF_2 deposits in the biofilm and can hamper bacterial metabolism (glycolysis) and growth (Buzalaf, 2018). The time beyond the 'critical pH' will diminish, and in this way, fluoride can prevent an unfavourable biofilm shift and support a symbiotic relationship with the host. Incorporation of systemically administered fluorides into developing (unerupted) enamel plays a minor role in caries prevention. It is, however, evident from clinical experience that effective fluoride-based caries prevention cannot be achieved without a somewhat increased risk of mild enamel fluorosis. The decision of what fluoride sources and levels should be recommended for children under 6 years must therefore always be balanced with the risk of fluorosis (Walsh et al., 2019).

TABLE 4.2 ■ **Example of a risk-based framework for primary and secondary prevention of caries in children**

Risk Category	Low risk and/or no detectable enamel demineralization	Moderate risk and/or clinical/radiographic enamel demineralization	High risk and/or detectable lesions, including risk behaviour
Plaque	• Reinforce importance of twice-daily toothbrushing, supervised at lower ages	• Demonstrate and reinforce twice-daily toothbrushing	• Repeated toothbrushing instructions and training with disclosing agent
Diet	• Reinforce good dietary habits and encourage healthy beverages	• Advise against high-amount and frequent intake of fermentable carbohydrates • Check intake of soft drinks and sports drinks	• Review food intake with a 3-day diet diary, including one weekend day • Advise reducing free sugars to less than 10% of the total energy intake. Provide achievable alternatives

Fluoride	• At least 1000 ppm toothpaste twice daily, no rinsing afterwards	• 1450 ppm toothpaste twice daily, no rinsing afterwards
		• Consider additional fluoride exposure:
		  • Weekly NaF mouth rinses (>6 years)
		  • Topical fluoride varnish, two times per year
			• Review fluoride toothpaste exposure. Consider high-fluoride toothpaste (>12 years)
			• Consider additional fluorides:
			  • Daily NaF mouth rinses (>6 years)
			  • Topical fluoride varnishes, four times a year
			  • Silver diamine fluoride (SDF) applications, two times per year, to arrest dentin lesions

Fissure sealants	• Apply selectively to deep, retentive fissures in permanent molars	• Apply to molars, especially those showing noncavitated lesions	• Apply resin-based fissure sealants to all molars and vulnerable premolars – use glass ionomer cement (GIC) for semi-erupted teeth • Selective (partial) caries removal and temporary/permanent restorations
Recall	• 12–18 months, if no life events occur	• 6–12 months for evaluation and renewed risk assessment	• 3–6 months for monitoring effect of treatment and secondary prevention

TOOTHBRUSHING

A thick and undisturbed (mature) dental biofilm is prone to ecological changes and needs to be periodically removed. There is strong scientific evidence for the efficiency of toothbrushing twice daily with fluoride toothpaste because it combines mechanical disruption of the biofilm with effective topical fluoride delivery (Walsh et al., 2019). Toothbrushing alone will not completely prevent caries, as it does not effectively remove biofilm from complex fissures and interproximal areas. Parents and children should be encouraged to adopt good, twice-daily brushing habits. Brushing should commence when teeth first erupt, as a part of everyday hygiene. Gauze

TABLE 4.3 ■ **Summary of the available evidence on caries-preventive measures for the primary and young permanent dentition**

Measure	Frequency	Certainty in the evidence[a]
Primary prevention: Self-care		
Fluoride toothpaste (1000–1450 ppm)	Two times daily	High
Fluoride mouth rinse (0.2% NaF)	Once weekly	Moderate
Fluoride tablets (0.25 mg)	Daily	Very low
Toothbrushing without fluoride	Two times daily	Very low
Flossing	Daily	Very low
Sugar substitutes (polyols, e.g., xylitol)	Daily	Low
Calcium-based agents: CPP-ACP/ CPP-ACFP	Daily	Very low/low
Primary prevention: Professional care		
5% Sodium fluoride varnish	Two to four times/year	Moderate
1.23% Phosphate fluoride gel	Two to four times/year	Moderate
Resin-based fissure sealants (occlusal)	Checked and maintained	Moderate
Chlorhexidine varnish	Four times/year	Low
Secondary prevention: Professional care		
5% Sodium fluoride varnish	Two to eight times/year	Moderate
1.23% Phosphate fluoride gel	Two to four times/year	Moderate
Fissure sealants (noncavitated lesions)	Checked and maintained	Low
Proximal resin infiltration	Regularly checked	Low
38% Silver diamine fluoride	Two applications/year	Moderate

[a]High ⊕⊕⊕⊕: very confident in a true effect; moderate ⊕⊕⊕O: moderately confident in a true effect but there is a possibility that it is substantially different; low ⊕⊕OO: the confidence in the effect is limited (the true effect may be substantially different); very low ⊕OOO: very little confidence in the effect (the true effect is likely to be substantially different).
CPP-ACP, casein phosphopeptide-amorphous calcium phosphate; *CPP-ACFP*, casein phosphopeptide-amorphous calcium fluoride phosphate.

or a facecloth on a finger, or a small very soft toothbrush, may help tooth cleaning in infants. It is beneficial when adults continue to assist with toothbrushing until children are around 8 years old and have developed the dexterity to remove plaque effectively by themselves. Electric toothbrushes remove biofilm more effectively than manual toothbrushing. The evidence for anticaries effects of flossing in the primary and permanent dentitions is very low and unreliable (de Oliveira et al., 2017; Worthington et al., 2019). Thus flossing cannot be a general recommendation but can be considered on individual indications for children with a fully erupted permanent dentition.

DIET MODIFICATION

Because the intake of sugar is considered the main driver of dysbiosis, the goal is to reduce the total carbohydrate consumption and to restrict the intake of sugary foods and drinks to mealtimes. The key messages are summarized in Box 4.2. Motivational interviewing provides a positive

---

BOX 4.2 ■ Diet and sugar recommendations to reduce caries

- The intake of free sugars shall not exceed 10% of total energy. This corresponds to 16–20 g per day for 2- to 7-year-olds (4 teaspoons), up to 30 g per day for 7- to 13-year-olds and 50 g per day for teenagers (maximum 10 teaspoons).
- The rule is five regular meals per day (three main, two small), but small children need to eat more frequently. At all ages, 'grazing' between meals should be discouraged.
- Limit high-energy intakes, sweets and soft drinks, including fruit juices and sports drinks. They are not only cariogenic but also erosive and highly caloric.
- Many foods labelled 'No added sugar' contain high levels of natural sugars.
- Increase intake of fruit and vegetables.

---

framework for counselling caregivers to support positive behaviour change in the family, although few studies have evaluated the effectiveness of this method (Harris et al., 2012). The delivery of chairside dietary advice is a complex issue that clinicians must adopt a systematic approach:

Record current sugar intake with a 3-day diet history and agree an agenda relating to the importance of sugar reduction.

Unveil sources of support for change, barriers to change and motivational factors.

Advise the parent and the child based on the outcome of the diet history. The information must be individual, practical and realistic in the context of family life and circumstances.

Dietary advice should not be all negative. Positive alternatives should be identified and start with small changes.

Arrange frequent follow-ups for evaluation and empowerment.

There is a need for policy advocacy to implement changes to support a population-level reduction in sugar consumption. Such initiatives could include sugar taxes on soft drinks, reformulation of products, limited marketing and reduced cup size. For example, it has been shown that the implementation of taxation on high-sugar products such as soft drinks reduces the sales of these products significantly and benefits oral health (Schwendicke et al., 2016).

FISSURE SEALANTS

Complex and deep pits and fissures are susceptible to caries also in low-caries communities. Evidence from numerous clinical trials show that resin-based sealants applied on targeted occlusal surfaces of permanent molars are effective for preventing caries in children and adolescents (Ahovuo-Saloranta et al., 2017). With the tight seal, bacterial substrate supply is 'locked out' and the remaining biofilm will be inactive and hibernating. Sealants must, however, be regularly checked and repaired/replaced when needed to maintain their efficacy.

ANTIMICROBIALS

Antibacterial regimes have a very limited role in preventive paediatric dentistry. Chlorhexidine-containing products (rinses or varnishes) may be considered for medically compromised children and those with an extreme caries risk as temporary help with the biofilm control.

EARLY CHILDHOOD CARIES

ECC is the presence of one or more decayed (noncavitated or cavitated lesions), missing (because of caries) or filled surfaces in any primary tooth of a child under 6 years of years (Tinanoff et al., 2019). Based on global studies, the mean caries prevalence is increasing from 17% in 1-year-olds to 36% and 55% for 2- and 4-year-olds, respectively. A systematic review has reported over 100 unique risk factors for ECC, but in principle, they are similar with caries development later in

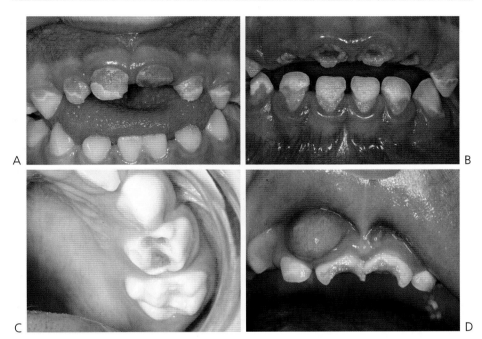

Figure 4.7 Early childhood caries (ECC). (A) ECC showing the characteristic pattern of decay. The upper anterior teeth and the molars are affected but the lower anterior teeth are spared. (B) A particularly rampant case of ECC where a pacifier had been dipped in honey. Both the upper and lower anterior teeth may be affected. (C) The first primary molars are carious because of a bottle habit at night. There is no interproximal decay (because of open contact points), and the canines that have erupted later are unaffected. (D) An abscess following pulp necrosis in carious upper incisors. Extraction is required, and the abscess will resolve following removal of the tooth and drainage of the pus.

life (Kirthiga et al., 2019). The progress rate and breakdown of the tooth structures are, however, faster in primary teeth (Figure 4.7). Typically, first affected are the upper anterior teeth and the first lower primary molars, reflecting the sequence of eruption and the feeding-related aetiology. In some countries, the term 'nursing bottle caries' is used because parents put their infants to sleep with a baby bottle containing fermentable carbohydrates or sweetened milk. Likewise, prolonged breastfeeding after 12 months of age may increase the risk for ECC.

Clinical management of early childhood caries

The preventive avenues for ECC are similar to caries later in life, albeit with a stronger focus on social aspects and feeding. Most important, the primary prevention should start early in life with timely delivery of educational information. Cooperation with physicians, nurses and other healthcare workers is beneficial, as they often have frequent contacts with the family in the first few years of the child's life for well-baby evaluations. Evidence shows the value of integrating the oral health with existing chronic disease management models within medical care settings.

PRIMARY PREVENTION OF EARLY CHILDHOOD CARIES

The essential messages are:

Limit free sugar intake in foods and drink for children, in particular for those under 2 years of age.

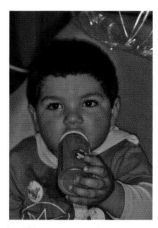

Figure 4.8 Parents should be encouraged not to use the bottle as a pacifier.

Avoid night-time bottle feeding with milk or drinks containing free sugars as pacifier (Figure 4.8).

Avoid baby bottle and breastfeeding beyond 12 months, especially if frequent and/or nocturnal.

Supervise toothbrushing with an age-appropriate amount of fluoride toothpaste containing at least 1000 parts per million (ppm) twice daily. Use a 'smear' layer (~0.125 mg F) for children under age 2 and a 'pea size' (~0.25 mg F) for children age 2 to 6 years (Toumba et al., 2019).

Review exposure to community fluorides (water, salt, milk) in countries where available.

SECONDARY PREVENTION OF EARLY CHILDHOOD CARIES

Early and periodic screening to detect early-stage lesions is the key component in the management of ECC. Dental check-ups can preferably be integrated with the child's general health examinations and vaccination programme. Dietary counselling focusing on sugar reduction can be coordinated with nondental primary caregivers to promote and support a healthy feeding behaviour with 'one voice'. To reverse and remineralize early noncavitated lesions, professional applications of fluoride varnish (2.26% NaF) every 3 to 6 months is best clinical practice. The varnish (~0.3 mL in total) is applied in a thin layer with a micro-brush on dry and clean tooth surfaces (Figure 4.9). The varnish sets in 60 seconds, and the child should refrain from eating within the

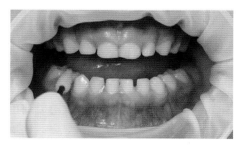

Figure 4.9 Topical application of fluoride varnish in a thin layer with aid of a micro-brush in a preschool child with increased caries risk. (Picture from Ivoclar Vivadent AG, Principality of Liechtenstein.)

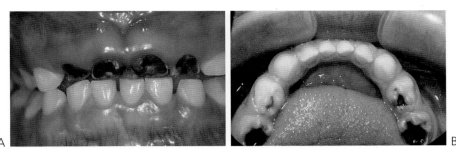

Figure 4.10 (A) Early childhood caries (ECC) in a child showing arrested caries. Removal of the cause of caries has allowed the process of demineralization to slow down. (B) When the carious process has resulted in an open lesion, it is possible to slow and arrest the process.

next hour. Fluoride varnish applications are safe even for infant and toddlers with a urinary excretion well below the maximal daily dose of fluoride intake (Twetman & Stecksén-Blicks, 2018). In fact, fluoride is the only professional high-fluoride product that is suitable for infants and small children. When the causes of ECC are removed, the protective factors are able to slow down or even arrest the caries process (Figure 4.10).

MANAGEMENT (TERTIARY PREVENTION) OF EARLY CHILDHOOD CARIES

The management of cavitated lesions should adhere to the minimum intervention philosophy to preserve tooth structures. Atraumatic restorative techniques, including selective (partial) caries removal with subsequent glass ionomer fillings, are effective treatment alternatives to conventional fillings. The peripheral part of the cavity must always be excavated to hard dentin, but current consensus reports state that nonselective (complete) caries removal in the pulpal area is overtreatment (Bjørndal et al., 2019). The selective removal to soft dentine can be performed in one or two visits (stepwise excavation) on asymptomatic teeth with no history of pain. For permanent restorations of moderate lesions, composites or compomers are the recommended options. Stainless steel crowns are sometimes required for extensive multiple-surface lesions in second primary molars (see Chapter 6). Biannual applications of 38% silver diamine fluoride (SDF) solution may be a temporary measure to arrest open lesions with exposed dentin, particularly in uncooperative children or in children with special needs. The proportion of arrested dentin lesions in preschool children is reported to be 66%, and the desensitizing effect may help children with hypersensitive teeth to eat and brush (Urquhart et al., 2019). A concern is the black staining, but parents may prefer this 'simple' option to advanced behavioural techniques such as sedation or general anaesthesia.

Extractions are often required in children with severe ECC. Extraction of the upper anterior teeth will not result in space loss if the canines have erupted and does not affect speech development. If posterior molars have to be extracted, an assessment should be carried out to determine if a space maintainer is appropriate. For extensive restorative treatment and multiple extractions, conscious sedation or general anaesthesia is generally recommended, but a comprehensive follow-up care plan must be established. Unfortunately, a large proportion of children continue to get new lesions even after the treatment, as the risk factors have not been altered (Twetman & Dhar, 2015). Educating caregivers and counselling with aid of the motivational interviewing methodology is effective for gaining positive behavioural change and shows promise for reducing caries relapse (Garcia et al., 2015; Moynihan et al., 2019).

Social aspects of night-waking and feeding

It is important to understand normal feeding routines or when these may be associated with habits contributing to ECC. Breastfeeding is encouraged; however, some mothers are unable to breastfeed, and there may be circumstances when babies have medical interventions that restrict their ability to breastfeed and so take bottle-feeds (such as cleft palate or in the early days of the neonatal intensive care admission). It is not recommended that children fall asleep with a bottle at night.

All infants wake at least once overnight and often resettle themselves. This may happen without the knowledge of the parents. Infants wake more often when they are unwell; when there are changes in their social and physical environment; or when learning a new developmental skill, such as pulling themselves up on the side of the cot to stand. If the parent offers milk or another feed to assist with resettling, then this night-waking behaviour will be reinforced and the infant will learn that the reward is the means to resettle. Unfortunately, this sets up conditioning for having feeds overnight that are not required developmentally (i.e., after 10–12 months of age). General recommendations for infant feeding routines are shown in Table 4.4. Babies that fill up with milk overnight may refuse their solid meals during the day. Children are best settled with comforts such as patting, cuddling and verbal reassurance. Unnecessary additional overnight feeds may reflect the parent's inability to cope with a wakeful, crying infant. Some reasons for offering feeds overnight include:

- Parental or infant illness.
- Maternal guilt, stress, anxiety or depression.
- Marital discord.
- Domestic violence.
- In these cases, the feeds are used as a quick fix to try to settle the infant.

It is important to give appropriate advice to the family about ECC. Blame should never be attributed; in many situations, the condition may have arisen out of ignorance, misinformation or tiredness and frustration of coping with an infant with poor sleeping habits. Elimination of an 'at risk' bottle habit can be achieved by gradually reducing the amount of sugar in the bottle by diluting with water, which may be done over several weeks. Alternatively, some parents find it easier to remove the bottle, immediately offering sips of water only. The only dentally safe fluid in a feeding bottle is water.

TABLE 4.4 ■ **General recommendations for infant feeding routines**

• Birth to 3 months	Breastfeeding up to 10 times in 24 hours or six to eight formula bottles in 24 hours.
• 3–6 months	Three to four hourly feeds, i.e., six to eight breast-feeds or five formula bottles.
	The early-morning 2 AM feed is ceased and usually the infant will have only one feed overnight.
• 4–6 months	Four to five milk feeds.
	Taste and texture of solids may be introduced from 4 months, although these recommendations may differ between countries.
• 6–12 months	Four milk feeds, last one before midnight.
	Three major solids meals: breakfast, lunch and dinner with morning and afternoon snacks.
• Over 12 months	No milk feeds required after bedtime but may have a bedtime ritual of milk feed, tooth cleaning, then a bedtime story in bed.

Understanding developmentally appropriate feed, sleep and play patterns will help both the parents and the dentist come to the conclusion that the family may require extra assistance with the infant's routine. Providing empathy and support for the challenges they are experiencing with night-waking is essential before offering education regarding ECC. Referral to community health nurses, lactation consultants or secondary parenting services is recommended to assist with the physical and psychological support necessary to change these behavioural patterns.

References and further reading

Dental caries

Ahovuo-Saloranta, A., Forss, H., Walsh, T., et al., 2017. Pit and fissure sealants for preventing dental decay in permanent teeth. Cochrane Database of Systematic Reviews 7, CD001830.

Bratthall, D., Hänsel Petersson, G., 2005. Cariogram – a multifactorial risk assessment model for a multifactorial disease. Community Dentistry Oral Epidemiology 33, 256–264.

Buzalaf, M.A.R., 2018. Review of fluoride intake and appropriateness of current guidelines. Advances in Dental Research 29, 157–166.

de Oliveira, K.M.H., Nemezio, M.A., Romualdo, P.C., et al., 2017. Dental flossing and proximal caries in the primary dentition: a systematic review. Oral Health Preventive Dentistry 15, 427–434.

Divaris, K., 2019. Searching deep and wide: advances in the molecular understanding of dental caries and periodontal disease. Advances in Dental Research 30, 40–44.

Dzidic, M., Collado, M.C., Abrahamsson, T., et al., 2018. Oral microbiome development during childhood: an ecological succession influenced by postnatal factors and associated with tooth decay. ISME J 12, 2292–2306.

Ekstrand, K.R., Gimenez, T., Ferreira, F.R., et al., 2018. The International Caries Detection and Assessment System – ICDAS: a systematic review. Caries Research 52, 406–419.

Featherstone, J.D.B., Chaffee, B.W., 2018. The evidence for caries management by risk assessment (CAMBRA®). Advances in Dental Research 29, 9–14.

Harris, R., Gamboa, A., Dailey, Y., et al., 2012. One-to-one dietary interventions undertaken in a dental setting to change dietary behaviour. Cochrane Database of Systematic Reviews 3, CD006540.

Kilian, M., Chapple, I.L., Hannig, M., et al., 2016. The oral microbiome – an update for oral healthcare professionals. British Dental Journal 221, 657–666.

Kassebaum, N.J., Smith, A.G.C., Bernabé, E., Fleming, T.D., Reynolds, A.E., Vos, T., Murray, C.J.L., Marcenes, W.; GBD 2015 Oral Health Collaborators. Global, Regional, and National Prevalence, Incidence, and Disability-Adjusted Life Years for Oral Conditions for 195 Countries, 1990-2015: A Systematic Analysis for the Global Burden of Diseases, Injuries, and Risk Factors. Journal of Dental Research 2017 Apr;96(4):380–387.

Marsh, P.D., 2018. In sickness and in health – what does the oral microbiome mean to us? An ecological perspective. Advances in Dental Research 29, 60–65.

Martignon, S., Pitts, N.B., Goffin, G., et al., 2019. CariesCare practice guide: consensus on evidence into practice. British Dental Journal 227, 353–362.

Mejàre, I., Axelsson, S., Dahlén, G., et al., 2014. Caries risk assessment. A systematic review. Acta Odontologica Scandinavica 72, 81–91.

Moynihan, P., Makino, Y., Petersen, P.E., et al., 2018. Implications of WHO guideline on sugars for dental health professionals. Community Dentistry and Oral Epidemiology 46, 1–7.

O'Mullane, D.M., Baez, R.J., Jones, S., et al., 2016. Fluoride and oral health. Community Dentistry and Health 33, 69–99.

Peres, M.A., Macpherson, L.M.D., Weyant, R.J., et al., 2019. Oral diseases: a global public health challenge. Lancet 394, 249–260.

Pitts, N.B., Zero, D.T., Marsh, P.D., et al., 2017. Dental caries. Nature Reviews Disease Primers 25, 17030.

Schwendicke, F., Thomson, W.M., Broadbent, J.M., et al., 2016. Effects of taxing sugar-sweetened beverages on caries and treatment costs. Journal of Dental Research 95, 1327–1332.

Twetman, S., 2016. Caries risk assessment in children: how accurate are we? European Archives of Paediatric Dentistry 17, 27–32.

Twetman, S., 2018. Prevention of dental caries as a non-communicable disease. European Journal of Oral Sciences 126 (Suppl 1), 19–25.

Walsh, T., Worthington, H.V., Glenny, A.M., et al., 2019. Fluoride toothpastes of different concentrations for preventing dental caries. Cochrane Database of Systematic Reviews 4, CD007868.

Worthington, H.V., MacDonald, L., Poklepovic Pericic, T., et al., 2019. Home use of interdental cleaning devices, in addition to toothbrushing, for preventing and controlling periodontal diseases and dental caries. Cochrane Database of Systematic Reviews 10, CD012018.

Zaura, E., Brandt, B.W., Prodan, A., et al., 2017. On the ecosystemic network of saliva in healthy young adults. ISME, pp. 1218–1231.

Early childhood caries

Bjørndal, L., Simon, S., Tomson, P.L., et al., 2019. Management of deep caries and the exposed pulp. International Endodontic Journal 52, 949–973.

Boustedt, K., Roswall, J., Twetman, S., et al., 2018. Influence of mode of delivery, family and nursing determinants on early childhood caries development: a prospective cohort study. Acta Odontologica Scandinavica 76, 595–599.

Garcia, R., Borrelli, B., Dhar, V., et al., 2015. Progress in early childhood caries and opportunities in research, policy, and clinical management. Pediatric Dentistry 37, 294–299.

Kirthiga, M., Murugan, M., Saikia, A., et al., 2019. Risk factors for early childhood caries: a systematic review and meta-analysis of case control and cohort studies. Pediatric Dentistry 41, 95–112.

Moynihan, P., Tanner, L.M., Holmes, R.D., et al., 2019. Systematic review of evidence pertaining to factors that modify risk of early childhood caries. JDR Clinical Translational Research 4, 202–216.

Tinanoff, N., Baez, R.J., Diaz Guillory, C., et al., 2019. Early childhood caries epidemiology, aetiology, risk assessment, societal burden, management, education, and policy: global perspective. International Journal of Paediatric Dentistry 29, 238–248.

Toumba, K.J., Twetman, S., Splieth, C., et al., 2019. Guidelines on the use of fluoride for caries prevention in children: an updated EAPD policy document. European Archives of Paediatric Dentistry 20, 507–516.

Twetman, S., Dhar, V., 2015. Evidence of effectiveness of current therapies to prevent and treat early childhood caries. Pediatric Dentistry 37, 246–253.

Twetman, S., Stecksén-Blicks, C., 2018. Urinary fluoride excretion after a single application of fluoride varnish in preschool children. Oral Health Preventive Dentistry 16, 351–354.

Urquhart, O., Tampi, M.P., Pilcher, L., 2019. Nonrestorative treatments for caries: systematic review and network meta-analysis. Journal of Dental Research 98, 14–26.

WHO Expert Consultation on Public Health Intervention Against Early Childhood Caries, 2017. Report of a meeting, Bangkok, Thailand 2016. World Health Organization, Geneva.

CHAPTER 5

Fluoride and dental health

Yasmi O. Crystal ▦ John Featherstone

Introduction

Fluoride has been instrumental in improving the oral health of millions of adults and children. Fluoride is a unique member of the halogen family in that it is termed a 'seeker of mineralized tissue'. It is this affinity with mineralized tissues which explains how fluoride can strengthen the teeth and prevent or heal dental caries.

Fluoride is naturally present in water sources across the world. To promote its caries prevention effects, optimal levels of fluoride exposure can be achieved through the various sources that will be discussed in detail in this chapter.

Mechanism of action

Concepts of how fluoride prevents caries have changed markedly since water fluoridation was first introduced in the United States in the late 1940s and early 1950s. When ingested systemically, fluoride is incorporated into developing tooth enamel. The fluoride ion displaces some hydroxyl groups in the carbonated hydroxyapatite crystals to form fluoridated-carbonated hydroxyapatite crystals (Featherstone, 2000; Featherstone, 2008). The smaller fluoride anion reduces crystal stress

73

and results in a less soluble material. Initially, researchers focused on the systemic effect of fluoride as the key factor in the reduction of dental caries. However, the evidence for the systemic effect has been superseded by the realization that the reaction of fluoride at the microenvironment of the plaque–enamel interface and within the early caries lesions, encouraging remineralization, is of major significance in terms of reducing the levels of dental caries (Centres for Disease Control and Prevention, 2001).

The important points to remember are:
- Fluoride acts primarily topically, inhibiting demineralization and enhancing remineralization.
- The mode of action is predominantly posteruptive, and prevention of caries requires lifelong presence of fluoride because fluoride works for adults as well as children.
- When remineralization takes place in the presence of fluoride, the remineralized enamel is markedly more resistant to further acid attack because the renewed surfaces of the crystals within the early caries lesion are essentially fluorapatite. These new crystal surfaces are manyfold less soluble than the original carbonated hydroxyapatite. Only low levels of fluoride are required at the plaque–enamel interface to promote effective remineralization, but higher levels of fluoride are even more effective.
- However, with a high and constant acid challenge, fluoride alone is not sufficient to prevent lesion formation.
- At higher concentrations, fluoride has some effect on the glycolytic pathway of oral microorganisms, reducing acid production and interfering with the enzymatic regulation of carbohydrate metabolism.
- Daily applications of fluoride are important to maintain a sustained and effective low concentration of fluoride at the plaque–enamel interface. Amounts and frequency required for each individual should be determined based on the caries risk level.

Community fluoridation

There are three ways to offer fluoride on a community-wide basis: using water, salt and milk.

WATER FLUORIDATION

The natural level of fluoride in drinking water is very variable. However, in reticulated community water supplies that are fluoridated in different parts of the world, the concentration of fluoride has been adjusted from 0.6 to 1 part per million (ppm). Because other sources of fluoride are now generally available (from toothpastes and other), in the United States, water fluoride content has been standardized to 0.7 ppm (2015 report of U.S. Department of Human Services), whereas other regions like Australia/New Zealand continue to maintain fluoride in the ranges of 0.6 to 1 ppm with variation within that range according to the mean maximum daily temperature to account for seasonal differences in water consumption (ARCPOH Fluoride Consensus Workshop 2012, at Adelaide.edu.au). These recommendations come after careful consensus considerations based on population studies and are an attempt to balance the benefits of caries prevention with reducing the prevalence of fluorosis.

The majority of International Health Agencies agree with the World Health Organization in support of the continuation of community water fluoridation, as it is an effective, efficient, socially equitable and safe population approach to caries prevention.

The reduction in dental caries in fluoridated communities ranges from 20% to 40%, which is considerably less than was the case when it was first introduced in the United States because of the general increase in availability of fluoride from other sources (Downer & Blinkhorn, 2007). However, when fluoridation programmes have been discontinued, there is rapid increase in dental caries within a short time frame (Burt et al., 2000).

There are a number of points which are important to stress to the public when considering the value of water fluoridation:

- Fluoride benefits adults as well as children.
- There is a decreased prevalence of root-surface caries in lifelong inhabitants of areas with fluoridated water.
- Fluoride from community water fluoridation benefits all the population and is a cost-effective intervention.

The market for bottled water has grown rapidly in the last decade, and for many individuals water consumption from this source may have fully replaced reticulated water. Consumers of bottled water should be advised that they may miss out on the benefits of fluoride from community sources and instructed that in some countries there is bottled water marketed with optimal levels of fluoride that is recommended for those with high caries risk.

In terms of infant fluoride exposure from milk formulas, several studies have shown the safety of consumption of both premixed and reconstituted infant formula regardless of presence of fluoride added to the water supplies (AAPD Fluoride Therapy Best Practice Recommendations, 2020).

Some water filters may remove fluoride, although this is mostly limited to those with reverse osmosis, bone or charcoal filters, distillation or ion exchange. Normal membrane filters will not remove a small ion such as fluoride. Ceramic and carbon filters retain fluoride in the filtered water.

SALT FLUORIDATION

Salt enriched with iodide has been used in many countries as an effective means of preventing goiter. It was a logical step to include fluoride in domestic table salt. It has the advantage of offering choice and does not encourage salt consumption, as it is marketed as an alternative to the standard product. The amount of fluoride added is 250 mg F^-/kg salt (250 ppm).

Switzerland was the first nation to pioneer salt fluoridation, and it is now available in more than 30 other countries. It is a practical alternative to water fluoridation, but the research base is limited on its absolute effectiveness, especially now that fluoride toothpaste is readily available. It is also likely that young children may not benefit as much from this source of fluoride because dietary recommendations for this age group favour low-salt diets.

MILK FLUORIDATION

Bovine milk is a common staple in the diet of babies and young children, and in many countries, free milk is offered to children at school. For these reasons, milk has been identified as a potential way to supplement children's fluoride intake. Typical fluoride concentrations in milk are usually in the range of 2.5 to 5.0 mg of F/L.

Despite its practical simplicity, milk fluoridation has not been implemented on a wide scale, mainly because of logistical difficulties and the fact that fluoride toothpaste is readily available. It may still be a valuable source of delivery in developing countries where children are at risk of caries and have limited access to other fluoride sources because the milk will improve nutrition as well as offer the benefits of fluoride.

Topical fluorides for home use

Lifetime protection against dental caries results from the continuous presence of fluoride in low concentrations that will (1) prevent formation of new caries lesions, (2) enhance the remineralization of noncavitated incipient lesions (white spots), (3) slow down the progression or even arrest dentin carious lesions and (4) limit lesions occurring around existing restorations for both adults and children (Adair, 2006; Lenzi et al., 2016; Scottish Intercolegiate Guideline Network, 2014). An optimal concentration of fluoride each day at both the plaque–enamel interface and in saliva will help minimize the risk of caries. An individual caries risk assessment should carefully evaluate risk and protective factors, as well as disease indicators and biological and social determinants that can allow the clinician to develop an individualized fluoride regime (CAMBRA handbook, 2019). Some of these factors include:

- Presence of active caries lesions.
- Patient's age.
- The frequency of consumption of sugary foods and drinks.
- Presence of visible plaque on the teeth (as a marker of heavy bacterial load).
- Medical conditions, especially those that directly or through their treatment may reduce salivary flow, or special needs that may limit successful home care routines.
- Current fluoride exposure considering all other sources.
- Patient's compliance with oral health advice.

FLUORIDE TOOTHPASTES

From all the different ways of providing topical fluoride for caries prevention, the simplest way in which to maintain effective fluoride concentrations at the plaque/enamel interface, is through the daily use of a fluoride containing toothpaste. Fluoride is added to toothpastes in one of the following forms:

- Sodium fluoride.
- Sodium monofluorophosphate (MFP).
- Stannous fluoride.
- Amine fluoride.

The typical strength of regular family toothpaste is between 1000 and 1500 ppm F, with some countries offering children's toothpastes with approximately 450 ppm F and 'training' infant toothpastes with no fluoride. Current systematic reviews confirm that brushing with a fluoride-containing toothpaste reduces dental caries compared with brushing with nonfluoride toothpaste in all age groups. A dose–response effect can clearly be found in all studies, which means that stronger fluoride toothpastes offer greater protection against dental caries, but they also increase the risk for fluorosis while teeth are developing. The exact magnitude of the caries-preventive effects of specific over-the-counter fluoride concentrations can be difficult to estimate in light of diverse background fluoride exposure and the limited number of studies available (Cochrane, 2019).

High-fluoride-concentration toothpastes and gels for home use (typically 5000 ppm F) are generally classified as a prescription-only medicine.

The use of fluoride toothpastes has led to a 25% reduction in the prevalence of caries in many countries (Davies et al., 2002). It is recommended that children should brush twice a day with toothpaste containing an appropriate concentration of fluoride, preferably last thing at night before bed and on one other occasion, ideally in the morning. It is essential to ensure that all parents are aware that supervising toothbrushing (Curnow et al., 2002), as well as spitting without rinsing after brushing, improves the preventive effects of fluoride toothpaste.

Advice on the type of toothpaste which young children should use, in terms of fluoride concentration, is problematic (Franzman et al., 2006), as international guidelines differ and availability of toothpastes with different concentrations varies among countries. Members of the dental team must familiarize themselves with the guidelines appropriate for their own country and practice location, taking into consideration all current sources of fluoride that could create a halo effect, as well as the caries risk of the patient. In Australia and the United States, for example, fluoridation of public water supplies is quite common, whereas in Europe there are only a few countries that provide community water fluoridation (Walsh et al., 2010).

There are a number of important factors that health professionals must consider when offering advice to parents on fluoride toothpaste usage, namely:

- There is a dose–response relationship between caries prevention and fluoride levels (Pretty, 2016). Therefore, low-fluoride toothpastes (<1000 ppm) are less effective in preventing caries than those with higher concentrations. Individuals who live in areas where the water supply is not fluoridated will ensure better caries preventive effects when using toothpastes that contain higher concentrations of fluoride (>1000 ppm).
- Parents should be encouraged to establish toothbrushing habits as soon as the first tooth erupts. The age when parents are advised to begin using fluoride toothpaste varies between countries, and members of the dental team should be familiar with the appropriate national policy.
- Current guidelines in the USA recommend that children younger than 36 months should use a smear of fluoride 1000 ppm F toothpaste (size of a grain of rice, approximately 0.1 g of toothpaste or 0.1 mg of fluoride) on the brush twice a day, whereas children aged 3 to 6 years use a pea-size amount (approximately 0.25 g of toothpaste or 0.25 mg of fluoride).
- Similarly, European recommendations were updated in 2019 so children from eruption of first tooth to 2 years of age, use a grain of rice size amount of 1000 ppm F toothpaste twice a day (0.125 g), children, while children aged 2-6 years should use a pea-size amount of 1000 ppm F twice a day (0.25 g), and children over 6 years should use up to full lenght of brush (0.5-1 g) of 1450 ppm F toothpaste. New guidelines also state that for children 2–6 years, 1000+ fluoride concentrations may be considered based on the individual caries risk (Toumba et al., 2019).
- In contrast, although Australia/New Zealand guidelines recommend that children younger than 17 months of age should brush without toothpaste, and children from 18 months to 5 years should brush with a pea-size amount of 500 ppm F toothpaste twice a day. The 2019 updated guidelines (Do, 2019) clearly state that for children at high risk of caries, the dental professional can recommend starting F toothpaste earlier, using 1000 ppm concentrations and brushing more often as determined by the child's individual needs.
- Brushing with fluoride toothpaste (1000–1450 ppm) before 12 months of age offers larger reductions in dental caries, staying within safe ranges of fluoride exposure for those children who are at high risk to develop caries lesions. To ensure these concepts, parents must supervise and only a smear of toothpaste should be placed on the brush twice a day.
- Children over 6 years of age should use a 'family' toothpaste (1000–1450 ppm). However, earlier use of a 'family' paste is indicated if children are at risk of developing dental caries.
- Young children (up to the age of 7 years) should be supervised when brushing, as this monitors toothpaste usage, has been associated with greater reductions in dental caries and reduces the chances of fluorosis in the upper anterior teeth.
- Children over 6 years of age and considered to be at high risk of developing caries or have active carious lesions may be prescribed a toothpaste or a gel containing more than 1400 ppm fluoride (i.e., 5000 ppm F). The availability of these high-fluoride toothpastes and gels varies from country to country. They may only be available by prescription in some locations, and parents should be provided with specific instructions for their use.
- Safe storage of all fluoride toothpastes is important to ensure that young children do not eat paste from the tube. This advice to parents should be reinforced on a regular basis.
- Brushing with a fluoride toothpaste is at the heart of any preventive programme. There is no 'right way' to brush. The important goal is to make sure the toothpaste is used at least twice a day with parental supervision and not washed away by rigorous rinsing.
- Many children dislike the strong flavours of many toothpastes, which is a barrier to regular use. Toothpastes are available without flavouring.

FLUORIDE MOUTH RINSES

In some countries, school-based daily fluoride mouth rinse (0.05% sodium fluoride) programmes have been successfully used to offer protection from dental caries. Although rinses do offer a benefit, their use as a public health measure has declined for a number of reasons:

- The widespread use of fluoride toothpaste has reduced the potential benefits for the average child.
- Rinse programmes are labour intensive because children need to be supervised while rinsing.
- Schools may not want the inconvenience of a daily rinsing programme.

Nevertheless, in some countries where people live in remote locations and toothpaste is expensive, local school-based fluoride rinsing programmes can be a very effective public health measure. Members of the dental team may also offer fluoride rinses to individual patients with active caries, provided they are over 6 years of age.

The three most common types of commercial rinses for home use are:

Daily

- 0.05% w/v neutral sodium fluoride (225 ppm F⁻). This is the most common 'over-the-counter' fluoride mouthrinse.
- Partly acidulated solution of sodium fluoride, phosphoric acid and sodium phosphate monobasic (200 ppm F⁻).
- 0.02% w/v acidulated sodium fluoride (90 ppm F). These products have recently become available 'over the counter' in several countries, have a low pH and usually include other ingredients for gingivitis control.

Weekly

- 0.2% w/v neutral sodium fluoride (900 ppm F⁻).

The most popular rinse is the daily one, as it is simpler to rinse on a regular basis than trying to remember to use a product just once a week. Also maintaining a low level of fluoride in the mouth on a daily basis fits in with our understanding of the mode of action of fluoride on the remineralization of enamel.

Recommending using the rinse at a different time to brushing with a fluoride toothpaste adds an additional protective exposure that could increase the caries preventive effects, especially in children at risk. A good time to rinse is when a child returns home from school because there will be plaque present which incorporates the fluoride and releases it slowly over time.

There are a number of patient groups at high caries risk who will benefit from the prescription of a daily fluoride rinse or a high-concentration (5000 ppm) fluoride toothpaste or gel:

- Children undergoing orthodontic treatment. The rinse or gel can prevent or reduce demineralization around the brackets.
- Patients with hyposalivation caused by medications or those with congenital absence of the major salivary glands.
- Children with medical problems for whom caries could be a serious problem, for example, cardiac patients and individuals with bleeding disorders.
- Children with active dental caries.
- Children who are assessed to be at high risk for developing future caries lesions.
- Some individuals who find toothbrushing difficult (but in many cases they will also find rinsing a problem).

Fluoride rinses are not recommended for children before the eruption of the permanent incisors because many younger patients will swallow the rinse, which may cause fluorosis. High-concentration F toothpastes and gels are preferable as the amount used is easier to monitor. These latter forms can be very valuable in children who have experienced decay on the primary dentition and for whom preventing decay from developing on their susceptible erupting permanent molars is of utmost importance.

TOOTH MOUSSE OR CASEIN PHOSPHOPEPTIDE-AMORPHOUS CALCIUM PHOSPHATE CRÈMES

CPP-ACP and CPP-ACPF (containing 900 ppm F) are available as crèmes for topical application at home (Tooth Mousse®, Tooth Mousse Plus®, also known as MI Paste and MI Paste Plus in some countries, GC Corp, Japan) to be applied to surfaces at risk of caries, erosion or with white spot lesions. CPP-ACPF releases fluoride, calcium and phosphate ions for local remineralization of enamel (Reynolds, 2008).

The crème is applied to the teeth after brushing by smearing across tooth surfaces with a clean finger or cotton-tipped applicator. The crème should not be rinsed out.

- Tooth Mousse Plus® contains 900 ppm F^-.
- The crème should not be used by people with a milk protein allergy.

FLUORIDE TABLETS

At one time, fluoride tablets were widely recommended as a useful caries preventive measure. However, they have been superseded because fluoride toothpastes are widely available and offer a better level of protection from dental caries. In addition, research has shown that compliance with tablet-taking regimes is very poor and the consumption of up to 1 mg of fluoride in one tablet is linked to fluorosis. Thus fluoride tablets are no longer routinely recommended in many countries (Ismail et al., 2008; Tubert-Jeannin et al., 2011).

STANNOUS FLUORIDE GEL

A stannous fluoride (SnF_2) treatment gel in a methylcellulose and glycerine carrier (marketed as Gel Kam® by Colgate Oral Care) can be used at home for the remineralization of white spot and hypomineralization lesions of enamel (e.g., molar or incisor hypomineralization). Anecdotal clinical reports support the efficacy of this product, for example, where localized remineralization is desirable before the placement of definitive restorations. The 0.4% stannous fluoride gel has also proved effective in arresting root caries and has been incorporated into a synthetic saliva solution to reduce caries in postirradiation cancer patients.

- Contains 1000 ppm F^- and 3000 ppm Sn^{2+}.
- A very small amount is placed on a cotton bud and applied to dried tooth surfaces by adult patient or for a child by the parent at home.
- The parent must fully understand the instructions given about the use of the gel.

Professionally applied fluoride products

FLUORIDE VARNISH (5% NaF)

Varnishes were developed with the rationale that products with higher viscosity would prolong the contact time between the fluoride and dental enamel. Most commercial products available today contain 50 mg NaF/mL (5% NaF, 22600 ppm F^-). This varnish remains on the teeth for up to 12 to 48 hours after application, slowly releasing fluoride into the plaque and saliva.

Numerous clinical trials have proven the efficacy of 5% sodium fluoride varnish (FV) for caries prevention, reporting estimated caries reductions of over 46% (Marinho et al., 2009). Systematic reviews of professionally applied fluoride products favour the use of FV applied twice a year in both primary and permanent teeth, and they are now the recommended form of topical agent for professional use on children younger than 6 (Weyant et al., 2013).

Sodium FV has also proven its clinical efficacy to remineralize early enamel caries, with recent systematic reviews and metaanalysis reporting an overall percentage of remineralized enamel lesions of 63.6% (Gao et al., 2016) when applied twice a year.

FV plays an important part in an effective individualized prevention plan for patients at risk of caries, and indications for their use are:

- Hypersensitive areas of enamel and dentine.
- Local remineralization of white spot lesions.
- As part of a preventive programme for children with active caries in the primary and/or permanent dentitions.
- A routine preventive measure for children at risk for caries, including medically compromised and other special needs patients, children with reduced salivary flow and children with orthodontic or prosthetic appliances.

Varnishes are simple to apply; prophylaxis of the teeth is not required routinely, as fluoride uptake is not reduced by surface plaque. In fact, plaque can serve as a recycling reservoir for fluoride and allow prolonged exposure to enamel. Drying teeth before application facilitates adhesion and may also be beneficial for fluoride uptake.

The age of the child and the number of teeth present should be considered when deciding the amount of FV to be used. In very young children without a complete set of primary dentition, only a small amount needs to be applied to present teeth. There are numerous brands in the market worldwide with different flavourings and presentations, and uni-dose dispensers with varied amounts are common. Recommendations for application include the following amounts present on common uni-dose presentations of varnish:

- Primary dentition: 0.25 mL (6 mg F^-).
- Mixed dentition: 0.40 mL (9 mg F^-).
- Permanent dentition: 0.50 mL (11 mg F^-).

CONCENTRATED FLUORIDATED GELS AND FOAMS

Concentrated fluoridated gels and foams with concentrations of 9000 to 12 300 ppm F^- were popularly used as professionally applied products delivered on fluoride trays during dental preventive visits. Variable dosage during application, followed by inadvertent swallowing, especially on young children, can result in the ingestion of large amounts of fluoride, which may result in acute symptoms like malaise, nausea and vomiting. There is also clinical evidence that concentrated fluoridated gels are more effective in the permanent dentition than the primary dentition, benefitting particularly the first permanent molars. In addition, there is limited evidence that fluoride foams are effective when applied for less than 4 minutes.

For all of these reasons, the use of these products on children has declined because FVs have a much simpler application that reduces danger of swallowing and are therefore safer, retaining higher levels of efficacy for caries prevention. Gel formulations available for older children and adolescents with specific fluoride needs are discussed in the next two sections.

ACIDULATED PHOSPHATE FLUORIDE GELS

- Acidulated phosphate fluoride (APF) gels, containing 12 300 ppm F^- (1.23% APF), consist of a mixture of sodium fluoride, hydrofluoric acid and orthophosphoric acid. The incorporation of a water-soluble polymer (sodium carboxymethyl cellulose) into aqueous APF produces a viscous solution that improves the ease of application using custom-made trays.
- Thixotropic gels in trays flow under pressure, facilitating gel penetration between teeth.

NEUTRAL HIGH-CONCENTRATION SODIUM FLUORIDE GELS FOR PROFESSIONAL APPLICATION

A neutral pH gel (e.g., 2% w/v neutral NaF gel, 9000 ppm F⁻) can be used for cases of enamel erosion, exposed dentine, carious dentine or where very porous enamel surfaces (such as hypomineralization) exist.

- Sodium fluoride is chemically very stable, has an acceptable taste and is nonirritating to the gingivae. It does not discolour teeth, composite resin or porcelain restorations, in contrast to APF or stannous fluoride, which may cause discolouration.
- A neutral pH fluoridated gel or solution is preferred where restorations of glass ionomer cement, composite resin or porcelain are present, as acidic preparations may etch these restorations.

SILVER DIAMINE FLUORIDE

Silver products (like silver nitrate) have been used in dentistry for over a century as dentin desensitizers and caries arrest agents. Silver fluoride was developed in Japan in the 1970s to combine the antibacterial effects of silver with the remineralizing effects of fluoride in a solution of ammonia as a stabilizer. Since then, it has been manufactured and used in several countries including Australia, South America and the United States in different concentrations, mainly 12%, 30% and 38%, respectively, where it has been used mainly for the arrest of cavitated caries lesions in primary dentition and root caries in the elderly. Silver diamine fluoride (SDF) 38% contains 5% F, or 44,800 ppm F. Although is it highly concentrated, one drop (estimated to measure 32.5 microliters and contain 1.7 mg of fluoride and 8.5 mg of silver) is enough to treat several teeth (Crystal et al., 2019). It is presented as a clear or blue tinted solution that:

- Is painless to apply with a micro-brush onto cleaned and dry dentin lesions.
- Does not require prior caries removal.
- Acts a desensitizer on the teeth applied.
- Arrests dentin lesions, making the lesion dark-black and hard within a few hours after application.
- This dark staining of caries lesions can be very visible depending on the location of the cavities and could be a deterrent for its use (Figure 5.1).

Many clinical trials conducted on over 4000 school children in different locations confirm its safety when used as indicated: one drop to treat four to five cavitated lesions using cotton rolls isolation (Crystal & Niederman, 2016). Several systematic reviews have confirmed that 38% SDF gets best results compared to lesser concentrations, and it arrests approximately 81% of lesions (from 68% to 89%) when applied twice a year and followed for 6 to 30 months (Gao, 2016). The range of the arrest is because anterior teeth have much higher rates of arrest than posterior

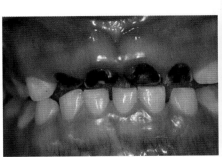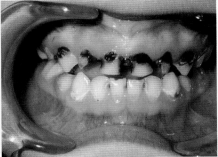

A   B

Figure 5.1 A child with early childhood caries before (A) and after (B) the application of silver diamine fluoride.

teeth (89% vs. 60%; from Fung et al., 2018), and large lesions and lesions with visible plaque at follow-ups have a lesser likelihood of becoming arrested. For this reason, current guidelines for its use (AAPD SDF guideline; Crystal et al., 2017) recommend using SDF for the arrest of dentin caries lesions on primary teeth, as part of a comprehensive caries management plan where there is adequate follow-up that includes appropriate re-application as necessary to achieve arrest, in combination with other preventive measures like FV and a plaque control program.

Because of its ease of application, low cost and safety, it is an ideal form of nonsurgical management of caries for children who are either too young, are medically compromised, have behavioural limitations to cooperate or lack the access to receive traditional restorative care. SDF is a reasonable alternative to delay or defer operative treatment that would require sedation or general anaesthesia to be completed. Even when the discoloration of the cavities can be a deterrent for its use, a study (Crystal et al., 2017) found that many parents are willing to compromise aesthetics to avoid more invasive and expensive interventions like general anaesthesia.

Lesions arrested with SDF can be restored with glass ionomer materials in the future, if necessary, when the conditions of the patient are more favourable for restorative interventions.

Contraindications:
- SDF should not be used on patients with silver allergies or on patients that have gingival irritations or ulcerations.
- SDF should not be used on teeth that are pulpally involved.
- Considerations:
- Because of the potential staining of tissues and surfaces, careful precautions should include protecting lips and cheeks with petroleum jelly before application.
- Minor side effects have been described as transient gingival irritation and metallic taste.
- Staining on the lesions can be very noticeable on anterior teeth, so an informed consent that includes pictures of typical cases should be carefully discussed with the parents.
- In some countries, SDF has restricted labelling, and its use for caries arrest is off label. Practitioners should be familiar with regulations in their country when using products obtained from foreign sources.

FLUORIDE DELIVERED THROUGH RESTORATIVE DENTAL MATERIALS

Fluoride has been incorporated into restorative materials, mainly glass ionomers, compomers and sealants, as a way to release fluoride into the surrounding tissues to promote remineralization of enamel and dentin and prevent recurrent decay; and into saliva and plaque to control biofilm formation and prevent new lesions.

Planning a preventive programme in the practice

Twice-daily toothbrushing with a fluoridated toothpaste beginning before 2 years of age, together with dietary advice to reduce the frequency of consumption of sugary foods and drinks, is the cornerstone of a preventive programme to ensure minimal caries activity. Reviews of epidemiological data in nonfluoridated communities indicate that the twice-daily use of a toothpaste containing fluoride will prevent new caries development in approximately 80% of children and an estimated 60% to 70% of adults.

Members of the dental team offer care to many different families with varying levels of dental disease. It is important to tailor advice to maximize the benefit for each individual child by making appropriate recommendations after a careful caries risk assessment has been performed. The aetiological factors leading to the development of caries are multifactorial, so risk assessment should involve all the likely key factors. Understanding the social, behavioural, microbiological, environmental and clinical factors still remains essential in the determination of caries risk during specific time periods. Commonly used caries risk assessment procedures (CAMBRA, Cariogram,

AAPD) subdivide risk in levels of low, moderate and high. Regardless of the method use to establish risk, it should be the basis for the establishment of a comprehensive caries management plan that includes a program for changing behaviour (to improve diet and promote home care measures) and prescribing appropriate preventive products for all children (Featherstone et al., 2021).

The scope of a preventive programme will be influenced by the following factors, which are part of a risk assessment protocol:

- White spot demineralization on cervical surfaces.
- Visible deposits of dental plaque and/or gingivitis.
- New carious lesions visible on clinical examination or on radiographs.
- Patients with orthodontic appliances.
- Individuals who have chronic medical problems.
- Children with special needs.
- Frequent consumption of sugary foods and drinks.
- Infrequent attendance for dental recall.
- Repeated attendance for emergency treatment.

Patients with these signs will likely fall on the high risk for caries category, which will alert clinicians to the importance of concentrating on preventive advice and therapies (Threlfall et al., 2007). Failure to guide and inform families on how to control and prevent caries may lead a child to suffer pain and require more clinical intervention. The preventive program can be a team effort utilizing the skills of the dentist, hygienist and dental therapist, each playing a part in the delivery of appropriate advice.

The preventive plan will have two themes:

- Prescription of preventive products.
- Behaviour change program.

Preventive products

It is well known that all preventive plans must include a fluoride component to successfully control or prevent dental caries. The specific products will depend on the severity of the caries problem and the age of the child.

Children 0 to 6

It is important to note that early childhood caries (ECC) in children under 3 years of age is primarily a dietary problem and fluoride products, whilst helpful, cannot overcome the constant intake of sugary foods and drinks. In addition, the fluoride products that one can safely use on children younger than 6 are limited. With those caveats in mind the preventive products at our disposal are:

- Fluoride toothpaste: Children must brush twice a day with a family toothpaste. Parents are advised to use a smear of paste on the brush for children under 3 years of age and the size of a pea for children ages 3–6 years. High-risk children, especially those who have current or recent caries experience, may benefit from a third brushing after the mid-day meal, that will help them through plaque removal and an additional exposure to fluoride toothpaste.
- FV applications: Children at risk of developing caries benefit from biannual application of FV. Those who have current or recent caries experience benefit from additional (every three months) applications as this will have a preventive caries effect, will arrest incipient enamel lesions and will offer the opportunity to reinforce the behavioural component of the preventive plan during that visit.
- Tooth Mousse Plus®: This product may have preventive benefits with ongoing use in controlling early enamel lesions as part of a comprehensive programme that includes the previous two options.
- Fissure sealants: These are of great value especially on the vulnerable surfaces of first and second adult molars.

Behaviour change

Although fluoride products have revolutionized the success of caries preventive programmes, it is still important to explain to parents/caregivers the multifactorial nature of the caries process. Our focus should be on diet and toothbrushing.

- Diet: Reducing the frequency of consumption of sugary foods and drinks is the dietary goal. How this is achieved is dependent on the age of the child and the cooperation of the parents. This chapter is essentially focusing on fluoride products, but dietary analysis is a key skill for the dental team, hence its being highlighted here.
- Toothbrushing: This is a behaviour which, if embedded early in a child's life, offers a proven benefit because it delivers fluoride toothpaste at least twice daily on a regular basis. In addition, as the child matures, removing plaque and controlling gingivitis become more important. For caries control, however, the dental team needs to make sure a child brushes at least twice a day. There are different strategies for achieving this, such as disclosing plaque, using toothbrushing charts and suggesting electric toothbrushes. The essential point is to make sure parents and caregivers monitor the brushing and that the appropriate amount of fluoride toothpaste is used.

However, dental caries for many of our child patients may not be a major problem, and our strategy should be to encourage healthy behaviour and highlight possible risk factors to parents and caregivers. These families can be classified as low risk but must be given advice to maintain a healthy lifestyle. The helpful pointers to low risk are:

- No new carious lesions within last 12 months.
- Little plaque noted on the cervical regions of the teeth.
- Parents report that child brushes twice a day with a fluoride toothpaste.
- Visits your practice once per year.
- Frequency of consumption of sugary drinks and foods is controlled.

Although a child may be at 'low risk' for future caries, there are some standard actions which will be helpful in maintaining the status quo:

- Reinforce diet advice concentrating on limiting sugary snacks and drinks between meals.
- Appropriate fissure sealants on newly erupted first and second permanent molars are helpful.
- Children over 6 years of age should be advised to use a family-strength fluoride toothpaste at least twice a day.

These simple behaviours will ensure that your patients remain at low risk of developing dental caries. Research suggests that a child with one carious lesion is five times more likely to develop further disease when compared with a child who is clinically caries-free, and as such, timely advice to parents is extremely important. This huge difference in risk highlights the importance of primary prevention and should be an essential part of the practice policy.

TECHNIQUES FOR TOOTHBRUSHING

There are many ways advocated to clean teeth and remove plaque. In reality, the horizontal 'scrub' technique is the one usually employed by most people. It should be simply put that the plaque should be removed from:

- The 'biting surfaces' (occlusal) using a vigorous scrubbing technique.
- All the gum margins (gingival margin) using a circular motion.
- Both sides of the teeth (labial/buccal and lingual/palatal) using a circular motion similar to earlier.

The area most poorly cleaned is the labial gingival margins of the lower anterior teeth. This is a naturally sensitive and difficult area to access, which children and parents need to be taught how to clean. It should be stressed that gingival tissues should not bleed following brushing at any age, and this sign highlights the need to clean these areas more effectively. Furthermore, the current recommendation should be that children do not rinse with water following brushing. They may spit out at the end of brushing but be encouraged to swallow the residue (Figure 5.2). This is based on the qualification that the appropriate amount of fluoride toothpaste has been placed on the brush.

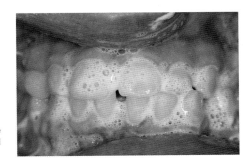

Figure 5.2 Allow children to spit out the toothpaste following brushing but try to avoid rinsing. The small amount of residue may be swallowed.

Fluoride toxicity

Overwhelming evidence corroborates the safety of fluorides at low concentrations, but a single exposure to high concentrations of fluoride can result in acute toxicity. It is important to use high-strength fluoride products with great care, especially in children under 4 years of age, but it is also prudent to advise parents about the safe storage of fluoride toothpastes.

PROBABLY TOXIC DOSE OF FLUORIDE (Table 5.1)

- Some 3 to 5 mg F⁻/kg of body weight can produce symptoms of gastrointestinal acute toxicity (nausea, vomiting, diarrhoea and abdominal pain), especially in young children and very frail adults.
- Some 5 mg F⁻/kg of body weight is accepted as the 'probably toxic dose' of fluoride and is defined as 'the minimum dose that could cause toxic signs and symptoms, including death, and that should trigger immediate therapeutic intervention and hospitalization' (Whitford, 1987). The 5 mg F⁻/kg of body weight 'probably toxic dose' corresponds to all the contents of a 45 g tube of 1000 ppm toothpaste ingested by a 10 kg child (small 2-year-old child) or less than one 90 g tube of 1000 ppm F toothpaste ingested by an average 4-year-old child (15 kg). Therefore, young children should not be allowed unsupervised access to fluoride toothpastes or fluoride supplements. Table 5.1 gives information on the amount of toothpaste that reaches the 'probably toxic dose'.

REPORTED LETHAL DOSE

- Reported lethal doses are 15 to 16 mg F⁻/kg of body weight (Whitford, 1992), and in addition to gastrointestinal (GI) toxicity symptoms, patients develop central nervous system (CNS) depression symptoms followed by cardiorespiratory arrest.

TABLE 5.1 ■ **Amount of toothpaste ingested to receive a probable toxic fluoride dose**

Age of child	Average weight	Probable toxic dose (at 5 mg/kg) F⁻	Amount of 1000 ppm toothpaste (90 g tube = 90 mg F⁻)		Amount of 400 ppm toothpaste (45 g tube = 18 mg F⁻)	
			Weight	Tube/s	Weight	Tubes
2 years	12 kg	60 mg	60 g	66%	150 g	3
4 years	15 kg	75 mg	75 g	85%	188 g	4
6 years	20 kg	100 mg	100 g	>1 tube	250 g	5 1/2

Probable toxic dose: 5 mg F⁻/kg.
ppm, Parts per million.

- A number of concentrated topical preparations could provide such levels for young children if used in a single dose.

The inappropriate prescription of home fluoride treatments with high-concentration fluoridated gels for very young children (e.g., in the management of ECC) and inappropriate use of high-fluoride products in the dental office are of concern (Evans & Stamm, 1991). For this reason, FV is the preferred form of professionally applied F product on young children, and its repeated controlled application is preferable to the prescription of high fluoride concentrations in very young children. It must be emphasized that fluoride cannot control ECC in very young children without a change in diet, especially modification of the use of a night-time bottle or the use of bottle during the day as a comforter.

The management of acute fluoride toxicity consists of:
- Estimating the amount of fluoride ingested.
- Minimizing further absorption. Products that limit absorption include milk, calcium carbonate and aluminium-magnesium based antacids.
- Removing fluoride from the body fluids.
- Supporting the vital signs.

If less than 5 mg F$^-$/kg of body weight has been ingested:
- Give as much milk as can be ingested or administer orally 5% calcium gluconate or calcium lactate or milk of magnesia.
- Inducing vomiting is not recommended.
- Keep the patient under observation until symptoms subside.

If greater than 5 mg F$^-$/kg of body weight has been ingested or if the amount is unknown:
- Immediate transport to an emergency facility for treatment and observation.
- If it does not delay transport, follow the procedures to minimize further absorption.

While this immediate action is being taken, the hospital should be advised that a case of acute fluoride poisoning is in progress so that preparation for the appropriate therapeutic intervention can be made. Notification to appropriate poison control centres should be done as required by national guidelines.

Clinical implications

Fluoride products are still the most valuable tool to prevent tooth decay. In our modern changing environment, the challenge for the clinician is to balance established measures of population health in their setting with the trend towards precision health and personalized treatments.

Dental caries is a multifactorial disease, so proper identification of the exact individual risk factors that contribute to the establishment and progression of the disease will lead to optimal interventions with specific targets with the aim of promoting and preserving health.

Clinicians are advised to:
- Be familiar with population health measures in their area, as well as local guidelines and fluoride products available.
- Do a careful caries risk assessment that allows specific identification of risk factors so a targeted-optimal treatment and preventive plan can be designed for the individual patient.

Further reading

Adair, S.M., 2006. Evidence-based use of fluoride in contemporary pediatric dental practice. Pediatric Dentistry 28, 133–142.

American Academy of Pediatric Dentistry. Fluoride therapy. The Reference Manual of Pediatric Dentistry. Chicago: American Academy of Pediatric Dentistry; 2020:288–291. https://www.aapd.org/research/oral-health-policies--recommendations/fluoride-therapy/ accessed April 10, 2021.

Burt, B.A., Keels, M.A., Heller, K.E., 2000. The effects of a break in water fluoridation on the development of dental caries and fluorosis. Journal of Dental Research 79, 761–769.

Centers for Disease Control and Prevention, 2001. Recommendations for using fluoride to prevent and control dental caries in the United States. MMWR 50 (RR14), 1–42.

Crystal, Y.O., Janal, M.N., Hamilton, D.S., Niederman, R. Parental perceptions and acceptance of silver diamine fluoride staining. Journal of the American Dental Association 2017 Jul;148(7):510–518.e4. doi: 10.1016/j.adaj.2017.03.013. Epub 2017 Apr 27. PMID: 28457477; PMCID: PMC6771934.

Crystal, Y.O., Marghalani, A.A., Ureles, S.D., Wright, J.T., Sulyanto, R., Divaris, K., Fontana, M., Graham, L. Use of silver diamine fluoride for dental caries management in children and adolescents, Including Those with Special Health Care Needs. Paediatric Dentistry 2017 Sep 15;39(5):135–145. PMID: 29070149.

Crystal, Y.O., Niederman, R. Silver Diamine fluoride treatment considerations in children's caries management. Paediatric Dentistry 2016 Nov 15;38(7):466–471. PMID: 28281949; PMCID: PMC5347149.

Crystal, Y.O., Rabieh, S., Janal, M.N., Rasamimari, S., Bromage, T.G. Silver and fluoride content and short-term stability of 38% silver diamine fluoride. Journal of the American Dental Association 2019 Feb;150(2):140–146. doi: 10.1016/j.adaj.2018.10.016. PMID: 30691572; PMCID: PMC6500427.

Curnow, M.M., Pine, C.M., Burnside, G., Nicholson, J.A., Chesters, R.K., Huntington, E. A randomised controlled trial of the efficacy of supervised toothbrushing in high-caries-risk children. Caries Research 2002 Jul–Aug;36(4):294–300. doi: 10.1159/000063925. PMID: 12218280.

Davies, G.M., Worthington, H.V., Ellwood, R.P., et al., 2002. A randomized controlled trial of the effectiveness of providing free fluoride toothpaste from the age of 12 months on reducing caries in 5–6 year old children. Community Dental Health 19, 13136.

Do, L.G.; Australian Research Centre for Population Oral Health. Guidelines for use of fluorides in Australia: update 2019. Australian Dental Journal 2020 Mar;65(1):30-38. doi: 10.1111/adj.12742. Epub 2020 Jan 26. PMID: 31868926.

Downer, M.C., Blinkhorn, A.S., 2007. The next stages in researching water fluoridation: evaluation and surveillance. Health Education Journal 66, 212–221.

Evans, R.W., Stamm, J.W., 1991. An epidemiologic estimate of the critical period during which human maxillary central incisors are most susceptible to fluorosis. Journal of Public Health Dentistry 51, 251–259.

Featherstone, J.D. The science and practice of caries prevention. Journal of the American Dental Association 2000;131(7):887–899.

Featherstone, J.D. Dental caries: a dynamic disease process. Australian Dental Journal 2008;53(3):286–291.

Featherstone, J.D.B., Crystal, Y.O., Alston, P., Chaffee, B.W., Doméjean, S., Rechmann, P., Zhan, L., Ramos-Gomez, F. Evidence-based caries management for all ages—practical guidelines. Frontiers in Oral Health 2:657518. doi: 10.3389/froh.2021.657518.

Franzman, M.R., Levy, S.M., Warren, J.J., et al., 2006. Fluoride dentifrice ingestion and fluorosis of the permanent incisors. Journal of the American Dental Association 137, 645–652.

Fung, M.H.T., Duangthip, D., Wong, M.C.M., Lo, E.C.M., Chu, C.H. Randomized clinical trial of 12% and 38% silver diamine fluoride treatment. Journal of Dental Research 2018 Feb;97(2):171–178. doi: 10.1177/0022034517728496. Epub 2017 Aug 28. PMID: 28846469; PMCID: PMC6429575.

Ismail, A.I., Hasson, H. Fluoride supplements, dental caries and fluorosis: a systematic review. Journal of the American Dental Association 2008 Nov;139(11):1457–1468. doi: 10.14219/jada.archive.2008.0071. PMID: 18978383.

Lenzi, T.L., Montagner, A.F., Soares, F.Z., de Oliveira Rocha, R. Are topical fluorides effective for treating incipient carious lesions? A systematic review and meta-analysis. Journal of the American Dental Association 2016 Feb;147(2):84–91.e1. doi: 10.1016/j.adaj.2015.06.018. Epub 2015 Nov 6. PMID: 26562737.

Marinho, V.C.C., Higgins, J.P.T., Logan, S., et al., 2009. Fluoride varnishes for preventing dental caries in children and adolescents. Cochrane Database of Systematic Reviews (1), CD002279.

Pretty, I.A. High fluoride concentration toothpastes for children and adolescents. Caries Research 2016;50 Suppl 1:9–14. doi: 10.1159/000442797. Epub 2016 Apr 22. PMID: 27101304.

Reynolds, E.C., 2008. Calcium phosphate based remineralization systems – scientific evidence. Australian Dental Journal 53, 268–273.

Scottish Intercollegiate Guidelines Network (SIGN). Dental interventions to prevent caries in children. Edinburgh: SIGN; 2014. (SIGN publication no. 138). [March 2014]. Available from URL: https://www.sign.ac.uk/media/1533/sign138.pdfhttp://www.sign.ac.uk.

Threlfall, A.G., Hunt, C.M., Milsom, K.M., et al., 2007. Exploring the factors that influence general dental practitioners when providing advice to help prevent caries in children. British Dental Journal 202 (4), E10; discussion 216–217.

Toumba, K.J., Twetman, S., Splieth, C. et al. Guidelines on the use of fluoride for caries prevention in children: an updated EAPD policy document. European Archives of Paediatric Dentistry 2019;20:507–516. https://doi.org/10.1007/s40368-019-00464-2.

Tubert-Jeannin, S., Auclair, C., Amsallem, E., et al., 2011. Fluoride supplements (tablets, drops, lozenges or chewing gums) for preventing dental caries in children. Cochrane Database of Systematic Reviews (12), CD007592.

Walsh, T., Worthington, H.V., Glenny, A.M., et al., 2010. Fluoride toothpastes of different concentrations for preventing dental caries in children and adolescents. Cochrane Database of Systematic Reviews (1), CD007868.

Weyant, R.J., Tracy, S.L., Anselmo, T., et al., 2013. Topical fluoride for caries prevention: executive summary of the updated clinical recommendations and supporting systematic review. Journal of the American Dental Association 144, 1279–1291.

Whitford, G.M. Fluoride in dental products: safety considerations. Journal of Dental Research 1987 May;66(5):1056–1060. doi: 10.1177/00220345870660051501. PMID: 3301934.

Whitford, G.M. Acute and chronic fluoride toxicity. Journal of Dental Research 1992 May;71(5):1249–1954. doi: 10.1177/00220345920710051901. PMID: 1607442.

CHAPTER 6

Restorative paediatric dentistry

Nicola Innes ■ Mark Robertson ■ Clement Seeballuck ■ Mariana Pinheiro Araujo

CHAPTER OUTLINE

Introduction

This chapter deals with restoration of the primary dentition, although some minimal approaches to the restoration of the permanent dentition are touched on. It aligns to the World Dental Federation (FDI) Policy Statement on Minimal Intervention in the Management of Dental Caries. The disease dental caries and the manifestation of the disease, the carious lesion, continue to be the main reasons for child patients to need dental treatment. This chapter is written around the management of the carious primary dentition that may or may not involve or require 'invasive' restoration. There are, of course, other dental problems that necessitate restorative solutions, such as dental trauma and developmental anomalies, that are covered in other chapters.

Managing dental caries and carious lesions in children

Children have the same right as adults to enjoy good oral health and high-quality dental care. Through laboratory studies and clinical trials, our ideas of the disease dental caries have evolved, and it is no longer considered an infectious disease but a biofilm-mediated and behaviourally-driven disease process.

Biofilm mediated means that the species of bacteria, and the proportions of each kind, present in the biofilm of dental plaque determine whether it is cariogenic, and how much so. In turn, this depends on different factors. These include:

- The length of time the biofilm has been able to mature
- The frequency and adequacy of toothbrushing and how effective it has been in plaque removal
- The type of nutrient source available to the bacteria and how favourable it is in supporting the acidogenic bacteria to thrive (high sugar diets promote more cariogenic species)

Behaviourally-driven means that the conditions that promote dental caries are strongly influenced by the person attached to the teeth! Their habits, such as toothbrushing, and the composition and frequency of their diet increase or reduce the cariogenicity of the biofilm.

The cariogenic plaque biofilm is fragile and dependent on its environment for its survival. Modern minimally invasive treatments often try to manipulate the biofilm's local environment to suppress its development. One way of doing this is to seal the carious lesion away from the oral environment using restorative solutions. Another way is to attack the lesion with a chemical that is harmful for cariogenic bacteria, such as silver diamine fluoride (SDF). These approaches to managing the disease aim to change the biofilm composition and virulence by manipulating the environment and making it less favourable for a cariogenic biofilm to thrive. The options can be grouped from more minimal to more invasive as follows:

1. Changing the behaviour that has led to/is promoting the disease (usually toothbrushing or diet)
2. Promoting remineralization of tooth tissue using chemicals, the most common being fluoride
3. Using topically applied chemicals that are damaging to the biofilm, such as SDF
4. Opening up dentinal lesions, where required, to make the lesions accessible to a toothbrush and cleansable, to remove the cariogenic biofilm
5. Separating the lesion from the oral environment using restorative solutions such as sealants, fillings or crowns
6. Restoring cavitations that are sheltered environments that would allow the biofilm to mature therefore preventing the biofilm from having a place to thrive

There are more options or children and primary teeth than are generally considered available for adults. The choice between them is driven by different priorities. Deciding on which option to choose depends on the carious lesion shape and state (e.g., active or inactive), tooth, mouth, child, family, habits, practitioner, practice and wider societal and economic characteristics. Although achieving good oral health and achieving a high standard of dental care are the same goals as for adults, the way to reach these goals may differ. This chapter will go through detecting and diagnosing dental caries, then talk through management options and finally summarize how to make decisions around each option, considering these characteristics as part of the decision-making process.

RESTORATIONS DO NOT CURE THE DISEASE

For children who have experienced dental caries, a restorative solution might work to prevent the disease from progressing quickly for an individual lesion or tooth, but it does not prevent further disease associated with other teeth. Unless there has also been a change in habits (e.g., diet, fluoride, plaque control), the factors that led to the disease occurring in the first place will still be present and the disease process is likely to continue. Restorations are not a solution to the disease dental caries; they manage its manifestation, the carious lesion. It is only by working at the child and family level that we will influence positive habits and stop the disease from progressing or recurring.

Effective management of the disease caries depends on:

- Ongoing prevention
- Early detection of lesions, that is, finding carious lesions when they are still limited to enamel and have not yet extended into dentine
- Accurate diagnosis of the carious lesions; their extent (depth) and activity
- Meaningful intervention to assist the adoption and maintenance of positive oral health behaviour changes
- The management of cavitated carious lesions, focusing on arresting or controlling (including restoring) existing lesions through minimally invasive restorative treatments (evidence informed), including repairing rather than replacing defective restorations

BEFORE BEGINNING ANY TREATMENT

Taking a history and carrying out an examination and investigations will lead to a treatment plan with several stages, probably carried out over more than one appointment. At the beginning of each appointment, check the following:

- The medical, social and clinical circumstances for any changes.
- The parent/carer and the child's understanding of the treatment to be carried out.
- The treatment steps have been explained to the child using appropriate language.
- Practice a 'STOP' signal between the patient and the clinician. The STOP signal involves an agreed-upon signal between the patient and clinician, often a raised hand, to indicate the patient requiring a break in proceedings. Once agreed upon, the clinician must be vigilant for the signal. The patient should be primed to raise the hand away from the side at which the clinician is working to prevent iatrogenic damage.

Detection and diagnosis of dental caries in children

Following a full social, medical and dental history, clinical and radiographic examinations should be carried out before treatment planning options are considered.

LESION DETECTION

Clinical detection of caries should not focus simply on finding cavitated lesions. The teeth must be closely examined for areas of demineralization and carious lesions that are at a precavitated stage, commonly known as white spot lesions. To do this, the surface of the teeth must be clearly seen. This means they must be:

- Clean and free from plaque: Where oral hygiene is suboptimal, dental plaque will conceal demineralized areas (sometimes called white spot, early or enamel lesions) – the very lesions that need to be identified before they progress to a cavitated state or to involve dentine and when they are readily remineralizable. Whenever it is not possible to observe the tooth surfaces because of poor oral hygiene, a prophylaxis, or toothbrushing, should be carried out for an accurate clinical examination.
- Dry: When optimally mineralized, enamel is translucent and microporous. Demineralized enamel interacts differently with light compared with optimally mineralized enamel. The first clinical sign of carious change in enamel is a change in translucency, that is, a white, matte enamel lesion (often called a white spot lesion), but it is visible only when the enamel has been dried. Water has a refractive index similar to enamel ($\sim$1); therefore, an enamel lesion at an initial stage (ideal for remineralising) will not be visible on a wet tooth. Further demineralization results in more micro-porosity and a further reduction in the refractive index of enamel. These lesions are seen when the tooth is wet and represent a more advanced lesion.
- Viewed under good lighting: Illumination of teeth will improve the clinician's ability to visualize teeth and their complex pit and fissure systems, while also assisting the detection of subsurface shadowing on teeth, indicative of dentinal caries.
- Magnified: This has also been shown to be useful in detecting the presence of early carious lesions.

DIAGNOSIS (Table 6.1)

- Lesion extent: The depth of the lesion can be judged clinically and recorded using a system such as the International Caries Detection and Assessment System (ICDAS). However, for assessing carious lesions, bitewing radiographs can supplement clinical information and lead the clinician toward a more accurate diagnosis and appropriate treatment options.
- Lesion activity: Assessing lesion activity gives a judgement on the current status of the lesions and future treatment successes. For example, if a preventive approach is being taken,

TABLE 6.1 ■ **Tactile and visual characteristics of enamel and dentinal lesion activity (active/inactive)**

Tooth tissue	Active or inactive lesion	Tactile features (by gently running a ball ended probe over the surface)	Visual appearance
Enamel	Active lesion	Rough	Dull, matte area although likely to be covered in biofilm (plaque)
	Nonactive/arrested lesion	Smooth	Shiny
Dentine	Active lesion	Soft	Often lighter in appearance, but this is not definitive. Likely to be covered in biofilm
	Nonactive/arrested lesion	Hard	Often darker in appearance, but this is not definitive. Likely to be free of biofilm

(From International Caries Detection and Assessment System-II classifications (Pitts, N.B., Ekstrand, K.R., 2013. International Caries Detection and Assessment System (ICDAS) and its International Caries Classification and Management System (ICCMS) – methods for staging of the caries process and enabling dentists to manage caries. Community Dentistry and Oral Epidemiology 41, e41–e52; Ekstrand, K.R., Gimenez, T., Ferreira, F.R., Mendes, F.M., Braga, M.M. 2018. The International Caries Detection and Assessment System – ICDAS: a systematic review. Caries Research 52, 406–419.)

and lesions are changing from active to nonactive lesions, then the treatment will be seen to be successful. However, if lesions remain active or there are new active lesions forming, then the treatment approach is not being successful, and needs to be reconsidered with a view to identifying and changing the elements that are preventing success.

Managing caries as a biofilm-mediated, behaviourally-driven disorder

Dental caries used to be considered an infectious disease that had to be 'cured' by removing bacteria or even a particular bacterial species. Instead, dental caries is now considered as a biofilm-mediated but behaviourally-driven disease that can only be fully managed by combining the dental restoration side with a behavioural intervention. This means a deep investigation to identify the habits and behaviours associated with the disease for each individual. Then controlling the causative factors, namely the supply of fermentable carbohydrates and the presence and maturation of bacterial dental biofilms.

Behaviour is often defined as an action undertaken as a result of stimuli or an observable act. It is part of our job as clinicians to ensure that our patients (or their families) have the necessary stimuli to support good dental and oral health. However, it can be challenging to find out what is going on in their lives.

In the case of prevention for dental caries, it can be helpful to think of there being three things necessary to allow our patients to successfully carry out preventive behaviours: knowledge, skills and attitude, with a fourth, opportunity, helping to ensure that the change is enacted regularly (Table 6.2). The behaviours can relapse and aspects will need to be reinforced regularly.

TABLE 6.2 ■ Changes to bring about preventive behaviours in patients

Behaviour change relating to...	Knowledge (following local guidelines or policy)	Skills	Attitude
Diet	Main messages: Limit sugar and eat a healthy diet	Related to shopping/ cooking and parenting skills to manage behaviour and expectations around food (outside of the scope of this chapter).	Assess how negative/ positive? Trying to move to positive with an internal locus of control. Using Motivational Interviewing or coaching to support positive habits related to sugar.
Plaque control	Twice-a-day brushing Conc.: >1000 ppm fluoride Amount: smear <2 years and pea-sized <7 years Supervised and assisted for under 7s Nothing after brushing at night Spit out excess toothpaste but no rinsing after	How to brush different ages of children's teeth. Dealing with difficult behaviour.	Negative or positive? Trying to move to positive with an internal locus of control. Using Motivational Interviewing or coaching.
Attending appointments	Why, how, where to go	Making appointments and keeping them, maybe some parental skills	Negative or positive? Trying to move to positive with an internal locus of control. Using Motivational Interviewing or coaching and work with the family to find the best times for attending and what they want from their dental appointments

- Knowledge can be defined as the condition of being aware of something. It includes the cognitive and mental abilities to process and retain information. Knowledge can be acquired through learning and experience, but being able to understand the facts and concepts related to a topic provides the foundation for carrying out a skill.
- Skills are the ability to perform a task and can be measured. Dexterity can be improved with practice, but the initial skills of toothbrushing and, where necessary, flossing need to be taught and assessed for children. Parents often also need to be shown how to brush younger children's teeth, how they can help teach their child toothbrushing skills and how they should go about supervising children until they are able to brush themselves.

■ Attitude is a way of thinking or feeling about something and influences the way we behave. It is one of the most important parts of learning because no matter how good your skill is and how much knowledge they have, it will not translate into an action unless there is a positive attitude toward it and a will to do it. Developing this can take time.

In addition to knowledge, skill and attitude, establishment and maintenance of a habit require social opportunity (i.e., access to an environment and the equipment to allow fulfilment of a task). Habit formation takes time and commitment and will require regular review from the healthcare professional to recognize and address relapse.

Deciding when to restore

The overall goals of restorative treatment are to preserve hard tissues as much as possible and retain the teeth long term.

■ Lesions that have been diagnosed as being confined to enamel (i.e., not extending in dentine) should be managed with preventive approaches, and there is no indication for removal of tooth structure or carious tissue or placement of a restoration (see chapter on prevention). Restorative interventions are indicated when cavitated carious lesions are either noncleansable, can no longer be sealed or are unlikely to arrest.

■ Lesions extending into dentine often need a restorative approach aiming to control caries progression. When a restoration is indicated, the priorities are to:
  ■ Preserve healthy and remineralizable tissue
  ■ Achieve a restorative seal
  ■ Maintain pulpal health
  ■ Maximize restoration success

Managing lesions limited to enamel (noncavitated, micro-cavitated and not extensive)

When a lesion is confined to enamel, it should not be removed and restored but managed using chemicals that promote remineralization (e.g., topical fluoride) or sealed using glass ionomer or resin-based materials. However, this action alone is not enough to stop the disease and must go hand in hand with any necessary change of habits (diet and oral hygiene). It is likely that a behaviour change intervention will be needed to support either home fluoride/toothbrushing and/or dietary change. It should be noted that fissure sealants may be used on both primary and permanent teeth depending on caries risk and activity in an individual child. Fissure sealants will be covered later in this chapter.

Fluoride to remineralize enamel lesions (see Chapter 5)

Effective use of fluoride toothpaste (containing at least 1000 ppm fluoride), combined with toothbrushing, in addition to being a successful preventive strategy, is by far the cheapest, most effective treatment available. However, the barrier in the treatment of younger children is the motivation of the parents. For the older child and young adult, it is their skills and motivation that must be activated and maximized (Walsh et al., 2019).

Clinically applied topical fluoride, where a high fluoride concentration (for example, containing 22,600 ppm fluoride) is applied to the teeth two to three times a year, has a strong evidence base to support its use for prevention and has been successfully used to arrest caries. There are guidelines for the quantity that should be applied, based on children's ages, to avoid fluoride toxicity: 0.25 mL should be used for patients aged 2 to 5 years, and 0.4 mL should be used for patients aged over 5 years.

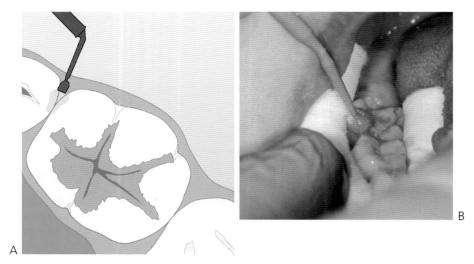

Figure 6.1 (A) Proximal surfaces of primary molars are particularly susceptible to dental caries, so should have fluoride varnish applied to these areas as well as the occlusal surface. (B) Application of fluoride varnish to occlusal surface with isolation.

PROCEDURE

1. Inspect the tooth when clean and dry under good light and clean the tooth if there is plaque/food in the fissures (using a prophy brush or toothbrush).
2. Isolate the teeth to achieve moisture control.
3. Use a microbrush to apply fluoride varnish to just below the contact points on proximal surfaces (Figure 6.1A).
4. Apply also to the occlusal surfaces (Figure 6.2B).
5. Instruct the child and parent/carer that the child should avoid eating and drinking for 30 minutes after application and to avoid brushing the teeth for at least 4 hours.

INDICATIONS

- Noncavitated lesions confined to enamel.

CONTRAINDICATIONS

- Fluoride varnish may be contraindicated in patients with an allergy to colophony and patients who have been hospitalized because of severe asthma or allergy (check product information sheet).
- Patients with ulcerative gingivitis/stomatitis.

Nonfluoride-based remineralizing agents

Over the last few decades, there have been extensive efforts to find new, more effective fluoride and nonfluoride-based remineralization agents. Many are widely advertised, but some have more supporting evidence than others. Evidence for casein phosphopeptide amorphous calcium phosphate with and without fluoride has been recently summarized as being inconclusive in effectiveness (Bijle et al., 2018), whereas the newer self-assembling peptide P11-4 (Alkilzy et al., 2018) has been more positively supported in clinical trials (although most are industry supported and not of the highest quality, so caution should be exercised in its adoption).

TABLE 6.3 ■ **Advantages and disadvantages of restorative materials used in paediatric dentistry**

	Advantages	Disadvantages
Glass ionomer cement	Adhesive Aesthetic Fluoride releasing	Brittle Susceptible to erosion and wear Technique sensitive
High-viscosity glass ionomer	Adhesive Aesthetic Simple to handle Fluoride releasing Higher compressive strength and wear resistance than conventional GICs	Water absorption Colour not as good a match as composite resins, compomers and other GICs Mechanical properties improving and approaching those of compomers or composites
Resin-modified glass ionomer	Adhesive Aesthetic – better translucency than conventional GICs Command set Simple to handle Fluoride releasing	Water absorption Significant wear Technique sensitive
Composite resin	Adhesive Aesthetic Reasonable wear properties Command set	Technique sensitive Good isolation and rubber dam required Expensive
Polyacid-modified composite resin (compomer)	Adhesive Aesthetic Command set Simple to handle	Technique sensitive Less fluoride release than GICs
Stainless steel crowns (also known as preformed metal crowns)	Durable Protect and support remaining tooth structure	Extensive tooth preparation in conventional approach but no tooth preparation when using the Hall Technique to place Patient cooperation required (moreso with the conventional technique than the Hall Technique) Unaesthetic
Zirconia crowns	Highly aesthetic Excellent biological properties Durable Protects and supports remaining tooth structure	Technique sensitive Excessive tooth preparation and often pulpotomy required Expensive

GIC, Glass ionomer cement.

Restorative materials

There are a variety of restorative materials available to restore carious lesions in the primary dentition. Given the large number of techniques and products available on the market, it is important for clinicians to understand the procedure they are using and to be aware that all approaches are operator and technique sensitive. Table 6.3 summarizes the main advantages and disadvantages of various dental restorative materials.

GLASS IONOMER CEMENTS

A glass ionomer consists of a basic glass and an acidic water-soluble powder that sets by an acid–base reaction between the two components. A principal benefit of glass ionomer cement (GIC) is that it will adhere chemically to dental hard tissues. A number of GICs are available on the market today, with different advantages and disadvantages.

CONVENTIONAL GLASS IONOMER CEMENTS

Conventional GICs are chemical-set glass ionomers with the weakest mechanical properties. The initial setting reaction is complete within minutes, but the material continues to 'mature' over the following months. It is important to protect these materials from salivary contamination in the hours following placement or the material may shrink, crack and even debond. Adhesion of all GICs may be enhanced by the use of a dentine-conditioning agent before placement. Today, chemically curing GICs are available as both restorative and protective sealant types of materials with high fluoride-releasing properties.

HIGH-VISCOSITY GLASS IONOMER CEMENTS

High-viscosity GICs (HVGICs) were developed for use with the Atraumatic Restorative Treatment (ART). These chemically cured materials have significantly better mechanical properties than the conventional GICs and are fast setting. Research suggests that these materials have a durability comparable with amalgam when used in occlusal restorations in primary teeth, although the success rate is much lower in occluso-proximal (multi-surface) restorations when other materials and crowns should be considered.

RESIN-MODIFIED GLASS IONOMER CEMENTS

Resin-modified GICs were developed to overcome the problems of moisture sensitivity and low initial mechanical strength of GIC. They consist of a GIC along with a water-based resin system which allows photopolymerization to occur before the acid–base reaction of the glass ionomer is complete. This reaction then occurs within the light polymerized resin framework. The resin increases the fracture strength and wear resistance of the GIC. Resin modified GICs are manufactured as restorative and lining materials for use in both primary and permanent teeth.

COMPOSITE RESINS

Photocuring bis-GMA (bisphenol A-glycidyl methacrylate) composite resins have become the mainstay of restorative dentistry in the permanent dentition, replacing amalgam. Over the past 40 years, their properties in relation to bonding, strength, bio-compatibility, colour stability and translucency have improved immensely, and with appropriate isolation and technique, they can be appropriate for the restoration of primary molar teeth. Placement of these materials is highly technique sensitive, patient compliance and adequate moisture isolation can prove difficult in the younger child.

COMPOMERS (POLYACID-MODIFIED COMPOSITE RESIN)

Polyacid-modified resin composite resins or 'compomers' are materials that contain a calcium aluminium fluorosilicate glass filler and polyacid components. They contain either or both essential components of a GIC. However, they are not water based, and therefore, no acid–base reaction can occur. As such, they cannot strictly be described as a glass ionomer. They set by resin photopolymerization. The acid–base reaction does occur in the moist intraoral environment and allows fluoride release from the material. Successful adhesion requires the use of dentine-bonding primers before placement.

STAINLESS STEEL CROWNS

Stainless steel crowns are preformed extra-coronal restorations that are particularly useful in the restoration of proximal dentinal lesions, multisurface cavities and grossly broken-down primary molar teeth. They cover the entire crown, and therefore, further caries is very unlikely. Placement of traditional stainless steel crowns is associated with considerable tooth preparation, which can be challenging for patient and clinician alike. However, the introduction of minimal intervention sealed restorations using crowns (known as the Hall Technique) has made the use of these restorations more realistic. There is strong evidence that stainless steel crowns are the most durable restoration in the primary dentition.

ZIRCONIA CROWNS

Zirconia crowns have been developed to address the demands of parents and patients for a more aesthetic full-coverage restoration rather than stainless steel crowns. Zirconia crowns are milled or injection moulded yttrium-stabilized tetragonal zirconia. They provide excellent aesthetics and a favourable tooth–tissue interface, being biologically inert. They are extremely strong, and much harder than enamel. However, their use is not without issues in relation to the amount of tooth preparation that is required, technique-sensitive placement and cementation procedures, retention, cost and clinical time required for the patient in comparison to the traditional metal crown.

Managing carious lesions extended into dentine

Dentinal carious lesions can be shallow (i.e., just beyond the enamel–dentine junction and confined to the outer third of dentine) or deeper and more extensive, extending to the inner third of dentine and close to the dental pulp. They can be noncavitated or cavitated.

There are some guiding principles for managing these lesions, with particular strategies given under each section related to different types of restorations.

GUIDING PRINCIPLES

For the noncavitated shallow lesions, it may be possible to seal and monitor them, but the integrity of the material used to seal and its margins must be maintained for this to be successful.

For deeper lesions, a portion of the carious tissue needs to be managed to stop the biofilm in the protected environment from destroying the tooth structure and/or reaching the dental pulp and promote a good seal when using the restorative material. Pulp vitality and health should be maintained wherever possible, and as little tooth substance that is healthy and liable to remineralization should be removed, with the aim to keep the tooth pain-free, in function and aesthetic as far as possible. The techniques used are selective carious tissue removal (generally used for primary teeth, although there is growing evidence to support this approach in permanent teeth), stepwise carious tissue removal (generally used for deep lesions in permanent teeth) and the Hall Technique (for primary teeth). Another technique, though still controversial is to use a nonrestorative cavity control (NRCC) approach which involves focussing on behaviour change to stop the disease overall and taking a cleaning and remineralising approach to the lesion. This is usually reserved for cavitated and cleansable lesions.

For cavitated lesions, they can either be accessible to cleansing (e.g., where the entire surface of the cavity is accessible to a toothbrush for cleaning) or the biofilm can be in a sheltered environment where it cannot be cleaned properly (where the lesion is more extensive than the cavity opening). These protected biofilm environments are the ones where restoration is usually necessary to stop the biofilm from remaining cariogenic and promoting continuation of the demineralization. It will also be necessary to place a restoration where a lesion cannot be arrested.

HOW MUCH CARIOUS TISSUE TO REMOVE?

When carious tissue removal is indicated, the location and extent of the lesion guide how much needs to be removed. Bacterially contaminated or demineralized tissue close to the pulp does not need to be removed just because it is there. Tooth tissue/carious lesion should only be removed to create conditions for long-lasting restorations. When a lesion has extended into dentine, the tooth preparation should be deep enough for the restorative material used to have enough bulk to withstand occlusal forces.

Where the carious lesion extends further than the depth needed for the restorative material to have sufficient strength, then selective caries removal (primary teeth) or stepwise removal (permanent teeth) is indicated. Selective caries removal involves the removal of enough soft carious tissue to place the material. Care must to taken to ensure that the cavity walls are clean of any decayed tooth tissue to allow optimal adhesion of the material. Caries-affected dentine can, and should, be left at the base of the cavity. Unsupported enamel is removed. The remaining carious tissue is sealed off from the oral environment with the restoration, preventing substrate access and arresting the caries process. This minimizes weakening the tooth and the risk of pulpal exposure.

HOW TO REMOVE CARIOUS TISSUE

There are three commonly used methods for the removal of carious tissue and preparation of the tooth. These are:

- Rotary instruments. These can be high-speed air rotors, slow or reduced-speed handpieces and they can be used with traditional burs or burs that are limited in their ability to cut hard tissue to reduce the chance of removing healthy tooth substance.
- Sharp hand instruments (usually linked to ART).
- Chemo-mechanical caries removal agents. These tend to be sodium hypochlorite or enzyme based. They are generally considered to be effective at caries removal but have the drawbacks of not allowing selective removal (i.e., all carious tissue is removed), requiring an open cavity (so sometimes, ART types of instruments or a rotary instrument is required to allow access to the dentine) and being time-consuming (Hamama et al., 2014).

Direct restorations for primary molars

Traditionally, direct restorations have been the most common treatment for managing carious lesions in primary molars and are most successful in single-surface cavities, with higher failure rates for multisurface. They offer aesthetic options compared with stainless steel crowns and are less invasive than providing a zirconia crown. However, with the evidence to support fissure sealants over noncavitated lesions, proximal infiltration and sealants and the high success rate with minimal intervention when using the Hall Technique, traditional restorations are carried out less often than they used to be for multisurface cavities.

The Minimata Convention (FDI, 2013) indicated that amalgam materials will be phased out. In many countries, these can no longer be used routinely in children. This means that there is a reliance on adhesive materials for primary teeth. Primary teeth present a number of challenges when trying to achieve moisture control and prepare a cavity that allows enough good-quality teeth to achieve good bonding. These have to be taken into consideration when preparing the tooth for the restoration.

The American Association for Paediatric Dentistry (AAPD) Guidelines 2020/21 recommend standard GICs for occlusal restorations and HVGICs for single surface ART restorations in primary and permanent teeth. It only recommends resin-modified GICs for multisurface cavities in primary teeth. The evidence supports stainless steel crowns as having better long-term survival whether used with a conventional technique or the Hall Technique.

CAVITY PREPARATION

The concepts behind conventional cavity preparation are based on evidence and the principle that cavity augmentation should be extensive enough to allow for adequate retention and bulk of restorative materials to maximize restoration longevity.

So the aims are to:

1. Establish cavity walls that are free of carious and soft dentine to allow good adhesion of the material to the tooth and reduce microleakage; and
2. Provide adequate depth of material for it to be strong enough to withstand the forces placed on it.

The carious tissue on the floor of the cavity is not removed. This minimizes iatrogenic damage to the dental pulp through pressure, vibration and heat (when using rotary instruments) from carious tissue removal. It also maintains the integrity of the tooth structure and reduces weakening the tooth. However, very soft tissue presenting biofilm should be removed from the floor of the cavity with caution.

The procedure of cavity preparation aims to create a cavity to facilitate the retention and function of whichever restorative material is used.

PROCEDURE FOR OCCLUSAL CAVITY (SIMILAR FOR OTHER SINGLE-SURFACE PREPARATIONS)

1. Place local anaesthesia, as it is likely that dentinal (sensitive) tooth tissue will need to be removed.
2. Access the carious lesion. Keep cavity preparation to a minimum and only remove the carious parts of the fissure pattern. The cavity shape is dictated by the carious lesion initially and then modified minimally to make a cavity suitable for a restoration (i.e., no sharp edges, corners, no overhanging unsupported enamel).
3. Prepare the cavity depth
   - For a shallow caries lesion (restricted to the outer one-half of dentine), ensure that the cavity allows adequate bulk of filling material. This may require removing all of the carious lesion and reaching hard dentine on the base.
   - For deep lesions (extending into the inner one-half of dentine), carry out selective caries removal. Keep the preparation as minimal as possible and avoid unnecessarily deepening the cavity. This helps maintain tooth structure/strength and avoids damaging or exposing the dental pulp. Caries affected dentine can be left on the floor of the cavity. Ensure that the walls of the cavity do not have soft dentine, as this will compromise bonding. There is no need to remove all carious tissue if an adequate seal can be achieved around the periphery of the cavity, as the seal will prevent the lesion from progressing and allow it to arrest.
4. Following the previous principles, use a high speed air rotor where necessary to remove enamel and remove any loose, soft carious tissue gently using hand excavators or a large slow-speed rosehead bur.
5. Place the chosen restorative material.
6. Check the occlusion with articulating paper and use floss to clean the proximal contacts.

PROCEDURE FOR OCCLUSO-PROXIMAL CAVITY (Figure 6.2)

It should be noted that there are numerous randomized control trials that have found the Hall Technique to last longer than multi-surface restorations. The Hall Technique or conventional crowns, should be the treatments of choice.

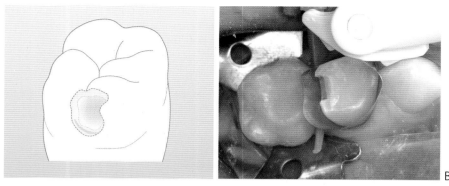

Figure 6.2 (A, B) Example of an occluso-proximal cavity design for the placement of resin-modified glass ionomer material to restore the tooth.

1. If the marginal ridge is intact, gain access to the carious tissue with a high-speed handpiece and diamond fissure bur, leaving a thin enamel wall at the proximal contact to protect the adjacent tooth. Although an idealised form is shown in Figure 6.2A, the cavity shape will be determined by the location and spread of the carious lesion.
2. The cavity will need to be of sufficient depth to give adequate bulk of filling material.
3. Remove soft dentine from the walls of the cavity using hand excavators or a large rosehead bur.
4. Prepare the proximal box margins and remove the remaining thin enamel wall with enamel/gingival margin trimmers. Take extreme care to avoid iatrogenic damage to the adjacent tooth.
5. Use a matrix band and wooden wedges to allow material packing (Figure 6.2B). This will aid in contouring the restoration and establish a contact point.
6. Place the restorative material. GIC does not perform well in multisurface cavities in primary molars, and composite, compomer or resin-modified/high-viscosity glass ionomer should be used.
7. Check the occlusion with articulating paper.

The longevity and success of any restoration are dependent on it being placed in line with manufacurer recommendations and with excellent moisture control. Patient age, behaviour management and cooperation will determine how this is best achieved and rubber dam can often provide isolation that ensures a dry field (Figure 6.3).

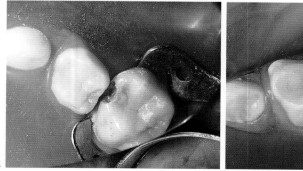
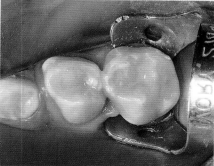

Figure 6.3 Two methods for using the rubber dam in children. (A) Traditional isolation of single teeth. (B) Split-dam technique, isolating the teeth from the canine to second primary molar with one large hole in the dam.

INDICATIONS

- Single-surface carious lesion.
- Multisurface carious lesions (although the success rate is lower and the Hall Technique should be the treatment of choice when treating primary teeth).

CONTRAINDICATIONS

- Lesions that have extended subgingivally and where moisture control would be difficult to achieve.
- Signs/symptoms of irreversible pulpitis, periradicular pathology/abscess/sinus.

Atraumatic Restorative Treatment

ART uses hand instruments; usually specially designed ones such as those in Figure 6.4 are used to access the lesion, if it is not already accessible, and remove selected amounts of carious tooth tissue to allow a glass ionomer restoration to be placed. Carious tissue removal in ART follows the same principle of selective caries removal with hand instruments only. ART has the aim of being a patient-friendly technique but is also useful for patients with anxiety/fear. However, on the base of the cavity only enough carious tissue is removed to allow sufficient depth of the material to withstand pressure from occlusal forces. This will usually leave soft or leathery dentine on the floor of the cavity, that is selectively removed to preserve pulpal health and tooth tissue but allows good adhesion of the restorative material.

It is recommended that HVGICs, originally developed for use with ART, are used to restore the cavity. These materials have better mechanical properties than conventional glass ionomer materials and are fast setting. There is wide variation in the reported success rates of ART restorations, but systematic reviews generally agree that these materials have a durability comparable with amalgam when used in occlusal (class I) restorations in primary teeth, although the success rate is significantly lower when used in multisurface restorations (De Amorim et al., 2018; Dorri et al., 2017; Jiang et al., 2020). For multisurface restorations, crowns, using either the conventional or the Hall Technique, should be the first option for treatment.

Although methods for traditional (rotary instrument) cavity preparation have been given earlier, it is possible, with the correct ART instruments, to prepare most cavities without the need for rotary instruments or the removal of live dentine. There are high success rates for ART with HVGIC single-surface restorations in both primary and permanent dentitions, with systematic reviews of the literature and meta-analyses showing annual failure percentages of 5% for primary molars over 3 years and 4.1% in permanent posterior teeth over 5 years.

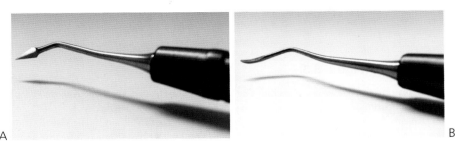

A   B

Figure 6.4 (A) Atraumatic restorative technique instrument for opening cavities. (B) A small excavator for removing caries.

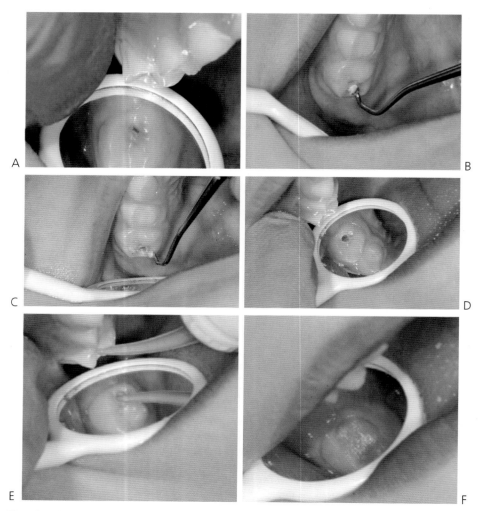

Figure 6.5 (A) Using Atraumatic Restorative Treatment (ART) to manage an occlusal lesion in an upper secondary primary molar. (B, C) Increasing occlusal access and caries removal of infected and/or heavily affected carious dentine with a sharp spoon excavator. Undermined enamel should also be removed. (D) ART principles have left minimally affected dentine over the cavity base, while cavity margins are caries-free, allowing for a satisfactory restorative seal to arrest the carious process. (E) Placement of a fast-setting glass ionomer into the cavity, which is then compressed with finger pressure (F).

PROCEDURE (Figure 6.5)

1. Explain to the parent and the child that when the carious tissue is being removed with the hand instruments ('tooth cleaners') (Figure 6.4B), it will sound 'scratchy'.
2. Ensure that the tooth is clean and dry. A clean, dry tooth will aid in the visualization of the extent and morphology of a caries lesion. Wet enamel has a similar refractive index to water, making it difficult to detect subsurface micro-porosities (white lesions) in the enamel matrix.

3. Remove plaque and/or food debris present in the cavity using a toothbrush or wet cotton pellet.
4. Isolate the tooth with cotton wool to keep it dry; moisture control should be maintained throughout the procedure and whilst placing the restoration (a 'dry guard' and suction may be helpful to maintain a dry field).
5. Widen the entrance to the carious lesion if the cavity is too small to allow the spoon excavator access by placing the spoon excavator or dental hatchet (Figure 6.5B) at the cavity entrance and turning around to one direction and then backwards, applying some pressure.
6. Remove carious tissue from the periphery of the cavity until clear, hard dentine is reached using a spoon excavator (Figure 6.5C–E). Excavators must be sharp and able to remove unsupported dental enamel. Only soft carious tissue on the floor of the cavity should be removed, using a 'scooping' motion, and care must be taken to avoid pressure for two reasons:
   - too much tissue removal could lead to exposure of the dental pulp; and
   - pressure on the dentinal tubules will cause dentinal fluid movement and cause pain.
7. Remove any remaining thin demineralized and unsupported overhanging enamel using the sharp spoon excavators or dental hatchets.
8. Clean the cavity and occlusal surfaces, including the pits and fissures, with wet cotton pellets.
9. Apply dentine conditioner (e.g., polyacrylic acid) to the entire cavity and adjacent fissures to promote a better bond between the GIC filling and the tooth using a disposable dental microbrush or cotton pellet, rubbing it against the dental tissues for 15 sec.
10. Wash the cavity immediately with wet cotton pellets or the triple syringe and dry with cotton pellets.
11. Use the HVGIC (encapsulated or powder/liquid) to slightly overfill the cavity, also placing it in the remaining pits and fissures.
12. Place a gloved finger to apply slight pressure on the filling surface (this allows the material to accommodate better to the cavity shape) for a full 2 minutes until the material has set (press-finger technique). Following slight overfilling of the cavity, prolonged (approximately 2 minutes) finger pressure allows for adequate conformity to the cavity margins.
13. Advise the patient to avoid eating for the next hour.

INDICATIONS

- Single-surface cavities in primary or permanent teeth.
- Multisurface cavity in primary teeth when no other option is available or if aesthetics are a concern.

CONTRAINDICATIONS

- Large-sized multisurface ART/HVGIC restorations in primary molars have lower success rates because of the limitations of the material rather than being related to the caries removal technique. However, ART may be a good interim strategy for large multisurface cavities or for stabilizing the dentitions before other restorative interventions.

Preformed stainless steel crown placement (the Hall Technique and conventional technique)

Preformed metal crowns are highly durable restorations and are recommended by the AAPD (2019). The preformed metal variety (often known as stainless steel) has been successfully used for the restoration of primary molars for around 80 years, with success rates of around 80–95% over 5 years. Efforts to make the preformed metal crowns more aesthetic by veneering materials to outside of them have, to date, been proven unsuccessful. However, over the last few decades, there have been major improvements in the nonmetal or white crowns by developing materials, commonly zirconia ceramic.

The preformed metal crown can be used in two ways. The original method involved placement of local anaesthesia and carrying out tooth tissue reduction to place the crowns over the teeth in a semi-passive fit, using cement to help retain them. However, the cariogenic activity of the biofilm can be arrested by sealing in the carious lesion and biofilm. This means that the bacteria are unable to thrive and their acidogenic activity stops, changing the biofilm to one with noncariogenic properties. The key to arresting the lesion is to have a thorough seal around the periphery of the restoration. It can be difficult to obtain a thorough seal with restorations on a multisurface cavity in primary molar because of the bulbous shape of the crown, the thin enamel and the small size of the tooth. Carious lesions occur just below the contact point between the teeth and when destruction of the enamel occurs to the extent that it breaks down and there is missing tooth tissue on the proximal side of the tooth, it leaves little sound tooth surface at the base, on which to place the restoration.

- Multisurface cavities
- Grossly broken-down teeth
- Primary molars that have undergone pulp therapy
- Hypoplastic or hypomineralized primary or permanent teeth
- Dentitions of children at high risk of caries, particularly children having treatment under general anaesthesia

The Hall Technique for primary molars

The Hall Technique is the name of a simplified method for using a standard preformed crown to seal carious lesions into a primary molar tooth. However, it differs from the conventional method for placing crowns, as it is placed by pushing it over the tooth and without the removal of any tooth structure or any carious tissue. It therefore does not require local anaesthetic or rotary instruments.

The Hall Technique has been shown in clinical trials and systematic reviews to last longer than plastic restorations (Badar et al., 2019) and as long as conventional crowns, showing a survival rate of 93% to 98% for 2- to 5-year follow-up (Innes et al., 2017). The Hall Technique is an effective treatment option for the management of asymptomatic dentin carious primary molars, especially for proximal or multisurface lesions (Araujo et al., 2020).

The idea of the crown can be introduced to the child as being like a 'a shiny helmet to protect the tooth', 'a precious, shiny, princess crown', the 'Ironman tooth' or it being a 'twinkle tooth'. It should be explained to the child and parent beforehand that the child might find the crown tight after it is placed (as there is no tooth preparation) and that there is an increase in the occlusal vertical dimension (OVD).

PROCEDURE

Crowns can be fitted most easily if the marginal ridge is still intact. Often, primary molar teeth have broad contact areas and there is sometimes spacing, which makes the crowns easier to place. However, for tight contacts where there is no space, it might be necessary to place orthodontic elastic separators and leave them in place for 2 days to a week to allow the space between the teeth to open and facilitate placing a well-fitting crown (Figure 6.6). When the child returns to have the separator removed, the crown is placed at the same appointment.

1. Measure and record the overlap of the canines to allow the increase in the OVD to be measured after the crown is fitted (Figure 6.6A).
2. Measure the occlusal surface of the tooth medio-distally and bucco-palatally (to help choose the correct size of crown (Figure 6.7B).

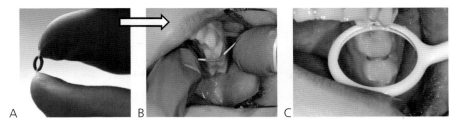

Figure 6.6 An orthodontic separator (A) is placed with dental floss (B) to provide tension and facilitate placement using a flossing action. Separator placement will allow sufficient interdental space for crown placement. N.B. the contact point should sit in the middle of the separator (C).

3. Choose the correct size of crown. It should cover the occlusal table and be able to be pushed toward the contact points on both the mesial and distal sides of the tooth.
4. Clean and dry the crown and the tooth.
5. The crown should be filled to at least two-thirds with the cement and placed over the tooth and pushed between the contact points to ensure that it will be seated evenly over the tooth (Figure 6.7E).

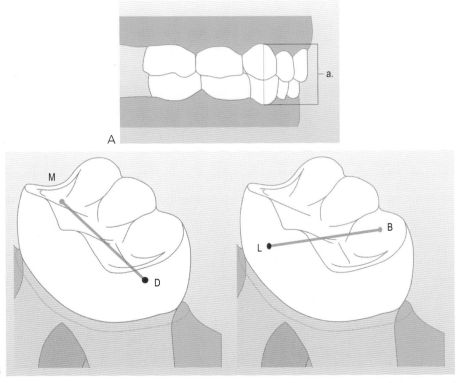

Figure 6.7 The Hall Technique for stainless steel crown placement. (A) Measure and record the overlap of the canines to allow the increase in the occlusal vertical dimension to be measured after the crown is fitted. (B) The tooth can be measured mesio-distally and bucco-lingually to help with choosing the correct size of crown. This can be done using a graded periodontal probe.

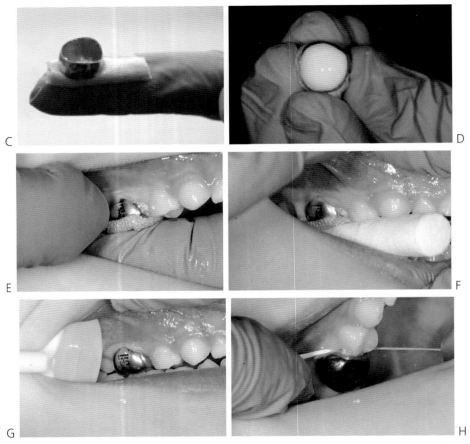

Figure 6.7 (Continued) (C, D) Airway protection is paramount during crown placement. A double-backed elastoplast on the operator's finger secures the crown; otherwise, a gauze swab should be placed in the patient's mouth to protect against a crown being swallowed or aspirated. (E, F). The first-stage of seating the crown will result in extrusion of cement. Cotton wool rolls should be used to remove as much of this as possible to prevent the patient tasting the cement. (G) Note the gingival blanching around the newly fitted crown. This is normal and will quickly resolve. (H) Ensure that contact points are cleared with floss following crown placement to ensure that the patient is able to effectively clean interdentally.

6. Check that the crown is going over the tooth evenly and not further on the buccal, lingual or proximal side.
7. Ask the child to bite down on the crown (Figure 6.7F). A cotton roll placed on the crown can help the child to bite hard, as they feel the soft cotton roll rather than the hard crown when they bite. If the child does not bite down, push the crown evenly down over the tooth.
8. Ensure that the crown has seated well. Excess GIC will flow out from under the margins of the crown (Figure 6.7G).
9. Ask the child to open his/her mouth and clear away the excess cement, trying not to let the child taste it.
10. Check that the crown has seated evenly, and if not, work out whether it was pushed on unevenly or it is the wrong size of crown, but do not delay in removing the crown while the cement is still soft, using the large spoon excavator.

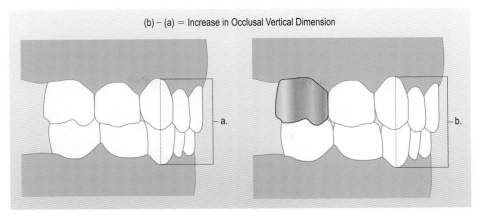

Figure 6.8 Following crown placement, the occluso-vertical dimension measured at the canines will likely increase. This will resolve after 2 to 4 weeks, by a combination of intrusion of the crowned tooth and intrusion of the opposing tooth.

11. Push the crown on again or ask the child to bite down again and hold the crown in place until the cement sets. The crown may need to be held firmly down. This stage is important, as it pushes the crown further so that it rests against the cusps and stops it from being forced up at all.
12. Check around the periphery of the crown using an excavator to clear away any excess cement.
13. Floss between the contracts (Figure 6.7H).
14. Measure the overlap or gap in the contact between the upper and lower canines and record the increase in the OVD (Figure 6.8).

Changes in tooth morphology often result from proximal carious lesions, causing marginal ridge breakdown, and the adjacent molar can migrate into the space. This leaves a narrower mesio-distal width to fit the crown compared with the ratio that would be expected relative to the bucco-lingual distance. This means that the crown may need to be adjusted to fit well, which can be done by trimming the base to reduce the height of the crown (although this is rarely necessary) or by using band-forming pliers to adapt the crown and create a concave area on the side of the crown, adapted to the shape of the tooth.

CLINICAL HINT (Figure 6.9)

Where there has been space loss because of mesial migration of the second primary molar into the space of a carious first primary molar, the following techniques may be useful:
- An upper first primary molar crown may be used to restore a contralateral lower first primary molar.
- A lower first primary molar crown can be rotated 90 degrees to restore an upper first primary molar. In this case, the crown requires trimming to remove the buccal projection of the tuberculum molare.

INDICATIONS

- Asymptomatic proximal or multisurface lesions (cavitated or noncavitated, active or inactive) and occlusal lesions (usually only if the patient is unable to accept a single surface restoration).
- The tooth should have sufficient sound tissue left to retain the crown.

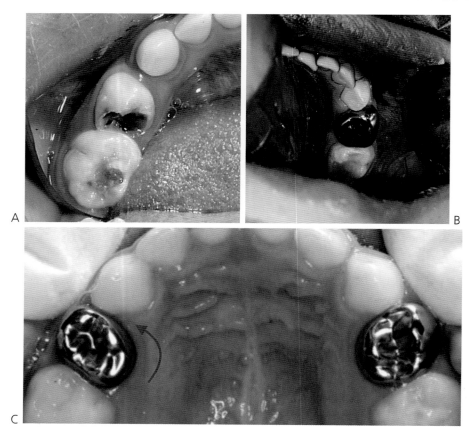

Figure 6.9 (A) Space loss (lower right) caused by mesial migration of the second molar owing to loss of the distal marginal ridge of the lower first primary molar. (B) Use of an upper first primary molar crown on the contralateral lower tooth. (C) A 90-degree rotation of a lower crown to restore an upper molar.

- Depth of the carious lesion: on a bitewing radiograph, a band of "normal" looking dentine should be visible between the pulp chamber or horn and the advancing edge of the carious lesion.
- No evidence of periapical pathology at the furcation or at the periapical area of the surrounding bone should be observed.
- Hypoplastic primary molars.
- Tooth vitality and dental pulp involvement: The pulp status judgement should be a combination of history (past and existing symptoms and main complaint), clinical extraoral examination and intraoral examination of the soft and hard tissues, including clinical tests such as palpation, percussion and tooth mobility.
- Dentally anxious children unable to tolerate more invasive restorative procedures.

CONTRAINDICATIONS

- Signs/symptoms of irreversible pulpitis, periradicular pathology/abscess/sinus.
- Where there is no band of dentine visible between the carious lesion and the dental pulp on a bitewing radiograph.
- Insufficient remaining tooth tissue for crown retention.

- A caries lesion extending apically to an extent that a preformed crown will not seal the lesion.
- Nickel or silver allergy.
- Radiographic signs of pulpal involvement or peri-radicular pathology.
- Lack of sufficient sound tissue to retain the crown.
- Atypical tooth shape, so that a crown cannot be easily fitted.

Conventional crowns for primary molars
PROCEDURE (Figures 6.10 and 6.11)

1. Place local anaesthesia (this is still needed if the tooth has had pulp therapy and is nonvital because when the tooth is being trimmed proximally, the bur needs to be passed subgingivally). Rubber dam is often recommended and makes access for trimming easier, but there is no evidence that it improves outcomes.

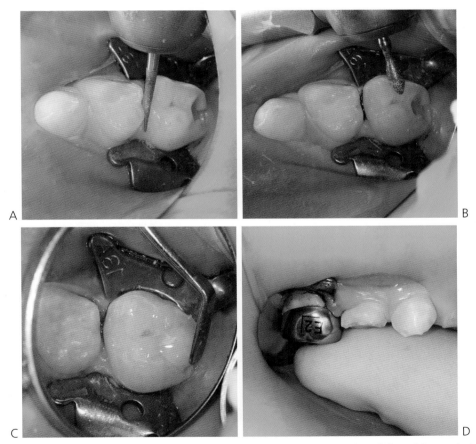

A   B

C   D

Figure 6.10   Placement of a stainless steel crown. This tooth had a large distal lesion with loss of the marginal ridge. (A) Aproximal reduction is completed with a fine tapering diamond bur, taking care not to damage the adjacent tooth. (B) Occlusal reduction of up to 1.5 mm is performed with a large diamond flat fissure bur, a small wheel or, in this case, a flame diamond bur. (C) Glass ionomer cement is used to build up the carious distal aspect of the crown. (D) Trial fit of the crown, by seating from the lingual/palatal onto the buccal surface.

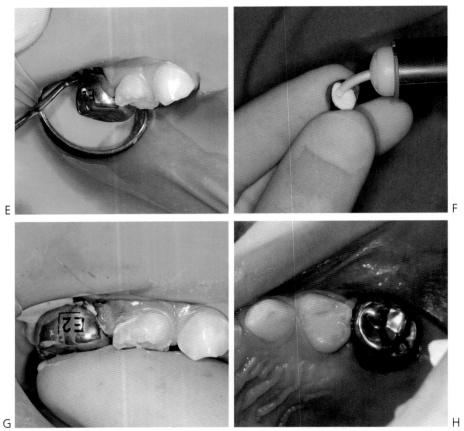

Figure 6.10 (Continued) (E) A large spoon excavator can be used to remove the crown. (F) The crown is filled with glass ionomer cement for luting and (G) the crown placed with finger pressure (H).

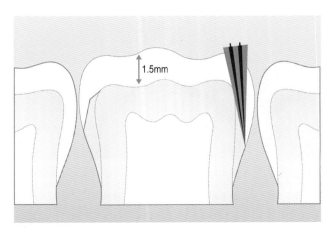

Figure 6.11 Coronal and proximal preparation required for the placement of a stainless steel crown. Note that in the proximal areas, there is a smooth contour without any ledge or step which would cause great difficulty in seating the crown.

2. If the tooth has lost a lot of structure (and sometimes following pulp therapy), it might be necessary to restore the tooth using a GIC or similar material, before preparation for the preformed metal crown.

3. Reduce the occlusal surface by about 1.5 mm using a flame-shaped or tapered diamond bur. Uniform occlusal reduction will facilitate placement of the crown without interfering with the occlusion.

4. Prepare the proximal sides of the tooth (mesially and distally) using a fine, long, tapered diamond bur, held slightly convergent to the long axis of the tooth. There should be sufficient removal of tooth tissue to allow a probe to be passed between the adjacent teeth (where the contact area was).

5. Reduce the tooth on the buccal and lingual surfaces; however, keep this to a minimum to aid retention. Reduction is usually only needed to shape the tooth for the crown if there are prominent anatomical features such as a Cusp of Carabelli or where there has been significant space loss and the proportions of the tooth have been distorted.

6. Choose the correct size of preformed crown by measuring the mesiodistal width.

7. Try the crown on the tooth to check the fit. It should sit around 1 mm subgingivally (look for blanching) and can be trimmed and smoothed with a white stone if necessary. Ideally, it should seat in a lingual/palatal to buccal direction with a 'snap' fit.

8. Cement the crown using GIC. If the crown of the tooth has been built up before the placement of the crown, a glass ionomer luting cement may be used; otherwise, glass ionomer designed for a restoration is recommended.

9. Clear away excess glass ionomer material. Care should be taken while holding the crown, as it can be easily dropped during placement. Excess cement should be wiped away and a layer of Vaseline placed around the margins while the cement is setting.

INDICATIONS

These are similar to the indications for the Hall Technique, but there are a few additional indications:
- Grossly broken-down teeth.
- Following pulp therapy.
- In very deep lesions where, radiographically, there appears to be no band of dentine between the lesion and the dental pulp or, clinically (or symptomatically), there is evidence of pulpitis or peri-radicular periodontitis, in which case all caries should be removed, a pulp therapy carried out (see Chapter 7) and a conventional crown preparation carried out.

Zirconia crowns for primary molars

The use of tooth-coloured ceramic crowns rather than traditional full metal crowns in the primary dentition is gaining popularity. They have excellent aesthetics, strength and biocompatibility and are often used to restore the primary dentition that has been affected by developmental disorders such as amelogenesis imperfecta or dentinogenesis imperfecta, in addition to those children with caries. They are useful when aesthetics are a concern. The main drawback of the ceramic, white material is that because the material has to be thick, a significant amount of tooth reduction is required to allow tooth-coloured ceramic crowns to be fitted; this means that pulp therapy is usually required. They are also significantly more expensive than stainless steel crowns.

PROCEDURE (Figure 6.12)

1. Remove all undermined enamel and carious, soft tooth tissue and complete pulp therapy as required. In first primary molars, the extent of tooth preparation may result in exposure of the distal pulp horn, and so careful assessment of the pulpal inflammatory status is important.

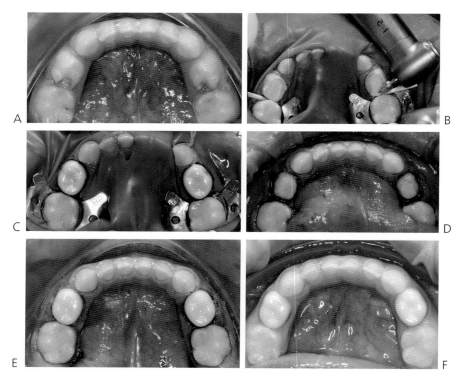

Figure 6.12   Placement of zirconia crowns on primary molars. (A) Initial situation in a 3.5-year-old child with reversible pulpitis in the lower first primary molars. (B) Isolation with rubber dam using a split-dam technique. Pulpotomies have been performed and the crowns rebuilt with glass ionomer cement. Occlusal reduction is achieved using a flame diamond bur. The mesial surfaces of the second molars are protected using wedges during aproximal reduction. (C) Size assessment using pink 'try-in' crowns. (D) Haemostasis is essential before cementation. Note the amount of tooth reduction and the smooth contours of the preparation. (E) Crown cementation. (F) Review at 24 months after crown placement showing excellent healing, marginal adaptation and stability of the restoration. (Courtesy of Dr. Tatyana Peshko, Kiev, Ukraine.)

2. Rebuild the core of the tooth if required with a GIC.
3. Reduce buccal and lingual cusps to the depth of central groove, maintaining cusp inclines using a pear (football)-shaped bur.
4. Reduce central groove by approximately 0.5 mm with the same bur.
5. Reduce the buccal and lingual occlusal third of the dental crown.
6. Create buccal and lingual depth cut to 0.5 mm.
7. Interproximal slice to 1.0 mm, being careful not to damage the adjacent tooth.
8. Level depth cuts and round facial lingual interproximal line angles.
9. Remove shoulder and extend preparation subgingivally to the feather edge. It is essential not to create any step that might impede placement of the crown.
10. Control haemorrhage with a haemostatic agent.
11. Place try-in crown to assess fit so there is good cervical fit and no rotational or rocking movement.
12. Cement the crown.

Direct restorations for anterior primary teeth

There are different techniques available to restore the anterior primary teeth, and the decision which one to choose is generally dictated by the clinical situation. The options range from simple small restorations for minimal dentinal carious lesions (small proximal or buccal) to hand build-ups for more loss of tooth tissue and crown forms for use where there is extensive tooth surface loss. There is also the option of aesthetic crowns (crowns with white facings, ceramic/zirconia crowns or other aesthetic materials) that can be used to restore anterior primary teeth usually following pulp therapy.

Small direct restorations for anterior primary teeth

Where there is minimal tooth loss such as a proximal or small buccal carious lesion, a simple restoration using composite, compomer or glass ionomer can be used. This should follow the principles of complete carious tissue removal. There must be adequate depth for the material to have sufficient bulk and enough tooth surface to give good adhesion. If the cavity is deep and there is a risk of pulp exposure, it is still good practice to leave carious tissue overlying the dental pulp on the base of the cavity.

Crown forms for restoring anterior primary teeth

Crown forms may be considered when restoring anterior primary teeth with significant loss of tooth structure. An advantage of this technique is that the shaping of the final restoration is undertaken extra-orally within the preformed crown matrix. This reduces procedural time intra-orally, therefore reducing the level of cooperation required, and enhances patient comfort.

PROCEDURE FOR USING A CROWN FORM (Figure 6.13)

1. Whilst the tooth is still wet with saliva, choose the appropriate shade of composite under natural light using a shade guide.
2. Access the carious lesion and establish a clean margin (using hand or rotary instruments) with adequate healthy tooth to bond to.
3. Use a high-speed tapered diamond bur to reduce the incisal edge, proximal sides and buccal surface of the tooth by 1.5 to 2 mm.
4. Choose the appropriately sized crown form. This is done by comparing the shape of the crown form to the tooth. Take into account space loss if teeth have moved.
5. Hold the crown form firmly using a locking instrument to make adjustments.
6. Trim the chosen crown to the appropriate size and shape to fit the tooth. The crown should be adapted to encompass the defects and circumscribing hard tissue to be bonded.
7. Place a pin hole with a diamond bur or a sharp probe at the corner of the incisal angles being restored to allow excess material to extrude and prevent the formation of air bubbles and voids.
8. Try the crown on the tooth following customization and adjust further if necessary.
9. Obtain moisture control using cotton rolls or rubber dam (consider a split-dam technique, if necessary, to avoid losing the orientation of the tooth in the mouth).
10. Etch the tooth structure to be bonded for 15 to 20 seconds, rinse off the acid etch and dry the tooth. Do not dessicate the dentine. Enamel 'frosting' should be visible.
11. Apply bond to the teeth, gently air thin and light cure, all following the manufacturer's instructions.
12. Away from the light, load the prepared crown form with the composite, firmly pressing the composite into the crown and ensuring that there are no voids. Further compact using a composite instrument if necessary. A small amount of composite will extrude from the hole at the incisal angle.

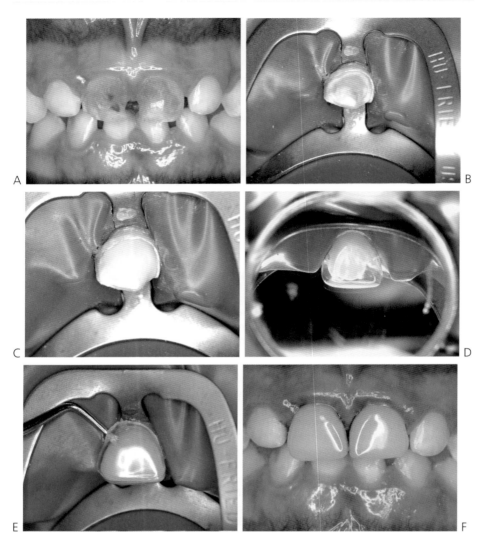

Figure 6.13 Placement of anterior strip crowns on the primary incisors. (A) Caries affecting the upper anterior teeth. (B) Initial reduction of incisal edge and caries removal under the rubber dam (butterfly clamp). Proximal reduction is achieved using a high-speed tapering diamond bur. (C) Placement of a glass ionomer cement base over the dentine. (D) Trial fitting of the cellulose acetate strip crown, which is then filled with composite resin. (E) Removal of the strip crown with a small excavator. (F) Final restoration after polishing. (Courtesy of Dr. E. Alcaino.)

13. Maintain moisture control, and if the child has difficulty cooperating for long periods, preload the crown before etching and bonding the tooth. However, the crown form must be covered to protect it from light. An opaque dappens dish is useful for this.
14. Firmly seat the crown onto the tooth.
15. Gently remove excess composite extruding beyond the crown form margins and incisal angle pinholes.

16. When the form of the tooth and restoration have been established, light cure, using digital pressure palatally. Once cured labially, cure palatally to ensure full setting has occurred.
17. Gently remove the crown form from the tooth using a flat plastic or hand excavator.
18. Assess the restoration for overhangs and with respect to aesthetics.
19. Use articulating paper to assess the occlusion in static and dynamic relations and floss to check the contact points.

INDICATIONS

■ Anterior teeth presenting with extensive carious lesions, or other conditions where there has been a considerable loss of tooth structure.

CONTRAINDICATIONS

■ Signs/symptoms of irreversible pulpitis, periradicular pathology/abscess/sinus.
■ Where there is insufficient patient cooperation.

Zirconia crowns for restoring anterior primary teeth

PROCEDURE (Figure 6.14)

1. Remove dental caries and complete pulp therapy if required.
2. Rebuild core if required to support remaining tooth structure.
3. Create incisal depth cuts to 1 mm as a guide (with tapered crown preparation bur).
4. Reduce incisal edge.
5. Create facial depth cut to 0.5 mm.
6. Carry out proximal reduction to 1.0 mm.
7. Complete level depth cuts and proximal reduction.
8. Reduce cingulum.

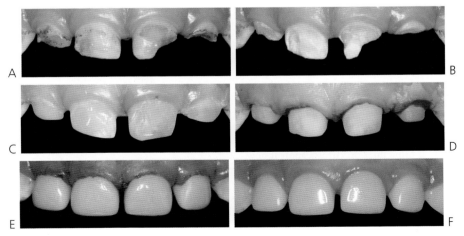

Figure 6.14 Placement of zirconia crowns on anterior teeth. (A) Initial presentation of a child 2 years 2 months old with early childhood caries. (B) Caries removal. (C) Crown build-up with composite resin. (D) Tooth preparation. Note the slightly tapered walls with no undercuts. Invariably, the preparation will extend subgingivally. (E) Placement of the crowns following cementation. (F) 12-month follow-up. Note the gingival adaptation and stability of the restoration. (Courtesy of Dr. Tatyana Peshko, Kiev, Ukraine.)

9. Remove shoulder and extend preparation to the feather edge (with fine-taper bur). It is important not to leave any margin that might impede the placement of the crown.
10. Control gingival haemorrhage.
11. Place try-in crown to assess fit so there is good cervical fit and no rotational or rocking movement and no major interference with the opposing occlusion.
12. Cement crown.

Other methods to manage dentinal lesions

SILVER DIAMINE FLUORIDE

38% Silver diamine fluoride (more correctly spelled silver diammine fluoride or SDF) is used to arrest and remineralize active carious dentinal lesions. It is a clear, odourless, metallic-tasting liquid that will stain most oxidizable surfaces black upon exposure to light, forming silver oxide. Surfaces that will be stained include carious lesions (enamel and dentinal), skin, soft tissues, clinic surfaces and clothes. There is growing evidence of its effectiveness for arresting active dentinal lesions (Seifo et al., 2019). SDF has a complex, multifaceted mechanism of action that involves the fluoride component remineralizing tooth tissue and the silver component damaging the bacteria and making them nonviable. It also forms a precipitate that occludes the dentine tubules. SDF has been in use in Japan for over 40 years and interest in it has grown over the last 5 to 10 years with its use now widespread.

Procedure

Ensure that the parent and child know that the lesion will go dark/black (consider a written consent procedure, particularly before use on anterior teeth).
1. Protect clothing and surfaces and ensure that the child has safety glasses and an apron on. SDF will stain anything it touches.
2. Ensure that the lesion is accessible/cleansable.
3. Apply barrier to the gingiva if the lesion is close and isolate the cheek and tongue. Alternatively, apply petroleum jelly to the patient's gingiva and lips to protect them if necessary and avoid staining.
4. Dry the carious lesion; triple syringe/cotton wool/gauze.
5. Dispense a few drops of SDF into a dish and apply directly onto the tooth surface using a microsponge/brush.
6. Allow it to be absorbed for up to 1 min; apply more if necessary.
7. Remove excess with cotton wool and rinse with water.
8. Dab a spot of toothpaste onto the child's tongue to avoid them tasting any metallic after taste.
9. If using potassium iodide, apply it now using a clean microsponge/brush, one to three times until no more white precipitate is seen to be forming (wait 5–10 seconds between applications)
10. If using fluoride varnish, apply it now.
11. Place gloves and all disposable equipment into a plastic waste bag.
12. Let the patient rinse.
13. Use twice per year and ensure that lesions are arresting and not progressing. If progressing, a different treatment may need to be instigated.

Silver diamine fluoride indications

- Asymptomatic cavitated dentine carious lesions in primary teeth that are, or can be, made cleansable.
- Patients at high risk of developing caries (xerostomia or severe early childhood caries).

- Patients with several carious lesions that may not all be treated in one visit.
- Molar incisor hypomineralization (to reduce sensitivity).
- Precooperative children, and those whose behaviour/medical conditions limit invasive restorative treatment and where there is a need to 'buy time' to avoid or delay treatment with sedation or general anaesthesia.
- Patients with high caries risk with medical or psychological conditions that limit other treatment approaches, for example, patients with dental phobia, medical conditions or disabilities.

Silver diamine fluoride contraindications

- Signs or symptoms of irreversible pulpitis, peri-radicular pathology/abscess/sinus.
- Infection or pain from pulp or food packing (unless the shape of tooth can be changed to become cleansable.
- Ongoing active lesions that are not arresting (only detectable over time).
- Silver allergy.

Silver-Modified Atraumatic Restorative Treatment (SMART) and Silver-Modified Hall Technique (SMART Hall)

Recently, there has been discussion and some case reports published which show clinicians combining SDF use with a restorative approach, using glass ionomer (so-called silver-modified ART, or SMART). This approach involves arresting the carious lesion using SDF and then restoring the form of the tooth with a restorative material to reduce cavitated areas and sheltered niches on the tooth that might harbour biofilm and allow it to reach a cariogenic state again. As Figure 6.15 shows, although the tooth is restored and the lesion is arrested with minimal loss of tooth substance and avoiding the use of local anaesthesia, the aesthetics are compromised.

In a similar way, 'SMART Hall' has been used to arrest the lesion and then follow up with placement of a crown. This is designed to tip the balance of demineralization/remineralization of the tooth with acidic activity in the biofilm away from progression and maximize the chance of arresting the lesion before it can progress toward the dental pulp and cause irreversible damage.

Although, empirically, these would seem to be sensible and indeed have some synergy, there are, as yet, no clinical trials that demonstrate superiority of these approaches over using only one at a time.

Table 6.4 presents a guide to options for managing carious lesions in primary molars.

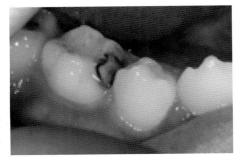

Figure 6.15 A tooth treated with silver diamine fluoride and then glass ionomer cement to remove the cariogenic sheltered environment and aid cleansability by the parent. Note that there is staining around the margins which compromises the aesthetics.

TABLE 6.4 ■ **A guide to choosing restorative and nonrestorative approaches for managing carious lesions in the primary dentition**

Depth of carious lesion	Occlusal	Multisurface/Proximal surface
Limited to enamel	• Active prevention including motivational interviewing and action planning • Topical fluoride • HVGIC fissure sealant	• Active prevention including motivational interviewing and action planning • Topical fluoride • Resin infiltration

Extending no more than the outer one-third to one-half of dentine	• Carious tissue removal[a]
	  - Atraumatic Restorative Treatment
	  - Chemo-mechanical caries removal
	  - Rotary instruments
	  Materials to restore:
	  - HVGIC
	  - Composite resin
	• Nonrestorative cavity control ± SDF
		• Hall Technique
		• Carious tissue removal[a]
		  - Atraumatic Restorative Treatment
		  - Chemo-mechanical caries removal
		  - Rotary instruments
		  Materials to restore:
		  - Composite resin
		  - HVGIC (if no other option available as low survival)
		  - Conventional SSC
		  - Zirconia crown
		• Nonrestorative cavity control ± SDF

Over one-half way through dentine	• Selective carious tissue removal[b]
	  - Atraumatic Restorative Treatment
	  - Chemo-mechanical caries removal
	  - Rotary instruments
	  Materials to restore:
	  - HVGIC
	  - Composite resin
	  - Conventional SSC
	  - Zirconia crown
	• Hall Technique
	• Nonrestorative cavity control ± SDF
		• Hall Technique (±SDF)
		• Selective carious tissue removal[b]
		  - Atraumatic Restorative Treatment
		  - Chemo-mechanical caries removal
		  - Rotary instruments
		  Materials to restore:
		  - Composite resin
		  - HVGIC (if no other option available, low survival)
		  - Conventional SSC
		  - Zirconia crown
		• Nonrestorative cavity control ± SDF

[a]Because the lesion is shallow, it is likely that complete carious tissue removal will be necessary to give adequate depth to the restorative material.
[b]Because the lesion is deeper, selective carious tissue removal can be carried out.
HVGIC, High-viscosity glass ionomer cement; *SDF*, silver diamine fluoride; *SSC*, stainless steel crown, •••.

Nonrestorative cavity control

NRCC is a controversial approach to managing dentinal carious lesions in the primary and permanent dentition. The evidence base for NRCC is not very robust, with some of the reports of its success being related to particular situations and carried out by dentists who support this technique, with different success rates ranging from 50% to 70% to 92% after 2.5 years (Mijan et al., 2014; Santamaria et al., 2017; van Strijp & van Loveren, 2018). The choice to use NRCC really depends on the skill of the dentist, or other dental care professional, in eliciting behaviour change in the parent of the child. It must be clarified that this approach is in no way a "watch and wait" approach but involves very proactive management of the disease in partnership with the child's family.

The technique can be considered to consist of three parts, which must be undertaken together.

- Working with the younger child's parent/carer to improve oral hygiene procedure and habits and to make plaque control more successful.

The patient or parent/carer (in the case of a young child) has to be ready to change behaviours that have led to the development of the disease in the first place. The success of an NRCC approach depends on the clinician's ability to change the individual's behaviour toward taking responsibility. So 'prevention' becomes very much more than simply providing instruction on what to do (knowledge) and how to do it (skills), but has to involve an aspect of refocusing the patient to feeling empowered to make a difference to their own oral health (attitude). Daily removal or disruption of this biofilm by brushing with a fluoridated toothpaste will slow down the carious process or even bring it to a halt.

- Creating a cavity shape where the carious biofilm/dentine is accessible to a toothbrush (lesion exposure). In some cases overhanging enamel has to be removed. To avoid aerosols by using rotary hand instruments, if possible, hand instruments can be used to gain access to the lesion (see ART).
- The application of 38% SDF and/or a 5% NaF varnish therapy to reduce carious activity and promote remineralization. However, it has been shown that even if these are not used, the treatment can still be successful (Mijan et al., 2014). The use of a remineralizing agent, in addition to creating a cleansable cavity, will improve the chance of success of the NRCC approach if the carious lesion is active or there is an increased risk that carious lesion activity will recur. It increases the patient's (or parent/carer's) awareness of their own responsibility and ability to make a difference to their oral health.

In the primary dentition, the goal is to avoid the lesion causing pain and/or infection until the tooth exfoliates. For the permanent dentition, with grossly broken-down teeth, root carious lesions or coronal smooth surface lesions, the main goal is to avoid the lesions leading to pain and/or infection whilst also avoiding the need for restoration.

INDICATIONS

- Individuals who already have a high standard of brushing or are likely to be responsive to measures to change behaviour to carry out frequent, high-quality toothbrushing or other methods to clean carious lesions.
- For those requiring assistance and/or supervision from a parent/carer, the responsible adult must be committed to working with the child to ensure that high-quality home-delivered plaque removal is sustained.
- Precooperative children for whom more invasive caries management strategies are contraindicated.
- Cleansible carious lesions or those that can be made cleansable.

CONTRAINDICATIONS

- Where there is likely to be a lack of compliance with toothbrushing (cavity cleaning).
- Signs/symptoms of irreversible pulpitis, periradicular pathology/abscess/sinus.
- Lesions that a patient cannot clean adequately, for example, subgingival caries lesions.

Management of occlusal caries in permanent teeth

The guidling principles for deciding how much caries to remove is the same as described earlier under the section about managing carious lesions. Carious lesions limited to enamel or where there is doubt that they extend into dentine should be sealed or remineralized. There is no need to remove the carious tooth tissue, and this is considered unnecessarily destructive (Assembly, 2009; Frencken, 2017; Pitts & Zero, 2016; Schwendicke et al., 2019; Urquhart et al., 2019) because the enamel can be repaired through remineralisation. Where the carious lesion has extended into dentine, carious tissue removal should be considered and a restoration should be carried out. For shallow lesions, all of the carious lesion may need to be removed to provide adequate depth of material for good adhesion, and in deeper lesions, it may be possible to carry out stepwise caries removal. The evidence is growing for selective caries removal for permanent teeth. Dental amalgam is no longer considered the most appropriate technique for the restoration of caries lesions in the occlusal surfaces of permanent molars. The need to incorporate mechanical retention into the cavity design can lead to undermining of marginal ridges and weakens the cusps, which will eventually fracture. Teeth restored in this manner often require further, even larger restorations with the risk of pulp disease, root canal treatment and, finally, full coverage restoration. Once placed, the glass ionomer or the resin restoration should have an unfilled resin seal placed over it and over all remaining fissures.

In previous times, clinicians would carry out so-called 'preventive' resin restorations for lesions confined to enamel. However, they are not preventive, and the contemporary treatment for caries limited to enamel should be a sealant or remineralization treatment with fluoride (both of which do prevent tooth destruction from disease and from the bur).

INDICATIONS

- Carious lesions extending into dentine but confined to the occlusal surface.

SUCCESS

Studies have shown good longevity and durability for resin composites in restoring occlusal cavities in permanent teeth and for high-viscosity glass ionomers too (Ahovuo-Saloranta et al., 2017; De Amorim et al., 2018), whether using an ART technique or rotary instruments to remove the carious tissue. They have been found to have equivalent outcomes to occlusal amalgam restorations and can be provided with less removal of sound tooth tissue as a retention form does not need to be created. However, as with all adhesive restorations, a sound hermetic seal must be achieved to avoid marginal leakage. Good technique is therefore essential.

METHOD FOR COMPOSITE OR GLASS IONOMER RESTORATION (SINGLE SURFACE) (Figure 6.16)

1. Use local anaesthesia and rubber-dam isolation if caries extends into dentine.
2. With a small high-speed diamond bur (or hand instruments if using an ART approach), obtain access to the caries.
3. Remove the carious dentine completely if there will not be adequate depth for the restoration without removing it all. If the caries extends beyond half of the dentine on the radiograph, then caries should only be cleared from the margins of the cavity to ensure that a good bond is achieved. Soft caries should be left on the base of the cavity to avoid removing more tooth tissue than necessary and weakening the tooth and to ensure the pulp is not stressed or exposed. At this time, either a temporary restoration, which is left in place for 6 to 9 months and then removed to place a permanent restoration (stepwise caries removal), or a permanent restoration (selective caries removal) can be placed.
4. Any dentinal caries that needs to be removed should be removed using a slow-speed round bur or had excavators to ensure that more is not removed than is essential.
5. Place either the glass ionomer restoration or the composite.

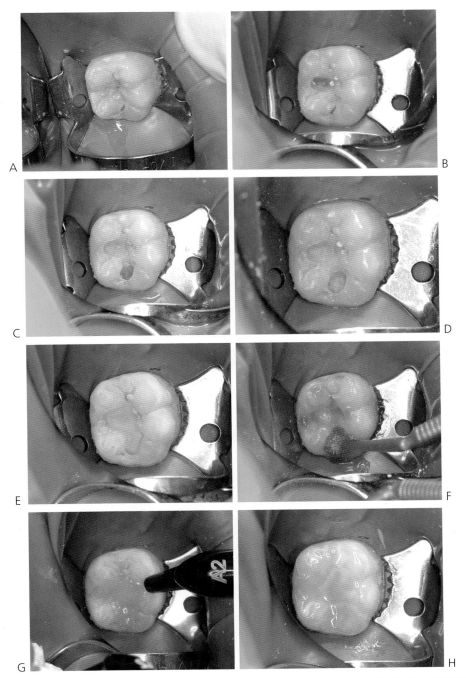

Figure 6.16 Technique for occlusal surface composite restoration in a permanent molar. (A) The true extent of the caries may not be visible without the aid of a radiograph. (B–D) Carious dentine is removed. (E) Placement of a glass ionomer base. (F) Etching. (G) Incremental placement with nano-filled composite resin. (H) Final restoration with sealant placed over surface. Note that the discoloured tissue seen in the lingual fissure in (B) and the distal extension in (C) could be left and sealed under the restoration.

6. Gel etchant is placed for 20 seconds on the enamel margins and occlusal surface and is washed and dried. It is not necessary to etch the liner; sufficient roughening of the surface of the GIC will result from the washing process.
7. Place a thin layer of bonding resin into the cavity and cure for 20 seconds. An excess of resin will produce pooling and reduce the integrity of the bond.
8. Incrementally fill and polymerize the cavity with hybrid composite resin until it is level with the occlusal surface.
9. Flow opaque unfilled fissure sealant over the restoration and the entire occlusal fissure pattern and cure for 20 seconds. There is no need to re-etch the occlusal surface before placing the fissure sealant.
10. Remove the rubber dam and check the occlusion.

Fissure sealants

Fissure sealants are primarily used to create a physical barrier and prevent carious lesion formation by 'filling in' deep pits and fissures. However, the presence of the fissure sealant will also treat existing carious lesions by 'sealing in'. This essentially cuts off the bacteria from their nutrient sources in the oral environment. The lesion stops progressing when bacteria no longer have access to nutrients. This is sometimes known as a microinvasive treatment. This has been shown to be a successful method for managing the lesions even where they are diagnosed to extend just into dentine (Wright et al., 2016). Fissure sealant materials, however, do not have good longevity when placed over more extensive lesions in primary teeth (Borges et al., 2012; Dias et al., 2018) or permanent teeth (Alves et al., 2017; Qvist et al., 2017), and selective caries removal is a better option.

Although resin-based sealants are the most widely used, HVGIC can also be used. These involve fewer clinical stages and do not generate any aerosol (as rinsing is not necessary). There is some evidence that they can be as successful as resin-based sealants. GICs might be suitable, therefore, for fissure sealants for patients with limited cooperation and in partially erupted teeth where moisture control is challenging.

PROCEDURE (GLASS IONOMER CEMENT FISSURE SEALANT) (Figure 6.17)

1. Inspect the tooth when clean and dry under good light and clean the tooth if there is plaque/food in the fissures (using a prophy brush or toothbrush).
2. Isolate the teeth to achieve moisture control. Cotton wool rolls may be used both buccally and lingually/palatally to achieve moisture control during fissure sealant application
3. Place enough GIC onto the occlusal surface to fill the fissure system when spread out. GIC fissure sealants may be placed by extruding GIC directly on to the tooth surface from an applicator or by extruding GIC on to a gloved finger before applying the finger directly to the surface being sealed. If the finger application technique is used, firm pressure should be applied to the surface of the tooth for 2 minutes to ensure coverage of the fissure system and to aid material curing.
4. Place and keep a gloved fingertip firmly placed over the occlusal surface and sealant for 2 minutes, to allow the glass ionomer to set. By applying pressure from a gloved finger, moisture is kept away from the material whilst it sets.
5. Remove the finger and remove any excess, whilst still maintaining moisture control.
6. Place the petroleum jelly over the sealant as a barrier against moisture.
7. Floss the adjacent contact points gently.
8. Check the occlusion with articulating paper and adjust if necessary.
9. Advise the patient not to eat for at least an hour.

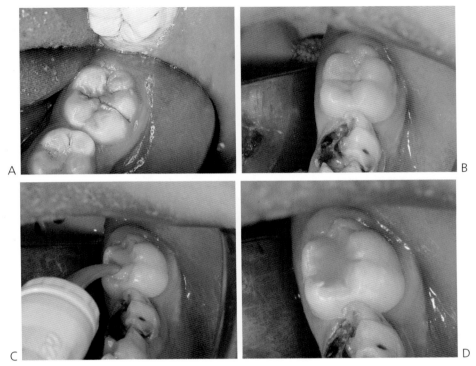

Figure 6.17 Glass ionomer cement fissure sealants. (A) Assess individual's caries risk. Not every molar requires sealing, but it is important to remember that risk can change. These fissures are caries-susceptible fissures, and sealing of the buccal pit in this child is essential. (B–D) Newly erupted first permanent molars can benefit from fissure protection and the placement of a high-fluoride-releasing glass ionomer cement. Note how the material extends into the high-risk areas of the buccal and distal fissures.

PROCEDURE (RESIN FISSURE SEALANT) (Figure 6.18)

1. Inspect the clean, dry tooth under direct vision or indirectly with a mirror, depending on the location of the tooth.
2. If there is debris within the fissure pattern, gently debride with a toothbrush or a blunt instrument such as a ball-ended probe.
3. Isolate the tooth to achieve moisture control and maintain moisture control throughout the procedure.
4. Apply acid etch to the tooth for 15 seconds.
5. Use an aspirator (suction) to remove most of the acid etch from the occlusal surface.
6. Rinse the tooth thoroughly to remove the remaining acid etch.
7. Dry the tooth.
8. Apply the resin sealant (a blunt instrument can be used to drag the material through the fissure system) and light cure.
9. Examine the circumference of the sealant using a sharp examination probe to ensure that the sealant is firmly bonded all around its peripherals and that the margins are smooth. Remove any parts of the sealant that are not adhering and replace.
10. Check the occlusion with articulating paper and adjust if necessary.
11. Floss the adjacent contact points.

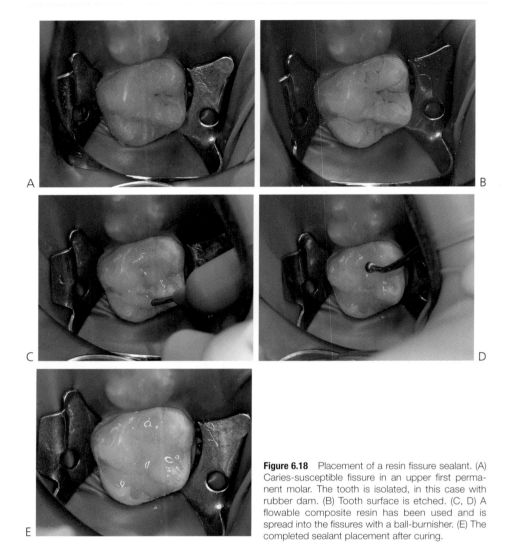

Figure 6.18 Placement of a resin fissure sealant. (A) Caries-susceptible fissure in an upper first permanent molar. The tooth is isolated, in this case with rubber dam. (B) Tooth surface is etched. (C, D) A flowable composite resin has been used and is spread into the fissures with a ball-burnisher. (E) The completed sealant placement after curing.

The sealant must be monitored regularly, at least every 6 months. Its integrity should be carefully checked using a sharp probe around its periphery, and it should be topped up regularly where it is deficient. There is a possibility that if the carious lesion being sealed is quite extensive (this can occur even when there is no large cavitation visible), then a 'trampoline' effect may be seen and the sealant material, being only an unfilled resin, may not be strong enough to withstand the forces from biting etc. This may lead to failure of the sealant, and a restoration will be required.

INDICATIONS

- Noncavitated or microcavitated carious lesions restricted to enamel on the occlusal surface.
- Noncavitated carious lesions even if the lesion can be seen clinically (through shadowing), or radiographically, to extend into the outer half dentine.
- GIC fissure sealants are indicated for patients with limited cooperation.

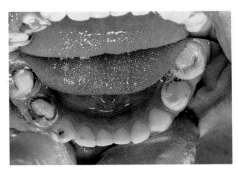

Figure 6.19 Breakdown of glass ionomer cement restorations following conservative (minimal intervention) dentistry. Note, however, that there has been a substantial slowing of the caries rate such that all the lesions are inactive and the teeth have been preserved in the mouth. Although it is easy to criticize the quality of these restorations, these had been placed in a young child who found it difficult to cope with more invasive treatment and where there was no access to general anaesthesia or other forms of sedation. Some arch length has been lost; however, because the crowns have not been restored to their natural contour, the majority of the space occupied by the teeth has been preserved. The question should be asked whether these restorations have 'successfully' retained the teeth. Is this treatment better than having no treatment or having all these primary teeth extracted and the child having to undergo the negative experience of a general anaesthetic?

CONTRAINDICATIONS

- Where there is a significant breach in the surface integrity of the tooth or there is frank cavitation.
- Lesions that have extended extensively into dentine, undermining the enamel (and therefore weakening the tooth structure).

SUCCESS OR FAILURE

The aim of minimal intervention approaches to dentistry is to allow the child to reach the stage where they are old enough and have the cognitive ability and confidence to cope with dental treatment without having to resort to chemical methods of management. Sometimes this means compromising on the intermediate stages in terms of the aesthetics. Figure 6.19 shows such a case which may not look like a traditional successfully restored dentition but where the long-term outcome meant the child had only positive dental experiences and could accept more invasive treatment as necessary. The ultimate goal, of course is a child who has a positive view of their oral health and the ability to care for their dentition.

Proximal sealants

There is evidence to support the use of proximal sealants to stop the progression of proximal carious lesions that are limited to enamel (Dorri et al., 2015). These can be difficult to place, even when an orthodontic separator or other method is used to create space.

One type of proximal sealant which is being more widely used is very-low-viscosity resin infiltration. This technique relies on the diffusion of resin into hydrochloric acid–created micro-porosities. The micro-porosities are then dehydrated by using ethanol, after which the resin is allowed to be 'sucked' into the dehydrated areas in the enamel and block them. There are kits available that allow targeted placement of the materials. For resin infiltration, lesions should be limited to enamel or extend no further than the outer third of dentine and must be noncavitated (Liang et al., 2018). Resin infiltration can also be used to camouflage the whitish appearance of decalcified and hypomineralized enamel on smooth surfaces (Borges et al., 2017; Höchli et al., 2017).

Behavioural change and motivational interviewing

There is considerable evidence that behaviour can be effectively modified through behaviour change interventions. However, evidence for the sustainability of behaviour change is limited (Kwasnicka et al., 2016). As healthcare professionals, empowering patients to adopt and maintain positive health behaviour changes must be our primary focus. In dentistry, patients practicing regular, high-quality oral hygiene routines combined with diets of low cariogenic potential will minimize caries risk and promote disease stabilization. Although behaviour change can be challenging, it is an integral part of our management of caries and must not be overlooked.

So, how can we aim to achieve this with our patients?

MOTIVATIONAL INTERVIEWING

Lack of motivation is a significant contributor to health behaviour change seldom being sustained. Motivational interviewing is a counselling process through which a patient is empowered to identify personal barriers preventing adoption and maintenance of particular health behaviour(s) with guidance from a healthcare professional. The patient is encouraged to consider their own reasons for change in an environment that is supportive and free from judgement. The goal is to work constructively around barriers to coproduce an individualized strategy for success (Copeland et al., 2015).

Summary

This chapter has focussed on a minimally invasive approach to restorative management of the carious dentition in the child. It has emphasized the partnership between treatment and prevention as restorative treatment alone does not address the problem that caused the disease of dental caries in the first place.

Further reading

Ahovuo-Saloranta, A., Forss, H., Walsh, T., et al., 2017. Pit and fissure sealants for preventing dental decay in permanent teeth. Cochrane Database of Systematic Reviews (7).

Alkilzy, M., Tarabaih, A., Santamaria, M., et al., 2018. Self-assembling peptide P11-4 and fluoride for regenerating enamel. Journal of Dental Research 97, 148–154.

Alves, L.S., Giongo, F.C., Mua, B., et al., 2017. A randomized clinical trial on the sealing of occlusal carious lesions: 3–4-year results. Brazilian Oral Research, 31.

Araujo, M.P., Innes, N.P., Bonifacio, C.C., et al., 2020. Atraumatic restorative treatment compared to the Hall technique for occluso-proximal carious lesions in primary molars; 36-month follow-up of a randomised control trial in a school setting. BMC Oral Health 20, 318.

Assembly, F.G., 2009. FDI policy statement: minimal intervention in the management of dental caries. Journal of Minimum Intervention in Dentistry 2, 101–102.

Badar, S.B., Tabassum, S., Khan, F.R., et al., 2019. Effectiveness of Hall technique for primary carious molars: a systematic review and meta-analysis. International Journal of Clinical Pediatric Dentistry 12, 445.

Bijle, M.N.A., Yiu, C.K.Y., Ekambaram, M., 2018. Calcium-based caries preventive agents: a meta-evaluation of systematic reviews and meta-analysis. Journal of Evidence Based Dental Practice 18, 203–217.

Borges, A., Caneppele, T.M.F., Masterson, D., et al., 2017. Is resin infiltration an effective esthetic treatment for enamel development defects and white spot lesions? A systematic review. Journal of Dentistry 56, 11–18.

Borges, B.C., de Souza Bezerra., Dantas, R.F., et al., 2012. Efficacy of a non-drilling approach to manage non-cavitated dentin occlusal caries in primary molars: a 12-month randomized controlled clinical trial. International Journal of Paediatric Dentistry 22, 44–51.

Copeland, L., McNamara, R., Kelson, M., et al., 2015. Mechanisms of change within motivational interviewing in relation to health behaviors outcomes: a systematic review. Patient Education and Counseling 98, 401–411.

Dias, K.R., de Andrade, C.B., Wait, T.T., et al., 2018. Efficacy of sealing occlusal caries with a flowable composite in primary molars: a 2-year randomized controlled clinical trial. Journal of Dentistry 74, 49–55.

Dorri, M., Dunne, S.M., Walsh, T., et al., 2015. Micro-invasive interventions for managing proximal dental decay in primary and permanent teeth. Cochrane Database of Systematic Reviews (11).

Dorri, M., Martines-Zapata, M.J., Walsh, T., et al., 2017. Atraumatic restorative treatment versus conventional restorative treatment for managing dental caries. Cochrane Database of Systematic Reviews (12).

FDI, 2013. Minimata Convention on Mercury, fdiworlddental.org. Available: https://www.fdiworlddental.org/what-we-do/advocacy/dental-amalgam/minamata-convention-on-mercury.

Frencken, J., 2017. Atraumatic restorative treatment and minimal intervention dentistry. British Dental Journal 223, 183.

Hamama, H., Yiu, C., Burrow, M., 2014. Current update of chemomechanical caries removal methods. Australian Dental Journal 59, 446–456.

Höchli, D., Hersberger-Zurfluh, M., Papageorgiou, S.N., et al., 2017. Interventions for orthodontically induced white spot lesions: a systematic review and meta-analysis. European Journal of Orthodontics 39, 122–133.

Innes, N.P., Evans, D.J.P., Bonifacio, C.C., et al., 2017. The Hall technique 10 years on: questions and answers. British Dental Journal 222, 478–483.

Jiang, M., Fan, Y., Li, K.Y., et al., 2020. Factors affecting success rate of atraumatic restorative treatment (ART) restorations in children: a systematic review and meta-analysis. Journal of Dentistry 104, 103526.

Kwasnicka, D., Dombrowski, S.U., White, M., et al., 2016. Theoretical explanations for maintenance of behaviour change: a systematic review of behaviour theories. Health Psychology Review 10, 277–296.

Liang, Y., Deng, Z., Dai, X., et al., 2018. Micro-invasive interventions for managing non-cavitated proximal caries of different depths: a systematic review and meta-analysis. Clinical Oral Investigations 22, 2675–2684.

Mijan, M., de Amorim, R.G., Leal, S.C., et al., 2014. The 3.5-year survival rates of primary molars treated according to three treatment protocols: a controlled clinical trial. Clinical Oral Investigations 18, 1061–1069.

Pitts, N., Zero, D., 2016. White paper on dental caries prevention and management. a summary of the current evidence and the key issues in controlling this preventable disease. FDI World Dental Federation, Geneva, Switzerland.

Qvist, V., Borum, M., Moller, K.D., et al., 2017. Sealing occlusal dentin caries in permanent molars: 7-year results of a randomized controlled trial. JDR Clinical & Translational Research 2, 73–86.

Santamaria, R.M., Innes, N.P., Machiulskiene, V., et al., 2017. Alternative caries management options for primary molars: 2.5-year outcomes of a randomised clinical trial. Caries Research 51, 605–614.

Schwendicke, F., Splieth, C., Breschi, L., et al., 2019. When to intervene in the caries process? An expert Delphi consensus statement. Clinical Oral Investigations 23, 3691–3703.

Seifo, N., Cassie, H., Radford, J.R., et al., 2019. Silver diamine fluoride for managing carious lesions: an umbrella review. BMC Oral Health 19, 145.

Urquhart, O., Tampi, M.P., Pilcher, L., et al., 2019. Nonrestorative treatments for caries: systematic review and network meta-analysis. Journal of Dental Research 98, 14–26.

van Strijp, G., van Loveren, C., 2018. No removal and inactivation of carious tissue: non-restorative cavity control. In: Caries excavation: evolution of treating cavitated carious lesions. Editors: F Schwendicke, J Frencken, N Innes. Karger Publishers, Basel, pp. 124–136.

Walsh, T., Worthington, H.V., Glenny, A.M., et al., 2019. Fluoride toothpastes of different concentrations for preventing dental caries. Cochrane Database of Systematic Reviews (3).

Wright, J.T., Tampi, M.P., Graham, L., et al., 2016. Sealants for preventing and arresting pit-and-fissure occlusal caries in primary and permanent molars. Pediatric Dentistry 38, 282–308.

CHAPTER 7

Pulp therapy for primary and immature permanent teeth

Erin Mahoney ■ Angus C. Cameron

CHAPTER OUTLINE

Introduction

Dental caries, trauma and the iatrogenic effects of conservative dental treatment all provoke a biological response in the pulpo-dentinal complex. This chapter is concerned with the cascade of therapeutic interventions used to promote an adaptive biological response in the pulpo-dentinal complex of the treated tooth and optimize subsequent growth and development. These therapeutic efforts are directed towards the retention of carious or traumatized teeth to maintain normal function by either resolving the pathology or maintaining the tooth free from clinical symptoms until it exfoliates.

Role of primary teeth

Premature loss of a primary tooth through trauma or infection has the potential to destabilize the developing occlusion with potential space loss, arch collapse and premature, delayed or ectopic eruption of the permanent successor teeth.

Effective pulpal therapy in the primary dentition must not only stabilize the affected primary tooth but also create a favourable environment for normal exfoliation of the primary tooth, without harm to the developing enamel or interference with the normal eruption of its permanent successor. Where these outcomes cannot reasonably be achieved over the clinical life of the primary tooth, it is appropriate to extract the affected tooth and consider alternative strategies for occlusal guidance and maintenance of arch integrity. Space maintenance will be considered in Chapter 8.

Evidence for current practice

The single biggest issue surrounding pulp therapy in the primary dentition is the lack of correlation between clinical symptoms and pulpal status. Hence, dependent on the different combinations of symptoms and clinical findings, there is a range of different pulp treatment protocols.

In general, it is appropriate to use the least invasive intervention that is predictably associated with a healthy, adaptive healing response in the affected primary or permanent tooth. Obviously, effective primary prevention and early intervention will obviate the need for many of the procedures and techniques described later in this chapter.

ANATOMICAL AND MORPHOLOGICAL CONSIDERATIONS IN PRIMARY TEETH

When considering the management of carious primary teeth, the status of the pulp and the restoration are linked inexorably. Primary teeth have significant morphologic differences that make their caries susceptibility and subsequent risk of pulpal pathology much greater when compared with permanent teeth. Importantly, the primary molars have:

- Less mineralization of the enamel than permanent teeth;
- A neonatal line that is less mineralized and makes up approximately 5% of the thickness of the enamel on the distal approximal surface;
- Pulp chambers that are proportionally much larger and closer to the dentino-enamel junction;
- Broad contact points interproximal with the adjacent primary molars;
- A floor of the pulp chamber that is porous, leading to inter-radicular rather than periapical pathology;
- The first primary molar has less than 0.5 mm of enamel on the distal approximal surface.

Clinical assessment and general considerations

Often, in the precooperative young patient, useful radiographs may be difficult to obtain, but through a careful history and clinical examination, the clinician will be able to determine the pulp status of the affected tooth.

TABLE 7.1 ■ Assessment of pulpal status

	Reversible pulpitis	Irreversible pulpitis
Pain	Stimulated pain Well controlled by analgesics	Spontaneous May not be controlled by analgesics
Swelling	None	Buccal/labial abscess Extraoral cellulitis
Mobility	Normal	Increased
Colour change in crown	No discolouration	Darkening of crown
Clinical caries	Marginal ridge intact	Destruction of marginal ridge consider possibility of irreversible changes
Radiographic caries	Less than 2/3 through dentine	Caries extends into pulp chamber
Radiographic pathology	No periapical of intraradicular changes	Periapical of intra-radicular rarefaction or loss

The important factor is to determine the pulp status and whether the pulp is reversible or irreversibly affected (Table 7.1). Unfortunately, there are at present no objective or definitive tests to determine the health of the pulpo-dentinal complex in the primary or immature permanent tooth and clinical signs and symptoms are poorly correlated with actual pulp histology.

Reversible inflammation should be managed conservatively:

■ Preventive therapies (including the Hall Crown technique, see Chapter 6)
■ Pulp capping
■ Pulpotomy

Irreversible inflammation can only be managed by extraction or pulpectomy.

IRREVERSIBLE PULPITIS: ACUTE VERSUS CHRONIC PULPAL PATHOLOGY

Clinical signs and symptoms to help determine pulp status include the following:

■ Acute pain

Discrimination between acute and chronic pain in young children is difficult. Infants and young patients frequently have difficulty communicating their experience of pain. It is often not until their pain is severe and prolonged that parents will become aware of this and seek treatment for their child. Symptoms of severe, prolonged, spontaneous or nocturnal pain suggest irreversible pulpitis or a dental abscess (i.e., a localized collection of pus resulting from a bacterial infection in the pulp chambers) (Figure 7.1B). A history of repeated need for analgesics is also suggestive of pulp necrosis. These episodes present often, immediately before pulp necrosis. Pain is caused by an increase in pressure within the pulp chamber and canals extending into the periapical or intraradicular bone.

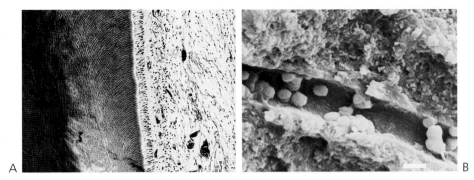

Figure 7.1 (A) Healthy pulp. The aim is preservation of tissue. (B) Ingress of oral streptococci into dentine tubules. (Courtesy of the Institute of Dental Research, SEM Unit WESTMEAD.)

- Chronic pain

  Most dental pain in children is episodic and represents acute exacerbation of chronic infection. The exact aetiology of 'tooth pain' is difficult to determine. Much of the discomfort from proximal dental caries in primary molars is a result of food impaction into the gingival tissues and not from any pathology within the pulp.

  Once an acute inflammatory process (dental abscess) has achieved drainage, by way of a sinus or spread into the superficial tissues, then pain subsides. However, the underlying pathology persists and must be resolved, despite the lack of obvious discomfort.

- Mobility

  Abnormal tooth mobility is associated with loss of bone from infection or imminent exfoliation. The acutely infected primary tooth is not excessively mobile as bone loss takes a number of days to occur; however, it may be exquisitely tender to percussion or apical pressure.

- Swellings

  Alveolar swellings, particularly involving the vestibular reflection and facial swellings, are indicators of pulp necrosis and abscess formation or spreading bacterial infection through tissue planes (cellulitis) (see Figure 7.1B).

Periapical or intraradicular abscess. An abscess is a collection of pus in a cavity. Children rarely present with large collections of pus in the face as adults do. However, they can develop large buccal abscesses that will drain spontaneously if no other treatment is provided. Pus will 'point' to the most dependent area, which fortunately is usually towards the buccal or labial sulcus.

Facial cellulitis, including spread of infection into the tissue planes that may involve the airway (see Chapter 10). This can be life threatening.

Anecdotally, a child with only a small number of carious teeth can present with a large facial cellulitis requiring inpatient, emergency treatment, whereas children who have multiple, extensively carious primary teeth only present with multiple intraoral sinuses (gum boils). These latter children may not even complain of pain. Typically, once 'drainage' has been established (i.e., with the formation of an intraoral sinus), the infection remains chronic. Rarely do these children develop a subsequent acute presentation with a significant extraoral swelling (an acute exacerbation of a chronic infection). Acute infections tend to develop first and then (often with the administration of antibiotics) become an ongoing chronic inflammation.

This may not be the case for those children who are immunosuppressed.

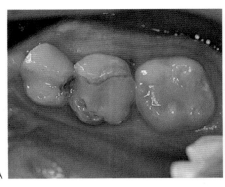
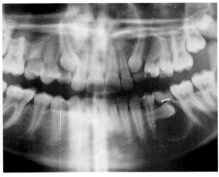

A   B

Figure 7.2 (A) Large multisurface glass ionomer restorations are inadequate to properly restore primary molars. Persistent coronal microleakage leads to pulp necrosis. (B) Panoramic radiograph showing the results of coronal microleakage and the formation of a large inflammatory follicular cyst associated with the second premolar.

OTHER SIGNS AND SYMPTOMS OF CHRONIC INFECTION AND IRREVERSIBLE PULPITIS

- Persistent infection with draining sinuses.
- Inflammatory follicular cyst (see Chapter 10).
- Failure of exfoliation of primary teeth.
- Apical fenestration.
- Ectopic permanent teeth (Figure 7.2).
- Coronal darkening.
- Significant loss of the marginal ridge in a first primary tooth is suggestive of carious pulpal inflammation in interproximal caries (Figure 7.3A).
- Loss of the occlusal triangular ridges or carious undermining of the cusps in occlusal caries in second primary molars also suggests carious pulpal involvement (Figure 7.3B).

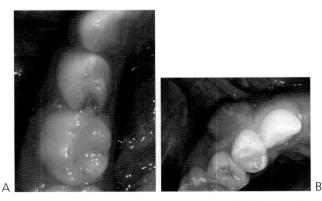

A   B

Figure 7.3 (A) Much of the pain that children experience may be caused by food impacting into a cavity. Even without radiographs, it is important to recognize that the pulp will always be involved when the carious lesion is of this size. (B) Buccal swelling indicates not only pulpal necrosis and pus formation but also the loss of bone and perforation of the cortical plate. It may also be difficult to initially determine which tooth is responsible for the swelling; in this case, both teeth should be removed.

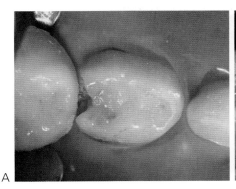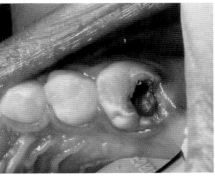

A   B

Figure 7.4 (A) Loss of marginal ridge of the first primary molar or (B) undermined triangular ridge or cusp suggests carious pulpal involvement.

- The external appearance of the carious lesion can in some cases be misleading (Figure 7.4). Persistent symptoms occurring soon after placement of a restoration usually indicate irreversible pulpal pathology.

CLINICAL INVESTIGATIONS TO DETERMINE PULP STATUS

- Pulp sensibility tests

  Standard techniques of pulp sensibility testing are of limited value in assessing the vitality of a primary tooth. These techniques rely on patient feedback in response to thermal or electrical stimulation. In the primary dentition, it is likely that children will not have achieved the cognitive development necessary to respond reliably to a potentially painful stimulus and response challenge. In the healthy immature permanent tooth, raised response thresholds to electrical stimuli are observed. These decrease with root maturation and apical closure.

- Radiographs

  A series of longitudinal radiographs showing normal dentine deposition within the pulp chamber and the roots suggests pulpal health. Irregular pulp calcification or pulpal obliteration suggests pulpal dystrophy, whereas failure of physiological pulp regression or arrested root development suggests pulpal necrosis. In a single radiographic examination, primary and young permanent individual teeth can be compared with their antimere to identify asymmetry.

  Clinical signs or symptoms that suggest carious involvement of the pulp warrant radiographic investigation. Radiographs will usually underestimate the extent of the carious lesion. However, they will show:

  - The presence of caries and an estimate of the extent of the lesion;
  - The position and proximity of pulp horns;
  - The presence and position of the permanent successor;
  - The status of the roots and their surrounding bone;
  - Periapical or intraradicular lesions (rarefactions).

  Radiographic examination should be considered essential before undertaking pulp therapy procedures. The presence of caries in the furcation, internal or external root resorption, including physiological root resorption, and periapical or furcation (radiolucencies) bone lesions are all contraindications to pulp treatment in the primary dentition. Primary teeth with these radiographic signs should be extracted.

  In young permanent teeth, radiographic examination is also essential for assessment of the stage of root development that might determine the appropriateness of retaining extensively carious teeth (see later).

Treatment planning and aspects regarding the decision to retain and restore or extract primary teeth

MEDICAL CONSIDERATIONS

A thorough medical assessment is essential before the commencement of any dental treatment, especially when contemplating pulp therapy. Medical issues may limit or change treatment options, as pulp therapy relies on the adaptive healing response after treatment, so patients with a significantly compromised immune system are considered poor candidates for pulp therapy.

Contraindications

- Immunosuppressed patients and those with poor healing potential (see Immunodeficiency, Chapter 12) should be treated more aggressively (e.g., extractions rather than pulp therapy).
- Congenital cardiac disease (see Appendix E). Guidelines for the management of children with congenital cardiac disease have changed significantly over recent years, with most children with cardiac anomalies not requiring antibiotics for standard paediatric dental treatment. Notwithstanding this, patients who are considered to be at risk of bacterial endocarditis should be free of oral infection, and any primary tooth with clinical signs of infection should be extracted. However, there is no evidence to suggest that a primary tooth with a large restoration is more or less likely to become infected if it has undergone pulp therapy according to established guidelines. Readers are advised to access the current guidelines in their country and, if in doubt, to liaise with the child's cardiologist.
- Other medical conditions: Generally, children with well-managed diabetes present no particular problem in relation to healing potential. The use of long-term corticosteroids for the management of asthma should not affect the decision to retain primary teeth.

Indications

- Bleeding disorders and coagulopathies (see Chapter 12). Current management protocols for patients with a bleeding diathesis (such as haemophilia) may use regular, often home-based, factor replacement. Where patients have access to such medical treatment, the decision to extract or retain a pulpally involved primary tooth should not be determined by the bleeding diathesis, but should be based on the same criteria used for any other patient. Consultation with the child's haematologist is essential.

BEHAVIOURAL CONSIDERATIONS

- Is the child manageable in the chair or is there a need for sedation or general anaesthesia?
- Effective pulp therapy requires a high level of patient compliance and the ability of the clinician to appropriately manage the child's behaviour. If a child is unable to cooperate with pretreatment diagnostic procedures such as radiographs, they are unlikely to cope with complex pulp therapy and associated restorative procedures.

Pulp therapy also requires effective pain control. Even with usually effective doses of local anaesthetic, a child may experience breakthrough pain. This is particularly seen on entry to the pulp chamber. The sedative effects of inhalation sedation (nitrous oxide) used in conjunction with local analgesia can facilitate patient comfort and compliance. The use of the rubber dam to isolate the tooth undergoing treatment and to protect the patient from instruments and medicaments is important.

- What management options are available in the event of failure of the pulp therapy? No clinical technique is without risk of failure, and although published studies report success up to 90% for pulpotomies and indirect pulp capping, these rely heavily on expert assessment and strict inclusion criteria. Considering behaviour management difficulties and our inability to accurately diagnose the true state of the pulp, it is unsurprising that day-to-day success is much lower.
- Most specialists would consider management under general anaesthesia to be more pragmatic and would elect to extract questionable teeth rather than risk complex endodontic and restorative procedures whose failure might necessitate another anaesthetic.
- Alternatively, a child might tolerate pulp therapy in the chair but not an extraction, which will lead to failure of a pulpotomy that might subsequently require a pulpectomy.

DENTAL CONSIDERATIONS

- Hypodontia (i.e., ectodermal dysplasia, Figure 7.5A; see also Chapter 11). In cases of congenital absence of teeth, the decision to extract or retain individual teeth will be influenced by the overall orthodontic strategy. In some cases, there is a requirement to extract primary teeth early to encourage occlusal drift and space closure. In these cases, timing of extractions can be critical and possibly necessitating an interim restoration with or without pulp therapy of the affected primary tooth. In other cases, it is necessary to maintain a primary tooth without a successor for many years.
- Tooth must be able to be restored after pulp therapy with a restoration, which provides an excellent seal from the oral cavity. The restoration of the tooth must be planned together with the pulp therapy. Long-term success in pulp therapy requires an effective coronal seal to prevent microleakage and the ingress of oral bacteria to the root canals. If the carious tooth is not restorable, it should be extracted. Pulpotomy and pulpectomy procedures require significant access cavity preparations, which have the potential to weaken the axial walls of the treated tooth. In general, full coverage restoration with a preformed metal or zirconia crown is performed. The lack of coronal seal will inevitably lead to pulpal pathology.

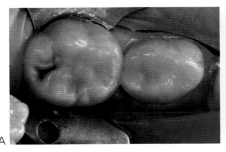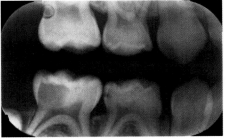

A   B

Figure 7.5 (A) Caries may be much more extensive than clinically visible. (B) The full extent of caries is only radiographically evident and shows pulpal involvement.

OTHER CONSIDERATIONS

Antibiotic usage to control acute infection (see Odontogenic infection, Chapter 10) may temporarily resolve some or all of these clinical signs mentioned earlier, but they will not resolve the underlying pathology. A primary tooth that cannot be saved requires extraction despite potential future orthodontic complications.

Chronic infection in the primary dentition can cause disturbances to enamel formation in the permanent dentition (Turner tooth, see Chapter 11) and malocclusion (Figure 7.2B) even in the absence of clinical symptoms or pain.

Pulp capping

INDIRECT PULP CAPPING

The basis of indirect pulp capping is to seal off the advancing carious lesion from the oral environment and promote pulpal healing with the formation of reactionary (secondary) dentine. Both primary and permanent teeth have the ability to 'heal'. Indirect pulp capping can occur in the Hall Crown technique.

It is uncertain whether the carious lesion in dentine will become sterile and remineralize, or if it merely becomes quiescent with the potential to reactivate if there is leakage around the final restoration; hence, there has previously been debate over the necessity of re-entering the tooth to remove the residual caries once there is clinical and radiographic evidence of pulpal healing. Regardless, because of the known service life of the primary tooth, there is no indication for re-entering the primary tooth to remove residual caries when the clinical response is favourable.

Silver diamine fluoride has been proposed as an adjunctive antimicrobial agent in conjunction with indirect pulp capping. At present, there is a lack of evidence to support its use.

Large carious lesions and associated cavity preparations alter the mechanical properties of the treated tooth, reducing the rigidity of the cavity walls in normal function, increasing the potential risk of microleakage. As indirect pulp capping relies on sealing off the residual caries from the oral environment, the residual tooth structure should be carefully evaluated, areas of unsupported enamel should be removed and weakened cavity walls, which are likely to flex in function (increasing microleakage), should be protected with full coverage restorations. This is of particular importance with approximal lesions where the buccal and lingual walls can be extensively undermined.

Indications

- Large carious lesion.
- Asymptomatic tooth or mild transient symptoms.
- Preoperative radiograph confirms the absence of radicular pathology.

TECHNIQUE

- Pain control and isolation.
- Remove superficial caries.
- Remove all peripheral caries, leaving the deep caries over pulp.
- Finalize cavity preparation.
- Restore tooth ensuring adequate coronal seal.
- Appropriate follow-up.

It is important to remember that there may be a fine balance between what is reversible and irreversible pulpitis. This can change with cavity preparation, and the use of rotary instruments, continual irrigation and desiccation of the dentine may shift this balance.

DIRECT PULP CAPPING

Primary teeth

Small pulp exposures can be broadly classified as mechanical (iatrogenic) or carious. However, the size of the pulp exposure in a primary molar does not affect prognosis.

Direct pulp capping of carious pulp exposures in primary teeth has a poor prognosis, with failure occurring as a result of internal root resorption. A pulpotomy, pulpectomy or extraction should be undertaken in such cases.

Immature permanent teeth

Direct pulp capping of pinpoint pulp exposures, either mechanical or carious, has a favourable prognosis in the immature permanent tooth. The use of calcium hydroxide, hard-setting calcium hydroxide cements and mineral trioxide aggregate (MTA) has been widely reported; however, there is limited evidence to support the use of other materials. The use of MTA in anterior permanent teeth is discussed in Chapter 9.

Pulpotomy in primary teeth

Pulpotomy is the most widely used pulp therapy in the primary dentition. The suffix *otomy* means 'to cut', so pulpotomy is 'to cut the pulp'. The aim of pulpotomy in the primary tooth is to amputate the inflamed coronal pulp and preserve the vitality of the radicular pulp, thereby facilitating the normal exfoliation of the primary tooth. A pulpotomy cannot be performed if the pulp is necrotic.

The contemporary pulpotomy traces its origins to nineteenth-century techniques for the mummification of painful, inflamed or putrescent pulpal tissue. Over the twentieth century, the pulpotomy technique changed with fewer stages and reduced duration of application and concentration of medicaments. Emphasis is now placed on the preservation of healthy radicular pulp rather than mummification.

GENERAL TECHNICAL CONSIDERATIONS

Caries removal

- The treated tooth must be rendered caries-free before proceeding with the pulpotomy.
  The recommendation to remove caries from the periphery to the pulp not only prevents contamination of the pulpotomy site with carious debris but also reduces the risk of inadvertent pulp exposure. Access to the coronal pulp requires complete removal of the roof of the pulp chamber. Amputation of the coronal pulp requires a clean cut at the level of the pulpal floor. Residual tissue tags at the amputation site will create problems with haemostasis. High-speed rotary instrumentation with copious water spray irrigation creates the optimal cut.
- If the floor of the pulp chamber is perforated, the tooth should be extracted.

Haemostasis

Haemostasis at the pulpotomy site must be obtained before application of the therapeutic agent. This is achieved with continuous irrigation and gentle dabbing with cotton wool pellets and should occur within 5 minutes. If bleeding cannot be arrested, the pulpal inflammation is considered to have spread to involve the root canal and is associated with a poor prognosis. This is referred to as the 'bleeding sign' or a 'hyperaemic pulp'. Pulpectomy or extraction should be considered in these cases.

Pulp medicaments

A therapeutic medicament can be applied to the pulpotomy site once haemostasis has been obtained. The pulpotomy site is then covered with a therapeutic base (see later). Traditionally, this has been a zinc oxide–eugenol-based cement. However, eugenol in direct contact with pulp tissue causes chronic pulpitis. It is reasonable to substitute eugenol-free cement as the therapeutic base. When MTA is used as the therapeutic medicament, it will also act as the therapeutic base. Finally, a core material should be used to seal the tooth before the final restoration.

Final tooth restoration

Earlier texts have suggested that teeth that require a preformed metal crown should also have a routine elective pulpotomy, regardless of whether they have a carious pulp exposure. This position is no longer tenable given the predictable success of indirect pulp capping. However, the reverse is true, in that all teeth that have had a pulpotomy should be restored with a preformed metal crown. With the advent of the zirconia crown, the amount of tooth preparation required, especially for first primary molars, may result in a pulp exposure, necessitating a pulpotomy. The concept of full coverage also applies to anterior teeth, where a full coverage restoration should also be used in those incisors in which a pulpotomy has been performed.

Indications

- A tooth with reversible pulpitis.
- Tooth asymptomatic or mild transient pain.
- Carious pulp exposure.
- Preoperative radiograph confirms the absence of radicular pathology and physiological resorption less than one third of the root.
- Restorable tooth.

TECHNIQUE (Figures 7.6 and 7.7)

1. Pain control and rubber-dam isolation.
2. Complete removal of caries from peripheral to pulpal.
3. Removal of roof of pulp chamber.

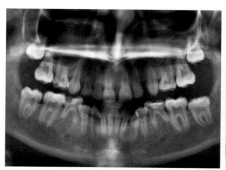
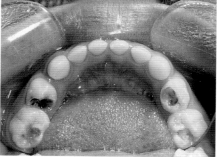

A   B

Figure 7.6 (A) Panoramic radiograph of a child with congenital absence of six premolars. Whereas three of the second primary molars are carious, it is important to retain these teeth. (B) It is important to consider the implications of space management when deciding on the most appropriate options in managing a cariously exposed primary molar. In this case, tooth 74 is pulpally involved, but restoration with a stainless steel crown has been made more difficult because of mesial migration of the second primary molar into the distal carious lesion.

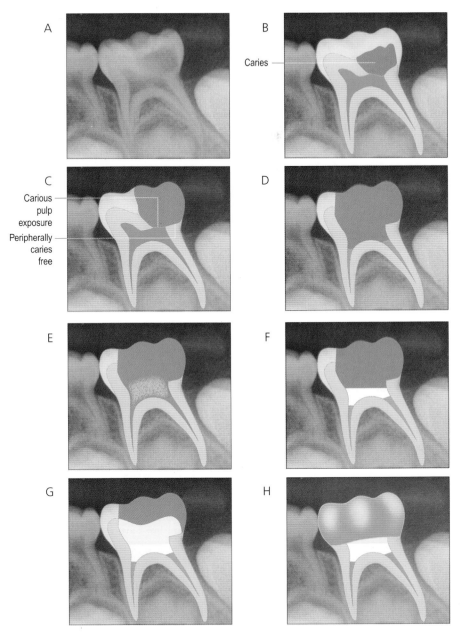

Figure 7.7 Method of performing a pulpotomy. (A) Preoperative radiograph shows deep carious lesion. Clinical history revealed intermittent symptoms on eating with no history of spontaneous pain. (B) Carious lesion identified relative to dental anatomy. (C) Cavity preparation showing complete removal of peripheral caries. (D) After the tooth is rendered free of caries, the roof of the pulp chamber is removed completely, and the pulp is amputated to the level of the pulpal floor. Haemostasis must be achieved at this point before proceeding. (E) The therapeutic agent is applied to the pulpotomy site. (F) Base is applied to completely seal the pulpotomy site. (G) The tooth is built up with a core material. (H) The tooth is restored with a preformed metal crown.

4. Amputation of coronal pulp.
5. Arrest of bleeding at amputation site (see discussion of 'bleeding sign' earlier).
6. Application of therapeutic agent (see Therapeutic agents used for pulpotomy in primary teeth).
7. Place base directly onto pulp amputation site.
8. Placement of a core, if required.
9. Restoration of the tooth with a preformed metal crown (molars) or a composite resin strip crown for anterior teeth or zirconia crown. Composite resin may be used if sufficient tooth substance remains to achieve a broad adhesive seal.
10. Appropriate follow-up.

Therapeutic agents used for pulpotomy in primary teeth

A diverse range of chemicals have been used as pulpotomy agents. As most of these have not been subject to rigorous clinical trials, their use has been based on expert opinion and retrospective studies. In their review for the Cochrane Collaboration, Smail-Faugeron and colleagues (2018) concluded that, based on the available randomized controlled trials:

- Pulp treatment for extensively decayed primary teeth is generally successful.
- The evidence suggests MTA may be the most efficacious medication to heal the root pulp after pulpotomy.
- Any future trials to determine the ideal pulpotomy material would require a very large sample size and a minimum of 1 year.

The available evidence suggests that formocresol, ferric sulphate, electrocautery and MTA have similar efficacy. Calcium hydroxide appears to have a consistently lower success rate in pulpotomies in primary teeth than these four agents. There are a number of other materials that are of historical significance, or have regional usage, and a number of experimental techniques including bone morphogenic protein and growth factors, which will not be discussed. All current therapeutic agents have toxic effects and must be correctly handled within their therapeutic range. Clinicians should carefully read the Materials Safety Data Sheet for these agents. Cases should be carefully selected within the guidelines recommended.

MINERAL TRIOXIDE AGGREGATE

MTA is a mixture of tricalcium silicate, bismuth oxide or zirconium oxide, dicalcium silicate, tricalcium aluminate and calcium sulphate. It is chemically similar to standard Portland cement mix. MTA powder reacts with water to form a paste, which is highly alkaline (pH 13) during the setting phase, then sets to form an inert mass. Clinical success rates for MTA pulpotomy are similar to formocresol and ferric sulphate but have improved radiographic success.

The MTA powder is mixed with water immediately before use. The resultant paste is applied to the pulpotomy site using a proprietary carrier or a plastic instrument and is left in situ to set. It is covered with a suitable base material before restoration of the tooth. The paste should only be applied after haemostasis has been obtained.

FERRIC SULPHATE

Ferric sulphate has been used widely in dentistry as a haemostatic agent. It was used initially in pulpotomies as an aid to haemostasis before placement of calcium hydroxide. However, as an independent therapeutic agent, ferric sulphate pulpotomy has a success rate of 74% to 99%. Ferric sulphate is thought to react with the pulp tissue, forming a superficial protective layer of iron-protein complex. The predominant mode of failure is the result of internal resorption.

Ferric sulphate is burnished onto the pulp stumps (pulpotomy site) using a micro-brush for 15 seconds, then rinsed off with water and dried. Persistent bleeding after the application of ferric sulphate is an indication for pulpectomy or extraction.

ELECTROSURGERY

Electrosurgery uses radiofrequency energy to produce a controlled superficial tissue burn. It is both haemostatic and antibacterial. Excessive energy or contact time causes a deep tissue burn with necrosis of the radicular pulp and subsequent internal root resorption, although electrosurgical pulpotomy has a success rate of 70% to 94%.

The electrosurgery unit should be set to coagulate, with a low power setting. A small ball or round-ended tip is applied to the pulpotomy site and briefly activated (Figure 7.8). The site should immediately be flooded with water to remove excess heat. Each pulp stump is treated in turn. If necessary, electrocoagulation can be repeated to control persistent bleeding, until the total cumulative application time is 2 seconds. Persistent bleeding after this time is an indication for pulpectomy or extraction. Electrosurgical equipment has the potential to interfere with pacemakers and implanted electronics.

FORMOCRESOL

Formocresol has been used in dentistry for over 100 years, and for pulpotomies in primary teeth for over 80 years. Its efficacy has been studied extensively, with clinical success rates ranging from 70% to 100%, making it the standard against which newer techniques are compared. The formaldehyde component of formocresol is strongly bactericidal and reversibly inhibits many enzymes in the inflammatory process. Originally, the aim of using formocresol was to completely mummify (fix) all residual pulpal tissue and necrotic material within the root canal. Techniques using dilute formocresol (Buckley solution) aim to create a small superficial layer of fixation over the amputated pulp, while preserving the vitality of the deeper radicular pulp.

In 2004, the International Agency for Research on Cancer concluded that chronic exposure to high levels of formaldehyde causes nasopharyngeal cancer in humans. Formaldehyde does not bioaccumulate. However, with the advent of MTA and other suitable alternatives, these should be used in preference to formocresol, if available.

Pulpectomy in primary teeth

Pulpectomy is the complete removal of all pulpal tissue from the tooth. Pulpectomy can only be considered for primary teeth that have intact roots. Any evidence of root resorption is an indication for extraction. The success rates following pulpectomy when used to manage severe infections including acute facial cellulitis associated with primary teeth is very low. Extraction is recommended in these cases.

Pulpectomy procedures in primary teeth are technically challenging and generally do not have as high a success rate compared with other forms of pulp therapy. Therefore, many paediatric dental specialists do not perform this technique routinely.

GENERAL TECHNICAL CONSIDERATIONS

Root canal morphology

Although the root canal morphology of primary incisors is relatively simple, the root canal morphology of multi-rooted primary teeth is often more complex than permanent teeth, with fins, ramifications and inter-canal communications. These anatomical factors inhibit complete chemo-mechanical debridement of the root canal space that is usually achievable in permanent teeth. The anatomical apex may be up to 3 mm from the radiographic apex and occurs frequently on

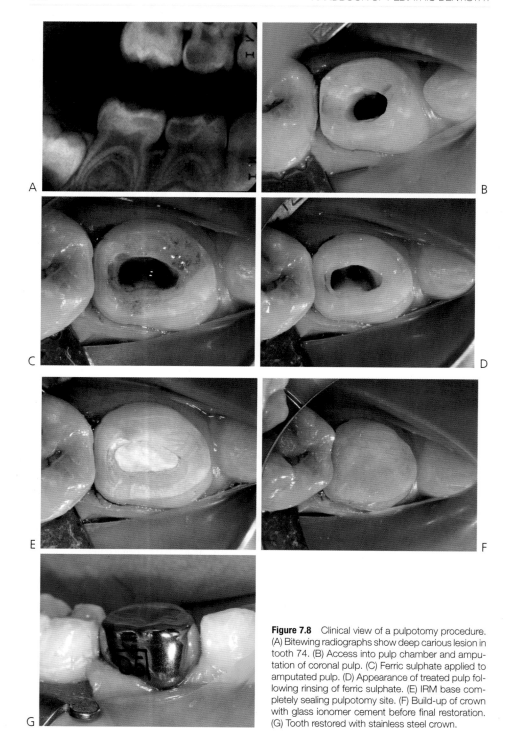

Figure 7.8 Clinical view of a pulpotomy procedure. (A) Bitewing radiographs show deep carious lesion in tooth 74. (B) Access into pulp chamber and amputation of coronal pulp. (C) Ferric sulphate applied to amputated pulp. (D) Appearance of treated pulp following rinsing of ferric sulphate. (E) IRM base completely sealing pulpotomy site. (F) Build-up of crown with glass ionomer cement before final restoration. (G) Tooth restored with stainless steel crown.

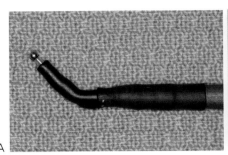
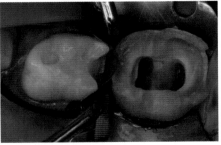

A   B

Figure 7.9   (A) Electrosurgical tip used in pulpotomy. (B) Appearance of root stumps following electrocautery.

the lateral surface of the root, making it difficult to determine the true working length. Over-instrumentation of the primary tooth root canal has the potential to damage the underlying permanent tooth. Electronic measurement of the root canal can assist with the location of the anatomical apex of a primary tooth.

Obturation

Obturation of the root canal space in a primary tooth must not interfere with normal exfoliation of the permanent successor. This requires a resorbable paste root filling. The exception to this would be where it is planned to retain a primary tooth that does not have a permanent successor. Suitable materials for obturation include unreinforced zinc oxide eugenol cement, calcium hydroxide paste and iodoform paste (Figure 7.9).

Indications

- Pulp necrosis in any primary tooth, or carious exposure of vital primary incisor.
- Restorable tooth.
- Preoperative radiograph confirms intact nonresorbed root with minimal bone loss.
- Retention of tooth is required.

TECHNIQUE

1. Pain control and rubber-dam isolation.
2. Complete removal of caries as for pulpotomy.
3. Chemo-mechanical cleaning and preparation of the root canal, taking care to force neither instruments nor debris beyond the anatomical apex. Copious irrigation with sodium hypochlorite.
4. Obturation with a resorbable paste (see earlier).
5. Restoration to ensure adequate coronal seal.
6. Appropriate follow-up.

Treatment planning for grossly carious or necrotic immature permanent teeth (Figure 7.10)

Gross caries involving the first permanent molars poses a difficult dilemma in treatment planning. The early presentation of the patient is essential in obtaining favourable results. The basic questions about whether these teeth should be removed or restored are:

- What tooth is affected?
- How old is the child and are they able to cooperate for possible lengthy dental treatment?
- What is the long-term prognosis for the tooth?

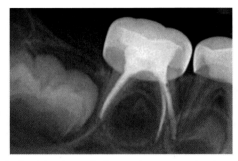

Figure 7.10 Radiograph of a pulpectomy of a lower primary second molar using a resorbable paste.

- What is the status of the pulp?
- Are the root apices fully formed?
- Are the third molars present?

GENERAL CONSIDERATIONS

- The decision to extract is often best made in conjunction with a paediatric dentist or orthodontist. For example, if a carious lateral permanent incisor has significant decay, then it may be removed as part of the orthodontic treatment plan and the space closed or held for implant placement.
- If the tooth is unrestorable, no matter what the occlusion, then it should be removed. Even if successful root canal treatment can be completed, the status of the crown is most important. Commonly, these teeth have extensive loss of tooth structure, with only an enamel shell remaining.
- If removal of a first permanent molar is contraindicated, severely carious or hypomineralized/hypoplastic first permanent molars (see Chapter 11) can be stabilized effectively with preformed metal crowns to allow time for maturation of the pulp and dentine before definitive restoration. With growth, pulpal regression occurs, giving increased dentine thickness for crown preparation and improved thickness of the radicular dentine, giving better root strength. At the completion of dental growth, the restorative options for these teeth can be re-evaluated.

Pulpotomy in the immature permanent tooth

All teeth are immature when they erupt. In addition to the important phase of posteruptive enamel maturation, the roots of newly erupted permanent teeth will take up to 3 years before their growth is completed. During this period, the roots are short, the root apices are wide open, the dentine is thin and the dentine tubules are relatively wide, increasing the permeability of dentine to bacteria. The open apex is associated with excellent pulpal vascularity and the potential for a favourable healing response. Therapeutic efforts are directed towards preserving the vitality of the pulpo-dentinal complex to facilitate normal root development and maturation (Figure 7.11).

The aim of pulpotomy in the immature permanent tooth is to amputate the inflamed coronal pulp and preserve the vitality of the remaining pulp to promote apexogenesis (see Chapter 8). Apexogenesis involves the continued normal development of the radicular pulp below the pulpotomy site, resulting in normal root length, thickness of radicular dentine and apical closure. Apexogenesis optimizes root anatomy and strength. The main risk of apexogenesis is the potential for dystrophic pulp calcification (root canal obliteration) in the event that subsequent pulpectomy is required. The biomechanical properties of the root are more favourable after apexogenesis than

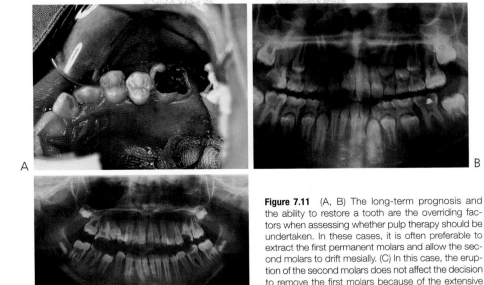

Figure 7.11 (A, B) The long-term prognosis and the ability to restore a tooth are the overriding factors when assessing whether pulp therapy should be undertaken. In these cases, it is often preferable to extract the first permanent molars and allow the second molars to drift mesially. (C) In this case, the eruption of the second molars does not affect the decision to remove the first molars because of the extensive carious breakdown in addition to the presence of the third molars.

after apexification. The use of haematogenous stem cells, revascularization and regenerative endodontics hold hope for the future management of these teeth.

Unlike the primary dentition, in which the pulpotomy is always at the level of the pulpal floor, a small carious exposure of the pulp horn of a permanent tooth can be managed by a superficial pulpotomy of only 1 to 2 mm. This is based on Cvek's pulpotomy technique (see Chapter 7). Where a large exposure is present, or multiple exposure sites, a deep pulpotomy is required to the opening of the root canals, or the level of the cemento-enamel junction in an anterior tooth. The exposure site is continuously irrigated until haemostasis occurs, before application of the therapeutic medicament. The therapeutic medicament can be calcium hydroxide powder or paste or MTA. Antibiotic/corticosteroid paste has also been used.

CLINICAL CRITERIA

- Carious pulp exposure.
- Asymptomatic tooth or episodes of mild, transient pain.
- Preoperative radiograph confirms immature roots with open apices.
- Absence of radicular pathology.
- Restorable tooth.

TECHNIQUE

1. Pain control and rubber-dam isolation.
2. Complete removal of caries.
3. Removal of roof of pulp chamber.
4. Amputation of coronal pulp, either superficially or deep to the opening of the root canal.
5. Arrest of bleeding at amputation site.
6. Application of therapeutic medicament (calcium hydroxide or MTA).

7. Place base directly over the therapeutic medicament (IRM® or Cavit®).
8. Restore tooth with adequate coronal seal.
9. Appropriate follow-up.

Endodontics versus extraction in immature permanent teeth

If pulp necrosis occurs in a permanent molar before root maturation, although the affected tooth can still be preserved using (nonvital) endodontic strategies, the tooth will be compromised with regard to strength, root length and apical development. It is important to consider whether the tooth itself is actually restorable in the long term. By definition, these teeth have already lost significant amounts of tooth structure. In addition, endodontic treatment will weaken an already compromised tooth, require apexification over many years (see Chapter 8) and involves significant operative challenges (i.e., isolation, obturation, restoration).

- Retention of a compromised immature permanent tooth with a poor long-term prognosis may still be beneficial for behavioural reasons, arch integrity and normal alveolar development during the period of dentofacial growth or may facilitate subsequent orthodontic treatment by holding space until the optimal time for extraction.
- Except in exceptional circumstances, these teeth should be removed.
- Consider the long-term costs to the patient comparing orthodontic treatment to align second permanent molars with the prospect of placing four ceramic crowns (or similar) that would require replacement several times during a lifetime.

Orthodontic considerations for first permanent molar extraction

The first permanent molar, because of its early emergence in the oral cavity and predisposition to dental anomalies such as enamel hypomineralization (see Chapter 11), is susceptible to large carious lesions. This, often in consultation with an orthodontist, will result in a decision to remove the tooth. There are a number of considerations, and briefly these are:

- If only the lower first permanent molars are removed, then the upper molars should be monitored closely and, if required, an upper fixed appliance such as a trans-palatal arch or a removable appliance such as a Hawley might be placed to prevent over-eruption of these teeth before the eruption of the lower second molars.
- The ideal time for lower first permanent molar extraction is before alveolar eruption of the second molar. These teeth will migrate mesially and assume the position of the first molar. Radiographic assessment is important to determine the appropriate time for removal to facilitate space closure.
- The presence or absence of third molars will influence a decision to extract the first molars, but ultimately it will be the long-term prognosis of the first molars that determines the final treatment plan. The goal is to have a long-term, functional occlusion with minimum maintenance.
- If three molars are grossly carious and require removal, it is usually better to keep the extractions symmetrical and extract all four teeth.

TIMING OF EXTRACTIONS

Although the timing of extractions will be determined in individual cases, some general rules should be followed if possible.

Class I (with no crowding)
- Extract teeth that are unrestorable on presentation.

Class I (crowding) or class II
- Extract the lower first permanent molars as early as practicable.

- Retain the upper first permanent molars until the second molars begin to erupt.
- Extraction of the upper first permanent molars should coincide with orthodontic treatment for crowding.

Class III

- No clear guidelines exist as to the best time to extract and unrestorable teeth should be extracted as dictated clinically.

It has been reported, generally, that the most ideal time at which to extract the lower first molars is when calcification of the bifurcation of the lower second molars is observed. More recently, this has been questioned and, in most cases, clinicians have little choice in the timing of extractions because of the dictates and urgency of treatment. Furthermore, if sedation or general anaesthesia is required to remove these teeth, it is better to plan for one procedure rather than two.

Tables 7.2 and 7.3 summarize the treatment options for primary and permanent teeth.

TABLE 7.2 ■ Treatment options for primary teeth

Clinical event	Signs or symptoms	Pulpal status	Treatment choice
Caries without exposure	No spontaneous symptoms	Healthy or reversible pulpitis	Restore tooth
Caries with possible or near exposure	No spontaneous symptoms	Healthy or reversible pulpitis	Indirect pulp capping
Caries with possible or near exposure	Occasional pain on stimulation	Reversible pulpitis	Pulpotomy
Caries with possible or near exposure	Close to exfoliation		Consider elective extraction
Iatrogenic/noncarious exposure	No spontaneous symptoms	Healthy	Pulpotomy
Carious exposure	Minimal history of pain No mobility No radiographic evidence of pathology	Reversible pulpitis	Pulpotomy
Carious exposure	Spontaneous pain	Irreversible pulpitis	Pulpectomy Intermediate dressing Extraction
Carious exposure	Draining sinus Swelling Mobility Radiographic pathology (inter-radicular or periapical, root resorption)	Necrotic pulp	Pulpectomy with resorbable dressing or Extraction
Gross caries	Caries through bifurcation Extensive root resorption Tooth not restorable Furcation periapical pathology	Necrotic pulp	Extraction

TABLE 7.3 ■ **Treatment options for immature permanent teeth**

Clinical event	Signs or symptoms	Pulpal status	Treatment choice
Caries without exposure	No spontaneous symptoms	Healthy or reversible pulpitis	Restore tooth
Caries with possible or near exposure	No spontaneous symptoms or Occasional pain on stimulation	Healthy or reversible pulpitis	Indirect pulp capping
Small pulp exposure	No spontaneous symptoms	Healthy	Direct pulp capping
Carious exposure	Minimal history of pain No mobility No radiographic evidence of pathology	Reversible pulpitis	Pulpotomy and apexogenesis
Carious exposure	Spontaneous pain	Irreversible pulpitis	Pulpectomy and apexification or Extraction
Carious exposure	Draining sinus Swelling Mobility Radiographic pathology	Necrotic pulp	Pulpectomy and apexification or Extraction
Gross caries	Tooth not restorable	Irreversible pulpitis or Necrotic pulp	Extraction

FOLLOW-UP

Regardless of the pulp therapy that is performed on primary or young permanent teeth, appropriate follow-up is important. Although pulp therapy treatments are successful, no treatment has 100% success rate, and so providing informed consent to young patients and their caregivers is important. Informed consent should include information about the likely success of the pulp therapy and what signs and symptoms they should be aware of that will indicate failure.

Children who require pulp therapy because of caries should, in most cases, be classified as 'high-caries-risk' patients, and the follow-up timing should be dictated by their caries risk status. At each follow-up appointment, a history of each pulp-treated tooth should be taken along with a yearly radiographic assessment of pulp-treated teeth. Pulp-treated teeth can become necrotic without any clinical symptoms, necessitating regular radiographic assessment.

Signs of pulp therapy failure include:

■ Pain on biting or tenderness to percussion or increased mobility.
■ Presentation of a draining sinus.
■ Redness of gingivae around full coverage restoration.
■ Intraradicular radiolucency on radiograph.
■ Other clinical signs of irreversible pulpitis or abscess formation (see earlier).

It is essential that these teeth are monitored regularly. Frequently, carious, primary teeth that have been quiescent for months or years suddenly become necrotic following restoration. Unfortunately, once a primary tooth becomes necrotic after pulp therapy, the tooth requires removal or a pulpectomy to be performed. Extraction, with the provision of a space maintainer if needed, is the preferred option in the majority of cases.

Further reading

American Academy on Pediatric Dentistry Clinical Affairs Committee – Pulp Therapy Subcommittee, 2009. Guideline on pulp therapy for primary and young permanent teeth. American Academy on Pediatric Dentistry Council on Clinical Affairs. Pediatric Dentistry 30 (7 Suppl), 170–174.

Casas, M.J., Kenny, D.J., Johnston, D.H., et al., 2004. Outcomes of vital primary incisor ferric sulfate pulpotomy and root canal therapy. Journal of the Canadian Dental Association 70, 34–38.

Fuks, A.B., 2008. Vital pulp therapy with new materials for primary teeth: new directions and treatment perspectives. Pediatric Dentistry 30 (3), 211–219.

Huth, K.C., Paschos, E., Hajek-Al-Khatar, N., et al., 2005. Effectiveness of 4 pulpotomy techniques – randomized controlled trial. Journal of Dental Research 84, 1144–1148.

Huth, K.C., Hajek-Al-Khatar, N., Wolf, P., et al., 2011. Long-term effectiveness of four pulpotomy techniques: 3-year randomised controlled trial. Clinical Oral Investigations 16 (4), 1243–1250.

International Agency for Research on Cancer (IARC), 2006. Formaldehyde, 2-butoxyethanol and 1-tert-butoxypropan-2-ol. IARC Monographs on the Evaluation of Carcinogenic Risks to Humans, Number 88.

Kahl, J., Easton, J., Johnson, G., et al., 2008. Formocresol blood levels in children receiving dental treatment under general anesthesia. Pediatric Dentistry 30 (5), 393–399.

Nadin, G., Goel, B.R., Yeung, C.A., et al., 2003. Pulp treatment for extensive decay in primary teeth. Cochrane Database of Systematic Reviews (1), CD003220.

Rodd, H.D., Waterhouse, P.J., Fuks, A.B., et al., 2006. UK National Clinical Guidelines in Paediatric Dentistry. Pulp therapy for primary molars. International Journal of Paediatric Dentistry 16 (Suppl 1), 15–23.

CHAPTER 8

Clinical and surgical techniques

Angus C. Cameron ■ Stephen Fayle

Extraction of teeth in children

The removal of teeth in children can be one of the most stressful procedures for both the operator and the patient. Although a tooth may be totally anaesthetized, the pressure felt during the extraction can be extremely upsetting and uncomfortable. As one of the most important aspects of clinical practice, dentists need to be skilled, efficient and sensitive in the removal of teeth in children. Teeth should be removed gently with good surgical technique rather than excessive force that may fracture roots or upset the patient.

General principles of tooth extraction in children
PREOPERATIVE ASSESSMENT

- Obtain thorough medical history and informed consent for the procedure.
- Evaluate the tooth to be extracted both clinically and radiographically.
- Identify potentially difficult root anatomy and the proximity of other important structures before extraction. Be aware of implications for the permanent successor.

- Clearly identify the tooth to be extracted and confirm again before extraction. Once confirmed against the patient's details, the treatment plan and the consent form, it is good practice to ensure that the tooth (teeth) to be extracted is (are) written on a board that is clearly visible to the operator and the assistant. Counting from the midline can be useful in positive identification of the tooth for extraction (LocSSIPS Toolkit, RCS England, 2017). Immediately before extraction, just as elevator/forceps are applied, a 'pause' is advisable where the treatment plan is rechecked; arch, side and tooth are verbally announced and confirmed (e.g., 'lower right six'), ideally with a second dental professional/assistant 'confirming' that the instrument is being applied to the correct planned tooth before proceeding with extraction. Adopting these steps can significantly reduce the risk of wrong tooth extraction.
- Profound local anaesthesia is vital. Explain the feeling of 'numbness' and the sensation associated with luxation of the tooth before commencing the procedure.
- If the child will be unable to cope with the extraction(s) under local analgesia alone, then sedation or general anaesthesia should be considered. Ideally, the decision to sedate a child should be made at the assessment appointment, not once the child has become upset during the procedure. Appropriate consent should be obtained before any treatment under sedation or general anaesthesia, and this should include explanation of the relative risks and benefits of these approaches. In some countries (e.g., the United Kingdom), consent for sedation or general anaesthesia must be obtained in writing.

OTHER PRINCIPLES

- Primary teeth do not require a 'primary drive' that is often recommended for permanent teeth.
- Children tolerate the use of luxators or elevators much better than application of forceps. The alveolar bone in children is soft and teeth can be elevated easily to a high degree of mobility before a final delivery with forceps.
- If small apical root fragments remain after an extraction, they may be left to resorb, as attempted removal may damage the permanent successor.
- Choose a pair of extraction forceps suited to the required procedure. A wide range of forceps designed for primary teeth is available (Figure 8.1).

Anterior teeth

- Primary incisors, especially if there is a fracture present, should be gently luxated rather than elevated to avoid damage to the permanent incisor.
- Single rooted teeth should be delivered with forceps utilizing a rotational movement (Figure 8.2).

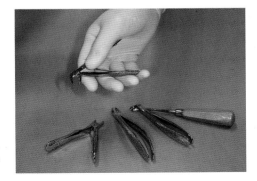

Figure 8.1 A selection of paediatric extraction forceps. It is important to use the appropriate-size forceps for the tooth to be removed.

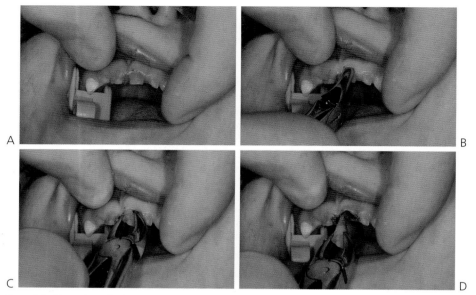

Figure 8.2 Extraction of primary anterior teeth. (A) The alveolus is supported and the upper lip retracted. (B) The beaks of the forceps engage the tooth root, not the crown. Notice the blanching of the attached gingiva. (C, D) The tooth should be delivered with a rotation movement and with minimal apical force that might damage the permanent tooth germ.

Premolars

- The removal of premolars is most commonly required for orthodontic reasons and may be the first dental intervention for some children. Extraction of the upper first premolar should be addressed with great care, as this tooth usually has two roots (buccal and lingual), and the root apices may be fine and easily fractured. Surgical removal of a retained root fragment usually involves loss of bone and may have implications for orthodontic treatment and the ability to move adjacent teeth into this space.
- The use of a 3-mm luxator is invaluable to expand the socket and avoid excessive bone damage before application of the forceps.
- Delivery with forceps should be made with gentle movements, avoiding excessive buccal forces that might fracture the buccal bone or fine root tips.

Molars

- Extractions should be clean and atraumatic.
- Avoid gingival injuries by freeing the gingival margin with a flat plastic, luxator or elevator (Figure 8.3).
- Second primary molars are sometimes difficult to remove because of the divergent spread of the roots. Sectioning the tooth vertically can facilitate extraction if the crown is considerably damaged or the roots encircle the crown of the underlying permanent tooth.
- Initial luxation/elevation may be valuable, especially for permanent molars (and is especially useful before upper first permanent molar extraction). Care should be exercised when elevating to avoid inadvertent application of force to adjacent teeth, which can lead to unintended damage or luxation.
- Support the alveolus on either side with fingers. This improves access, protects adjacent soft tissues and can provide valuable proprioceptive 'feedback' to the operator.

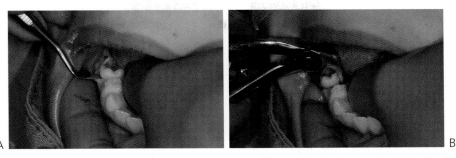

Figure 8.3 (A) When extracting primary posterior teeth, it is useful to free the gingiva from the tooth with a flat plastic or a similar blunt instrument to protect it from tearing. (B) Avoid excessive buccal movement that will damage the thin, buccal, cortical plate and the attached gingiva when delivering these teeth.

- Multi-rooted permanent teeth can be extracted by using alternating, slow, buccal and palatal/lingual force or a 'figure of 8' motion to expand the alveolar bone. Although many oral surgery texts recommend the buccal delivery of lower molars, the most dense bone is found on the buccal aspect, and excessive movement of a lower permanent molar buccally may result in root fracture, particularly in teeth missing significant amounts of coronal structure.
- 'Cow-horn' pattern forceps are extremely useful in removing lower permanent molars, especially those with little or no crown remaining on the lingual aspect (Figure 8.4). A 'cow-horn' pattern is also available for upper molars.

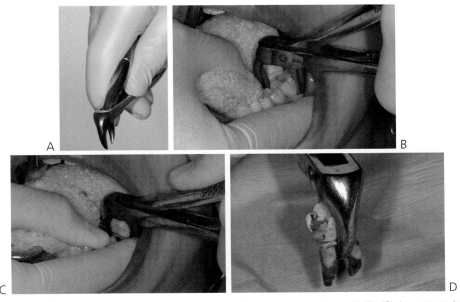

Figure 8.4 (A) 'Cow-horn' pattern forceps engage the bifurcation of a molar tooth (B). (C) As pressure is applied, the beaks are worked further apically and the tooth will rise out of the socket, usually with minimal rotation or buccal movements. These forceps are very useful for badly broken-down molars. Although fractures of the crown may occur, the level of the fracture is more coronal and tends to section the tooth, allowing easy delivery of the roots with an elevator. Note the finger support of either side of the alveolus. (D) The beaks of the forceps engage the furcation.

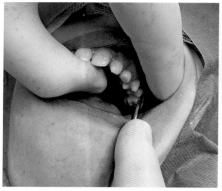
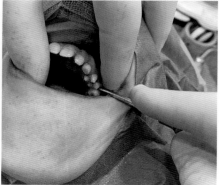

A

B

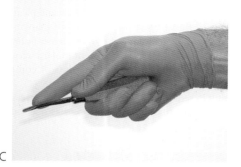

C

Figure 8.5 (A) Luxators are delicate and sharp instruments, designed to shear the periodontal attachment and enlarge the tooth socket. The application of the luxator should be vertical along the long axis of the roots. (B) Elevators should be applied at an angle to the long axis of the root, similarly to a screwdriver, so their application on the tooth root is more horizontal between the embrasure. (C) The index finger should run along the blade and serves to protect the patient if the instrument slips.

Avoiding and managing root fractures

- Avoid root fractures by first luxating or elevating the tooth to a high degree of mobility before the application of forceps (Figure 8.5).
- If the delivery of the tooth becomes difficult during the extraction, stop and reassess rather than applying more force that may break the roots.
- Always assess where a permanent tooth germ is positioned before elevating the roots of primary teeth. If a root is fractured when extracting an ankylosed primary molar, this can usually be left in situ, especially if it is below the interseptal bone.
- Cryer elevators are used to remove interseptal bone between mandibular permanent molar roots to gain access to the roots and then can be used to deliver the root. Cryer elevators should be used with care, as they can generate high forces. Care is also required during removal of interseptal bone surrounding primary molar roots so as to avoid damage to the permanent successor.
- If it appears impossible to deliver a tooth without a root fracture, then the procedure should be performed as a surgical removal. Ideally, this assessment should be made before starting the procedure.

Following the extraction

- Examine the extracted tooth carefully.
- If any granulation tissue remains in the socket, it should be removed, whilst taking care of the developing tooth germ.
- Obtain haemostasis before discharging the child.
- Suture any areas of gingiva or mucosa that may have been torn or damaged.

POSTOPERATIVE INSTRUCTIONS FOLLOWING EXTRACTIONS FOR CHILDREN

Always give clear and lucid instructions to the child and caregiver:

- Allow the blood clot to stabilize by avoiding rinsing on the day of extraction.
- The next day, the mouth may be gently rinsed with water. There is little evidence that warm saline or antiseptic mouthwashes are of any real benefit following tooth extraction in children, but good oral hygiene is essential, and gentle toothbrushing can start the day after the extraction. Parents should be advised that halitosis often occurs following extraction or oral surgery.
- Prescribe appropriate analgesics and, if required, antibiotics.
- Warn that there should be no sport or excessive play for the remainder of the day.
- Warn the parent and child against lip biting or sucking whilst soft tissue anaesthesia persists.
- Explain to the parent how to identify significant haemorrhage and how to manage it with appropriate local measures such as pressure from biting on a sterile gauze.
- Give instructions about what to do if prolonged bleeding, excessive pain or infection occurs.

Repair and suturing of soft tissue injuries

Generally, soft tissue wounds should be closed within 24 hours. Good closure of wounds allows for more rapid healing by primary intention. Suturing may reduce the sequestration of displaced bony fragments and may prevent bacterial contamination of the gingival sulcus. Furthermore, there is much less pain from the wound if exposed bony defects are well covered with periosteum and gingival tissues. Deeper lacerations of the lip will involve the muscle layer, and it is important to close this, as a separate layer to prevent the formation of a 'dead space' will easily become infected (Figure 8.6). It is essential that the wound is properly debrided and free of contamination from foreign bodies or bony spicules before apposition of tissues. Any wound involving skin, including those crossing the vermillion border of the lip, requires precise and expert skill to facilitate the best possible result. Often this requires timely referral to an appropriate surgeon.

Cyanoacrylate (tissue glue) (Figure 8.7) is now commonly used for closure of smaller soft tissue wounds on the face and scalp in children without having to give local anaesthetic or remove sutures. Currently, the literature is equivocal as to whether suturing or gluing produces better outcomes, although it is clear that gluing is far less traumatic for the child, provides a water-resistant coating and is much faster.

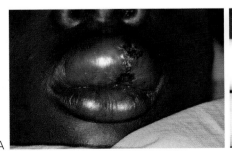
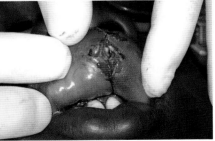

A   B

Figure 8.6   (A) When closing any wound, it is essential not to leave a dead space. This laceration to the upper lip was closed only superficially, leaving the muscle layers open. A large abscess developed within 12 hours, requiring reopening of the wound, drainage and debridement, and reclosure including the muscle and the mucosa (B).

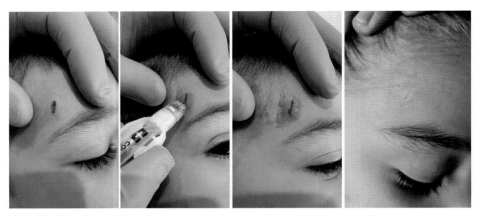

Figure 8.7 Use of tissue glue to treat a deep but short laceration in the forehead. (A) The wound is separated and cleaned; and ensure that the surrounding tissue is clear of debris. Ensure that the skin is dry. (B) The wound edges are opposed with finger pressure, and then three layers of glue are applied over the surface. (C) The wound is held until the glue sets. Maximum strength is achieved within 2½ min. (D) Healing after 3 months.

CHOICE OF MATERIAL (Table 8.1)

The choice of suture material and needle will depend on the following.

The type and location of the wound to be closed

- Reverse-cutting-edge needles should be used in sites involving keratinized gingiva.
- Tapering needles are suitable for nonkeratinized gingiva and more friable mucosa.
- Monofilament materials such as nylon must be used for skin to minimize tissue reaction (Figure 8.8A).
- Internal (muscle) closure must use resorbable materials.
- Suturing of torn or lacerated gingival tissues should be conducted using a fine suture, such as a 4-0 or 5-0 resorbable suture. Vicryl® (polyglactin), Dexon® (polyglycolic acid) or Monocryl® (poliglecaprone) sutures have good traction strength for at least 3 weeks and have far less tissue reaction than catgut. They are resorbable, but because they comprise braided material, they are not nearly as clean as monofilament sutures. Where strength is required and removal of the sutures is not an issue, monofilament nylon is preferable.

The required strength and length of time required

- Keratinized and thick tissue such as the palate requires thicker suture material (3-0).
- Large but thin, friable flaps may still need the strength of a thicker material without the risk of the suture tearing the mucosa.

Whether the material needs to be removed: resorbable or nonresorbable

- Resorbable sutures such as chromic gut, polyglactin, polyglycolic acid or poliglecaprone (4-0 or 3-0) are preferable for use in young children or where behavioural issues are a concern (Figure 8.8B).

SUTURE NEEDLES (Figure 8.9)

A wide variety of needle sizes and curvatures are available, and it is up to the individual surgeon as to which type is preferred. The most commonly used needles are 1/2 or 3/8th circle (Figure 8.8B).

TABLE 8.1 ■ Some indications for the selection of suture materials in paediatric dentistry

Suture	Indications	Size	Needle	Absorption	Tissue reaction	Notes
Surgical gut	Extraction suture	3/0	Cutting	Completely digested by 70 days. Effective strength for 2–3 days in the oral cavity	Moderate	Used for tissue closure where strength is required for 1–2 days
Chromic catgut	General closure	3/0, 4/0	Taper	Completely digested by 110 days, but in the oral cavity, it has effective strength for up to 5 days	Moderate but less than plain gut	Excellent for oral tissue closure when longer life is required compared with plain gut
Polyglycolic acid (Dexon®)/ polyglactin (Vicryl®)	Alveolar mucosa Attached gingiva Large flaps where strength is required but a resorbable suture is desirable Subcuticular skin closure	4/0 5/0 3/0, 4/0 5/0	Taper Cutting Cutting	Completely absorbed by hydrolysis after 90 days. Faster absorption when exposed to the oral environment. Good strength for least 2 weeks. Vicryl Rapide® is resorbed after 42 days	Mild	Polyglactin has great advantages for use in the oral cavity in children. It has good strength over 7 days and is resorbable. It is often retained for longer periods, however, and has a tendency to accumulate plaque because of its braided nature. Tapering needles are useful where tissues are friable
Poliglecaprone (Monocryl®)	Attached gingiva or palate Larger flaps where strength is required	4/0, 5/0 3/0, 4/0	Cutting	Completely resorbed by 100 days, but generally it loses half its tensile strength after 2 weeks	Minimal	Being monofilament, there is excellent tissue reaction and they are much cleaner than a braided suture
Monofilament nylon prolene	Large flaps where strength is required (i.e., palate) Skin	3-0 4-0 6/0	Cutting	Essentially nonresorbable materials, but degrades at 15%–20% per year	Extremely low	Excellent tissue reaction and strength. Monofilament material is extremely clean and allows good wound healing but needs to be removed Skin closure must be performed with 6-0 sutures should be removed before 7 days

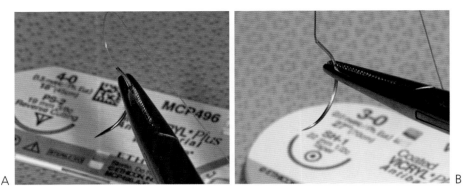

Figure 8.8 (A) Surgical nylon 4-0 on a reverse cutting needle. This monofilament suture material has excellent tissue reaction and strength. The reverse cutting needle has its cutting edge on the convex surface, which avoids tearing. Cutting needles are used for thick, keratinized tissue such as attached gingiva or palatal mucosa. (B) Vicryl® is a resorbable, braided material. It also has good tissue reaction but tends to accumulate plaque and can become quite dirty in the mouth before their loss after 2 weeks. The taper needle (usually 16–22 mm) is excellent for friable or thin alveolar mucosa.

INSTRUMENTS

Although each surgeon will have their own individual preference of surgical instrumentation, the following instruments are those commonly used in many oral surgical suturing situations.

Needle holders

Many different patterns of needle holders are available. The most convenient holders are around 15 cm in length with tungsten carbide beaks and a locking, ratchet handle. For very fine

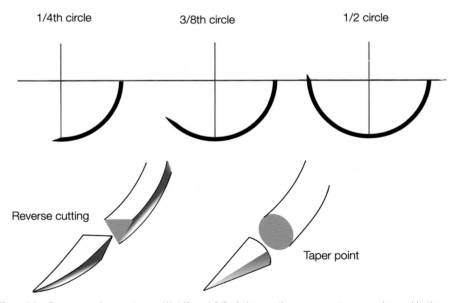

Figure 8.9 Suture needle curvatures. (A) 1/2 and 3/8 circles are the ones most commonly used in the oral cavity. (B) Shape of needle points.

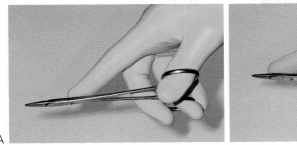
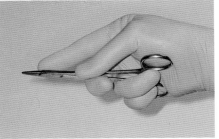

A   B

Figure 8.10 (A) Suture needle holders may be held in a scissors or (B) palm grip, with the index finger supporting the instrument.

suturing, iridectomy-type (microsurgical) needle holders may be useful. Needle holders can be held in a scissors or a palm grip, but in either case, the index finger should support the blades (Figure 8.10).

Toothed tissue forceps

Always use toothed forceps to hold tissue that would otherwise be crushed with a nontooth pattern. A straight pattern such as Gillies or McIndoe is sufficient for most procedures, but for fine procedures, a smaller Adson-type is used. Tissue forceps are held in a pen grip.

Fine suture scissors

Almost all scissors are made for use in the right hand, and any surgical assistant will be aware of how difficult it is to cut sutures using the left hand. Good suture scissors must be of adequate length to reach into the mouth, and although the blades can be short, they must be sharp and maintained. Do not use dissecting scissors that are designed for tissue cutting to cut suture material.

Skin hooks

The use of skin hooks is usually confined to extraoral work but is invaluable for mobilizing and everting flap and tissue margins.

SUTURING TECHNIQUES

- Simple interrupted: This is the most common suture used in the oral cavity. It is used for interdental suturing of flaps and relieving incisions (Figure 8.11).
- Horizontal mattress: The horizontal mattress suture applies force across the wound margin and can be placed across an extraction site. It can also be used to evert wound margins (Figure 8.12).
- Vertical mattress: This is frequently used to evert skin margins or in deep muscle closure in the lip. This suture can provide more tension than a simple interrupted suture.
- Haemostatic: This suture crosses over the tooth socket and can help retain packs for haemorrhage control.
- Continuous: An interlocking continuous suture is used for long wounds, particularly in the buccal vestibule. It has the disadvantage that if there is a break at any point, then the whole wound may open.
- Subcuticular: This is a form of running suture where a skin closure is hidden below the epidermis.

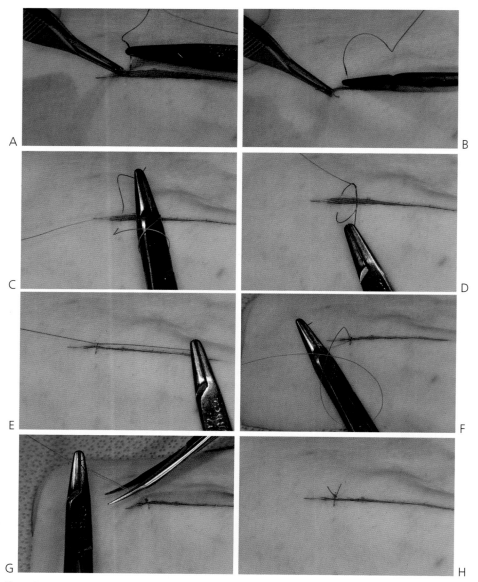

Figure 8.11 Technique for simple interrupted suture. (A, B) Each side of the flap is held and everted with toothed tissue forceps as the needle is passed in an arc from one side of the wound to the other. (C, D) A double throw knot is made and is tightened and locked by pulling on the long (or needle) end of the suture (E). Avoid pulling on the short end (held by the needle holder), as this will create a long tag end. (F) A reverse throw knot is made and the suture is cut short with fine scissors (G). (H) Note that the knot is sitting on tissue and not overlying the wound.

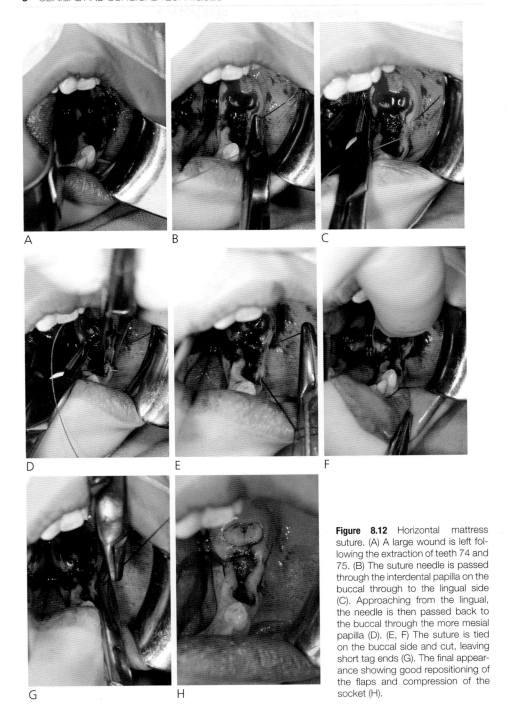

Figure 8.12 Horizontal mattress suture. (A) A large wound is left following the extraction of teeth 74 and 75. (B) The suture needle is passed through the interdental papilla on the buccal through to the lingual side (C). Approaching from the lingual, the needle is then passed back to the buccal through the more mesial papilla (D). (E, F) The suture is tied on the buccal side and cut, leaving short tag ends (G). The final appearance showing good repositioning of the flaps and compression of the socket (H).

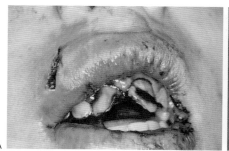
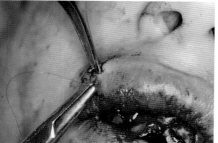

A

B

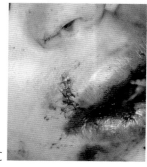

C

Figure 8.13   (A) When closing skin lacerations, it is essential that the key suture (the positioning suture) is at the vermilion border (B). A fine monofilament nonresorbable suture such as 6-0 nylon is used to minimize scarring (C).

CLINICAL HINTS

- Before suturing a site, examine it thoroughly for tooth fragments. If in any doubt, radiograph the site.
- Remove any jagged, damaged and necrotic soft tissues tags and freshen up old wound margins with a scalpel.
- Suture with adequate stress and tension, achieving complete haemostasis.
- Leave suture ends short if using resorbable materials, but longer if the material is to be removed. Very short tag ends often become buried and are difficult to remove.
- Remove skin sutures on the face within 5 days to prevent scarring of puncture sites (Figure 8.13).

Surgical removal of supernumerary teeth or impacted canines

IDENTIFICATION OF THE TOOTH

- Identify the tooth indicated for removal before surgery. It is good practice to confirm with the surgical assistant which teeth are to be removed by noting them on the radiographs, on a board visible to the whole surgical team and then on the patient.
- Most maxillary supernumeraries lie in the palate or in the midline between the central incisors. Midline inverted, conical supernumeraries often lie adjacent to the anterior nasal spine and are best removed via a labial approach. Tuberculate teeth are commonly palatal and inferior to the unerupted central incisor.
- Supernumeraries in the premolar region lie lingual and inferior to the premolars.
- Canines may be impacted buccally or palatally, although invariably, the root apex lies in close approximation to the floor of the sinus.

Radiology

Where the tooth (teeth) to be removed is (are) unerupted, clinical signs such as palpation and noting any abnormal angulation of adjacent erupted teeth can be useful, but radiographic investigation is always necessary. Often the position of the tooth in relation to adjacent structures will need to be determined as accurately as possible requiring specific types of radiographic views:

- Parallax radiographic views. This is commonly achieved by obtaining parallax radiographic views, where at least two radiographs are taken of the unerupted tooth position from significantly different angles (at least 30 degrees or more tube-shift). Objects further away from the x-ray source (tube) will tend to move WITH the direction of tube shift when compared with objects closer to the tube (conversely, objects closer to the x-ray tube will appear to move in the opposite direction to the tube-shift). The tube-shift between views can be either horizontal (usually two periapical views) or vertical (e.g., between an image on a standard anterior occlusal radiograph and a panoramic tomograph).
- Cone-beam computerized tomography (CBCT). A small-volume CBCT, if available, can be extremely useful where the relationship between adjacent structures is more difficult to determine. When prescribing a CBCT, the extra value of the enhanced diagnostic yield of a CBCT needs to be balanced against its higher x-ray radiation dose when compared with conventional radiography (Figure 8.14).
- Palatally impacted canine crowns will appear to be larger on panoramic films than teeth in the line of the arch or placed buccally.

SURGICAL TECHNIQUE

Anaesthesia

- Good anaesthesia is essential (Figure 8.15A). Many younger children will be managed under general anaesthesia; however, perioperative local anaesthesia is still required. A local anaesthetic with a vasoconstrictor can minimize postoperative pain and be an aid to haemorrhage control at the surgical site.

Mucoperiosteal flaps

- A large flap will heal in the same amount of time as a small flap. Therefore, an appropriately sized flap should be raised to ensure adequate access to remove the tooth (Figure 8.15B).

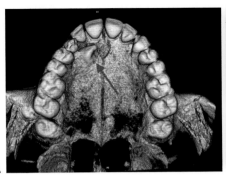
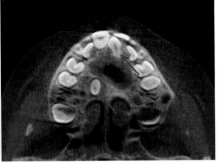

A   B

Figure 8.14 (A) Three-dimensional reconstruction of cone-beam computerized tomography images can give the surgeon a precise visualization of the position of an impacted tooth, in this case a palatally impacted 13 tooth (arrow). They can be of great benefit in showing the patient and parent what is planned in surgery. Although they may look impressive, it is important to analyse each section in each plane (axial, coronal and saggital) to determine exact relationships with associated structures. (B) This case shows an axial section of a child with two maxillary supernumerary teeth (arrow).

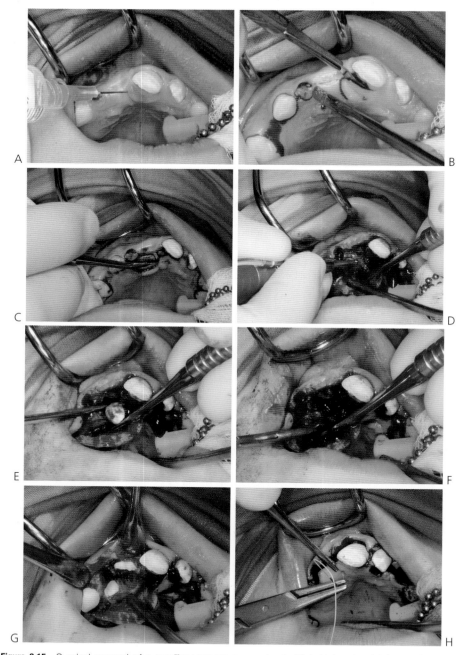

Figure 8.15 Surgical removal of a maxillary supernumerary tooth (A) Labial and palatal anaesthesia. (B) Crestal incision from at least the distal of the canine to the contralateral side. (C) Elevation of a full-thickness mucoperiosteal flap. (D) Removal of bone with bur. Note how the flap is protected by the periosteal elevator. (E) Exposure of the supernumerary and elevation with a Warwick James elevator. (F) Removal of the supernumerary tooth follicle with a pair of haemostats. (G) The socket is thoroughly irrigated, and in this case, bone overlying the impacted upper right central incisor is removed to encourage eruption. (H) Closure of the flap with a resorbable suture.

- When removing a palatal supernumerary tooth, a full-thickness palatal flap should be raised at least from the distal of the canine and beyond the midline (Figure 8.15C). Preserve the architecture of the palatal interdental papillae. The neurovascular bundle should be retained if possible, but if division is necessary to extend the flap, then a haemostat can be applied and the nerve bundle sectioned proximal to the forceps.
- When the tooth is labially impacted, a labial or buccal approach is indicated. A crevicular incision preserving the interdental papilla will be aided by the use of a relieving incision to reflect the flap.

Bone removal

- Access to the tooth can be made with hand instruments such as a 3-mm bone chisel or surgical drills (Figure 8.15D). The overlying bone is normally removed with a round bur and then the crown is more fully exposed by guttering around the crown to enable the application of an elevator.

Tooth removal

- Apply an appropriate elevator to the root to deliver the tooth (Figure 8.15E). The tooth should be luxated without placing any additional force on the adjacent teeth. The surgeon's fingers should support the adjacent teeth and will enable any inadvertent application of force to them to be detected.
- Occasionally, sectioning of the tooth may be required to facilitate removal. Never attempt to section a tooth without first elevating and establishing some movement within the socket.
- Remove the dental follicle carefully with a pair of haemostats or gentle curette with Mitchell's trimmer (Figure 8.15F).

Closure

- Irrigate the socket and operating site copiously, checking for any bony spicules or jagged margins (Figure 8.15G).
- Smooth off the bony margins with a bone file or bone rongeurs.
- Close the flap with an appropriate suture material (see earlier). Ensure that complete haemostasis is achieved (Figure 8.15H).

Postoperative care

- Provide adequate analgesia perioperatively and postoperatively. Depending on the amount of bone removal and the size of the bony defect, postoperative antibiotics are often not required. If antibiotics are required, a single perioperative administration is preferable.
- Give good clear oral hygiene instructions.
- Arrange an appropriate postoperative recall appointment.

Incision and drainage of abscess

Any collection of pus requires drainage (Figure 8.16). Fortunately, children usually attend the dentist (or doctor) early with odontogenic infections that have spread to involve the fascial planes of the face, and typically these present as a cellulitis. When treated inappropriately with repeated antibiotics and without removal of the cause (i.e., extraction of the offending tooth), or with particularly virulent organisms, then an abscess may develop. An abscess is a collection of pus within a cavity. An abscess will not resolve by itself, and pus will track to the most dependent point, which in the case of some head and neck infections will be extraorally or between tissue planes.

Spread between tissue planes may be life threatening, and any posterior spread of pus from a tooth in the upper arch may spread from the canine fossa to the antrum, the pterygopalatine fossa,

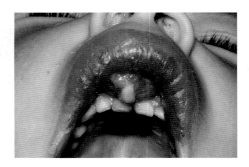

Figure 8.16   Any collection of pus requires drainage, whether that occurs spontaneously or surgically.

the orbit, the cavernous sinus and the brain. A submandibular abscess may spread to the floor of mouth, the buccal spaces, the pterygomandibular space, the parapharyngeal spaces and neck, and ultimately the mediastinum.

The following cases represent surgical emergencies and require urgent and immediate care and/or referral:

- A floor of mouth swelling, particularly those that have crossed the midline.
- Dysphagia or respiratory obstruction.
- Trismus.
- A fluctuant enlarging swelling in the head and neck.
- An enlarging swelling associated with acute fever, particularly a spiking temperature.

CLINICAL PRESENTATION

Cellulitis

- A hard, brawny swelling.
- Diffuse and tender.
- Warm to touch.

Abscess

- A soft, warm and painful swelling, usually fluctuant.
- Usually circumscribed, may be very well localized in the mouth or more diffuse if extraoral.

Surgical technique

Remember that such infections are serious and potentially life threatening and prompt referral to a suitably experienced surgeon is warranted.

Anaesthesia

Obtaining adequate anaesthesia may be difficult, so block injections are preferable. Where there is a significant swelling either intraorally or extraorally, general anaesthesia will be required to adequately manage and protect the airway and to undertake the procedure.

Intraoral (Figure 8.17)

- Protect the airway with gauze from pus or irrigating solutions that may go down the throat.
- Extract the tooth.
- Raise a flap and allow drainage of subperiosteal pus.
- An incision into the buccal or labial sulcus may also be required to establish drainage of any pus above periosteum.

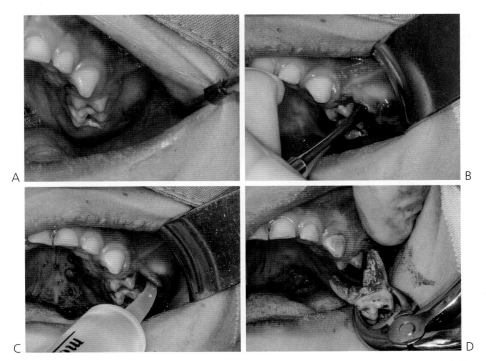

Figure 8.17 Management of an intraoral abscess. (A) A large fluctuant swelling associated with tooth 65. (B) Elevation of a flap to drain subperiosteal pus. (C) Irrigation of the abscess cavity. (D) Extraction of the offending tooth.

- Irrigate with copious sterile saline or a 50:50 mixture of povidine iodine and water.
- Suturing a drain through the incision may be required to maintain drainage.

Extraoral (Figure 8.18)

Extraoral drainage is typically only required for mandibular swellings.
- Prepare and drape the skin.
- Incise over the most dependent point of the abscess with the No. 15 blade. Hilton's method is used to incise into the abscess along any skin folds and along a line inferior to (if possible) the lower border of mandible. The incision must avoid the marginal branch of the facial nerve, the facial artery and the lower lobe of the parotid gland.
- Enter the abscess cavity with a pair of haemostats, opening the beaks of the forceps to bluntly dissect and establish a flow of pus. It may be necessary to investigate other tissue spaces such as the sublingual, submasseteric or pterygomandibular spaces.
- Take a sample of pus for culture and antibiotic sensitivity testing.
- Copiously irrigate the cavity.
- Suture a drain into the depth of the cavity and place a dressing over the skin.

Management of oral frenula

The management of oral frenula has become a highly controversial topic over the last decade, with concerns that the procedure is prescribed inappropriately and over-performed without due regard for the clinical indications, benefits and possible complications. This has been exacerbated

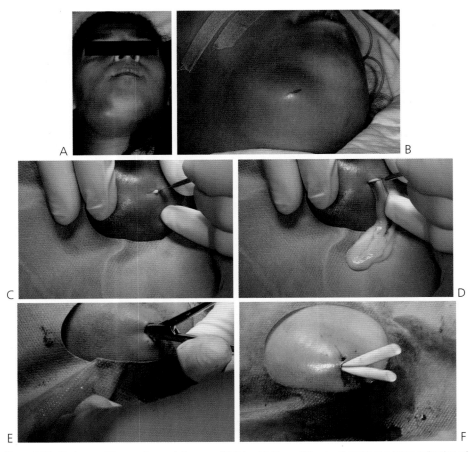

Figure 8.18   Drainage of large extra-oral abscess. (A) This child is acutely unwell and has a large collection of pus in the submandibular space with dysphagia. (B, C) The swelling is fluctuant, and an incision is made into the abscess. (D, E) Drainage is established with a pair of haemostats opening into the cavity and exploring the tissue space. (F) The cavity is kept patent with a flexible drain.

by claims made and debates in social media. Although there are many anecdotal gradings in the lay media, unfortunately there are no standardized, reproducible classifications describing severity that would lead the clinician to decide on a treatment strategy and, ipso facto, a reproducible and documented outcome. Recently, the Australian Dental Association and the American Academy of Pediatric Dentistry have both released policy guidelines on these procedures.

MAXILLARY LABIAL FRENULA

It is common for infants to present with an upper anterior diastema. As more teeth erupt and with the transition to the permanent dentition, especially with the eruption of the maxillary canines, the majority of diastemas will close spontaneously. The upper lip is passive during breastfeeding and bottle feeding and there is no evidence that the labial frenum will affect feeding. There is little involvement in the upper lip during speech. Hence, there are few indications for the early surgical treatment of a thick or short maxillary labial frenum. Furthermore, in the case of persistent anterior diastemas,

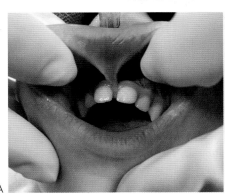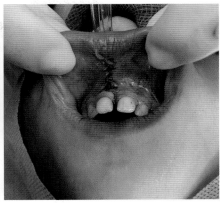

A   B

Figure 8.19 (A) Labial frenectomy with pulling of the frenum into the gingival margin and difficulty for this child to maintain oral hygiene. There is an extremely broad base into the upper lip with a thick frenum extending into the incisive papilla. (B) Postoperative surgical result showing the extent of the dissection but maintenance of the depth of the labial sulcus.

there is general agreement from both paediatric dentists and orthodontists that any surgery is best performed after the eruption of the maxillary canines. If surgery is performed early, then the scar tissue that forms between the central incisors can make space closure more difficult to retain long term; however, if performed in conjunction with orthodontic treatment, the scarring may assist retention.

However, an exception to this recommendation might include pulling of the attached gingiva if the insertion of the frenum is into the gingival margin (Figure 8.19) or an inability of the child to maintain oral hygiene in those cases where the frenum is particularly short and thick. When surgery is required to remove a supernumerary tooth or exposure of an impacted central incisor necessitates raising of a labial mucoperiosteal flap, then a labial frenectomy might be also required to reposition the flap correctly.

MANDIBULAR LABIAL AND BUCCAL FRENULA

Unless there are specific periodontal (gingival) problems caused by the insertion of the freunum (Figure 8.20), there is no indication for surgery.

There is no evidence to support the release of buccal frenula.

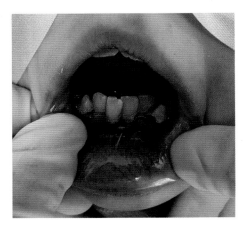

Figure 8.20 High insertion of the lower labial frenum into the free gingival margin resulting in a periodontal defect and subgingival calculus. The child is unable to maintain this area and a frenectomy is indicated.

Lingual frenotomy

A lingual frenotomy (simple cutting of the frenulum) is a procedure indicated in those infants where a tongue-tie is significant, affecting breastfeeding. The mere presence of tongue tie, no matter how 'anatomically' severe, without feeding issues is not an indication for performing this procedure. Interestingly, research has shown that the anatomical severity of tethering has little correlation with the feeding issues, or nipple damage, for example.

In line with current recommendations, a lactation consultant or speech pathologist must assess attachment and feeding practices to determine the need for surgery.

The procedure is performed normally on babies from birth to 4 months of age. Local anaesthesia is not required; however, sucrose (24% solution) may be given for analgesia. There is good evidence for the use of sucrose in managing pain in infants requiring minor surgical or invasive procedures such as newborn screening tests and repeated venesection.

Breastfeeding problems associated with ankyloglossia include:

- Difficult attachment onto the breast.
- Prolonged feeding times, up to 1 hour.
- Frequent feeding, more than every 2 hours.
- Nipple pain or damage.
- Recurrent mastitis.
- Low weight gain or failure to thrive.

Bottle-feeding problems associated with ankyloglossia may include:

- Clicking sounds made by the tongue during feeding.
- Poor saliva control and drooling.
- Swallowing of air while feeding.
- An inconsolable 'colicky' child.

A lingual frenotomy is simple and quick, with few complications. The frenum is usually a very fine translucent tissue in babies, although clinicians should be aware of the risk of a small amount of bleeding and possible postoperative infection. To minimize the risk of infection, parents are advised to sterilize/disinfect any nipple shields, pacifiers and bottles adequately. The tongue is examined by placing two fingers on either side of the frenum in the floor of the mouth (Figure 8.21).

CLINICAL PROCEDURE (Figure 8.22)

- The infant is wrapped (swaddled) to minimize movement.
- A Brodie probe (Figure 8.22A) may be used to retract the ventral surface of the tongue and to stretch the lingual frenulum.

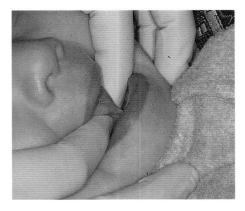

Figure 8.21 Examination of an infant with a severe tongue tie. It is easier to swaddle the child and perform the examination from behind, retracting the tongue with two fingers either side of the frenum.

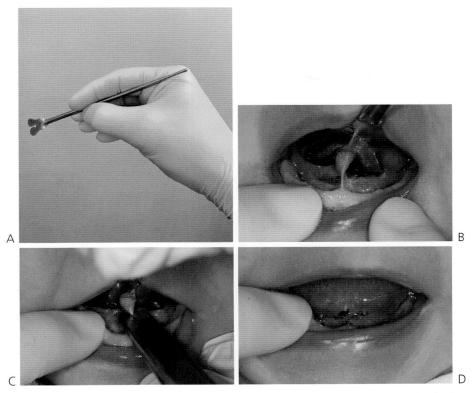

Figure 8.22 Lingual frenotomy. (A) A Brodie probe is useful in retracting the tongue and protecting the floor of the mouth. (B) The tongue is retracted with the Brodie probe. (C) An incision is made in the frenum with blunt-ended dissecting scissors. (D) There is minimal bleeding and the infant can commence breastfeeding immediately.

- Blunt-ended scissors (Metzenbaum, curved blunt 140 cm) are used to release the lingual frenulum, taking care not to injure the submandibular ducts or the ventral surface of the tongue. The cut is made superior to Wharton's (submandibular) duct extending posteriorly but not involving muscle.

The frenum may also be released using a soft tissue laser.

- Once the frenum is released, the baby is immediately placed on the breast/bottle to begin feeding. Postoperative feeding helps to comfort the baby and assists in haemostasis.
- Once haemostasis is achieved, the baby can be discharged.

Reports indicate that this simple procedure, with the addition of appropriate lactation support, leads to successful breastfeeding in most cases. Postoperative stretching should not be performed. There is no evidence as to its efficacy, and at best it may lead to oral aversion.

Lingual frenectomy

A frenectomy is normally carried out under local anaesthesia in older children and under general anaesthesia in younger children. Frenectomy involves surgical excision of the frenum, establishing haemostasis and suturing of the wound. In cases where there is a very short frenum and the floor

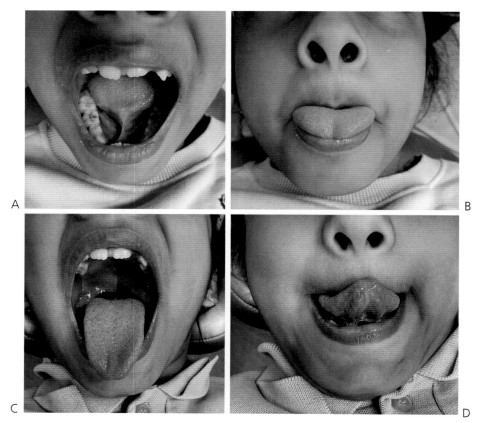

Figure 8.23   (A) A relatively short lingual frenum with the insertion into the tongue tip and a broad gingival origin. (B) The tongue is slightly bifid on protrusion, although the child is not able to protrude past the vermilion border. (C) Postsurgery, there is excellent extension and eversion of the tongue tip (D).

of the mouth is shallow, a Z-plasty is sometimes performed. Indications for lingual frenectomy in the age group older than infancy include:

- A documented restriction of the tip of the tongue, where there is limitation of tongue movement, an inability to evert the tip of the tongue, inability to protrude past the vermilion border or an inability to lateralize the tongue (Figures 8.23 and 8.24).
- Articulation disorders (see Chapter 15), following consultation and referral from a speech pathologist.
- Young child with severe feeding disorders or issues during transition to solids with poor weight gain and a failure of conservative feeding therapies.
- Periodontal problems where the frenum is inserted into the attached gingival margin causing a pulling of the around the tooth (see also Chapter 15, Figure 15.1D).
- Issues of a social nature.

There is no evidence that tongue-ties will result in abnormal growth of the jaws, temporomandibular joint (TMJ) dysfunction, obstructive sleep apnoea, open mouth posture or migrane.

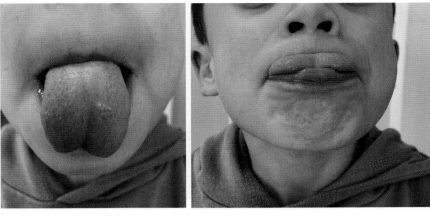

A   B

Figure 8.24 This child has a severe tongue tie that is bifid on protrusion. Although he is able to protrude to the level of the mental fold, he is unable to evert or elevate the tongue tip, resulting in his articulation errors in his speech.

CLINICAL PROCEDURE (Figure 8.25)

- Local anaesthesia is administered into the tip of the tongue and the floor of the mouth on either side of the frenum.
- The tongue may be secured with a large stay suture through the dorsal surface to mobilize, retract and control the tongue.
- A small curved haemostat is clamped parallel to the tongue from the insertion of the lingual frenulum at the tongue tip to a point at the greatest depth and most inferior aspect of the tongue. Iris scissors are used to cut along the jaws of the haemostat, releasing the frenum. A small transverse (horizontal) incision at the base of the haemostat allows for an extension of the incision and lengthening of the base of the tongue.
- The haemostat is then removed and the surgical site is closed with 4-0/5-0 resorbable sutures on the ventral surface of the tongue.
- Postoperative instructions should include analgesia if required. Tongue-tie exercises as prescribed by the speech pathologist are commenced 2 to 3 days postoperatively.

Biopsy of soft tissue lesions (Figures 8.26 and 8.27)

A definitive diagnosis of soft tissue lesions can only be made following histopathological examination; however, biopsy procedures in children are not without potential complications. Consideration must therefore be given as to how the procedure is to be performed, with younger children usually requiring general anaesthesia. There is a risk of damage to adjacent structures, possible scarring and the excessive removal of tissue. Fortunately, life-threatening pathology in the oral cavity of children is rare, and there may be little benefit to the patient in removing tissue simply to confirm the diagnosis of a benign condition. Therefore, if a malignancy or other serious condition is suspected, then the child must be referred to a clinician who is able to manage or treat the patient appropriately.

- An excisional biopsy is recommended for small lesions to completely excise the lesion and to confirm the diagnosis. The biopsy must include a border of normal tissue.

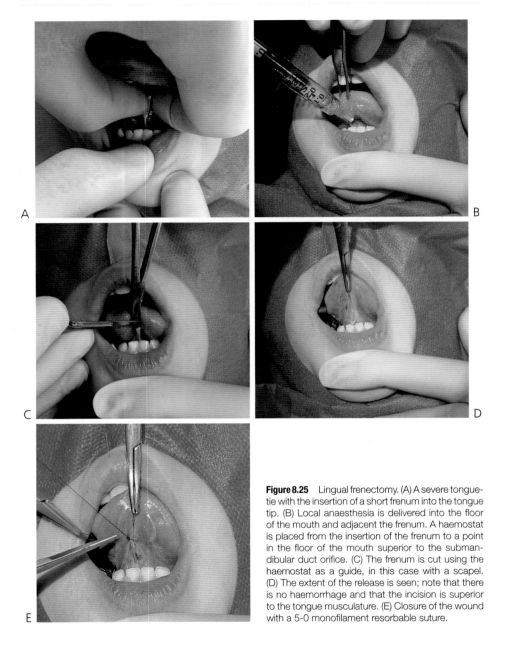

Figure 8.25 Lingual frenectomy. (A) A severe tongue-tie with the insertion of a short frenum into the tongue tip. (B) Local anaesthesia is delivered into the floor of the mouth and adjacent the frenum. A haemostat is placed from the insertion of the frenum to a point in the floor of the mouth superior to the subman-dibular duct orifice. (C) The frenum is cut using the haemostat as a guide, in this case with a scapel. (D) The extent of the release is seen; note that there is no haemorrhage and that the incision is superior to the tongue musculature. (E) Closure of the wound with a 5-0 monofilament resorbable suture.

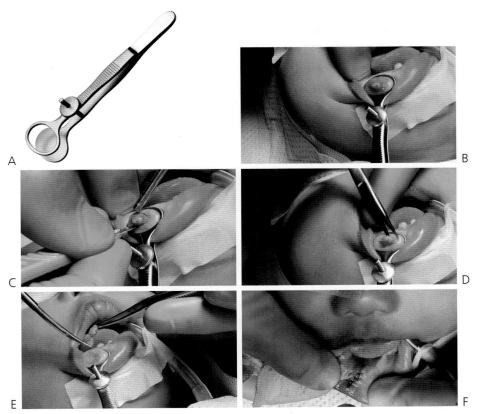

Figure 8.26 Excisional biopsy of exophytic lesions. (A, B) Chalazion forceps are useful for holding and protecting soft tissues when performing biopsies. They allow for stabilization of the tissue but also limit bleeding. A mucocoele on the lower lip of a 9-month-old infant. (C) Elliptical incision through the epithelium. (D) Blunt dissection with fine scissors. The beaks of the scissors are inserted into the incision and then opened to stretch and tear through tissue planes rather than cutting. (E) Removal of the mucoele with the associated accessory salivary glands. (F) Wound closure with a fine resorbable suture.

- An incisional biopsy is performed on larger lesions before complete resection. Incisional biopsies must include the most representative areas of the lesion together with a border of normal tissue to allow study of the margins.

SURGICAL PROCEDURE

- Adequate anaesthesia is essential. Although block anaesthesia may be beneficial, infiltration around the lesion aids haemostasis and provides a dry operating field.
- Elliptical (semi-lunal) incisions surrounding the lesion and tapering to meet at a point under the lesion are placed using a scalpel and No. 15 blade.
- Tissue is carefully dissected out and placed in an appropriate reagent, usually buffered formalin, for transfer to the pathology lab.
- Primary closure is preferred and the biopsy site is sutured with a 4/0 or 5-0 resorbable suture.
- It is essential that the histopathological report is reviewed and the patient followed up with appropriate treatment.

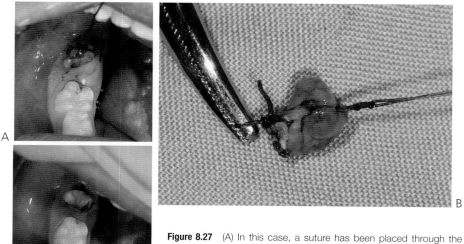

Figure 8.27 (A) In this case, a suture has been placed through the lesion to mobilize it and another (B) around the base in case of haemorrhage. The excised lesion is then sent for histopathological examination. (C) The operculum overlying the erupting 46 tooth has been removed, and haemorrhage has been controlled with diathermy.

Placement of a rubber dam (Figures 8.28 and 8.29)

The use of a rubber dam in restorative procedures is invaluable in restorative dentistry. Although there is reluctance by many clinicians to use a rubber dam, once the technique has been mastered, it becomes a simple and time-saving procedure.

ADVANTAGES

- Protection of the airway from aspiration of instruments, materials or medicaments.
- Provides retraction and protection of soft tissues.
- Improved infection control.
- Improves efficiency because of maintenance of a dry field.
- Superior access and visibility.
- Some evidence to suggest longer restoration survival (Cochrane review).
- Patient compliance.
- Enhanced inhalation and exhaust gas control with inhalation sedation (N_2O).

Modern adhesive restorative materials do not tolerate moisture contamination, and preformed metal crowns can be easily aspirated or ingested by accident in a reclining child patient.

PROCEDURE

When applying a rubber dam, it can be referred to as a 'raincoat for the tooth'. Clamps can be called a 'tooth ring' and introduce the idea that 'it hugs the tooth tightly'. It is important not to place the clamp on the gingiva, as this often causes bleeding and unnecessary discomfort.

Clamps

Rubber dam clamps come in a wide variety of designs to suit various circumstances and preferences. There are two main naming/classification systems for identifying clamps: the Ivory system (based primarily on numbers) and the Ash system (based primarily on letters). Different

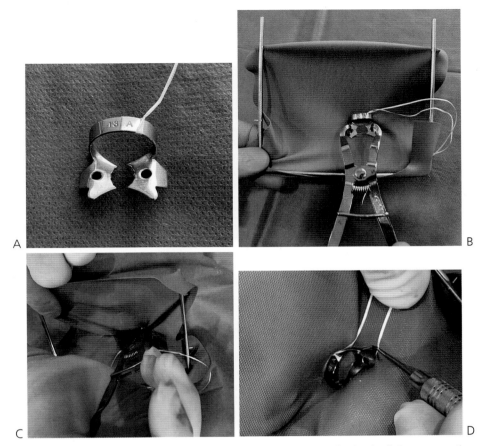

Figure 8.28   Placement of a rubber dam over a single tooth. (A) Winged 'tiger' or 'toothed' clamps are particularly useful on primary molar teeth. The clamp should be secured with dental floss. The rubber dam, frame, the clamp and clamp forceps are arranged (B) and then placed over the tooth in one step (C). (D) The rubber is then lifted from the wings with a flat plastic instrument to seal the tooth.

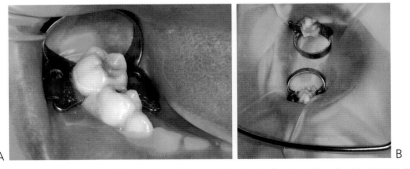

Figure 8.29   (A) The split-dam technique where a large hole (or two holes joined together) is stretched from the most distal clamped tooth to the mesial of the canine. (B) In the operating room, often, two arches can be isolated in this manner.

manufacturers will tend to use one or the other, with the Ivory system being most widely used but there being many equivalent patterns (e.g., Ivory clamps No. 26N and No. 27N, which are often choices for primary molars, are very similar in pattern and usage to Ash BW and DW, respectively).

- Remember to always secure the clamps with dental floss, which should be positioned towards the buccal, to minimize the risk of ingestion/aspiration.
- When selecting a clamp, the aim should be to achieve a stable four-point contact with the cervical area of the crown (two points for each jaw). Once positioned, this can be checked for by trying to rock the clamp gently with a fingertip.
- Clamps with toothed jaws can sometimes grip effectively lingually or palatally without impinging significantly in the gingival margin. For example, the No. 13A clamp is ideal for quadrant 1 and 3 (odd numbered quadrants), and the No. 12A for quadrants 2 and 4. A No. 9 anterior clamp is perfect for anterior strip crowns. The larger circumference of the clamp should be directed towards the buccal aspect.
- Place the clamp on the tooth surface and guide it down the tooth until it is well seated below the bulbosity of the crown. Winged clamps are useful if the rubber dam, clamp and frame are to be placed in one step.
- Rubber dam clamps occasionally fracture, usually across the 'bow' section. The risk of this happening while in the mouth can be minimized by expanding and clamps to the required dimension and locking the clamp forceps outside the mouth before attempting to place the clamp.

Placement (Figure 8.28)

- Local anaesthesia is generally required when the clamp is placed below the gingival margin or the beaks of the clamp impinge into the interdental papilla. A standard buccal infiltration, supplemented with an intra-papillary injection, is usually sufficient.
- A split-dam technique (sometimes known as a 'trough') is frequently used in children using one hole that extends from the second molar (or first permanent molar) to the mesial of the canine. This can be achieved by punching three adjoining overlapping holes in the rubber dam sheet and allows quadrant dentistry to be completed with ease (Figure 8.29A).
- Alternatively, cut one hole for each tooth to be isolated and then stretch the rubber dam sheet over the clamp and individual teeth. Dental floss can be used to guide the rubber through the contact point. Rubber strips or tubes can aid with retention when dealing with open contacts. Finally, stretch the rubber dam onto a frame.
- The whole rubber dam apparatus can be removed by removing the clamp.
- For procedures under general anaesthesia, the double-dam technique is ideal, as it reduces the treatment time (Figure 8.29B).
- Latex-free rubber dam is now widely available and is essential for use in cases where latex allergy is confirmed or suspected.

Space maintainers

The best space maintenance treatment is the preservation of the primary molars until natural exfoliation; however, early loss of carious primary teeth remains one of the most common controllable causes of malocclusion. There is a natural tendency for teeth to drift mesially into space. However, the relative importance of each primary tooth diminishes over time closer to normal exfoliation and, with it, the relative risk of losing space. Currently, there is only poor long-term evidence and a lack of consensus for the use of space maintainers to prevent or reduce the severity of malocclusion. Generally:

- Use of the leeway space: The combined mesiodistal width of the deciduous molars is greater than that of the premolars. This residual space can be used to relieve mild crowding (1–2 mm) elsewhere in the arch.

- More space is lost from early loss of a second primary molar than a first primary molar.
- More space is lost when the second primary molar is extracted before the eruption of the first permanent molar.
- Children who already have crowding may lose more space; however, space maintenance is more important in those children who have a normal arch length.
- Any appliance should be placed within the first few months following tooth loss.

Before a decision is made to provide a space maintainer, it is often essential to critically evaluate its merits, the need and the benefit it would provide to the development of normal occlusion. Although theoretically ideal and preferable to maintain arch space following the premature loss of a primary tooth, there are many factors to consider:

- Placement of a space maintainer requires care of the appliance and oral hygiene maintenance. A child with poor oral hygiene and high caries risk is not the ideal case for such appliance therapy.
- Will the appliance prevent a malocclusion? In many countries, the provision of and access to orthodontic treatment have increased substantially over the last decades, and for those children who will ultimately receive orthodontics and who already have space issues, space loss can be corrected later.
- For what period of time will the appliance be required, and if it fails, can it be easily recemented or replaced? Many children require their treatment to be performed under sedation or general anaesthesia. With such behaviour management problems, will it be possible to manage the child in the dental chair following failure of the maintainer?
- Balancing extractions (i.e., removal of a similar primary tooth of the opposite side of the arch) can help to make any space loss symmetrical and to avoid affecting the dental midline. Balancing extractions may be considered where subsequent space maintenance may not be possible or advisable, where there is a poor prognosis tooth on the other side of the arch, where treatment is being carried out under general anaesthesia or where the risk of further caries progression is deemed to be high (in this circumstance, balancing extraction of, for example, a first primary molar will eliminate posterior primary contacts, improve self-cleansing and minimize approximal caries-risk). If a primary canine is to be extracted, without either space maintenance or a balancing extraction, the risk of centre-line shift is significant, especially where there is significant crowding. In common with space maintenance, the evidence base supporting the value of balancing extractions is relatively weak, and consequently, opinions vary on the relative merit of this technique.

FAILURE OF SPACE MAINTAINERS

Any appliance should last until eruption of the succedaneous tooth. However, the literature reports high failure rates for all such devices. Retrospective studies showed that over 60% of appliances will fail and that the mean survival rate was between 7 and 20 months.

- Fibre-reinforced composite resin has up to 80% failure within 12 months.
- Band and loop maintainers have the longest survival rate (up to 13 months).
- Most are lost because of issues with cementation.
- Distal shoe appliances may cause issues with eruption of the permanent tooth, plaque retention and tissue irritation.
- Lower lingual arches have the poorest long-term survival.
- It is better to remake rather than recement.

TYPES OF SPACE MAINTAINER

Removable space maintainers have shortcomings similar to all removable appliances:

- They may be worn at the whim of the patient.
- May be broken.
- Easily lost when removed by the patient.

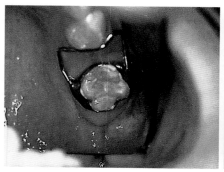
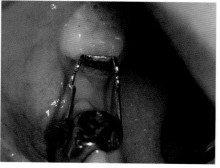

A   B

Figure 8.30   (A) A band and loop space maintainer. The placement of a space maintainer must not compromise the permanent tooth. Bands should be cemented with a luting glass ionomer as a protection against caries and the appliance reviewed regularly. As the premolar erupts, the appliance is removed when there is interference with normal emergence. (B) A distal shoe space maintainer is place following early loss of the second primary molar before the eruption of the first permanent molar. It prevents mesial migration of the permanent tooth.

A removable space maintainer that is worn only at night is often sufficient to hold space and prevent the mesial drift of permanent molars. Night-only wearing of the appliance also reduces the risk of loss or breakage by the patient. The appliance should be washed and inserted in place before going to bed, then removed, washed and placed in a safe place when not worn. A Hawley appliance is a typical example.

Fixed space maintainers have the advantage that they are worn continuously and do not require patient cooperation in wearing them.

- It should be noted that the placement of a fixed appliance in a child at high risk of caries may compromise those teeth which are banded as well as adjacent teeth.
- Band and loop appliance (Figure 8.30A) is typically used in cases of unilateral loss.
- Distal shoe appliances (Figure 8.30B) are used when a second primary molar has been extracted before the eruption of the first permanent molar.
- A transpalatal arch is used in the maxilla.
- A lingual arch is used in the mandible.
- Nance appliance or lingual arch can be used if the loss is bilateral.

Further reading

American Academy of Pediatric Dentistry, 2019. Policy on management of the Frenulum in pediatric dental patients. Available: https://www.aapd.org/globalassets/media/policies_guidelines/p_mgmt_frenulum.pdf.

Australian Dental Association, 2020. Ankyloglossia and Oral Frena consensus statement. Available: https://www.ada.org.au/Dental-Professionals/Publications/Ankyloglossia-Statement/Ankyloglossia-and-Oral-Frena-Consensus-Statement_J.aspx.

Sasa, I.S., Hasan, A.A. & Qudeimat, M.A., 2019. Longevity of Band and Loop Space Maintainers Using Glass Ionomer Cement: A Prospective Study. European Archives of Paediatric Dentistry 10, 6–10. Available: https://doi.org/10.1007/BF03262659.

Stevens, B., Yamada, J., Ohlsson, A., et al., 2017. Sucrose for analgesia (pain relief) in newborn infants undergoing painful procedures. Cochrane Database of Systematic Reviews 7, CD001069.

Royal College of Surgeons of England, 2017. LocSSIPS toolkit dental extraction. Available: https://www.rcseng.ac.uk/dental-faculties/fds/publications-guidelines/locssips-toolkit-dental-extraction/.

Wang, Y., Li, C., Yuan, H., et al., 2016. Rubber dam isolation for restorative treatment in dental patients. Cochrane Database of Systematic Reviews 9, CD009858.

CHAPTER 9

Trauma management

Angus C. Cameron ▓ Richard P. Widmer ▓ Marc Semper ▓
Andrew A.C. Heggie ▓ Paul Abbott

Pulp necrosis and infection of the coronal fragment

Pulp necrosis and infection of both the apical and coronal fragments

Crown/root fractures

Uncomplicated crown/root fracture

Complicated crown/root fracture (i.e., with pulp exposure)

Crown/root fractures in immature teeth

Luxations in the permanent dentition

Concussion and subluxation

Lateral and extrusive luxation

Intrusion

Dentoalveolar fractures

Pulp status

Avulsion of permanent teeth

First aid advice

Management in the dental surgery

Complications in endodontic management of avulsed teeth

External inflammatory root resorption

External replacement root resorption

Questions concerning the long-term management of avulsed teeth

Other considerations and options for management of the resorbing incisor

Autotransplantation

Indications

Success rates

Procedure for autotransplantation

Reasons for an unfavourable outcome

Internal bleaching of root-filled incisors

Method

Soft tissue injuries

Alveolar mucosa and skin

Attached gingival tissues

Prevention

Education of parents and caregivers

Introduction

The management of dentoalveolar trauma in children is distressing for both the child and the parent (Figure 9.1), and it is often difficult for the dentist. However, trauma is one of the most common presentations of young children to a paediatric dentist. The patient's emergency must be the dentist's routine. The child should be carefully assessed regarding treatment needs before commenting to parents, because many cases are not as bad as they first appear. Initial reassurance to both parent and child is of great value. Trauma not only compromises a previously healthy dentition but may also leave a deficit that affects the self-esteem and quality of life, and it commits the patient to lifelong dental maintenance.

Guidelines for the management of dental injuries

The International Association of Dental Traumatology (IADT) published guidelines in 2020 with recommendations for the management of dental injuries based on a review of the literature and consensus opinions. These guidelines provide views on care based on the published evidence and the opinions of professionals who practice in this field. As is stated in the guidelines, there is no guarantee of success, and as further research is published, clearly the recommendations in these guidelines will be updated. The practitioner should be aware that clinical judgement is still required, depending on the presentation of each case. An internet-based set of suggestions of treatment approaches based on published research has also been developed in conjunction with the University Hospital of Copenhagen and the IADT (www .dentaltraumaguide.org). This is a website that practitioners can use to quickly and easily access information about how to manage dental injuries, the prognosis of the teeth and many other details.

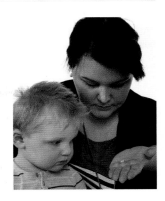

Figure 9.1 The presentation of a child with trauma is distressing for parent and child. The child in other instances may be oblivious to what has happened and is happily playing in the surgery.

Aetiology

Most injuries are caused by falls and play accidents. Luxation injuries to the upper anterior teeth predominate in toddlers because of their frequent falls during play and attempts at walking. Injuries are generally more common in boys. Blunt trauma tends to cause greater damage to the soft tissues and supporting structures, whereas high-velocity or sharp injuries cause luxations and fractures of the teeth. Data differ from various published sources; however, in Australia, where the use of mouthguards is mandatory for most organized contact sports, the frequency of dental injuries from this area tends to be lower. Consistently, the maxillary incisors are those most affected.

PREDISPOSING FACTORS

- Class II division 1 malocclusion.
- Overjet 3–6 mm: double the frequency of trauma to incisor teeth compared with 0–3 mm overjet.
- Overjet greater than 6 mm: threefold increase in the risk.

The study summarized in Table 9.1, by Warren et al. (2014), from The Children's Hospital, Westmead, in Sydney, shows that falls and play accidents account for the majority of injuries. Importantly, although accounting for only 1% of all injuries, over 80% of child abuse occurs in the very young child. Dog bites account for a significant number of injuries, and every year several children are killed by dogs. It is common that the dog is known to the child, and it cannot be stressed too highly that children must be supervised when around even the most timid of animals.

FREQUENCY

- 90% of dental trauma occurs before the age of 20 years.
- 10%–30% of children suffer trauma to the primary dentition. This figure may represent up to 20% of all injuries in preschool children.
- 22% of children suffer trauma to the permanent dentition by the age of 14 years.
- It is estimated that 1 billion people living in the world have suffered a dental injury (Petti et al., 2018).
- Children who sustain trauma to their dentition are more likely to have multiple dental injuries over their childhood. 45% have damaged the same tooth.
- Male : female ratio is 2 : 1.
- Peak incidence is at 2 to 4 years and rises again at 8 to 10 years.

TABLE 9.1 ■ **Causes of maxillofacial injuries in children presenting after-hours at a children's hospital emergency service (The Children's Hospital, Westmead)**

Cause of injury	Total, %
Accident during play	33.2
Fall (on ground)	31
Non-motorized vehicle accidents	19.0
Fall (from height)	6.8
Water-related accidents	6.3
Organized sport	5.8
Other	2.6
Motor vehicle accidents	1.6
Unknown by carer	0.5
Total	100

(From Warren, M., Widmer, M., Arora, R,. et al., 2014. After hours presentation of traumatic dental injuries to a major paediatric teaching hospital. Australian Dental Journal 59, 172–179.)

- Most paediatric dental injuries occur before or after lunch, and more commonly outdoors on weekends. There is a tendency of injuries to occur in spring and autumn rather than in summer or winter months
- The upper anterior teeth are the most commonly involved teeth, especially the central incisors (in both the primary and permanent dentitions).
- Usually only a single tooth is involved, except in cases of motor vehicle accidents and sporting injuries.

Child abuse

Child abuse is defined as those acts or omissions of care that deprive a child of the opportunity to fully develop his/her unique potential as a person either physically, socially or emotionally. There are four types of child abuse:
- Physical abuse
- Sexual abuse
- Emotional abuse
- Neglect

Dental neglect is the knowing failure of a parent or guardian to access treatment of orofacial conditions for a child. When left untreated, such conditions may adversely affect a child's normal growth and development.

The true incidence of child abuse and neglect is unknown, and although there is increasing awareness and reporting, professionals are still reluctant to deal with it. The first step in preventing abuse is recognition and reporting. Dentists are in a strategic position to recognize and report mistreated children because they often see the child and parent/caretaker interacting during multiple visits and over a long period of time.

The orofacial region is commonly traumatized during episodes of child abuse (Figure 9.2). Injuries that do not match the given history, bruising of soft tissue not overlying bony prominences, injury that takes the shape of a recognizable object and multiple injuries of different ages

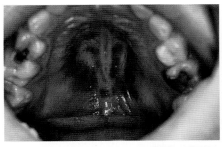
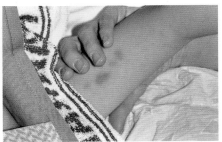

A   B

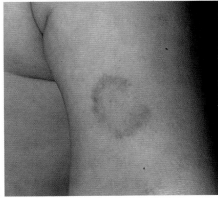

Figure 9.2 (A) Child abuse caused by sexual assault by a family member. Commonly, the perpetrator is known to the child. (B) Bruising on the arm of an infant discovered during routine dental treatment under general anaesthesia. (C) An 18-month-old infant who was bitten by an older child. Good photographic records are required, and the wounds should not be washed until specimens for DNA testing of saliva are taken. The child assault team will organize appropriate input from social workers, paediatricians and the police, if necessary. The dentist should also be aware of the legal requirements for recording of evidence (i.e., standardized photography with measuring scale).

C

may be the result of nonaccidental trauma. Bite marks in children represent child abuse until proven otherwise. The characteristics and diagnostic findings of child abuse, and the protocol of reporting such cases, should be familiar to the dentist so that appropriate notification, treatment and prevention of further injury can be instituted.

Whenever injuries are inconsistent with the history, the patient must be investigated for abuse. There is a legal obligation in some countries or states to report the suspicion of child abuse or sexual assault. In Australia, child abuse teams are available at all paediatric hospitals or through the departments of family and community services.

History

As dental injuries may become the subject of litigation or insurance claims, a thorough history and examination are mandatory. Where possible, injuries should be photographed. An accurate history gives important information regarding:

- Status of the dentition at presentation.
- Prognosis of injuries.
- Other injuries sustained.
- Medical complications.
- Possible litigation.

QUESTIONS TO ASK

- When, where and how did the trauma occur?
- Were there any other injuries?
- What initial treatment was given?

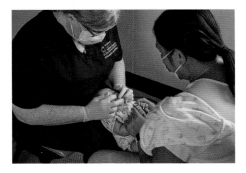

Figure 9.3 One of the most convenient ways to examine young children is with the child's head in the dentist's lap. The child can see the parent, who gently restrains the arms. This gives an excellent view of the upper teeth and jaws, where most trauma occurs.

- Have there been any other dental injuries in the past?
- Are immunizations up to date?

Examination

Examination should be undertaken in a logical order. It is important to examine the whole body, as the patient may present first to the dentist and other injuries may also have occurred (Figure 9.3).

TRAUMA EXAMINATION AND RECORDS

- Extraoral wounds and palpation of the facial skeleton (Figure 9.4).
- Injuries to oral mucosa or gingivae.
- Palpation of the alveolus.
- Displacement of teeth.
- Abnormalities in occlusion.
- Extent of tooth fractures, pulp exposure, colour changes.
- Mobility of teeth.
- Reaction to pulp sensibility tests and percussion.

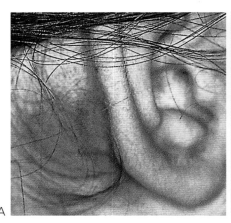
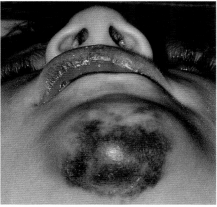

A   B

Figure 9.4 (A) The 'battle sign', or bruising of the mastoid region, is associated with a base-of-skull fracture. Examination must include all areas of the head and neck, which often requires parting the hair to detect lacerations and bruising. (B) Bruising is a collection of blood which will fall to the most dependent point. The chin-point ecchymosis shown here is often associated with gingival degloving, laceration and/or a mandibular fracture.

TABLE 9.2 ■ Assessment of cranial nerves involved in facial trauma

	Cranial nerve	Function	Deficit following injury
I	Olfactory	Olfaction	Inability to smell
II	Optic	Vision	Visual deficit, blindness
III	Oculomotor	Movements of the globe	Ptosis, strabismus and diplopia Inability to open eyelid Open pupil
IV	Trochlear	Superior rectus	Inability to turn globe downwards and medially
V	Trigeminal	Muscles of mastication	Loss of sensation to face. Weakness or paralysis of muscles of mastication
VI	Abducent	Lateral rectus	Inability to abduct the eye: strabismus and diplopia
VII	Facial	Muscles of facial expression	Paralysis of muscles of facial expression
VIII	Vestibulocochlear	Hearing and balance	Loss of hearing and balance during mobilization
IX	Glossopharyngeal	Sensation of posterior third of tongue, parotid secretion	Diminished gag reflex Asymmetric elevation of palate
X	Vagus	Contraction of larynx	
XI	Spinal accessory	Rotation of head and shoulder function	Inability to shrug shoulders
XII	Hypoglossal	Tongue movement	Deviation of tongue to the affected side

HEAD INJURY

Closed head injury is the most common cause of childhood mortality in accidents. Between 25% and 50% of all accidents in children aged up to 14 years involve the head. If there is any suggestion that a head injury has been sustained, the child should be immediately medically assessed, preferably in a paediatric casualty department. An assessment of cranial nerve function should be performed, and a summary is shown in Table 9.2.

Signs of closed head injury

- Altered or loss of consciousness.
- Bleeding from the head or ears.
- Disorientation.
- Prolonged headache.
- Nausea, vomiting, amnesia.
- Altered vision or unilateral dilated pupil.
- Seizures or convulsions.
- Speech difficulties.

Dentoalveolar injuries may take second place if there is central nervous system involvement. As a head injury may be long-lasting, initial management and replantation may be possible in consultation with other medical practitioners. If there is any loss of consciousness, hourly neurological observations should be commenced. The Glasgow Coma Scale is commonly used in accident and emergency departments to assess the severity of head injury and prognosis (see Appendix G).

Investigations

RADIOGRAPHS

The request for radiographs should only be made after a thorough history and clinical examination. There is great value in using extraoral films in young children, for example, panoramic radiographs. In the very upset or difficult child, it may be the only way that some clinical information can be gained in the acute phase of management.

When taking intraoral radiographs, several periapical images from different angulations should be taken for each traumatized tooth, plus an anterior occlusal radiograph. These are especially important to determine the presence of root fractures and tooth luxations. As a baseline, all traumatized teeth should be radiographed to assess:

- The stage of root development.
- Injuries to the roots and supporting structures.
- The degree and direction of luxation or displacement.

GUIDE TO PRESCRIPTION OF RADIOGRAPHS (see Appendix I)

Dentoalveolar injuries

- Periapical radiographs.
- Anterior maxillary occlusal or anterior mandibular occlusal.
- Panoramic radiograph.
- True lateral maxilla for intrusive luxations of primary anterior teeth and alveolar fracture (Day et al., 2020).
- Cone-beam computed tomography (CBCT).

There is now sufficient published evidence that CBCT enables an enhanced visualization of traumatic dental injuries with regards to the localization and extent and the direction of specific injuries such as root fractures, crown/root fractures and lateral luxations. With these specific injuries, three-dimensional (3D) imaging can be useful and should be considered (Bourguignon et al., 2020; Cohenca & Silberman, 2017; Cohenca, Simon, Mathur, et al., 2007; Cohenca, Simon, Roges, et al., 2007).

Condylar fracture (Figure 9.5)

- Panoramic radiograph, closed and open mouth.
- CBCT or computed tomography (CT) scan.

Mandibular fracture

- Panoramic radiograph.
- True mandibular and anterior mandibular occlusal (for parasymphyseal fractures).
- CBCT or CT scan.
- Lateral oblique (this is rarely used today except in cases where a CT is unavailable).

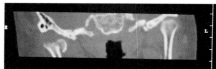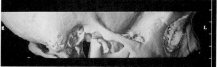

A   B

Figure 9.5 Use of computed tomographic reformatting to visualize fractures to the mandibular condyle. (A) Coronal section showing an intracapsular fracture with medial displacement of the condylar head owing to the pull of medial pterygoid muscle. (B) Three-dimensional reconstruction showing the degree of displacement of the condylar head following chin-point trauma.

Maxillary fractures

- CBCT or CT scan.

New imaging technologies have superseded older-style views such as the lateral oblique, the reverse Towne and Waters (occipitomental 30 degrees) projections. Although such radiographs may be valuable in particular cases, contemporary practice indicates the use of fine-slice CT or CBCT for an accurate assessment of middle third fractures in children.

PULP SENSIBILITY TESTS

Pulp sensibility tests provide an essential baseline measure of the pulp status. It is common that there may be no response to pulp tests at the initial presentation following trauma; however, it is important that results are recorded for later comparison. The results of pulp sensibility tests performed immediately following trauma are also very useful predictors of the prognosis of traumatized teeth. Teeth that do respond to these tests are more likely to recover than teeth that do not respond. Young children often find it difficult to discriminate between the touch of the tester and the actual stimulus itself, so the clinician must be aware of the possibility of false results. In cases that are difficult to diagnose, isolation of individual teeth under rubber dam may be required.

Pulp sensibility tests are used to help assess the status of the pulp. Previously and erroneously termed 'vitality tests', the contemporary terminology (i.e., sensibility tests) stresses the fact that the neural and vascular components of the pulp tissue need individual consideration. Sensibility is defined as the 'ability to respond to a stimulus' – which is what is tested with thermal and electric pulp tests. It is important to understand that a tooth may not respond to a thermal or electric pulp test but it may still have an intact blood supply. Such discrimination of the health of the pulp is important in planning treatment.

Thermal pulp tests

Responses to cold stimuli give the most reliable and accurate results in children (even with immature teeth). The carbon dioxide (dry ice) pencil is regarded as the most convenient. Cold sprays may also be used but are not as accurate or as reliable. Cold tests have the advantage that assessment of the pulp is possible while temporary crowns and splints are in place.

Electric pulp tests

Electric pulp tests may give a graded response to stimuli. When using these instruments, the current should be slowly increased so that sudden painful stimulation of the tooth is avoided.

Laser Doppler flowmetry and pulse oximetery

New technologies offer the potential for more accurate measurement of pulp vitality. Laser Doppler flowmetry provides a direct measurement of pulp blood flow and assesses vitality but not sensory function. It has been researched extensively in traumatized teeth to assess the extent of revascularization. Pulse oximetry could be a more reliable method of assessing vitality by measuring oxygen saturation levels within the pulp. These are emerging devices and their uses will increase over time.

Percussion

There are two reasons to percuss teeth:

- Tenderness to percussion gives information about the extent of damage to the periapical tissues and the periodontal ligament. Tenderness to percussion can also indicate that a tooth has been concussed or subluxated. The percussion of luxated teeth will usually be painful, but there is no need to percuss teeth that are obviously luxated on visual examination.

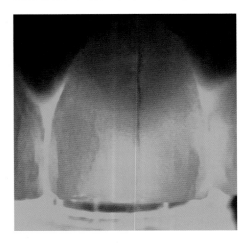

Figure 9.6 Transillumination to detect enamel infarctions.

- The sound in response to percussion, especially during follow-up examinations, is also an important indicator of the presence of ankylosis.

Transillumination (Figure 9.6)

This is an extremely useful, noninvasive technique to assess the presence of cracks and/or fractures and subtle alterations in crown colour which may indicate a change in the pulp status.

Other considerations in trauma management

Having carefully assessed the patient, the only treatment necessary may be to reassure the child and parent, and to discuss the various possible sequelae such as pulp necrosis, resorption, infection and facial swelling.

FASTING REQUIREMENTS

If the patient requires extensive work under general anaesthesia, it is important to check fasting details. A child over 6 years of age must be fasted for at least 6 hours without solids or liquids. Children under the age of 6 years must be fasted for 6 hours without solids and 2 hours without liquids. If it is anticipated that treatment under general anaesthesia will be required, then inform the parents or carers early so that the child does not eat (while awaiting treatment), necessitating a delay in access to surgery.

IMMUNIZATIONS

If a child has sustained an injury that involves contamination of the wound with soil, especially from a farm area, their tetanus immunization status must be determined. If the child has completed their normal immunization schedule, under normal circumstances, boosters are not required.

Maxillofacial injuries

Fractures of the facial bones are uncommon in children and account for less than 5% of all maxillofacial fractures. Consequently, fewer surgeons have extensive experience in managing these cases that require an understanding of the implications of such injuries for the growing child (Figure 9.7).

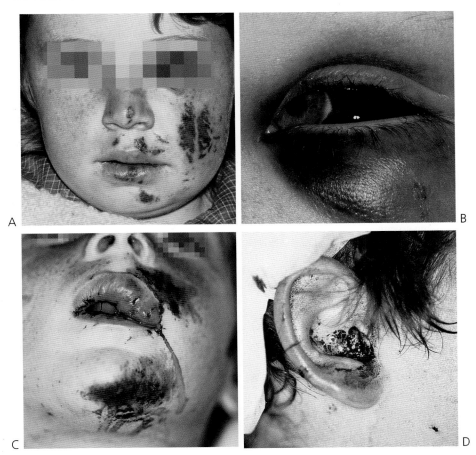

Figure 9.7   (A, B) This girl fell from a Tarzan rope onto her face. There is extensive ecchymosis and subconjunctival haemorrhage. Although many of the signs of a zygomatic fracture are present, the immaturity of the frontozygomatic suture allowed for some displacement and there was no fracture evident. (C, D) Many children suffer chin-point trauma, and it is important to check the mandibular condyles. This boy sustained a right subcondylar fracture. There was bleeding from the external meatus, as the condyle had perforated the anterior wall of the meatus. Under no circumstances should the ear be suctioned because the ossicles may be removed if the tympanic membrane is ruptured.

With younger patients having a relatively greater upper-to-lower facial ratio, the pattern of fractures changes with the development of the maxilla-mandibular complex into adolescence.

PRINCIPLES OF MANAGEMENT

The management of maxillofacial trauma in a child is influenced by factors such as the difficulty of taking a history, parental anxiety, the unerupted dentition and the more common association of closed head injuries that may delay definitive treatment. The use of internal fixation such as mini-plates and screws must be undertaken with care because of the potential for damaging developing tooth buds. Although arch bars may be used if there are sufficient teeth, acrylic cap splints may be still used effectively. Many undisplaced fractures can be managed conservatively.

For displaced fractures, accurate reduction, fixation and immobilization will result in union within 3 weeks. Prophylactic antibiotic treatment and strict oral care must be maintained, but fortunately, nonunion or fibrous unions are rare.

FRACTURED MANDIBLE

Most mandibular fractures involve the parasymphyseal region (owing to the position of the unerupted canine and the paucity of bone) and the condyle either in isolation or in combination.

Clinical signs

- Pain, swelling.
- Trismus.
- Occlusal discrepancies.
- Stepping at the lower border.
- Sublingual/buccal ecchymosis (Figure 9.8).
- Chin asymmetry.
- Paraesthesia of the mental nerve distribution.

Management

- Reduction and fixation using arch bars with dental 'bridle' wires or elastic intermaxillary fixation. Lower-border mini-plates or resorbable plates may be indicated to maintain reduction.
- Occlusal or lingual splints may be attached with glass ionomer or retained with circum-mandibular wiring.

CONDYLAR FRACTURES

Fractures of the mandibular condyle are under-diagnosed in children and comprise up to two-thirds of all mandibular injuries. This injury usually results from trauma to the chin at the lower border. If a subcondylar fracture occurs, the condylar head is usually displaced antero-medially by the action of the lateral pterygoid muscle. Depending on the displacement of the fragments and the compensatory posturing of the mandible, there may be deviation of the chin to the affected side or there may be no occlusal disharmony. Bleeding from the external meatus may occur because of perforation of the anterior wall of the auditory canal by the condylar head (see Figure 9.7C, D).

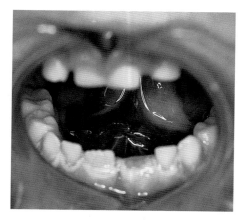

Figure 9.8 The sublingual haematoma is pathogno-monic for a fractured mandible in the symphysis or in the canine region of the body.

Bleeding or discharge from the ear should be investigated by an otolaryngologist, but suctioning of the external meatus is contraindicated because of the potential for disturbance of the ossicular chain should there be a perforation of the tympanic membrane. Displacement of the condylar head into the middle cranial fossa has been reported but is a rare event.

As a general rule, the younger the child, the higher the fracture will occur within the condyle, and in young children there is a higher incidence of intracapsular fractures that may occur either in the sagittal or coronal planes.

Management

Treatment is almost always conservative, with a short period of rest followed by the encouragement of active movement to prevent temporomandibular joint ankylosis. Fractures of the condylar neck, involving telescoping of the condyle and distal fragment, may be successfully treated with functional appliances for 2 to 3 weeks or longer, allowing better remodelling. Bilateral subcondylar fractures may result in a posterior mandibular displacement with an anterior open bite. A short period of intermaxillary fixation with posterior bite blocks to distract the fragments may be indicated in such cases, to minimize the consequent malocclusion. For patients with a low, displaced subcondylar fracture and who are nearing the completion of growth, an open reduction and plate fixation may be indication for an accurate reduction, if sufficient bone volume enables fixation of the proximal fragment.

As the condylar neck is relatively broader in the child with a greater volume of cancellous bone, fractures of the articular surface are more common than in the adult, and the resulting haematoma formation may prevent normal function and growth. In cases of intracapsular fracture (Figures 9.5 and 9.9), follow-up for several years will enable detection of any growth disturbance. Should there be a progressive limitation of opening or bony ankylosis, early intervention to mobilize and/or reconstruct the mandible is recommended.

MAXILLARY FRACTURES

Middle-third fractures are rare in children and usually present in severe cranio-maxillofacial injuries. Mid-facial fractures tend not to follow the typical 'Le Fort' level lines, as the immature skeleton results in more greenstick and incomplete fractures.

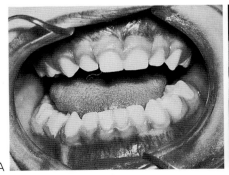
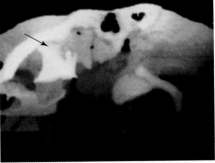

A   B

Figure 9.9 (A, B) Mandibular asymmetry caused by a dislocation of the left condyle after play equipment fell on this young girl. Imaging of these injuries can be difficult, and in this case, a computed tomography (CT) scan was performed with three-dimensional reconstruction to detail the injury. The CT demonstrates the dislocation, with the condylar head (*arrow*) anterior to the articular eminence and lying under the zygomatic arch. As is common with these injuries in children, an intracapsular fracture-dislocation is present, which remodelled itself without treatment. Normal function was achieved within 6 months.

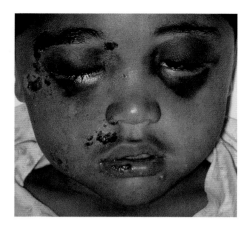

Figure 9.10 Middle-third fracture of the face in a child involved in a motor vehicle accident. Note the bilateral periorbital ecchymosis and swelling resulting in closure of the eyes. Despite the appearance, there was only minimal displacement of the maxilla, although external fixation was required to reduce the depressed nasal fracture.

Orbital floor 'blow-out' fractures also occur because of bony displacement and elasticity. Orbital contents, such as fascia and the inferior rectus muscles, herniate into the sinus and remain incarcerated in the fracture line, thus preventing normal ocular movements accompanied by vagal symptoms. Urgent reduction is usually required.

Clinical signs

- Facial swelling and periorbital ecchymosis (Figure 9.10).
- Periorbital surgical emphysema.
- Subconjunctival haemorrhage, with no posterior limit.
- Diplopia.
- Nausea, vomiting and photophobia often occur with inferior rectus muscle entrapment.
- Orbital rim contour deformities.
- Mid-facial mobility.
- Infraorbital paraesthesia (Figure 9.11).
- Cerebrospinal fluid rhinorrhoea.
- Epistaxis.
- Malocclusion.

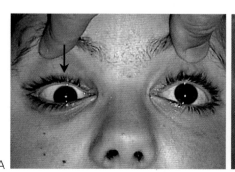
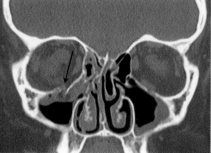

A   B

Figure 9.11 (A) Limitation of upward gaze associated with right orbital floor 'blow-out' fracture. (B) Coronal computed tomography scan demonstrating 'trapdoor' orbital floor fracture with tissue entrapment.

Management

- Conservative management is usual unless there is significant displacement of the mid-facial complex. In this situation, open reduction with or without semi-rigid internal fixation is required.
- Maxillary dentoalveolar fractures are managed with arch bars or bonded orthodontic appliances after reduction. More severe displaced fractures will require reduction and mini-plate fixation.
- More severe and displaced maxillary fractures will require reduction and mini-plate fixation.
- Orbital 'blow-out' fractures with soft tissue entrapment are a surgical emergency and must be explored as soon as possible for release of orbital contents for recovery of muscle function.

Sequelae of fractures of the jaws in children

CLOSED HEAD INJURY

Children who sustain middle-third facial injuries usually have concomitant head injuries. Head injuries occur in 25% of cases of facial trauma. These children spend extended periods in intensive care units, may undergo personality changes, suffer posttraumatic amnesia and may have episodes of neuropathological chewing.

TOOTH LOSS

Approximately 10% of children who sustain fractures of the jaws will also have loss of permanent teeth.

DEVELOPMENTAL DEFECTS OF TEETH

In addition to the damage caused by displacement of primary teeth into the crypts of permanent successors (see 'Sequelae of trauma to primary teeth' later in the chapter), unerupted teeth in the line of jaw fractures may also be damaged. Defects may include:
- Hypoplasia or hypomineralization of enamel.
- Dilaceration of crown and roots.
- Displacement of the developing tooth within the bone.
- Arrest of tooth development with pulp canal calcification.

INTRA-ARTICULAR DAMAGE TO THE TEMPOROMANDIBULAR JOINT (Figure 9.12A–C)

There is always a risk of ankylosis of the temporomandibular joint after significant displacement of the condylar head, intracapsular fracture or a failure to achieve early mobilization of the joint. Treatment of the ankylosis involves condylectomy and joint reconstruction with a costochondral graft in later childhood.

GROWTH RETARDATION

Maxillary (Figure 9.12D) and mandibular growth retardation may occur following major trauma. Significant scarring of soft tissues and/or tissue loss may inhibit jaw growth. Mandibular asymmetry with antegonial notching may occur on the affected side after subcondylar fracture. The key to management is to correct asymmetries early to avoid secondary maxillary deformity.

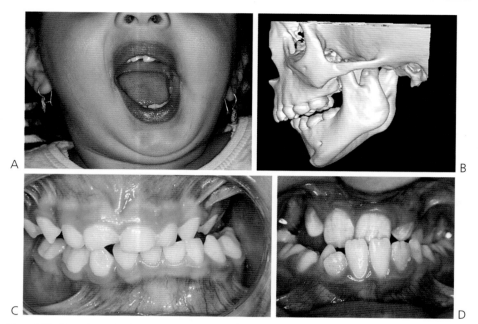

Figure 9.12 Sequelae to jaw fractures in children. (A) Left intracapsular and condylar neck fracture in a 4-year-old girl. There is deviation of the chin-point on opening to the affected side. (B) Remodelling of the left condyle has resulted in shortening of the neck. (C) The intraoral view shows the midline shift in centric occlusion and the left posterior crossbite. (D) Maxillary hypoplasia and growth retardation, following in a child, 8 years after sustaining a middle third fracture.

Luxations in the primary dentition

GENERAL MANAGEMENT CONSIDERATIONS

There is general agreement that most injuries to the primary dentition can be managed conservatively and heal without sequelae. Up to 2 years of age, the most common injuries to the primary teeth are luxations involving displacement of the teeth in the alveolar bone.

As a general rule, either leave and observe or extract the tooth. Although there is a desire to save every tooth, a pragmatic approach to treatment is essential. Severely luxated primary teeth may be splinted; however, these splints need also to be removed, and the cooperation at the first appointment may not occur at subsequent visits. It is always advised that treatment be performed by those with experience in trauma management in a child-centred environment (Figure 9.13).

Immunization

If the child is not fully immunized, then a tetanus booster is required: tetanus toxoid 0.5 mL by intramuscular injection.

Antibiotics

Unless there are significant soft tissue or dentoalveolar injuries, antibiotics are not usually required. Antibiotics are prescribed empirically as a prophylaxis against infection, but they are not a substitute for proper debridement of wounds. All drugs should be prescribed according to the child's weight (see Appendix H).

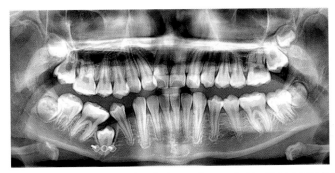

Figure 9.13 Orthopantomogram demonstrating the issue of unerupted teeth occurring in paediatric mandibular fractures. This child suffered a fracture to the right body of mandible 2 years before this radiograph. The fracture would have occurred in the area of greater weakness of the bone because of the unerupted and impacted 45 tooth. There is no contraindication for leaving developing teeth within lines of fractures, but the miniplate and screws used for fixation are too close to the tooth. Dental understanding is required for the best management because, in this case, the tooth and plate should have been subsequently removed to facilitate orthodontic treatment. Leaving a tooth in this position will always compromise the mandible and leave a periodontal defect on the mesial of the 46 tooth. (Courtesy Dr. Deepika Katragadda, Queensland.)

Homecare

A soft diet is recommended; however, most children will avoid biting hard foods if their teeth are mobile. The traumatized area should be kept clean. Toothbrushing might prove difficult in the younger child, but the area can be swabbed with gauze, moistened with alcohol-free chlorhexine. Parents and carers should be warned about possible sequelae.

CONCUSSION AND SUBLUXATION (Figure 9.14)

Concussion is an injury to the tooth and periodontal ligament without displacement or mobility of the tooth. Subluxation occurs when the tooth is mobile but is not displaced. Both involve minor damage to the periodontal ligament. Teeth with these injuries will be tender to percussion. There will be haemorrhage and oedema within the ligament, but gingival bleeding and mobility only occur if the teeth have been subluxated.

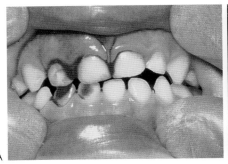
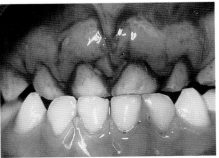

A   B

Figure 9.14 (A) Subluxation of the upper right incisors with minimal displacement. (B) Palatal luxation of the upper incisors resulting in an occlusal interference. These teeth can be repositioned by digital pressure, only to relieve the interference. Further anterior movement may damage the permanent teeth.

Management

- Periapical radiographs as baseline in cases of subluxation, but are not required in cases of suspected concussion.
- Soft diet for 1 week.
- Advice to the parents of possible sequelae, such as pulp necrosis and infection.
- Individualized follow-up.

INTRUSIVE LUXATION

Intrusive injuries (Figure 9.15) are the most common injuries to the upper primary incisors. Newly erupted incisors often take the full force of any fall in a toddler. There is usually a palatal and superior displacement of the crown, which means that the apex of the tooth is forced away from the permanent follicle.

Management

- If the crown is visible and there is only minor alveolar damage, leave the tooth to re-erupt.
- If the whole tooth is intruded, extract.

The tooth should be extracted in cases where there will be an unfavourable outcome, such as when there are symptoms and signs of pulp necrosis and/or infection, a cessation of further root development of the succedaneous tooth or a negative impact on the development or eruption of the permanent successor (Day et al., 2020).

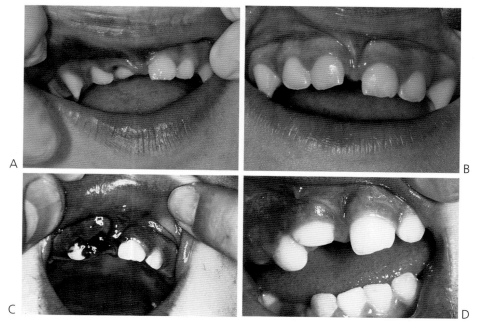

Figure 9.15   (A) Many intruded primary teeth will re-erupt (B). (C) The decision as to whether or not to extract is dependent on the degree of displacement and direction of displacement of the crown and the amount of gingival and alveolar damage. An intrusive luxation of the upper right central incisor in a 12-month-old child is shown. Note the displacement of the gingiva, indicating that the tooth has not been avulsed. (D) The tooth partially re-erupted within a month.

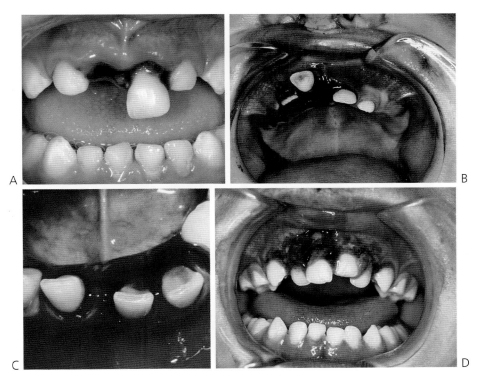

Figure 9.16 (A) Extrusive luxations result in increased mobility necessitating removal of the tooth. There is no indication for repositioning such teeth. (B) Similarly, lateral luxations of this magnitude require removal of the tooth. (C) This child presented 1 week following lateral luxation of the lower primary incisors with continued gingival oozing. He was subsequently diagnosed with Christmas disease (factor IX deficiency). (D) Gross displacement of all upper anterior teeth with gingival degloving and loss of the labial plate. This child had the displaced teeth extracted, and debridement and suturing of the gingiva under general anaesthesia.

EXTRUSIVE AND LATERAL LUXATION (Figure 9.16)

Treatment is dependent on the mobility and extent of displacement. If there is excessive mobility or extrusion, interference with the occlusion or an unfavourable outcome, the tooth should be extracted (Day et al., 2020).

AVULSION (Figure 9.17)

- Avulsed primary teeth should not be replanted.
- Replanting an avulsed primary tooth may force the blood clot in the socket, or the root apex itself, into the developing permanent tooth. The other main reason is lack of patient cooperation. There are cases in which the parent or caregiver has replanted the tooth and it appears to be stable; in these cases, the tooth could be left in situ, but it should be splinted to prevent it being inhaled or swallowed.
- Unless significant soft tissue damage is present, antibiotics are not required.
- Splinting of primary teeth may be difficult in young, traumatized children, and if successfully placed, the splint must then also be removed later when the child may be less compliant.

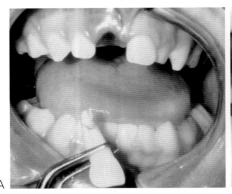 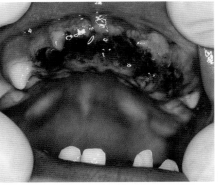

A   B

Figure 9.17 (A) There is almost no indication for the replantation of an avulsed primary tooth. There is more risk of damage to the permanent tooth than there is benefit gained by replanting the tooth. (B) A child involved in a motor vehicle accident resulting in six avulsed primary teeth, but with surprisingly very little dentoalveolar damage. A chest radiograph was required to ensure that no teeth were swallowed or aspirated.

Fractures of primary incisors

RESTORABLE CROWN FRACTURES NOT INVOLVING THE PULP (Figure 9.18A)

Unlike the permanent dentition, primary teeth are more commonly displaced rather than fractured. Enamel and dentine fractures may be smoothed with a disc and, if possible, the dentine can be covered with glass ionomer cement or composite resin. Paediatric strip crowns are often useful. A possible sequel is grey discolouration and/or pulp necrosis. If the pulp does become necrotic, then it may subsequently become infected, leading to an apical abscess requiring removal of the tooth.

RESTORABLE COMPLICATED CROWN/ROOT FRACTURES

'Complicated' fractures involve the pulp. More commonly, fractures of primary teeth involve the pulp and extend below the gingival margin. Commonly, there are multiple fractures in individual teeth. In these cases, it is not feasible to adequately restore the tooth, and therefore it should be extracted. Often the fracture is not evident immediately, but the child may present several days after the trauma with a pulp polyp which is causing separation of the fragments. Such a proliferative response is a protective mechanism and is not painful. Management of such a case should be by extraction of the tooth.

Management

- Most of the discomfort results from the movement of fractured pieces of tooth that are still held by the gingiva or periodontal ligament. In the emergency management of such teeth, these loose tooth fragments should be removed.
- The remaining tooth can be extracted when convenient. This may necessitate the use of sedation or a short general anaesthetic.
- If a root fragment remains in the socket after a fracture, it may be safely left in situ where it will be resorbed as the permanent tooth erupts. It is important to keep parents adequately informed in these situations.

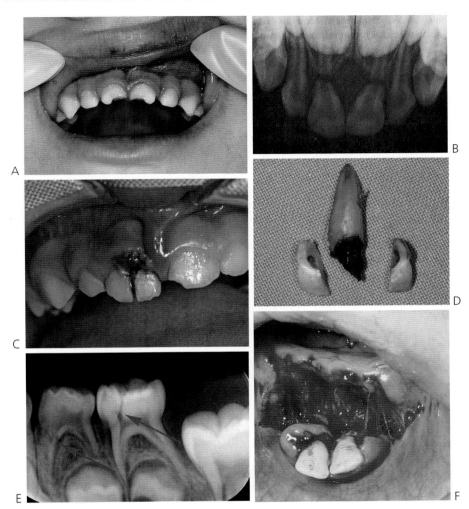

Figure 9.18 (A) Minor enamel/dentine fractures can be smoothed with a disc or left untreated. (B) Root fractures require no treatment unless the coronal fragments are excessively mobile. The pulp in the apical portions remains normal and the roots will resorb normally. (C) A complex crown/root fracture involving the upper left primary central incisor. These teeth are not suitable for restoration and need to be extracted. The extent of the subgingival fracture can be seen in (D). These teeth are often difficult to remove, and care must be taken to avoid damage to the permanent teeth if using elevators or luxators to remove large fragments of root. (E) Complicated crown and root fractures of the first and second primary molars. (F) A dentoalveolar fracture in a 6-month-old infant. In these cases, it is important to reposition the bone, with or without the teeth. A thick (2-0) nylon suture passed through both labial and lingual plates can be used to provide fixation for the fragment. Teeth usually survive this trauma, and there are few untoward sequelae for the permanent teeth.

ROOT FRACTURES (Figure 9.16B)

As mentioned earlier, when children fracture primary incisors, there is usually a complex crown/root fracture that extends below the gingival margin that makes restoration impossible or inappropriate, and so extraction is indicated. Isolated, subcrestal root fractures in primary incisors are uncommon. Normally, no treatment is necessary for primary incisors with horizontal or transverse root fractures. If, at regular review, the pulp shows signs of necrosis and infection, with excessive mobility or sinus formation, the coronal portion should be extracted. The apical root fragments are usually removed by resorption as the permanent tooth erupts.

UNRESTORABLE FRACTURES (Figure 9.18C–E)

These teeth should be removed.

DENTOALVEOLAR FRACTURE (Figure 9.18F)

This is more common in the mandible with the anterior teeth being displaced anteriorly with the labial alveolar cortical plate. In young children, it is often desirable to reposition and splint the teeth and the bony complex to maintain the alveolar contour. Unless there is a significant displaced bony segment, this can be achieved with a thick monofilament, resorbable suture (such as 2-0 PDS or Monocryl®) passed through the labial and lingual plates of the bone (remembering that the bone is very thin and soft). Teeth that are excessively mobile should be carefully dissected out of the sockets, preserving the labial plate, which should be repositioned and sutured.

SEQUELAE OF TRAUMA TO PRIMARY TEETH (Figures 9.19 and 9.20)

It is important to discuss with parents the sequelae of luxated or avulsed primary incisors. Although it may be difficult to accurately predict the prognosis for the unerupted permanent teeth, parents appreciate having an idea of the possible outcomes. Studies have shown that up to 25% of children are left with some developmental disturbance of the permanent tooth.

Damage to the unerupted permanent dentition occurs more often with intrusive luxation and avulsion in very young children. It is important to warn parents of the possible problems with permanent teeth but also to reassure them that, with modern restorative materials, minor defects are easily repaired. Sequelae in the permanent dentition depend on the following:

- Direction and displacement of the primary root apex (Figure 9.21).
- Degree of alveolar damage.
- Stage of formation of the permanent tooth.
- Treatment provided to the primary tooth.

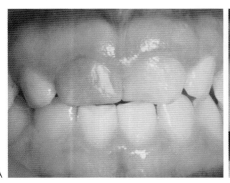
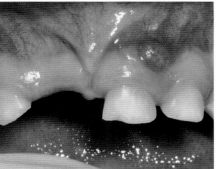

A   B

Figure 9.19   (A) Discolouration of the crown following trauma to the primary incisors. Unless an abscess is present (B), these teeth do not require treatment other than monitoring and reassurance of the parents.

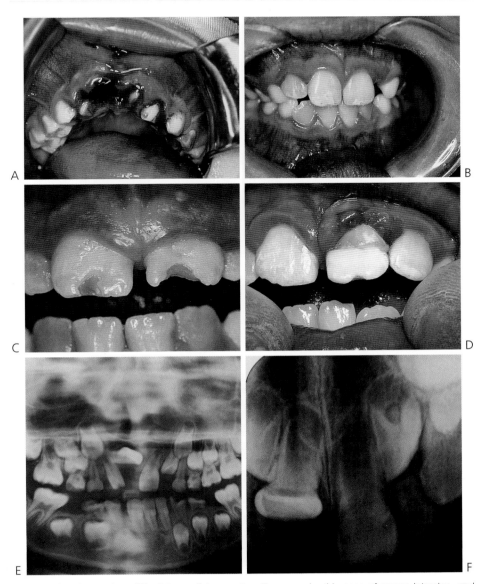

Figure 9.20 (A) It is often difficult to predict sequelae. For example, this case of severe intrusion, and alveolar disruption, has caused little damage other than mild hypocalcification of the permanent incisors (B). (C) Hypoplasia of the permanent central incisors resulting from trauma in the primary dentition. (D) Restoration of dilacerated teeth is extremely difficult, especially when the defect involves the gingival margin. (E) Displacement and dilaceration of the upper-right permanent central incisor, following avulsion of the primary precursor tooth, at 18 months of age. (F) Severe dilaceration of the crown of the upper left central incisor.

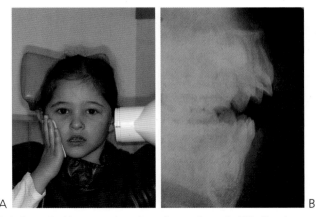

Figure 9.21 (A) Technique of taking a true lateral maxillary radiograph. This film gives a good localization of the position of the primary root apex in relation to the central incisors. (B) The root apex is clearly visible, just underneath the anterior nasal spine, having perforated the labial plate. In this situation, damage to the unerupted permanent tooth is less likely.

POSSIBLE SEQUELAE TO PRIMARY AND PERMANENT TEETH FOLLOWING TRAUMA

- Discolouration of the crown. In primary teeth, grey discolouration may not represent pulp necrosis. Discolouration that occurs early may improve over time.
- Pulp necrosis and possible infection of the root canal system followed by abscess formation (Figure 9.18). Initially, this may be an aseptic necrosis.
- Internal resorption of the primary tooth.
- Ankylosis of the primary tooth. Commonly, intruded primary teeth will fail to fully erupt but will exfoliate normally. In rare cases, extraction may be required just before eruption of the permanent incisor.
- Hypomineralization (Figure 9.20B) or hypoplasia (Figure 9.20C, D) of succedaneous teeth (see also Chapter 11).
- Dilaceration of the crown, or root of the permanent tooth; varies by the developmental stage of the permanent tooth at the time of trauma (Figure 9.20E, F).
- Resorption of the permanent tooth germ.

TREATMENT OPTIONS

- If the primary tooth is discoloured but asymptomatic, no treatment is usually indicated. Masking a discoloured tooth with composite resin may be an option if aesthetics are a concern. If an abscess is present, pulpectomy (and subsequent treatment of the root canal system) or extraction is indicated.
- Hypoplasia and hypomineralization of the permanent teeth can be restored with composite resin.
- Dilaceration of the crown or root of the permanent tooth often necessitates surgical exposure and bonding of chains or brackets for orthodontic extrusion (see Chapter 11 for details of surgical procedure). Severe cases may be untreatable, and such teeth may need to be removed.

Crown and root fractures of permanent incisors

CROWN INFRACTIONS

When there is an infraction (or crack) of the enamel, there is no loss of tooth structure. Infractions do not usually cross the dentino–enamel junction and usually require transillumination or indirect light to be identified (see Figure 9.6). However, it is impossible to determine the depth or extent of an infraction and whether it involves dentine or not.

Management

- Pulp sensibility tests.
- Periapical radiographs taken from several angulations to exclude other injuries.
- Anterior maxillary occlusal radiograph to exclude other injuries.
- Cover the infractions with two coats of light-cured resin bonding liquid as a temporary means of protecting the pulp by preventing bacterial penetration during the early healing phase.

Review

- No particular reviews are required if there is certainty that this is the only injury. Pulp sensibility testing is prudent at normal 6- and 12-month visits for regular oral care.
- Periapical radiographs are only recommended if signs or symptoms present.

UNCOMPLICATED CROWN FRACTURES

Uncomplicated crown fractures are confined to the enamel only or may involve the enamel and dentine, but they do not involve the pulp. The most common presentation is an oblique fracture of the mesial or distal corner of an incisor.

Management

- Account for any missing tooth fragment.
- Baseline pulp sensibility tests.
- Baseline periapical radiographs taken from several angulations to exclude other injuries.
- Anterior maxillary occlusal radiograph to exclude other injuries.
- Enamel-only fractures: smooth over the sharp edges with a disc or restore with composite resin if required.
- Enamel and dentine fractures: cover the dentine with glass ionomer cement and then restore the crown with composite resin either immediately or at review (Figures 9.22 and 9.23). Tooth fragments may be bonded back on to the tooth.

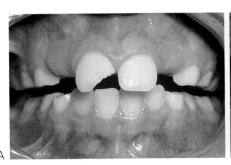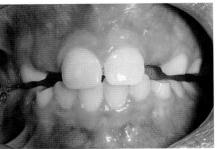

A   B

Figure 9.22 (A, B) Composite resin restoration on a proximal fracture. Retention is aided by using a long bevel over the labial surface. The dentine is protected with a glass ionomer base.

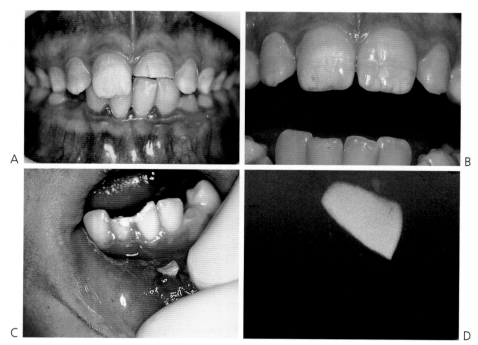

Figure 9.23 Restoration of a fractured enamel fragment by bonding the fragment back on to the tooth. (A) A chamfer or bevel is placed around the fragment and remaining crown and the dentine covered with glass ionomer cement. (B) Composite resin is then used to bond the fragment to the crown. It is often impossible to re-create the subtle hypocalcific flecks in a crown with composite resin alone; the replacement of the fractured piece is a good alternative technique if the fragment can be found. (C) Always look for fragments of tooth in the soft tissues. It is essential that they are removed at the time of the trauma, as they are extremely difficult to find once the tissues have healed. (D) Radiographs are useful in localizing tooth fragments within the lip.

Review

- Pulp sensibility testing after 6 to 8 weeks and then at 12 months.
- Periapical radiographs at each review.

CLINICAL HINT

It is extremely important to cover the exposed dentine of permanent incisors as soon as possible. This is to prevent direct irritation of the pulp caused by entry of bacteria via the dentinal tubules. Parents often save the fractured piece of a permanent incisor that can sometimes be used to restore the tooth by being bonded back onto the tooth with composite resin (Figure 9.22). Soak the fragment in water for 20 minutes.

In the very immature tooth, where there is a questionable pulp exposure, an elective Cvek pulpotomy (see later) may be indicated. This will ensure normal development of the root and prevent the need for any possible open apex endodontic procedure (apexification).

Prognosis

Pulp necrosis after extensive proximal fracture:
- No protective coverage of dentine: 54%.
- With dentine coverage: 8%.

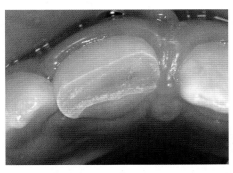

Figure 9.24 Assessment of any pulp exposure is essential, especially when the tooth is immature. The exposure of the mesial pulp horn is quite small and there is no haemorrhage, so it may be easily missed. Immediate coverage and dressing will help to prevent pulp necrosis and infection and the subsequent need for an open apex endodontic procedure.

COMPLICATED CROWN FRACTURES (Figure 9.24)

- Fractures involving the enamel, the dentine and exposure of the pulp.
- Involves laceration of the pulp and its exposure to the oral environment and bacteria within the mouth.
- Healing does not occur spontaneously, and untreated exposures will result in pulp necrosis and subsequent infection of the root canal system, leading to apical periodontitis and possible apical abscess.

The time elapsed since the injury and the stage of root development will influence treatment. If the tooth is treated within several hours of the exposure, conservative management is appropriate. After several days, microabscesses may occur within the pulp, and more radical pulp amputation will be required.

Management

- Baseline pulp sensibility tests, to assess adjacent teeth for possible injury.
- Baseline periapical and occlusal radiographs taken from several angulations to exclude other injuries.
- The aim of managing the exposed pulp is to preserve the non-inflamed pulp tissue and for it to be biologically walled off by a hard tissue barrier (Cvek, 1978).

In almost all situations, if the pulp tissue can be covered with a calcium hydroxide or a non-staining calcium silicate dressing, it is possible for a dentine bridge to form over the exposed pulp. It is undoubtedly preferable to preserve the pulp rather than to do root canal treatment.

IMMATURE ROOT WITH A CLINICALLY NORMAL PULP

Cvek pulpotomy (apexogenesis) (Figure 9.25)

The Cvek pulpotomy procedure involves the removal of contaminated pulp tissue with a clean, round, high-speed diamond bur, using saline or water irrigation. A nonsetting calcium hydroxide paste is then placed directly onto the uncontaminated pulp tissue (see step 5). The steps are as follows:

1. Administer local anaesthesia.
2. Place rubber dam to isolate the operating field; this is mandatory.
3. Remove 1 to 2 mm of pulp using a high-speed diamond bur, as described earlier.
4. Wash the pulp with saline until the haemorrhage stops. Any blood clot should then be gently rinsed away.
5. Place a nonsetting calcium hydroxide paste over the remaining pulp and then cover this paste with a hard-setting calcium hydroxide cement or liner. It is essential that the calcium hydroxide is placed over pulp tissue, and not over a blood clot.

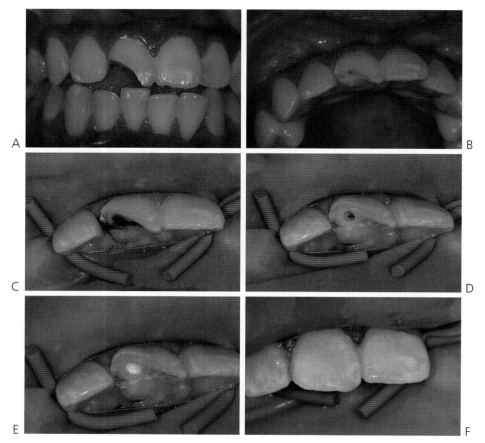

Figure 9.25 Cvek pulpotomy. (A, B) Large proximal fracture of tooth 11 resulting in a pulp exposure. (C) Isolation and obtaining access to the pulp chamber with a high-speed diamond bur with copious saline irrigation. (D) Removal of 2 mm of pulp tissue to a level with no contaminated pulp tissue and achieving haemostasis. (E) Placement of nonsetting calcium hydroxide dressing over the pulp tissue. (F) Cementation of the fractured tooth portion to restore the tooth.

    6. Place a glass ionomer cement base over the calcium hydroxide and restore the tooth with composite resin.

    This technique does not need to be limited to the coronal pulp. A 'partial pulpotomy' may be performed at any level of the pulp space because there are great benefits in preserving the apical part of the pulp in traumatized incisors.

Review

- Review 6 to 8 weeks and then at 6 and 12 months with pulp sensibility tests.
- Periapical radiographs at each review to check for continued root development and narrowing of the root canal space as the root develops (Figure 9.26).

Prognosis

- Favourable pulp healing, 80% to 96%.

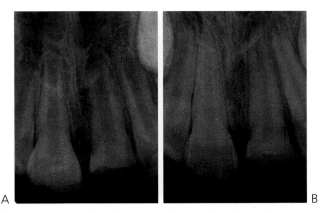

A   B

Figure 9.26 (A) Pulp exposure in an immature central incisor. (B) A Cvek pulpotomy (apexogenesis) has allowed normal root development with a dentine barrier in the crown. This significantly strengthens the root, especially at the cemento–enamel junction.

Immature root with a necrotic and infected pulp (Figure 9.27)

Pulp necrosis is unlikely to occur immediately after trauma that results in a complicated crown fracture. It is more likely to be diagnosed at follow-up examinations. If the pulp of a tooth with a complicated crown fracture becomes necrotic and infected, then removal of the pulp and subsequent root canal treatment are required. Although there is no difference in the prognosis of root canal treatment in immature teeth compared with mature teeth, the long-term survival of a tooth with an open apex may be compromised. This is caused by the thin dentine walls of the root, especially in the cervical third, and a shortened root which make the tooth susceptible to fracture during function or if there is further trauma to the tooth. Endodontic treatment of immature anterior teeth is complicated because of the inability to create an apical seat, the thin dentinal walls and the difficulty in filling the root canal by traditional methods such as lateral compaction of gutta-percha.

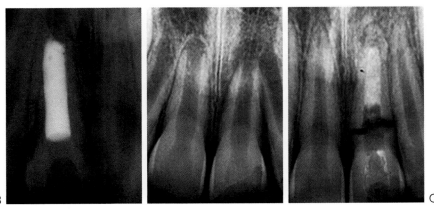

A, B   C

Figure 9.27 (A) Open apex root canal treatment requiring an apexification procedure. (B, C) The long-term prognosis of these teeth is not ideal with some sustaining subsequent root fractures because of inherent weakness in the cervical region.

Management

The aim of management is to create an apical hard tissue barrier against which the root canal filling can be placed. The formation of this apical hard tissue barrier is stimulated by using long-term intra-canal calcium hydroxide dressings (apexification).

Technique (apexification)

1. Administer local anaesthesia.
2. Place rubber dam; this is mandatory for all root canal treatments.
3. Prepare an access cavity through the palatal or lingual surface of the crown.
4. Remove any necrotic pulp tissue from the canal with a barbed broach.
5. Biomechanically prepare the canal to a level 1 mm short of the radiographic apex.
6. The canal should be carefully instrumented to completely remove necrotic tissue and debris, while also preserving as much tooth structure as possible. The apical root, being very thin, is weak and may fracture if undue pressure is exerted. Very little instrumentation of the canal walls is required.
7. Irrigate thoroughly with 1% to 3% sodium hypochlorite and ethylene diamine tetra-acetic acid (EDTA) to dissolve pulp tissue remnants and to disinfect the root canal system (Galler et al., 2016).
8. Calcium hydroxide paste or, alternatively, a corticosteroid/antibiotic paste should be placed as the initial dressing. The latter is very effective at reducing periapical inflammation, reducing pain and controlling infection within the root canal. The pastes can be inserted into the root canal using a spiral root filler in a low-speed handpiece, run at a very low speed.
9. Place a small pledget of cotton wool, foam pellets or Teflon in the coronal pulp chamber and then place a temporary restoration in the access cavity using a temporary filling material such as Cavit® or a double-layer temporary restoration using Cavit and IRM® (Naoum & Chandler, 2002).
10. After 4 to 6 weeks, the patient should be reviewed. If there are no symptoms or other problems, then under rubber dam isolation, the temporary filling material should be removed and the canal should be thoroughly irrigated to remove the previous dressing. After drying the canal, it should be re-dressed with a nonsetting calcium hydroxide paste.
11. Compress the calcium hydroxide with a cotton wool pellet, or foam pellet, to ensure good condensation in the canal and to allow contact with the apical tissues. Another temporary restoration should then be placed in the access cavity.
12. Review the child every 3 months and change the calcium hydroxide dressing each time in the manner described earlier. The formation of an apical hard tissue barrier typically takes about 12 months, but it may take up to 18 months. Once the barrier has formed, the canal should be filled with gutta-percha and cement. Root canal filling with gutta-percha is performed using either a warm vertical compaction technique or lateral compaction. An impression of the apical seat may be made with heat-softened gutta-percha, which is then cemented into the canal with root canal cement. Whichever technique is used, it should be stressed that gentle pressure must be applied to avoid splitting the root or breaking the hard tissue barrier off the root and pushing it into the periapical tissues. Thermoplasticized gutta-percha delivery systems are often invaluable in these cases.
13. Remove the gutta-percha and cement from within the crown part of the tooth. Gutta-percha can be easily removed with a hot instrument and then the remainder should be vertically compacted into the coronal third of the canal while it is still warm. The access cavity should be thoroughly cleaned by wiping it out with cotton pellets soaked in alcohol

to remove the root canal cement. This should be repeated 2 to 3 times to ensure complete removal of the cement to avoid discolouration of the tooth.

14. Restore the access cavity with a base of Cavit, followed by a glass ionomer cement to replace dentine and finally composite resin. The Cavit will facilitate any further access to the root canal system should it become necessary in the future.

In immature teeth, occasionally, a small root apex may develop, although the pulp otherwise appears necrotic. This is caused by surviving remnants of the Hertwig epithelial root sheath. Such a situation requires no management or change to the treatment being provided for the tooth.

Review

- Review 6 months after the root filling has been completed and then annually for at least 5 years to monitor the tooth and the periapical tissues.
- Periapical radiographs at each review.
- Adjacent teeth should also be monitored in the usual manner following trauma.

Obturating an open apex tooth without apexification

The approach that has been advocated in recent years is the use of mineral trioxide aggregate (MTA) to fill the apical few millimetres of an open apex tooth without first having to use long-term dressings of calcium hydroxide. Although sometimes called 'MTA apexification', it is not an apexification procedure because an apical hard tissue barrier is not formed before root filling the tooth. It is more accurate to consider this procedure as placing an "apical plug" to fill an open-ended root canal.

Initially, the root canal system must be cleaned and disinfected. This can be achieved through the use of irrigating solutions such as sodium hypochlorite and ethylene diamine tetra-acetic acid plus cetrimide (EDTAC), plus the use of an appropriate intracanal medicament. The medicament chosen will depend on the presenting condition of the pulp or root canal system. A corticosteroid/antibiotic paste may be used if there has been irreversible pulpitis, or calcium hydroxide alone should be used if the root canal system had been infected.

Once the canal has been disinfected and dried, the MTA can be placed in the apical few millimetres of the canal. Special instruments and magnification are required to achieve an adequate filling, as it is very technique-sensitive and difficult to do. The remainder of the canal can then be filled with conventional materials (such as gutta-percha and cement) and techniques (such as lateral compaction) (Kaur et al., 2017).

It is claimed that this technique reduces the chances of root fractures occurring later because the dentine is not exposed to long-term calcium hydroxide. However, MTA releases calcium hydroxide, and therefore the effects of this need further investigation. The other disadvantages of this procedure are the high costs of the material, the need for two appointments to do the root canal filling, the slow setting time and the technical difficulties of placing the material without any of it being pushed into the periapical tissues.

New methods to manage open apex teeth with pulp necrosis and infection

An emerging prospect for the management of teeth with incomplete root development where the pulp has necrosed and become infected is the concept of regenerative endodontics (Figure 9.28). The aim is to achieve revascularization of the root canal system and regeneration of tissue that is capable of producing what radiographically appears to be dentine. Cases have been documented in the literature showing that this is feasible, especially in premolar teeth that had developmental defects such as dens evaginatus. The prospect of using this approach for traumatized teeth with an open apex is being researched and shows promise. Protocols are being updated constantly; however, the initial approach is to:

1. Disinfect the root canal system by using sodium hypochlorite and/or EDTA irrigating solution.

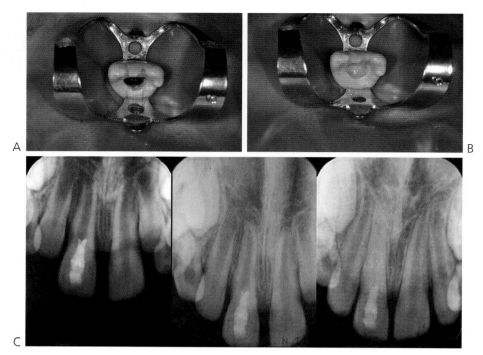

Figure 9.28 Pulp revascularization. (A) Haemorrhage is induced into the canal by passing a file through the apex of this immature tooth. (B) Mineral trioxide aggregate is placed over the clot at the level of the cemento–enamel junction. (C) Periapical radiographs of an open apex tooth treated with this new technique. Over 3 and 12 months, there have been further development and closure of the root apex.

2. Place antibiotics as an intracanal dressing. A triple antibiotic paste (ciprofloxacin, metronidazole and minocycline) has been advocated, but some authors have reported using only one or two antibiotics to avoid the use of tetracyclines (minocycline is a tetracycline antibiotic) that might result in staining of the tooth.
3. At the next appointment, the antibiotic paste is removed and bleeding is induced in the periapical tissues by instrumenting through the apical foramen with a root canal file. The aim of this is to fill the canal with blood that will then clot and organize to form a matrix for cell regeneration (Figure 9.28A).
4. Once the clot has formed in the canal, a cement such as MTA is placed in the coronal part of the root canal, followed by restoration of the crown of the tooth (Figure 9.28B).

The tooth should then be reviewed after 6 and 12 months to determine whether there is further root development and hard tissue formation along the canal walls (Figure 9.28C). Research is currently being carried out to determine whether the procedure can be more predictable if stem cells, growth factors, tissue scaffolds or other tissue-engineering techniques are used.

It is important to understand that these procedures for regeneration are largely based on case reports at present, and clear guidelines need to be established. Current recommendations are that regenerative procedures in traumatized, infected, incompletely developed permanent teeth should be performed only if the tooth is not suitable for apexogenesis or root canal treatment and apexification.

MATURE ROOT

If the pulp of a permanent anterior tooth is exposed by trauma, and the period of exposure is short, it need not be removed, regardless of the stage of root development. The Cvek (partial) pulpotomy can be used to attempt to preserve the pulp. If there are restorative considerations (i.e., the need for a post), it may be better to remove the pulp and perform root canal treatment immediately.

Root fractures (Figure 9.29)

- A fracture involving the enamel, dentine and cementum may or may not involve the pulp. Pulp necrosis occurs in about 25% of teeth with root fractures and is related to the degree of displacement of the coronal fragment. External inflammatory and replacement root resorption are rare.
- To check for horizontal root fractures, alter the vertical angulation of periapical radiographs. When looking for vertical root fractures, change the horizontal angulation; however, the range of angulation where a fracture is visible is only between 4 degrees and 6 degrees. CBCT may be useful and therefore indicated in all cases.
- Sometimes, a horizontal root fracture is not initially evident. This is because the fracture site opens up under the influence of the inflammatory reaction several days after the injury. Thus, for all traumatized teeth, it is important to take a subsequent radiograph within 2 weeks.

FREQUENCY

- Permanent dentition: 2% to 4%.

TISSUE RESPONSES FOLLOWING ROOT FRACTURES

- Healing by hard tissue union with calcified tissue (osseodentin).
- Healing by interposition of bone and connective tissue.

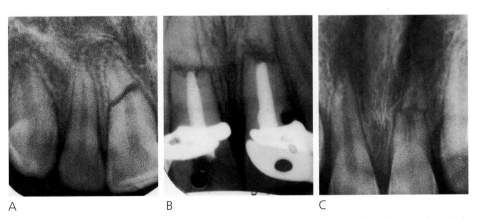

A   B   C

Figure 9.29 (A) Root fractures near the apex of the root often require no treatment. In most cases, the pulp in the apical fragment remains normal. (B) When the coronal fragments become necrotic and infected, root canal treatment should only be performed up to the fracture line. Long-term calcium hydroxide treatment is required because the root canal at the fracture site will be wide open. In this case, bone is interposed between the two fragments. (C) Not all pulps in the coronal fragments become necrotic. Healing of an apical third root fracture is shown. The pulp in the apical fragment is normal and there has been pulp canal calcification in the coronal two-thirds. In this case, there is probably bone interposed between the two fragments.

- Healing by interposition of connective tissue.
- Granulation tissue in the fracture line, indicating coronal pulp necrosis and infection.

MANAGEMENT

- Radiographs: several vertical and/or horizontal angulations of periapical radiographs plus an occlusal radiograph are usually required to adequately determine the extent of the fracture.
- Reposition the coronal fragment.
- Place a splint with composite resin and wire or passive orthodontic appliances for 4 weeks if the coronal fragment is mobile. If the fracture is located cervically, then up to 4 months of fixation may be required (Bourguignon et al., 2020).
- Root fractures in the apical few millimetres often require no treatment.

REVIEW

- Review at 4, 6 to 8 and 16 weeks with pulp sensibility testing and radiographs.
- Review at 6 and 12 months and then annually for 5 years.
- Take periapical radiographs at all review appointments.

PULP NECROSIS AND INFECTION OF THE CORONAL FRAGMENT (Figure 9.29B)

It is uncommon for the apical fragment to develop pulp necrosis, and it will usually undergo pulp canal calcification, which requires no treatment. If pulp necrosis and infection of the coronal fragment occur, there will be radiographic signs of bone loss at the level of the fracture. Symptoms, such as pain, excessive mobility, gingival swelling or a draining sinus, may also indicate that the coronal pulp has necrosed and become infected. These problems will not be evident at the time of the trauma, so endodontic treatment should not be commenced then. These problems will only become evident during the review of root-fractured teeth and may take several months or even longer to occur. If they occur, then the tooth should be managed as follows:

- Remove the pulp from the coronal fragment. Never advance an endodontic instrument through the fracture line.
- Take a periapical radiograph to determine the 'working length' at approximately 1.0 mm coronal to the fracture line.
- Biomechanically prepare the root canal to the working length.
- Place a nonsetting calcium hydroxide paste as an initial dressing to control the infection and reduce the inflammation in the fracture line.
- Place a temporary restoration in the access cavity and arrange to review the patient in about 4 weeks.
- At the 4-week review appointment, open the access cavity and irrigate the root canal to remove the initial dressing. Then, replace the nonsetting calcium hydroxide paste to induce the formation of a hard tissue barrier at the end of the coronal fragment (Figure 9.24B). The nonsetting calcium hydroxide dressing should be replaced every 3 months until the hard tissue barrier has formed. This may take up to 18 months.
- Place a root canal filling using gutta-percha or MTA once the barrier has formed, using a similar technique to that described previously following apexification. The access cavity can then be restored, also as described earlier for apexification cases. Be aware of potential issues with staining from MTA.

PULP NECROSIS AND INFECTION OF BOTH THE APICAL AND CORONAL FRAGMENTS

When the apical fragment shows signs of pulp necrosis and infection, the prognosis is poor. However, fortunately, it is very rare for the pulp in the apical fragment to necrose. Root canal treatment of the coronal fragment should be performed, followed by surgery to remove the apical fragment. There have been case reports of intraradicular splinting and endodontic implants, but both have a very poor long-term prognosis.

Crown/root fractures

The coronal fragments should always be removed to fully assess the extent of the fracture (Figure 9.30).

UNCOMPLICATED CROWN/ROOT FRACTURE

Where the fracture extends just below the gingival margin (Figure 9.30A), cover the dentine with glass ionomer cement initially and then restore the tooth with composite resin or a crown. Only the crown part of the tooth should be restored to allow re-attachment and new cementum formation on the fractured root surface; that is, do not restore the root portion.

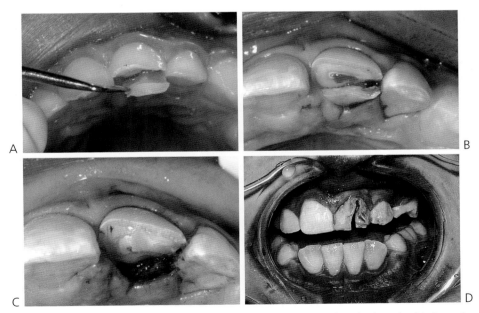

Figure 9.30 Crown/root fractures. (A) The coronal fragment of a crown/root fracture should always be removed to investigate the full extent of the fracture. (B) This case shows a complicated crown/root fracture (i.e., pulp exposed) with the fracture extending just above the alveolar crest on the palatal aspect. (C) The fractured portion has been removed, and it is clear that the fracture extends approximately 3 mm below the gingival margin. The pulp was capped and the access cavity filled. Treatment will involve periodontal-flap surgery and placement of a crown with an extended shoulder. Alternatively, orthodontic extrusion may be required. (D) Unfortunately, vertical crown/root fractures are untreatable, and such teeth should be extracted. Retention in the short term may be valuable to preserve bone while planning for possible orthodontics, or implants, when growth has finished.

COMPLICATED CROWN/ROOT FRACTURE (I.E., WITH PULP EXPOSURE)

If the fracture extends below the crestal bone and the root development is complete, remove the coronal fragment(s) to assess the extent of the fracture(s) (Figure 9.30B). Root canal treatment is required. Calcium hydroxide or a corticosteroid/antibiotic paste may be placed as the initial endodontic dressing (Bourguignon et al., 2020).

A Cvek (partial) pulpotomy may be performed (Figure 9.30C) at any depth even if the fracture extends below the crestal bone. The decisions as to how such teeth are restored are really dependant on the individual circumstances for each case. These types of fractures may be restored with composite resin, whereas deeper fractures may need a cast restoration or may require surgical treatment to expose the margins for restoration.

Unfortunately, the long-term prognosis for a tooth with a complicated crown/root fracture is poor.

Options for management

- Gingivectomy to expose the fracture margin. If the fracture is minimal, and just below the gingival margin, then restoration of the root surface may be performed with glass ionomer cement and a crown build-up in composite resin.
- Crown with extended shoulder with or without periodontal flap procedure.
- Orthodontic or surgical extrusion of the root to expose the fracture margin.
- Extraction.
- Root burial (decoronation).
- Autotransplantation in conjunction with an orthodontic treatment plan.

Orthodontic extrusion. This may be a viable option, provided there is adequate root length to support a crown. However, because of the narrower emergence profile of the root compared with the crown of a normal tooth, a satisfactory aesthetic result may be difficult to achieve. A gingivoplasty will almost always be required to reposition the gingival margin after the tooth has been extruded and then retained for an adequate period of time. Fixed appliances are placed to extrude the root so that the margin is exposed. A pericision is often advisable.

Root burial (Figure 9.31). In cases of subalveolar root fracture, root burial (decoronation) may be an alternative to extraction to preserve the alveolar bone. The root is 'buried' below the alveolar crest (i.e., the root is reduced in length from a coronal direction until it is entirely within bone) and a coronally repositioned flap is raised to cover the defect with periosteum. In this way, it is possible for bone to grow over the root surface (Figure 9.31E, F). The pulp may be normal or root canal treatment may be necessary. This technique is valuable in the preservation of the labio-palatal width of the alveolus, which may be essential if an osseointegrated implant is required later because it may negate the need for ridge augmentation.

CROWN/ROOT FRACTURES IN IMMATURE TEETH

When complex crown/root fractures occur in teeth with incomplete root formation, consideration should be given to maintaining the pulp, where possible, to allow continuation of root development. However, if the pulp has undergone necrosis and infection, then endodontic treatment including apexification will be necessary. It is worth noting, however, that complicated crown/root fractures tend to occur in mature teeth, where consideration of apical development is unnecessary. As a general comment, if the complex fracture extends below the crestal bone, then the prognosis is poor.

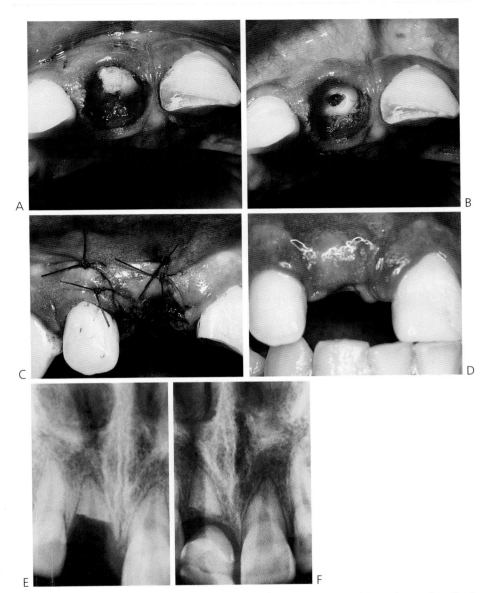

Figure 9.31 Root burial of a tooth fractured below the alveolar crest. Root burial may be an alternative to extraction in these cases. (A) This root has been traumatized with the fracture extending from the gingival margin on the labial to a level below the alveolar crest on the palatal. (B) The root was sectioned 1 to 2 mm below the crestal bone and (C) covered with a coronally repositioned mucoperiosteal flap. (D) Healing after 2 weeks. (E, F) Bone growth has been stimulated over the root. This preserves the alveolar height for later prosthodontic work. The original crown has been contoured and attached to adjacent teeth with composite resin.

Luxations in the permanent dentition

CONCUSSION AND SUBLUXATION

These teeth are treated symptomatically. Concussed teeth will have a marked response to percussion, but the tooth will be firm in the socket. A subluxated tooth (Figure 9.32A) will exhibit increased mobility but will not have been displaced and there are no radiographic abnormalities. They are tender to percussion and show bleeding from the gingival margin.

Management

- Pulp sensibility tests and radiographs (several periapical views plus an anterior maxillary occlusal view).
- Relieve from occlusion; flexible splinting for up to 2 weeks is not usually required unless there is excessive mobility.
- Soft diet for 2 weeks.

Review

- Pulp sensibility testing at 3, 6 and 12 months.
- Radiographs at each review.
- It is important to follow up these teeth for at least 12 months (to check the pulp status, colour, mobility) and radiographically, to assess changes in the size of the pulp chamber and root development, as both of these indicate that the pulp has recovered and returned to a clinically normal state.

Prognosis

- Pulp necrosis in 3% to 6% of cases; will depend on any concurrent injuries (e.g., infractions, crown fractures, etc.).

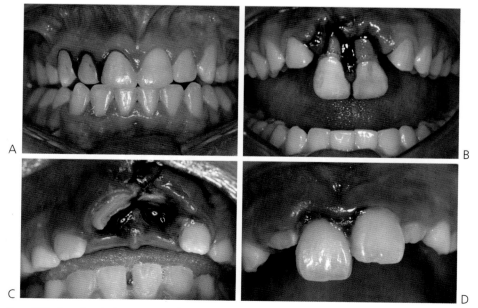

Figure 9.32   Luxations in the permanent dentition. (A) Subluxation. (B) Extrusion. (C) Intrusion. (D) Lateral luxation. Often, there is a combination of injuries, for example, a lateral and intrusive luxation.

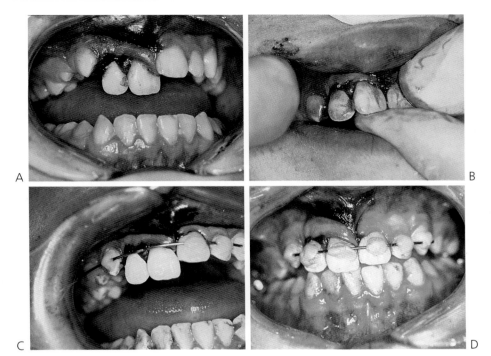

Figure 9.33   (A) Lateral luxation (palatal) with a dentoalveolar component involving the upper right central and lateral incisors. (B) The block of teeth and bone is manually repositioned with finger pressure. (C, D) A rigid composite resin and wire splint is placed. When placing a splint, attach and stabilize uninvolved teeth before splinting the displaced segment.

LATERAL AND EXTRUSIVE LUXATION (Figure 9.33)

Teeth may be luxated in any direction and will usually need repositioning and splinting. It is common to have a combination of injuries. Repositioning can be achieved with digital pressure. Ideally, forceps should not be used because they can damage the root surface, and this predisposes the tooth to root resorption. Luxated teeth are easily identified by visual examination, as the tooth is obviously displaced, potentially mobile and with radiographic changes to the periodontal ligament. Pulp sensibility tests may give negative results initially.

Management

1. Reposition under local anaesthesia. Early repositioning is important (Figure 9.33A, B) because it is often extremely difficult to reposition the tooth if the patient presents later (especially after 24 hours) owing to the presence of a blood clot in the original socket space.
2. Suture gingival lacerations: particularly check for 'degloving' of the palatal gingivae with all luxated teeth by using an instrument (e.g., flat plastic instrument) to check whether the tissue is still attached or not. They may visually appear to be attached but may not actually be attached. If in doubt, it is better to suture the tissues to ensure that the ideal conditions for healing are created.
3. Place a flexible splint using composite resin and wire or passive orthodontic appliances for 10 to 14 days for extrusive luxation. Lateral luxation cases should be splinted with a more

rigid splint for 4 weeks (because of concomitant alveolar bone fracture) by using wire and composite resin or passive orthodontic appliances.

4. Prescribe antibiotics, tetanus prophylaxis and aqueous 0.2% chlorhexidine mouthrinse.

Lateral luxations always have a fracture of the alveolar socket wall, and hence it is important to mould the bone back into the correct position. Fragments of bone attached to the periosteum should be retained. In case of an alveolar fracture, the splinting time should be about 6 weeks for both types of luxations (Bourguignon et al., 2020).

Review

- Review every 2 weeks while the splint is in place, and then after 1, 3, 6 and 12 months. Subsequently, annual reviews for up to 5 years.
- Perform pulp sensibility tests at each review.
- Take radiographs at each review.

Prognosis

- Depends on the degree of displacement and apical development, with excellent healing in immature teeth. Also depends on whether there are any concurrent injuries such as a crown fracture.
- Pulp necrosis and infection occur in 15% to 85% of cases and are more prevalent in teeth with closed apices. Also depends on whether there are any concurrent injuries such as a crown fracture.
- Pulp canal calcification often occurs in immature teeth.
- Resorption is rare.
- Transient apical breakdown (2%–12%) is a repair process where the apical foramen appears to 'open up' via a resorptive process to allow revascularization of the pulp to occur. There is also an expansion of the apical periodontal ligament space. Essentially, there is some resorption followed by repair so the process is really a remodelling process. There is no indication for root canal treatment unless there are other indicators of infection of the root canal system.

INTRUSION

Intrusion results from forcing the tooth into the alveolar bone and is an injury with one of the poorest prognoses (Figures 9.32C and 9.34). There is extensive damage to the supporting structures (i.e., crushing of the periodontal ligament and bone) and the neurovascular bundle that supplies the pulp.

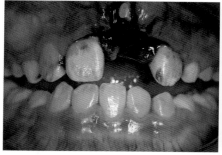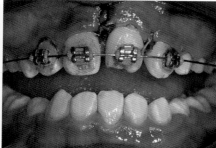

A   B

Figure 9.34   (A) Intrusion of the upper left central incisor. Early mobilization is essential to prevent ankylosis and to allow access to the palatal surface to perform root canal treatment. (B) The tooth was repositioned surgically and splinted with orthodontic appliances.

Management

There is much discussion about whether intrusively luxated teeth should be repositioned or allowed to re-erupt on their own. Treatment may well depend on the state of root development, but as a general rule, all intruded teeth should be monitored for a period of 4 weeks to observe if there is spontaneous re-eruption, except where the tooth has been intruded more than 3 mm and the root development is complete. Incompletely developed teeth have more eruptive potential than those that have immature apices (Bourguignon et al., 2020). However, there is always a risk for intruded teeth to undergo rapid external resorption because of pulp necrosis and damage to the periodontal ligament and root surface. The aims of subsequent repositioning are to disimpact the tooth to avoid ankylosis, minimize pressure necrosis of the periodontal ligament and allow access to the palatal surface of the tooth to remove the pulp immediately. It is highly unlikely that the pulp will survive, and therefore its removal is important, as this will help to reduce the possibility of external inflammatory resorption occurring.

Repositioning

Teeth with incomplete root formation

- Allow re-eruption independent of the amount of intrusion for up to 4 weeks.
- If the crown remains visible and there is a very wide immature apex (>2 mm), the tooth may be allowed to re-erupt spontaneously.
- Monitor closely every 2 weeks.
- If there is no improvement in position over 3 to 4 weeks, then rapid orthodontic repositioning is required.

Teeth with complete root formation

- Immediate repositioning is preferred for mature teeth if the tooth has been intruded more than 3 mm (see previously).
- Gently reposition the tooth with fingers or with forceps applied only to the crown. Avoid rotating the tooth in the socket.
  Or
- Fixed orthodontic appliances can be used to apply traction to the intruded tooth over a 2-week period (Figure 9.34B).
- Extrusion should be rapid enough so that the palatal surface is exposed and an access cavity can be made as soon as possible.

Endodontic treatment

- Removal of the pulp is essential in almost all cases. The only exceptions are partially intruded, extremely immature teeth that are being left to re-erupt (with regular monitoring).
- A corticosteroid/antibiotic paste should be placed as the initial dressing for 6 weeks (change the dressing after 6 weeks to ensure adequate concentrations within the canal) to reduce the chances of external inflammatory resorption. This can then be followed by a nonsetting calcium hydroxide for 2 to 3 months before obturating the canal (Abbott et al., 1989).
- If the apex is immature, then a further period of nonsetting calcium-hydroxide therapy will be required for apexification before root canal filling.

Review

- It is essential that these teeth are regularly reviewed. External inflammatory resorption can occur very rapidly if preventive measures have not been used (such as immediate root canal treatment with a corticosteroid/antibiotic paste dressing). External replacement resorption may also occur very rapidly because of the damage to (especially crushing of) the root surface and periodontal ligament during the injury, and an immature tooth may be lost within a number of weeks.

- Review every 2 weeks during the splinting phase, then at 6 to 8 weeks, 6 months, 12 months and yearly for at least 5 years.

Prognosis

- Mature teeth undergo pulp necrosis in almost all cases (>96%), especially if there are also concurrent injuries such as a crown fracture, and there is a high prevalence of replacement resorption and ankylosis if not treated as previously mentioned because of the damage to the root surface.
- Immature teeth that re-erupt show pulp necrosis in 60% of cases and ankylosis in up to 50% of cases.
- Teeth treated early have a much better prognosis.

DENTOALVEOLAR FRACTURES

With luxation of teeth, the alveolar plate can be fractured or deformed. Use firm finger pressure on the labial/buccal and lingual/palatal plates to reposition. It should be remembered that alveolar fractures may occur without significant dental involvement. These alveolar fractures should be splinted for 4 weeks in children (or 6–8 weeks in adults). Laterally luxated, intruded and avulsed teeth always have some alveolar bone fracture and/or displacement. Firm pressure is needed to realign the bony fragments once the tooth has been repositioned. Splinting may be rigid or semi-rigid and is dependent on the degree of injury and the number of teeth involved (Figure 9.32).

PULP STATUS

Pulp sensibility tests only test the ability of the pulp's nerves to respond to the stimulus that is applied; they do not provide any information about the presence or absence of blood supply or the histological status of the pulp. When determining the status of the pulp in luxated permanent teeth, beware of false test results. The pulp may not respond to a stimulus because of damage to the sensory nerves of the pulp, even though the tooth's vascularity is maintained. It may take up to 1 year (or never) to obtain a response from such a pulp. Thus, one must be careful to judge the patient's signs and symptoms before commencing root canal treatment. Regular radiographs are required to assess root development and growth, evidence of external or internal root resorption and changes in the size and shape of the pulp chamber. Clinically, changes in colour, excess mobility, tenderness to percussion and a draining sinus are important diagnostic signs of an infected root canal system. A necrotic pulp does not cause apical periodontitis; it is only when the necrotic pulp becomes infected that a periapical response occurs. Hence, the most important thing to assess is whether the root canal system is infected or not.

Remember that when teeth have been luxated, they may also have sustained a crown or root fracture. Crown fractures are obvious usually; however, root fractures may be hidden or not yet apparent. Therefore, radiographs are always essential and a narrow-field CBCT should be considered.

Avulsion of permanent teeth (Figure 9.35)

If a permanent tooth is avulsed, the chance of successful retention is enhanced by minimizing the extraoral time. Even if the tooth has been out of the mouth for an extended period, it is usually still better to replant the tooth, with the knowledge that the tooth may ultimately be lost. In the mixed dentition, this is important, as replantation of even questionable teeth will allow normal

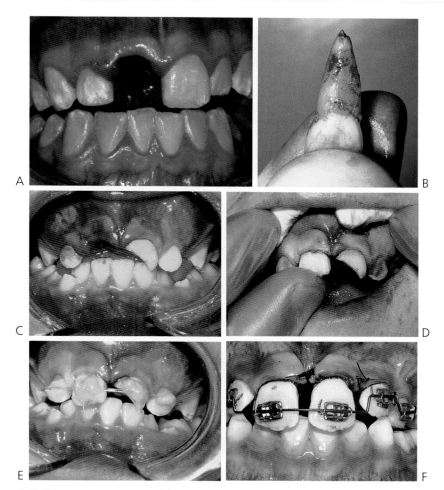

Figure 9.35 Management of avulsion. (A) With avulsions, there may be few other injuries. In other cases, there may be extensive damage to the supporting tissues. (B) Always hold the tooth by the crown and gently debride the root surface with saline. (C) The socket should be irrigated and clear of debris. (D) Replant with firm pressure. The tooth will usually click back into position. (E) Splint with a flexible splint, such as composite and nylon fishing line, to allow some physiological movement. (F) Orthodontic appliances are extremely useful when splinting traumatized teeth. The wire should be passive and allow physiological movement. Placement of a wire through orthodontic brackets allows the splint to be removed and the mobility of the tooth can be assessed.

establishment of the arch, occlusion and aesthetics. Furthermore, orthodontic treatment planning is simpler if the tooth remains in the socket. These teeth are usually lost by replacement resorption, which has the benefit of preserving the alveolar bone height and width, making prosthodontic replacement much simpler.

FIRST AID ADVICE

It is important that parents, caregivers and teachers have access to appropriate advice on the management of avulsed teeth. Timing is essential, and this information can be given over the telephone:

- Keep the child calm.
- Do not allow the child to eat or drink. If sedation or anaesthesia is required for extensive injuries, then the child may need to be fasted.
- Locate the tooth and hold by the crown only. Always check the patient's clothing for avulsed teeth that are thought to be lost.
- Replant the tooth immediately if clean. If the tooth is dirty, it should be washed (preferably with milk if available, otherwise saline or the patient's saliva). As a last resort, very briefly rinse under cold water (10 seconds only).
- Hold the tooth in place by biting gently on a handkerchief or clean cloth, or use aluminium foil or similar material, and seek urgent dental treatment.
- If unable to replant the tooth, store it in isotonic media to prevent dehydration and death of the periodontal ligament cells.
- Use:
  - Milk (the preferred and most available solution).
  - Saline.
  - Saliva.
  - Wrap in plastic cling wrap (with some saliva to keep it moist).
  - Avoid using water because this will result in hypotonic lysis of the periodontal ligament cells.
- Seek urgent dental treatment.

Time is essential! The long-term prognosis of the tooth is severely reduced after 10 minutes of being dry and out of the mouth. Do not waste time searching for the ideal storage medium; replant the tooth!

MANAGEMENT IN THE DENTAL SURGERY

The following are guidelines for replanting avulsed permanent teeth.

If the tooth has been replanted before arrival at the dental surgery/office do not extract, just clean the mouth if needed and splint.

Mature tooth (closed apex) maintained in storage solution with extraoral time less than 60 minutes

1. Gently debride the root surface under copious saline, milk or tissue-culture media (Hanks balanced salt solution) irrigation. When holding teeth, always do so by only holding the crown with a wet gauze square (teeth can be very slippery; see Figure 9.35B).
2. Give local anaesthesia (preferably without a vasoconstrictor) and gently debride the tooth socket with saline to remove any blood clot, but do not curette the bone or remaining periodontal ligament (Figure 9.35C).
3. Replant the tooth gently with finger pressure (Figure 9.35D). The tooth usually 'clicks' back into the correct position if there has not been too much bone damage and there is no blood clot left in the socket.

Mature tooth is dry or extraoral time is more 60 minutes (not in storage media)

1. Check the tooth and remove debris from the root surface by gently agitating it in saline, or by using a syringe to provide a stream of saline to the root surface. It is important to avoid damage to the root surface so do not use any mechanical means to clean the root. Keep the tooth in saline whilst taking a history, doing the clinical examination, taking radiographs, etc. It is essential that the tooth be rehydrated before replantation.

2. Give local anaesthesia and gently debride the tooth socket with saline to remove the blood clot; do not curette the bone or remaining ligament.
3. Replant the tooth gently with finger pressure.

Management of avulsed teeth with open apices

The ultimate aim should be to achieve pulp revascularization (see later). Careful monitoring is essential as external inflammatory root resorption may occur very quickly.

Management following replantation

1. Splint for 14 days with a flexible passive wire splint or passive orthodontic appliances (Figure 9.35E, F).
2. Reposition and suture any degloved gingival tissues and suture all lacerations.
3. Ideally, immediately after replantation and stabilization with a splint, or otherwise within 2 weeks and under rubber dam isolation, cut an endodontic access cavity and remove the pulp. Irrigate the canal with 1% sodium hypochlorite solution and then dry it. Place a corticosteroid/antibiotic paste dressing in the canal to reduce the chance of external inflammatory root resorption for 1 month, then replace with calcium hydroxide. Continue root canal treatment as outlined earlier for intruded teeth.
4. Prescribe a high-dose, broad-spectrum antibiotic (e.g., amoxicillin) for one week, and check current immunization status.
5. Account for any lost teeth. A chest radiograph may be required.
6. Normal diet and strict oral hygiene including an aqueous chlorhexidine gluconate 0.2% mouthwash.

Splinting of avulsed teeth

- Orthodontic brackets with a light archwire (0.014″). Orthodontic appliances are particularly useful, as the time taken to apply the brackets is half that to set composite resin (Figure 9.35F), or
- Composite resin and nylon fibre (0.13–0.25 mm diameter) such as fishing line (20 kg breaking strain).

Splints should be flexible to allow normal physiological movement of the tooth. This helps to reduce the development of ankylosis and replacement resorption; however, if there is a bone or root fracture present, then a rigid splint must be used so that there is no movement of the teeth or bone segments.

Splints should generally stay in place for 10 to 14 days if there are no complicating factors such as alveolar or root fractures. When bone fractures are present, the splint should be retained for 4 to 6 weeks. The occlusion may need to be relieved when the degree of overbite or luxation is such that the tooth will receive unwanted masticatory force. This can be achieved by minimal removal of enamel, or construction of an upper removable appliance, or placement of composite resin on the molars to open the bite. However, some physiological movement is necessary.

As a general rule, all teeth should be replanted, whether wet or dry. Although the prognosis of a dry tooth may be poor, it is usually preferable to have the tooth present during growth than not at all. Always keep options open for future treatment.

Orthodontic splinting is always preferable but obviously requires suitable training and access to equipment. It does not matter which orthodontic bracket system is used. The most important point is that any arch wire placed for splinting is passive and will not move adjacent teeth. There are certain advantages over the use of a composite resin splint, in particular:

- Easier and quicker to place.
- Allows the splint to be readily removed and replaced so that the mobility of the teeth can be monitored.

- Easier to maintain oral hygiene.
- Less time to remove and less chance of damage to the teeth following removal of composite resin (often used to excess).

If composite resin splints are used, then choose a distinct shade of resin, avoid filling embrasures and try to minimize the amount of resin used. All these points assist in the later removal of the splint. It is more comfortable to delay removal of the splint until after any endodontic procedures have been commenced.

Endodontic management of avulsed teeth

Open root apex. If a tooth has been avulsed, replanted within a short period, the apex is extremely immature (>2 mm) and the child is under 8 years of age, then root canal treatment is needed only if symptoms and clinical signs indicate that the pulp space has become infected. Hence, such teeth should not have root canal treatment commenced immediately after the replantation; instead, they should be monitored to see whether the pulp revascularization occurs.

If the canal becomes infected, the root canal should be dressed with a corticosteroid/antibiotic paste, placed initially for 6 weeks followed by calcium hydroxide. Calcium hydroxide treatment can then be used to induce apexification (see previously). This is changed every 3 months until an apical hard tissue barrier has formed and root canal filling is possible.

Closed root apex

> #### CLINICAL HINT: AVULSED IMMATURE PERMANENT INCISORS
>
> Sometimes, there is a reluctance for clinicians to intervene and begin endodontic treatment in these cases. Unfortunately, this well-meaning conservative approach may lead to eventual tooth loss. The risk of infection-related (inflammatory) root resorption should be weighed against the realistic chances of obtaining pulp space revascularization. Such resorption is very rapid in children (Fouad et al., 2020). Furthermore, it is almost impossible to reliably assess the pup status, and once signs and symptoms occur, it is may be too late to intervene.

In all other situations, in which the apex of the avulsed tooth is less than 2 mm open or closed, root canal treatment should be commenced immediately after replantation to prevent external inflammatory root resorption. The initial dressing should be a corticosteroid/antibiotic paste for 6 weeks each followed by calcium hydroxide. The root canal filling can usually be completed after 5 to 6 months.

Generally, it is best to always replant avulsed teeth even if they have a poor prognosis. Even with appropriate treatment, these teeth will often be lost by progressive external replacement resorption, but the positive benefit being that the alveolar bone is maintained. The only exceptions are those cases where avulsed teeth have very immature roots and where ankylosis will prevent alveolar bone growth which may complicate future orthodontic and prosthodontic management.

Complications in endodontic management of avulsed teeth

EXTERNAL INFLAMMATORY ROOT RESORPTION (Figure 9.36A)

This is the progressive loss of tooth structure by an inflammatory process caused by the presence of bacteria in the root canal system following necrosis of the pulp and damage to the root surface.

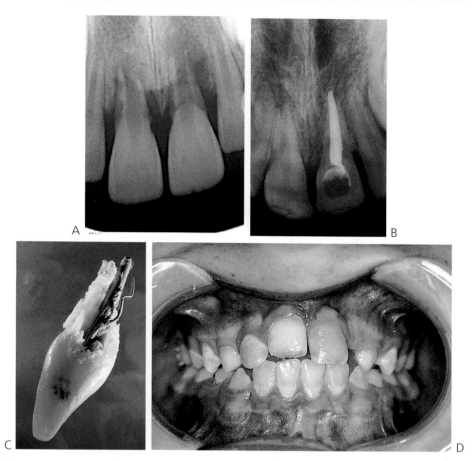

Figure 9.36 (A) External inflammatory root resorption of both central incisors resulting from a failure to adequately disinfect and medicate the root canal systems. (B) External replacement resorption where the root is being replaced by bone around the gutta-percha root filling. Note the slight infraocclusion of this tooth. (C) Loss of an avulsed central incisor because of external replacement resorption. Note the ankylosis on the labial aspect of the root. (D) Ankylosis and subsequent infraocclusion is a significant problem when permanent teeth are traumatized before the cessation of growth. There is retardation of alveolar growth and the tooth will ultimately be lost.

This resorption can be prevented or managed with appropriate treatment. Factors in prevention and management include the following.

- Prophylactic antibiotics: A broad-spectrum antibiotic (e.g., tetracycline, amoxicillin or penicillin V) should be given as soon as possible after avulsion and continued for 1 week. Although tetracyclines are preferred, they should be avoided in children up to 12 years of age where staining of other teeth may occur.
- Pulp removal: This should be done as soon as possible after the replantation: that is, on the day of the injury, once the tooth has been replanted and stabilized.

Medicaments such as calcium hydroxide may cause inflammation in the first 3 months after trauma. A corticosteroid/antibiotic paste is an ideal first-dressing medicament, as it has been shown to prevent inflammatory root resorption and inhibit the action of clastic cells.

Management

If inflammatory resorption is detected, the canal must be thoroughly instrumented, irrigated and then dressed with a corticosteroid/antibiotic paste for 3 months, but with a change of the dressing every 6 weeks. Calcium hydroxide can then be placed for a further 3 months, after which time, if there is no progression of the resorption, the root canal can be filled.

EXTERNAL REPLACEMENT ROOT RESORPTION (Figure 9.36B–D)

This is the progressive resorption of tooth structure and replacement with bone, as part of continual bone remodelling. It results from damage to the cementum and/or periodontal ligament or from replantation of dry teeth. It cannot be treated, so the aim must be to prevent ankylosis and replacement resorption. Factors in prevention and management include:

- Extraoral time: Prognosis decreases dramatically after 15 minutes if the tooth is dry. Approximately 50% of the periodontal ligament cells are usually dead after 30 minutes and all are usually dead after 60 minutes.
- Storage media
    - Milk is usually the best available medium (although not superior to Hanks balanced salt solution) and may keep cells viable for up to 6 hours. It has the advantage that it is pasteurized with few bacteria, is readily available and is cold. There appears to be no difference between low-fat and skimmed milk, but yoghurt and sour milk should be avoided because of their low pH (Osmanovic et al., 2018).
    - Saliva is suitable for up to 2 hours.
    - Saline and plastic cling wrap will maintain cells for 1 hour.
    - Water is hypotonic and causes cell lysis, so it should be avoided.
    - Tissue culture media such as Hank's balanced salt solution or RPMI 1640 (Roswell Park Memorial Institute tissue culture medium) is also appropriate, if available, and may give up to 24-hour cell survival.
- Mechanical damage: Ankylosis will result if the cementum has been removed or damaged.
- Risk increases with increased handling during transport and replantation.
- Splinting: Flexible splinting allows physiological movement and results in less ankylosis and less replacement resorption.
- Extraoral root canal treatment should be avoided since it will increase the likelihood of replacement resorption and ankylosis because of the prolonged extraoral time, damage during treatment and the effects of toxic substances such as irrigating solutions and root canal cements.

Management

- No treatment modality has been able to successfully arrest progressive replacement resorption.

QUESTIONS CONCERNING THE LONG-TERM MANAGEMENT OF AVULSED TEETH

Despite a plethora of literature supporting the different procedures for managing avulsed teeth, the clinical reality remains that teeth that have been out of the mouth for more than 30 minutes have a poor prognosis (Figure 9.37).

- There is good evidence to support the use of specialized storage media; however, they are rarely available at the scene of an accident. Many dental injuries occur on weekends during sport. It would be interesting to research the average time taken to get a traumatized child to a dentist on a Saturday afternoon.

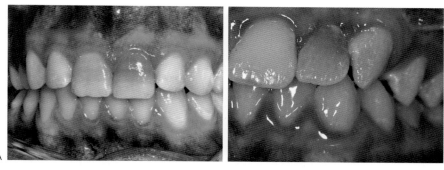

Figure 9.37 Complications post-trauma. (A) Discolouration of the crown of a previously luxated upper left central incisor attributed to breakdown of the temporary restoration in the access cavity. (B) External invasive resorption following trauma to the upper left lateral incisor.

- There is a social cost following trauma, including absence from school (for the child) and work (for the parent) in attending multiple appointments, and loss of self-esteem. There are also financial considerations of complex restorative and endodontic treatment for teeth that often have a very poor outcome.
- Parents and children should be given a clear indication about the probable outcomes of treatment. Heroic work is often performed with all good intentions when the prognosis is questionable (Barrett & Kenny, 1997).
- In some cases, it may be preferable to retain hopeless teeth where replacement resorption will preserve bone. In other cases, the retardation of alveolar bone growth accompanying ankylosis in a growing child may necessitate early removal.

Always keep the options open and consider the following questions:
- What is the long-term prognosis of the tooth?
- Are there orthodontic considerations such as the implications of ankylosis or space loss?
- Is the tooth important in the development of the occlusion?
- What are the prosthodontic options available to restore aesthetics and function?

OTHER CONSIDERATIONS AND OPTIONS FOR MANAGEMENT OF THE RESORBING INCISOR

Each case is unique and should be managed individually. Options include:
- Allowing the tooth to resorb and exfoliate, then prosthodontic replacement.
- Surgical repositioning of the submerging tooth.
- Dento-osseoss (segmental) osteotomy.
- Decoronation.
- Autotransplantation.

A resorbing tooth may be retained for quite a number of years. This of course delays the need for a prosthetic replacement and keeps options open. There is controversy as to whether more bone is lost by retaining such teeth compared with extracting them. In both situations, there will be a loss in alveolar height. More importantly, however, when teeth are completely removed, there is also a loss in alveolar width. There is general agreement that implants should not be placed in patients who are still growing. Some boys will continue growing into their early 20s. Consequently, any treatment should be directed at trying to preserve as much alveolar bone as possible. There is little evidence to support segmental osteotomies or surgical repositioning. Decoronation and autotransplantation provide better options. Decoronation has been shown to increase bone levels if performed in children before puberty. There was also no impediment to the later placement of implants.

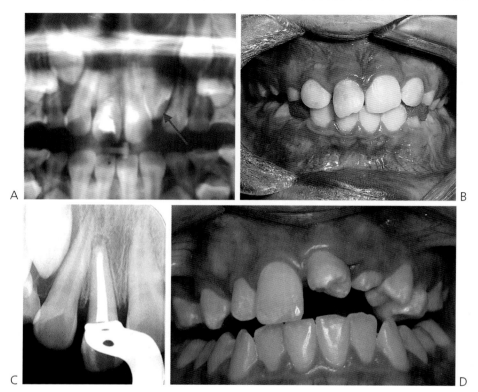

Figure 9.38 Autotransplantation. (A) The upper right central incisor in this boy was avulsed and undergoing resorption. A supernumerary lateral incisor was present lying palatal to the upper left central incisor. This tooth was autotransplanted into the socket of the traumatized central incisor. (B) Healing after 2 months. (C) Completion of root canal treatment at 6 months following transplantation showing good bone and periodontal healing. (D) Autotransplantation of a premolar. Notice the rotation of the crown by 45 degrees to improve the emergence profile of the tooth before restoration with a composite resin strip crown.

Autotransplantation (Figure 9.38)

Autotransplantation has been successfully used in the management of tooth loss following trauma. It may be used in the management of complicated crown/root fractures, replacement of the missing anterior teeth and after avulsion injuries.

Good case selection is essential.

INDICATIONS

- Traumatized anterior tooth with poor long-term prognosis.
- Donor tooth is favourable with respect to the stage of root development, size and shape of crown, etc.
- Cases with class I or class II malocclusion with moderate to severe crowding involving extraction of premolars.

Autotransplantation must be considered as part of an overall treatment plan for the patient, and other alternatives such as orthodontic space closure, fixed and removable prosthodontics and osseointegrated implant placement must be considered.

SUCCESS RATES

There is a difference between success and survival rates in published literature. Some recent papers have reported survival up to 100% using varying criteria for success and over differing time periods. This compares favourably with the published survival of anterior maxillary single tooth implants of 94% to 97% over 12 months. Nonetheless, overall survival rates for autotransplantation are approximately:

- 90% to 98% success rate for open apex teeth.
- Lower success rates for teeth with closed apices.

PROCEDURE FOR AUTOTRANSPLANTATION

1. Selection of donor tooth (Table 9.3) (usually a premolar)-consider:
   - The stage of root development.
   - The optimal time for transplantation is when the root is one-half to three-fourths formed.
   - In these cases, a 3D analysis is mandatory, including printing transplantation dummies and surgical guides.
2. Analysis of recipient site:
   - Size and shape of the recipient area.
   - Need for socket expansion or instrumentation.
   - Need to partially rotate the donor tooth.
3. Surgical procedure:
   - Remove the traumatized incisor as carefully as possible to minimize alveolar damage.
   - Prepare the socket: The socket can be enlarged if required and then irrigated with saline. Any necrotic or foreign debris such as gutta-percha, intracanal medicaments or granulation tissue must be removed. Surgical guides are available that mimic root dimensions of donor teeth. Further, a surgical dummy can be 3D printed from CBCT data and combined with a surgical guide, and the donor site can be prepared to the exact required dimensions to receive the donor tooth.
   - Make an incision into the periodontal ligament of the donor tooth through the gingival margin; a collar of attached gingiva may be included with the graft.
   - Gently extract the tooth, avoiding damage to the root surface.
   - Position the donor tooth into the recipient site. This usually involves rotation of a premolar tooth about 45 to 90 degrees.
4. Splint with a flexible splint.
5. Follow up as per protocols for avulsed teeth.

TABLE 9.3 ■ Selection of donor tooth for autotransplantation

Donor tooth	Recipient site
Third molars	First molars
Lower first premolar	Upper central incisor
Lower second premolar	Upper lateral incisor
Supernumerary/supplemental teeth	Upper incisors
Lower incisors	Upper lateral incisor
Upper premolars	Depends on root shape

The need for root canal treatment will depend on the degree of root development (Table 9.3) and recovery of the pulp after the transplantation.

REASONS FOR AN UNFAVOURABLE OUTCOME

- Inflammatory resorption or ankylosis and replacement resorption:
  - Closed apex: 20% root resorption.
  - Open apex: 3% root resorption.
- Pulp necrosis and infection.
- Infraocclusion.
- Incomplete root formation.
- No primary healing.

Details of healing and prognoses are shown in Table 9.4.

TABLE 9.4 ■ **Healing and prognosis after autotransplantation of premolars**

| Root development | Root resorption | | Pulp revascularization | Root formation |
	Inflammatory resorption	Replacement resorption		
Stage 1 Initial root formation				77% normal root length
Stage 2 One-fourth root formation	3%	6%	100% pulp revascularization	66% arrested root formation
Stage 3 One-half root formation				88% normal root length
Stage 4 Three-fourths root formation			87% pulp revascularization	Up to 98% normal root length
Stage 5 Root formation complete with apical foramen wide open				
Stage 6 Root formation complete with apical foramen half closed	9%	18%	No revascularization	Up to 98% normal root length
Stage 7 Root formation complete with apical foramen closed	25%	38%	0% pulp revascularization	Complete root development

(From Andreasen et al. 1990.)

Internal bleaching of root-filled incisors

One consequence of trauma is tooth discolouration (Figure 9.37A). Internal bleaching is a common procedure following root canal treatment. The integrity of the root canal filling is paramount and, above all, bleaching should not be carried out below the cemento–enamel junction because of the risk of initiating external invasive resorption.

METHOD

1. Bleaching must be carried out under rubber dam isolation.
2. Ensure adequate root canal filling and remove the gutta-percha to a level 3 mm below the cemento–enamel junction.
3. Place Cavit as a base at the level of the cemento–enamel junction (Abbott, 1997; Abbott & Heah, 2009).
4. Ensure that the access cavity is clean and free of all debris.
5. Acid etch the access cavity to open the dentine tubules and then rinse with water.
6. Place a thick, dry mixture of sodium perborate and hydrogen peroxide into the cavity and then place a temporary filling using Cavit. The bleaching mixture should remain in the tooth for 1 week, after which the tooth colour is evaluated. The procedure may be repeated several times if required.
7. Once good colour modification has been achieved, the access cavity can be restored. Cavit can be left as a base over the gutta-percha and also on the labial wall of the access cavity. This will facilitate further access to the root canal system if endodontic re-treatment becomes necessary. Leaving Cavit on the labial wall of the cavity will allow further internal bleaching in the future if the tooth discolours again, and it avoids the removal of dentine at that time. The remainder of the pulp chamber should be filled with glass ionomer cement followed by a layer of composite resin.

Soft tissue injuries

ALVEOLAR MUCOSA AND SKIN

Bruising (Figure 9.39)

The simplest and most common type of soft tissue injury is bruising (contusion). This will often be present without any dental involvement. Treatment is symptomatic. However, be careful to

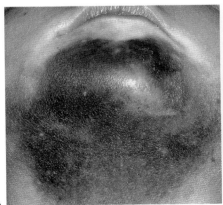
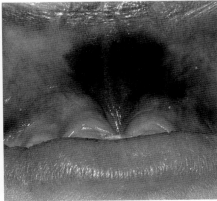

A   B

Figure 9.39 (A) Bruising of the chin is usually associated with severe degloving (see Figure 9.41B). (B) Bruising of the labial frenum may occur from a blow across the face; child abuse should always be suspected.

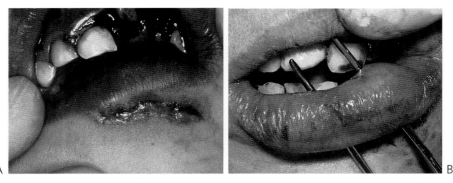

Figure 9.40   (A) When upper teeth are intruded, the lower lip is often bitten and it should be assessed for a through-and-through laceration. (B) These lacerations must be closed in three layers: the muscle, mucosa and skin. Always check lip lacerations for the presence of any tooth fragments if there are fractured teeth.

check in the depths of the labial and buccal sulci for any other deep soft-tissue wounds (e.g., lacerations) or degloving-type injuries.

Lacerations (Figures 9.40–9.42)

- Often, a full-thickness laceration of the lower lip can be undetected because of the natural contours of the soft tissues or the tentative examination of an upset child. If there has been a dental injury, always look for tooth remnants in the lips.
- Careful suturing of skin wounds will be needed to avoid scarring and should be performed only by those who are competent to do so. Skin wounds must be closed within the first 24 hours and preferably within 6 hours.
- Any debris, such as gravel and dirt, must be removed by scrubbing with a brush and an antiseptic surgical solution such as 2.5% povidone iodine or 0.5% chlorhexidine acetate.
- Ideally, skin edges should be excised with a scalpel to remove necrotic tags and irregular margins.

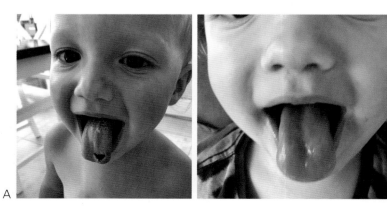

Figure 9.41   (A) Laceration of the tongue. Despite common opinions that tongue lacerations do not need to be sutured, best practice is that deep lacerations involving the muscle need primary closure. Deep suturing with slowly resorbing monofilament suture material is preferable, and more superficial closure may be performed with a softer material such as Vicryl. A common issue is that tongue wounds tend to open unless tightly sutured. (B) Healing of the same wound with minimal scarring.

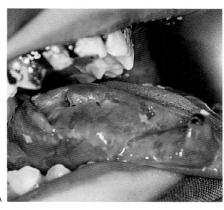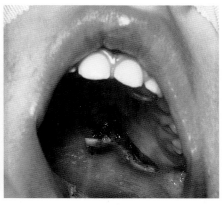

A B

Figure 9.42 (A) Lacerations may be caused by self-mutilation. This child has a peripheral sensory neuropathy (congenital indifference to pain). Attempts to make splints that would stop her behaviour failed, and after much agonizing, a full clearance was performed. (B) A severe laceration of the palate was caused by this child falling with a straw in her mouth. In many cases, small lacerations will granulate and heal without intervention. However, large lacerations require suturing.

- Muscle closure and deep suturing are achieved with a fine resorbable material such as 5-0 polyglactin or polyglycolic acid or Monocryl®.
- Final skin closure is with 6-0 monofilament nylon on a cutting needle.
- Tongue lacerations require closure unless very superficial (Figure 9.41)

ATTACHED GINGIVAL TISSUES

Degloving (Figure 9.43)

One of the most common injuries is degloving, which is when a full-thickness mucoperiosteal flap is stripped off the bone, with the separation line usually being the mucogingival junction (Figure 9.42A). These injuries tend to occur after blunt trauma, and a common presentation is a large collection of blood in the submental region (Figure 9.39A). The flap should be tightly sutured and a pressure dressing placed if the lower arch is involved. This prevents the pooling of blood and prevents swelling in the submental region, which may compromise the airway.

Interdental suturing of displaced gingival tissue is very important, especially where palatal tissue is involved (e.g., with lateral luxation). The close re-adaptation of tissues to the tooth surface will help preserve alveolar bone especially interdentally. Suturing will also help keep the tooth in position.

Suturing (see Chapter 8)

Prevention

EDUCATION OF PARENTS AND CAREGIVERS

- Seat belts and child restraints.
- Helmets for bike riding.
- Mouth guards.
- Face guards.
- Supervision of pets, especially dogs.

Although seatbelts and child restraints are covered by legislation, and helmets for bike riders are mandatory in many countries, the failure of parents to observe these regulations often results in unnecessary childhood craniofacial trauma. It has been the authors' experience that there is

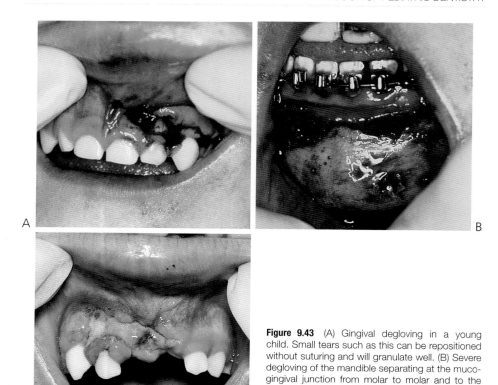

Figure 9.43 (A) Gingival degloving in a young child. Small tears such as this can be repositioned without suturing and will granulate well. (B) Severe degloving of the mandible separating at the muco-gingival junction from molar to molar and to the level of the hyoid. The mental nerve on the left was severed. (C) Inadequate repositioning of a degloving injury has resulted in delayed healing and soft tissue loss. It is essential that these injuries be treated early.

often little trauma seen from sports, as most children are wearing mouthguards; nevertheless, there is a disproportionate amount of trauma seen from leisure activities such as skateboarding, swimming and other 'noncontact' sports.

Educating parents, caregivers and teachers about primary care for dental trauma is essential. The correct protocols for dealing with avulsed teeth should be available to all schools and sporting clubs.

Further reading

Assessment

Gassner, R., Tuli, T., Hächl, O., et al., 2004. Craniomaxillofacial trauma in children: a review of 3,385 cases with 6,060 injuries in 10 years. Journal of Oral and Maxillofacial Surgery 62, 399–407.

Kopel, H.M., Johnson, R., 1985. Examination and neurological assessment of children with orofacial trauma. Endodontics and Dental Traumatology 18, 252–268.

Lam, R., Abbott, P.V., Lloyd, C., Lloyd, C.A., Kruger, E., Tennant, M., 2008. Dental trauma in an Australian rural centre. Dental Traumatology 24, 663–670.

Facial fractures in children

Ferreira, P., Marques, M., Pinho, C., et al., 2004. Midfacial fractures in children and adolescents: a review of 492 cases. British Journal of Oral and Maxillofacial Surgery 42, 501–505.

Posnick, J.C., Wells, M., Pron, G.E., 1993. Pediatric facial fractures: evolving patterns of treatment. Journal of Oral and Maxillofacial Surgery 51, 836–844.

Rowe, N.L., Williams, J.W., 1985. Maxillofacial injuries, vols. I, II. Churchill Livingstone, Edinburgh.

Zachariades, N., Mezitis, M., Mourouzis, C., et al., 2006. Fractures of the mandibular condyle: a review of 466 cases. Literature review, reflections on treatment and proposals. Journal of Craniomaxillofacial Surgery 34, 421–432.

Zimmermann, C.E., Troulis, M.J., Kaban, L.B., 2006. Pediatric facial fractures: recent advances in prevention, diagnosis and management. International Journal of Oral and Maxillofacial Surgery 35, 2–13.

Child abuse

American Academy of Pediatrics Committee on Child Abuse and NeglectAmerican Academy of Pediatric DentistryAmerican Academy of Pediatric Dentistry Council on Clinical Affairs 2005–2006, 2005. Guideline on oral and dental aspects of child abuse and neglect. Paediatric Dentistry 7 (Reference Manual), 64–67.

Cairns, A.M., Mok, J.Y., Welbury, R.R., 2005. Injuries to the head, face, mouth and neck in physically abused children in a community setting. International Journal of Paediatric Dentistry 5, 310–318.

Trauma to primary teeth

Brin, I., Ben-Bassar, Y., Zilberman, Y., et al., 1988. Effect of trauma to the primary incisors on the alignment of their permanent successors in Israelis. Community Dentistry and Oral Epidemiology 16, 104–108.

Christophersen, P., Freund, M., Harild, L., 2005. Avulsion of primary teeth and sequelae on the permanent successors. Dental Traumatology 21, 320–323.

Flores, M.T., 2002. Traumatic injuries in the primary dentition. Dental Traumatology 18, 287–298.

Flores, M.T., Onetto, J.E., 2019. How does orofacial trauma in children affect the developing dentition? Long-term treatment and associated complications. Dental Traumatology 2019 Dec 35 (6), 312–323.

Sennhenn-Kirchner, S., Jacobs, H.G., 2006. Traumatic injuries to the primary dentition and effects on the permanent successors – a clinical follow-up study. Dental Traumatology 2, 237–241.

Spinas, E., Melis, A., Savasta, A., 2006. Therapeutic approach to intrusive luxation injuries in primary dentition. A clinical follow-up study. European Journal of Paediatric Dentistry 7, 179–186.

Trauma to permanent teeth

Abbott, P.V., Hume, W.R., Heithersay, G.S., 1989. The release and diffusion through human coronal dentine in vitro of triamcinolone and demeclocycline from Ledermix paste. Endodontics and Dental Traumatology 5 (2), 92–97.

Andreasen, J.O., Andreasen, F.M., Bakland, L.K., et al., 2003. Traumatic dental injuries: a manual, second ed. Munksgaard, Copenhagen.

Cvek, M.J., 1978. A clinical report on partial pulpotomy and capping with calcium hydroxide in permanent incisors with complicated crown fracture. Journal of Endodontics 4, 232–237.

Petti, S., Glendor, U., Andersson, L., 2018. World traumatic dental injury prevalence and incidence, a meta-analysis-One billion living people have had traumatic dental injuries. Dental Traumatology 34 (2), 71–86.

Options for management

Akhlef, Y., Schwartz, O., Andreasen, J.O., Jensen, S.S., 2017. Autotransplantation of teeth to the anterior maxilla: a systematic review of survival and success, aesthetic presentation and patient-reported outcome. Dental Traumatology 34, 20–27.

Barrett, E.J., Kenny, D.J., 1997. Survival of avulsed permanent maxillary incisors in children following delayed replantation. Endodontics and Dental Traumatology 13, 269–275.

Campbell, K.M., Casas, M.J., Kenny, D.J., 2007. Development of ankylosis in permanent incisors following delayed replantation and severe intrusion. Dental Traumatology 23, 162–166.

Cohenca, N., Stabholz, A., 2007. Decoronation – a conservative method to treat ankylosed teeth for preservation of alveolar ridge before permanent prosthetic reconstruction: literature review and case presentation. Dental Traumatology 23, 87–94.

Humphrey, J.M., Kenny, D.J., Barrett, E.J., 2003. Clinical outcomes for permanent incisor luxations in a pediatric population. I. Intrusions. Dental Traumatology 19, 266–273.

Kafourou, V., Tong, H.J., Day, P., Houghton, N., James Spencer, R., Duggal, M., 2017. Outcomes and prognostic factors that influence the success of tooth autotransplantation in children and adolescents. Dental Traumatology 33, 393–399.

Kenny, D.J., Barrett, E.J., Casas, M.J., 2003. Avulsions and intrusions: the controversial displacement injuries. Journal of the Canadian Dental Association 69, 308–313.

Lee, R., Barrett, E.J., Kenny, D.J., 2003. Clinical outcomes for permanent incisor luxations in a pediatric population. II. Extrusions. Dental Traumatology 19, 274–279.

Nguyen, P.M., Kenny, D.J., Barrett, E.J., 2004. Socio-economic burden of permanent incisor replantation on children and parents. Dental Traumatology 20, 123–133.

Nikoui, M., Kenny, D.J., Barrett, E.J., 2003. Clinical outcomes for permanent incisor luxations in a pediatric population. III. Lateral luxations. Dental Traumatology 19, 280–285.

Guidelines

Bourguignon, C., Cohenca, N., Lauridsen, E, et al., 2020. International Association of Dental Traumatology guidelines for the management of traumatic dental injuries: 1. Fractures and luxations. Dental Traumatology 36, 314–330.

Cohenca, N., Silberman, A., 2017. Contemporary imaging for the diagnosis and treatment of traumatic dental injuries: a review. Dental Traumatology 33, 321–328.

Cohenca, N., Simon, J.H., Mathur, A., Malfaz, J.M., 2007. Clinical indications for digital imaging in dento-alveolar trauma. Part 2: root resorption. Dental Traumatology 23, 105–113.

Cohenca, N., Simon, J.H., Roges, R., Morag, Y., Malfaz, J.M., 2007. Clinical indications for digital imaging in dento-alveolar trauma. Part 1: traumatic injuries. Dental Traumatology 23, 95–104.

Day, P., Flores, M.T., O'Connell, A., et al., 2020. International Association of Dental Traumatology guidelines for the management of traumatic dental injuries: 3. Injuries in the Primary Dentition. Dental Traumatology 36, 343–359.

Fouad, A.F., Abbott, P.V., Tsilingaridis, G., et al., 2020. International Association of Dental Traumatology guidelines for the management of traumatic dental injuries: 2. Avulsion of permanent teeth. Dental Traumatology 36, 331–342.

Levin, L., Day, P., Hicks, M.L, et al., 2020. International Association of Dental Traumatology guidelines for the management of traumatic dental injuries: General Introduction. Dental Traumatology 36, 309–313.

Internal bleaching

Abbott, P.V., 1997. Aesthetic considerations in endodontics: Internal bleaching. Practical Periodontics & Aesthetic Dentistry 9, 833–842.

Abbott, P.V., Heah, S., 2009. Internal bleaching of teeth: an analysis of 255 teeth. Australian Dental Journal 54, 326–333.

CHAPTER 10

Paediatric oral medicine, oral pathology and radiology

Anastasia Georgiou ▦ Angus C. Cameron ▦ Richard P. Widmer

Cyclic neutropenia
Leucocyte adhesion defect
Papillon–Lefèvre syndrome
Chédiak–Higashi disease
Human immunodeficiency virus–associated
    periodontal disease in children
Langerhans cell histiocytosis

Metabolic disorders
Hypophosphatasia
Ehlers–Danlos type IV and type VIII
Erythromelalgia
Acrodynia (pink disease)
Acatalasia
Scurvy

Oral pathology in the newborn infant
Differential diagnosis
Cysts in the newborn
Congenital epulis
Melanotic neuroectodermal tumour of infancy

Diseases of salivary glands
Differential diagnosis
Mucocoele
Ranula
Sialadenitis
Salivary gland tumours
Diagnostic imaging of the salivary glands
Aplasia of salivary glands

Radiographic pathology in children
Periapical radiolucencies
Radiolucencies associated with the crowns of
    teeth
Separate isolated radiolucencies
Multiple or multilocular radiolucencies
Generalized bony rarefactions
Mixed lesions with radiopacities and
    radiolucencies
Radiopacities in the jaws

Introduction: how to diagnose pathology

Diagnosis is a puzzle, and the clinician must be a detective. A correct diagnosis leads to appropriate treatment and predictable outcomes for the patient. Unfortunately, not all the pieces of the puzzle may be at hand. Although some disorders are confined to the mouth, oral lesions may be a sign of a systemic medical disorder. The majority of oral pathology seen in children is benign; however, it is essential to identify or eliminate more serious conditions. The presentation of pathology in children is often different from adult pathology, and the subtleties of these differences are often important in diagnosis. In addition, many lesions change in form or extent with growth of the body. In this chapter, conditions will be grouped according to presentation, followed by a review of the most common causes and management of orofacial infections. Many of the lesions presented in this book and in other texts will show the most common presentation; however, it is important to remember that one disease entity may have different presentations while one presentation – for example, an ulcer – may be representative of many different diseases. Furthermore, lesions in the mouth may be representative of systemic pathology that will be discussed later in Chapter 12, and it is important to differentiate between a local isolated lesion and one that might be part of a generalized disease process. The process of arriving at a diagnosis must be conducted in a systematic way. History and initial examination lead to the development of a differential diagnosis. This is a list of possible diagnoses. Most medical specialties teach the use of a surgical or diagnostic sieve. This is a conceptual process by which all possibilities of a diagnosis may be considered by grouping the lesion or condition under standard subcategories. There are many such sieves; one example is shown in Figure 10.1. With further investigations, the differential list is refined to a form a provisional diagnosis. A definitive diagnosis is only possible following histopathological examination.

The decision to undertake a biopsy in a young child must be carefully considered. There will always be questions about management that might necessitate general anaesthesia or at least some form of sedation and the relative risks involved in both the operation and the surgery itself. These

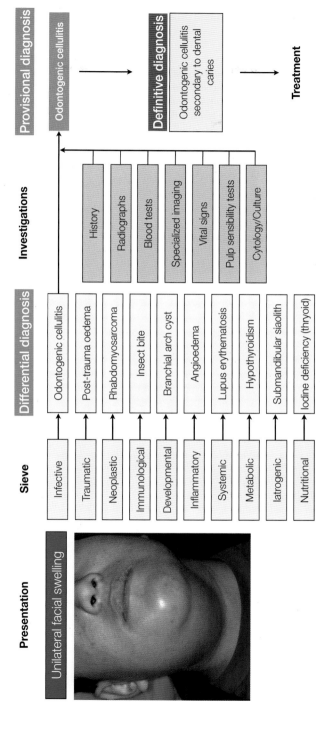

Figure 10.1 A surgical or diagnostic sieve. The sieve presents a number of different possible diagnoses from groupings of conditions. This forms the differential diagnosis. With further investigations and examinations, this is refined to form a provisional diagnosis which will form the basis of the treatment to be undertaken. The definitive diagnosis may only be determined following biopsy and pathological examination.

need to be balanced against the urgency and/or importance of finding an answer against the morbidity of surgery in a young child. The clinical procedures were covered in Chapter 8.

DEFINITION OF LESIONS

Clinical terms are often used to describe mucosal lesions, and it is important to understand the definitions or associated descriptions of these terms. Lesions can be broadly categorized as primary or secondary (Table 10.1A). A primary lesion originates from previously normal mucosa, such as a vesicle or a bulla. A secondary lesion originates from a primary lesion, for example, an ulcer which results from rupture of a vesicle or bulla. Certain terms have specific or implied meaning with clinical application and are listed in Table 10.1B.

When describing a lesion, it is important that certain features are noted:

- Location.
- Type (see Table 10.1).

TABLE 10.1A ■ Definitions of oral mucosal and skin lesions

Term	Description
Primary lesions	
Macule	A flat, discoloured lesion neither raised nor depressed <10 mm in size with well-circumscribed borders
Papule	A circumscribed solid elevated lesion <0.5 cm
Nodule	An elevated, circumscribed solid mass >0.5 cm with a depth extending into underlying tissue
Polyp	A small growth protruding from the mucosa which can either be broad-based 'sessile' or be on a stalk, or 'pedunculated'
Plaque	A flat, solid raised lesion
Vesicle	Small, fluid-filled elevation <0.5 cm
Bulla	A blister, fluid-filled >0.5 cm. May be intra- or subepithelial
Pustule	A vesicle filled with pus
Abscess	A localized collection of pus
Secondary lesions	
Scale	Thin or thick flake of skin varying in colour, usually secondary to desquamated epithelium
Crust	Dried exudate on skin surface
Fissure	Linear crack of skin surface
Desquamation	Loss or shedding of epithelial cells
Atrophy	A thinning of the epithelium with a decreased number of epithelial cells. Usually presents with red appearance. May present on the tongue as a loss of papillae
Erosion	A partial-thickness loss of epithelium
Ulcer	A full-thickness loss of epithelium that extends below the basement membrane, extending into the connective tissue

TABLE 10.1B ■ **Definitions of oral mucosal and skin lesions with specific clinical criteria**

Term	Description
Epulis	A nonspecific term for a raised lesion on the gingiva or alveolar mucosa
Tumour	A nonspecific term for any neoplastic lesion that may be benign or malignant
Fistula	An abnormal pathway connecting two anatomical spaces (i.e., oro-antral fistula)
Sinus	A channel opening from a blind end (i.e., a draining dental infection from a tooth)
Cellulitis	A spreading bacterial infection involving layers of the skin or fascia
Petechia	Pinpoint or small haemorrhagic spots. They do not blanch on pressure
Purpura	A collection of blood beneath the skin caused by extravasation of blood from the microvasculature that is not caused by trauma. It does not blanch on pressure
Ecchymosis	A bruise resulting from a large accumulation of blood in the tissues caused by trauma
Erythroplakia	An abnormal red patch or plaque that cannot be characterized clinically or pathologically as any other condition. Surface often described as 'velvet-like', and lesions have a high risk of malignant change
Leukoplakia	A whitish patch or plaque that cannot be characterized as any other definable lesion. It has a questionable risk of malignant change. They can be homogeneous or nonhomogeneous (speckled or nodular leukoplakia) with an irregular texture
Naevus	Any localized area of pigmentation or vascularization. Can be congenital
Cyst	A closed capsule or sac-like structure that can be filled with fluid, semisolid or gaseous material in soft-tissue or bone that may be lined or unlined by epithelium

- Size.
- Shape and symmetry.
- Colour and pigmentation.
- Surface features.
- Distribution over the tissue (diffuse or well demarcated).
- Findings on palpation (superficial, deep, fixed, mobile/movable, tender, etc.).

Orofacial infections

DIFFERENTIAL DIAGNOSIS

- Bacterial infections:
  - Odontogenic.
  - Scarlet fever.
  - Tuberculosis.
  - Atypical mycobacterial infection.
  - Actinomycosis.
  - Syphilis.
  - Impetigo.
  - Osteomyelitis.
- Viral infections:
  - Primary herpetic gingivostomatitis.
  - Herpes labialis.
  - Herpangina.

- Hand, foot and mouth disease.
- Infectious mononucleosis.
- Varicella.
- Fungal infections:
  - Candidosis.

ODONTOGENIC INFECTIONS

The basic signs and symptoms of oral infection should be familiar to all clinicians.
Acute infection usually presents as an emergency:
- A sick, upset child.
- Raised temperature.
- Red, swollen face.
- Anxious and distressed parents.
Chronic infection typically presents as an asymptomatic or indolent process:
- A sinus may be present (usually labial or buccal).
- Mobile tooth.
- Halitosis.
- Discoloured tooth.

Presentation

- When presenting as an acute infection, children tend to present with facial cellulitis rather than an abscess with a large collection of pus that might be seen in an adult. The child is usually febrile. Pain is common, although if the infection has perforated the cortical plate, the child may not be in pain. The mainstay of treatment is removal of the cause of the infection. Too often, antibiotics are prescribed without consideration of extraction of the tooth or extirpation of the pulp.
- Maxillary canine fossa infections are predominantly Gram-positive or facultative anaerobic infections (Figure 10.2A). Posterior spread may lead to cavernous sinus thrombosis and a brain abscess.

  Maxillary odontogenic infections may be misdiagnosed by medical practitioners as a periorbital or preseptal cellulitis, which are typically caused by *Haemophilus influenzae*, *Streptococcus pneumoniae* or *Staphylococcus aureus* from haematogenous spread, local trauma, a sty or chalazion or from sinus infection. Periorbital cellulitis is managed usually with second- or third-generation cephalosporins or flucloxacillin. These antibiotics are too narrow in their spectrum to adequately manage dental infections.
- Mandibular infections which spread inferiorly may compromise the airway, and there is the possibility of mediastinal involvement.
- Young patients may be dehydrated at presentation. It is important to ask about their fluid intake and ascertain whether the child has urinated during the previous 12 hours (see Appendix B).

Management

The treatment of infection follows two basic tenets:
- Removal of the cause.
- Local drainage and debridement if pus is present.

Criteria for hospital admission

- A child who is septic and clearly unwell.
- A significant infection present or spiking temperatures over 39° C.

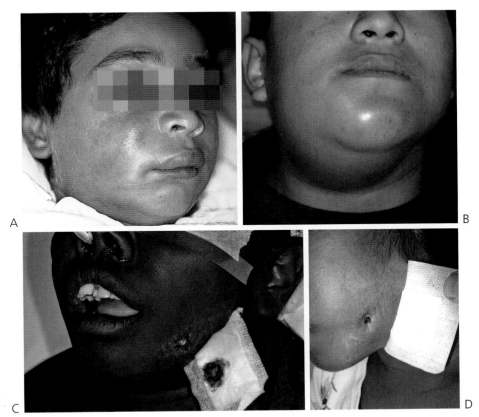

Figure 10.2 Severe facial swellings associated with odontogenic infections. (A) The right eye was almost closed from the spreading infection. (B) This child required extraoral drainage of the facial swelling, which was caused by involvement of the floor of mouth as well as the submandibular and sublingual spaces. He required hospitalization and was placed on high-dose intravenous penicillin supplemented with metronidazole. (C) Extraoral drainage of a long-standing abscess. Although this child was placed on repeated courses of antibiotics, no attempt was made to remove the cause of the infection, namely a carious tooth. (D) Healing 24 h after removal of the mandibular left first permanent molar tooth and debridement of the sinus tract draining sinus.

- Floor-of-mouth swelling or a swelling that crosses the midline.
- Dehydration.

Use of antibiotics

- Antibiotics should not be considered automatically as a first-line treatment unless there is systemic involvement. In a child, a temperature of 39° C or higher should be considered a significant rise (normal ~37° C).
- If a child has a systemic infection resulting from a local focus of dental infection – that is, a sick child with a high temperature – an obvious spreading infection of the face and regional lymphadenopathy, then antibiotics should be administered.
- Immunosuppressed patients or those with cardiac disease should receive antibiotics if infection is suspected.

General considerations

- Extraction of involved teeth.
Or
- Root canal treatment for permanent teeth if it is considered important to save particular teeth (see Chapter 7).
- Oral antibiotics if systemic involvement.

  A synthetic penicillin such as amoxicillin is usually the oral drug of first choice. This has the advantage that it is given only three times a day, achieves higher blood levels and is a more effective antibiotic than, for example, phenoxymethylpenicillin (penicillin VK). Often, the extraction of the abscessed tooth alone will bring about resolution without antibiotic treatment.

SEVERE INFECTIONS

- Hospital admission.
- Extraction of involved teeth. It is impossible to drain a significant infection solely through the root canals of a primary tooth.
- Drainage of any pus present. If the diagnosis or the correct management of an infection in the mandible has been delayed and the swelling has crossed the midline, or if there is swelling of the floor of the mouth, then extraoral drainage with a through-and-through drain should be considered (Figure 10.2B). If a flap is raised, any granulation tissue should be removed and the area well irrigated. Flaps should be apposed but not tightly sutured. Soft flexible drains such as Penrose drains are better tolerated in children than are corrugated drains.
- Swabs for culture and sensitivity. It is important to take specimens for culture, even though empirical antibiotic treatment needs to be commenced immediately. Should the infection not respond to the initial antibiotic treatment, the results of the culture and sensitivity tests can be used to determine subsequent management.
- Intravenous antibiotics. Benzylpenicillin is the drug of first choice (up to 200 mg/kg per day).
- First-generation cephalosporins may be used as an alternative. However, if the child is allergic to penicillin, there may be cross-allergenicity, and in these cases it would be prudent to avoid cephalosporins; clindamycin would be a better choice.
- In severe infections, particularly deep-seated infections and those involving bone, metronidazole can be added. The flora of most odontogenic infections is of a mixed type, and anaerobic organisms are thought to have a significant role in their pathogenesis.
- Combination antibiotics such as Augmentin Duo provide additional antimicrobial coverage and have the advantage of being more palatable orally than metronidazole.
- For any antibiotics administered, adequate doses must be used. Treat infections in the head and neck seriously.
- Maintenance fluids, adding 10% to 12% for every degree over 37.5° C, until the child is drinking of their own accord.
- Use 0.2% chlorhexidine gluconate mouth rinses.
- Give adequate pain control with paracetamol suspension (orally), 15 mg/kg, every 4 hours, or by suppository (rectally).
- If the eye is closed because of collateral oedema, it may be appropriate to apply 0.5% chloramphenicol eye drops or 1% ointment to prevent conjunctivitis.

Osteomyelitis

Very rarely, odontogenic infection may lead to osteomyelitis, most commonly involving the mandible. Radiographically, the bone has a 'moth-eaten' appearance. Curettage of the area is required to remove bony sequestra, and antibiotics are given for at least 6 weeks, depending on the results of microbiological culture and sensitivity test results. A variant of osteomyelitis has been reported in children and adolescents, termed 'juvenile mandibular chronic osteomyelitis'. In this condition, there is often no obvious odontogenic source of infection; there is limited response to a number of different treatment modalities.

Garré osteomyelitis (periostitis ossificans)

This is a usually painless, nonsuppurative, chronic osteomyelitis caused by a low-grade odontogenic infection in the mandible in children secondary to caries. The radiographic appearance is characteristic showing a reactive proliferative periostitis where new bone is laid down on the periphery of the cortical bone at the angle or lower border of mandible in response to mild infection.

PRIMARY HERPETIC GINGIVOSTOMATITIS (HUMAN HERPES VIRUS 1 AND 2) (Figure 10.3)

Many viral infections resulting in ulceration in children present similarly with a prodromal period of malaise and fever followed by vesicular eruption that often break down rapidly to form painful shallow ulcers. Often the history, location, number and presentation of ulcers will aid diagnosis.

Primary herpes is the most common cause of severe oral ulceration in children. It is caused by herpes simplex type 1 virus (HHV-1). These form different types of the human herpes viruses (HHVs). Occasional cases of HHV-2 (the usual cause of genital herpes) infection have been reported and should not immediately indicate a case of sexual abuse. The clinical appearances of the two different strains of herpes simplex virus are, however, clinically identical in the orofacial

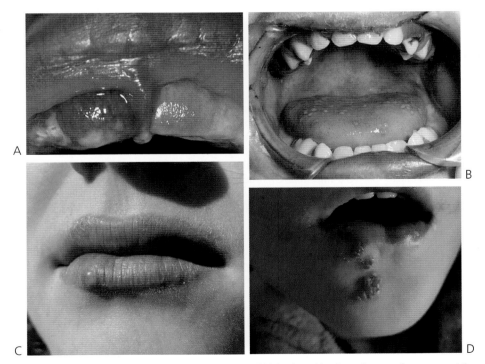

Figure 10.3   Different presentations of herpetic infection. (A) Infection with primary herpes often occurs at the time of eruption of primary teeth but not before. (B) Common presentation with multiple small ulcers on the tongue, the fauces and gingival inflammation. (C) Recurrent herpes labialis secondary to ultraviolet exposure. A classic, isolated vesicle on the lower lip. (D) Primary herpes involving the lips and chin but not the oral cavity with coalescence of multiple vesicles. (Courtesy Dr. M. Wilson, Sydney.)

region. Although majority of the population has been infected with the virus by adulthood, less than 1% manifest an acute primary infection. This usually occurs after 6 months of age, often coincident with the eruption of the primary incisors. The peak incidence is between 12 and 18 months of age. Incubation time is 3 to 5 days, with a prodromal 48-hour history of irritability, pyrexia and malaise. The child is often unwell, has difficulty in eating and drinking and typically drools. Stomatitis is present, with the gingival tissues in particular becoming red and oedematous.

Small intraepithelial vesicles appear and rapidly break down to form painful, shallow ulcers. Vesicles may form on any part of the oral mucosa, including the skin around the lips. Solitary ulcers are usually small (1–2 mm) and painful with an erythematous margin, but larger ulcers with irregular margins often result from the coalescence of individual lesions. The disease is self-limiting, and the ulcers heal spontaneously without scarring, within 10 to 14 days.

Diagnosis

- History and clinical features.
- Exfoliative cytology showing the presence of multinucleated giant cells and viral inclusion bodies can be used for rapid diagnosis if laboratory support is at hand.
- Viral antigen can be detected by polymerase chain reaction amplification. This can sometimes be useful in early confirmation of the diagnosis.
- Viral culture can take days or weeks to yield a result.
- Viral antibody detection in blood samples during the acute and convalescent phases. A rise in antibody titre can only provide late confirmation of the diagnosis.

Management

- Symptomatic care.
- Encourage oral fluids.
- If oral fluids cannot be taken, then hospital admission is mandatory and intravenous fluids must be commenced.
- Analgesics: paracetamol, 15 mg/kg, every 4 hours.
- Mouthwashes for older children: chlorhexidine gluconate, 0.2%, 10 mL every 4 hours. In children over 10 years of age, tetracycline or minocycline mouthwashes may be beneficial, but must be avoided in younger children to prevent possible tooth discolouration.
- In young children with severe ulceration, chlorhexidine can be swabbed over the affected areas with cotton wool swabs. Much of the pain from oral ulceration is probably because of secondary bacterial infection. Chlorhexidine 0.2% mouthwash has been shown to be beneficial in the management of oral ulceration. A mouthwash containing benzydamine hydrochloride 0.15% and chlorhexidine 0.12% (Difflam C®) may offer some advantages over chlorhexidine alone.
- Topical anaesthetics: lignocaine viscous 2% or lignocaine (Xylocaine®) spray.
  Note: Topical anaesthetics are often advocated; however, the effect of a numb mouth in a young child can be more distressing than the pain from the illness and can lead to ulceration from the decrease in sensation and subsequent trauma. In addition, it is often difficult to initiate swallowing with a soft palate that has been anaesthetized.
- Antiviral chemotherapy. Aciclovir oral suspension or intravenously for immunosuppressed patients. This treatment is only worthwhile in the vesicular phase of the infection, that is, within the first 72 hours.
  Children <2 years of age: aciclovir oral suspension 100 mg 5 times/day for 7 days
  Children >2 years of age: aciclovir oral suspension 200 mg 5 times/day for 7 days
  Note: the use of antiviral medications is contentious and usually reserved for children who are immunocompromised. There is some evidence to suggest, however, that the administration of aciclovir in the first 72 hours of the infection may be beneficial.

- Adequate pain control is also required with regular administration of paracetamol.
- Antibiotics are unhelpful.
- Severely affected young children often present dehydrated, being unable to eat or drink. Hospital admission is required for these cases with maintenance intravenous fluids.

CLINICAL HINT

An obviously ill child with a febrile illness for a few days and presenting with puffy erythematous gingivae is most likely to have primary herpetic gingivostomatitis. Frank ulceration may not be present.

HERPANGINA AND HAND, FOOT AND MOUTH DISEASE

These infections are caused by the Coxsackie group A viruses. As with primary herpes, both of these conditions have a prodromal phase of low-grade fever and malaise that may last for several days before the appearance of the vesicles. In herpangina (Figure 10.4A), a cluster of four to five vesicles is usually found on the palate, pillars of the fauces and pharynx, whereas in hand, foot and mouth disease, up to 10 vesicles occur at these sites and elsewhere in the mouth, in addition to the hands and feet (Figure 10.4B). The skin lesions appear on the palmar surfaces of the hands and plantar surface of the feet and are surrounded by an erythematous margin. The severity of both diseases is usually milder than primary herpes and healing occurs within 10 days. Both diseases occur in epidemics, mainly affecting children.

Diagnosis

- Clinical appearance and history.
- Known epidemic.
- Viral culture from swab.

Management

- Symptomatic care, as for other viral infections.

INFECTIOUS MONONUCLEOSIS (HUMAN HERPES VIRUS 4) (Figure 10.5A)

- This infection is caused by the Epstein–Barr virus (EBV) and mainly affects older adolescents and young adults. EBV is now recognized as one of the human herpes family and is known as HHV-4. The disease is highly infective and is characterized by malaise, fever,

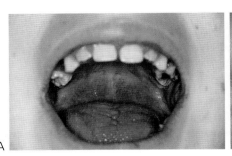
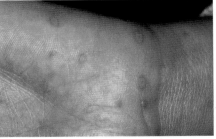

A   B

Figure 10.4 Infections caused by Coxsackie group A viruses. (A) Herpangina with characteristic palatal and pharyngeal ulceration and inflammation. (B) Cutaneous lesions in hand, foot and mouth disease.

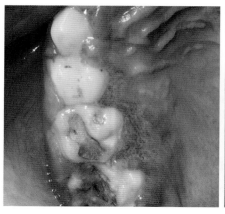
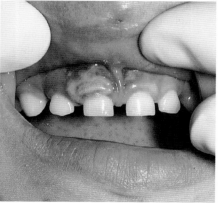

A   B

Figure 10.5 (A) Gingival ulceration and stomatitis during an acute episode of infectious mononucleosis. (B) Gingival ulceration in chickenpox infection.

lymphadenopathy and acute pharyngitis. In young children, ulcers and petechiae are often found in the posterior pharynx and soft palate. The disease is self-limiting.

Diagnosis

- History and clinical features.
- Monospot test (Mononucleosis spot test) or Paul–Bunnell agglutination test and atypical monocytes on blood film.

VARICELLA (HUMAN HERPES VIRUS 3) (Figure 10.5B)

This is a highly contagious virus causing chickenpox in younger subjects and shingles in older individuals. There is a prodromal phase of malaise and fever for 24 hours followed by macular eruptions and vesicles. In chickenpox, oral lesions occur in around 50% of cases, but only a small number of vesicles occur in the mouth. These lesions may be found anywhere in the mouth in addition to other mucosal sites such as conjunctivae, nose or anus. Healing of oral lesions is uneventful.

Diagnosis

- History and clinical features.

MEASLES

Measles is a highly contagious paramyxovirus infection (*Morbillivirus*), predominately of childhood that presents as an acute febrile illness, a maculopapular rash, keratoconjunctivitis, malaise, cough and the characteristic oral lesions; Koplik spots. These are small white papules surrounded by an erythematous margin and cover the buccal mucosa. They usually precede the typical measles rash by up to 4 days. The incubation period is 8 to 12 days, with a prodromal phase of malaise, fever, cough and oral signs. Healing of oral lesions is uneventful. Worldwide immunization programs have seen a 95% reduction in the disease; however, some children may suffer other complications of the disease such as pneumonia (5%) or encephalitis (0.1%). Subacute sclerosing panencephalitis is a rare, progressive and ultimately fatal complication of measles, caused by reactivation of the virus or an inappropriate immune response. The majority of deaths caused by measles (0.2%) are usually secondary to pneumonia.

Diagnosis

■ History and clinical features.

CANDIDOSIS

Acute pseudomembranous candidosis

The most common presentation of candidal infection in infants is thrush. White plaques are present, which on removal reveal an erythematous, sometimes haemorrhagic, base. In older children, thrush occurs when children are immunocompromised, such as in acquired immune deficiency syndrome (AIDS) or in diabetes, or when prescribed antibiotics or corticosteroids, or during chemotherapy and radiotherapy for malignancies.

> **CLINICAL HINT**
>
> Soft white lesions which can be rubbed off, leaving a red base, are typical of thrush.

Median rhomboid glossitis

This characteristic but uncommon lesion is a candidosis (rather than a developmental anomaly as was thought for many years) presenting as an erythematous, depapillated well-delineated area on the midline of the dorsal surface of the tongue anterior to the circumvallate papillae, often in children in response to the use of antibiotics and inhaled corticosteroids (for management of asthma).

Diagnosis

Some 50% of children will have *Candida albicans* as a normal commensal, and culture is of little benefit. Smears or scrapings for exfoliative cytology reveal hyphae when disease is present, but the clinical picture may be diagnostic.

Management

■ Antifungal medication for 2 to 4 weeks. Most antifungal treatment is unsuccessful because of poor compliance or instruction by the clinician.
■ Amphotericin B lozenges or nystatin drops.
■ Fluconazole orally (100 mg daily for 14 days) for cases of mucocutaneous candidosis.
■ Systemic antifungal medication may need to be used for children who are immunosuppressed or where the organism does not respond to topical treatment as described earlier.
■ Chlorhexidine 0.2% mouthwash or swabs.

Ulcerative and vesiculobullous lesions

Clinicians are often confused regarding the terminology of these lesions (see Table 10.1A). An ulcer is regarded as localized loss of the full thickness of the epithelium. Partial-thickness loss is termed an 'erosion'. Clinically, it can be challenging to distinguish between an ulcer and an erosion. A vesicle is a small, fluid-filled blister, whereas a bulla is a larger blister, generally measuring greater than 5 mm. Different conditions arise from cleavage of the epithelium at different levels (i.e., intraepithelial or subepithelial) and are important in determining a diagnosis. When these lesions burst, they leave an ulcer. A thorough history noting the number, frequency, duration and site of occurrence is very important.

DIFFERENTIAL DIAGNOSIS

- Traumatic:
  - Postmandibular block anaesthesia (Figure 10.6A).
  - Chemical or thermal burns (Figure 10.6C, D).
  - Riga–Fedé ulceration (traumatic ulceration of tongue) (Figure 10.7).

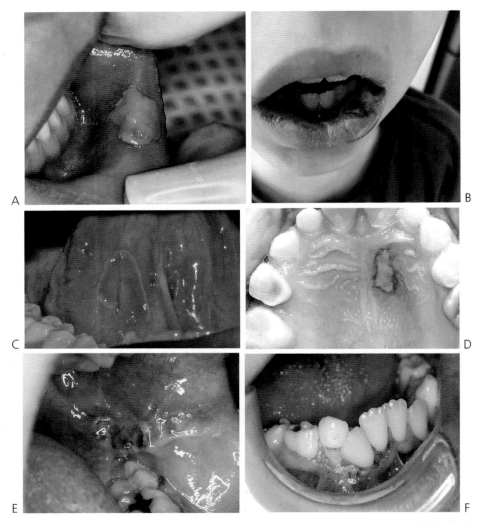

Figure 10.6 Traumatic ulceration (A) Traumatic oral ulceration from biting the lip after a mandibular block injection. (B) Lip-biting may be extensive leaving significant damage to mucosa and the underlying muscle. (C) Chemical burn from an antihistamine tablet placed under the tongue in an adolescent. (Courtesy Ms. Leanne Smith, Uni Newcastle.) (D) Early stages in the healing of a thermal burn on the palate caused by hot food. Note the well-defined inflammatory border while the defect is covered by a yellow pseudomembranous slough. (E) Pericoronitis does not only occur with the third molars in younger children; in this case, it occurs with the eruption of the second permanent molar. (F) The loss of tissue around tooth 83 has been caused by the child picking at the gingiva with his fingernail. Such episodes of self-mutilation warrant further investigation into the child's psychological situation and may be an indicator of anxiety, depression, attention seeking or even abuse.

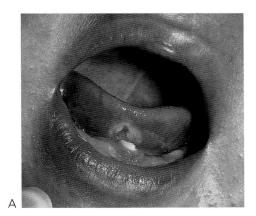

Figure 10.7 (A) Riga–Fedé ulcer on the ventral surface of the tongue arising from rubbing on the solitary mandibular incisor. (B) There may be extensive loss of tissue into the tongue musculature. A

- Infective (see orofacial infections differential diagnosis on p. 245):
  - Primary herpetic gingivostomatitis.
  - Herpangina.
  - Hand, foot and mouth disease.
  - Infectious mononucleosis.
  - Varicella.
- Others:
  - Recurrent aphthous ulceration (RAU).
  - Erythema multiforme.
  - Stevens–Johnson syndrome.
  - Behçet syndrome.
  - Epidermolysis bullosa (EB).
  - Lupus erythematosus.
  - Neutropenic ulceration.
  - Orofacial granulomatosis/Crohn disease.
  - Pemphigus.
  - Drug-induced (chemotherapy) lesions.
  - Lichen planus.

LIP ULCERATION AFTER MANDIBULAR BLOCK ANAESTHESIA

This is one of the most common causes of traumatic ulceration. Parents should be warned and children reminded not to bite their lips after mandibular block anaesthesia (Figure 10.6A).

RIGA–FEDÉ ULCERATION

This is ulceration of the ventral surface of the tongue caused by trauma from continual protrusive and retrusive movements over the lower incisors (Figure 10.7A, B). Once a common finding in cases of whooping cough, it is now predominately seen in children with cerebral palsy, although children with no other medical comorbidity may present with this condition.

Management

Smoothen sharp incisal edges or place domes of composite resin over the teeth. Rarely, in severe cases, extraction of the teeth might be considered (see also Chapter 13).

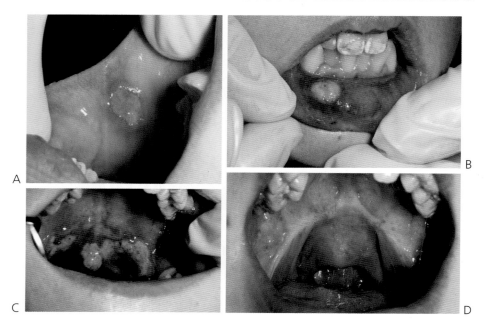

Figure 10.8 (A) Minor recurrent aphthae in an adolescent girl. These lesions were extremely painful. Haematological investigations revealed a low folate level, which, when corrected, eliminated further ulceration. (B, C) Major recurrent aphthous ulceration is a debilitating condition and heals with scarring. This girl's ulcers were managed with systemic steroids. (D) Over time, there was extensive scarring leading to tissue loss with obliteration of the uvula and shortening of the palate resulting in velo-palatine incompetence.

RECURRENT APHTHOUS ULCERATION (Figure 10.8)

RAU has been estimated to affect up to 20% of the population. Lesions are classified according to size, duration and severity. Two clinical groups have been described:

- Simple
  - Minor aphthae.
  - Major aphthae (Figure 10.8B).
  - Herpetiform ulceration.
- Complex
  - This fourth form, complex aphthous stomatitis, has recently been described.

Minor aphthae account for the majority of cases, with crops of two to five shallow ulcers measuring up to 5 mm and occurring on nonkeratinized mucosa. There is a typical central yellow slough with an erythematous halo. Ulcers heal within 10 to 14 days without scarring. The cause of RAU is contentious, although it is commonly believed to be precipitated by stress and local trauma. There is some evidence for a genetic basis for the disorder, with an increased incidence of ulceration in children when both parents have RAU. Some studies have suggested that RAU is associated with nutritional deficiency states, and so haematological investigation can be helpful. In major aphthae, the keratinized mucosa may also be involved, and the ulcers are larger, last longer and heal with scarring.

Complex aphthous stomatitis accounts for less than 5% of cases that are recurrent, with multiple lesions that are extremely painful and slow to heal. The differences between simple and complex forms are summarized in Table 10.2. Aphthous-like ulceration can be noted as an oral

TABLE 10.2 ■ **Presentation of aphthous stomatitis**

	Simple	Complex
Frequency	Episodic; <6 episodes per year	Continuous rather than episodic; >6 episodes per year
Duration	Short-lived	Persistent
Number	Few/limited number of lesions	Many rather than few lesions
Healing	Rapid healing and generally heal without scarring except for major aphthae	Slower to heal with scarring
Location	Generally confined to nonkeratinized mucosa	Can involve both keratinized and nonkeratinized mucosa
Pain	Minimal pain/discomfort with minimal disability	Extremely painful and disabling
Geography	Limited to oral mucosa	May have genital involvement Need to exclude Behçet disease

(Modified from Rogers, R.S. 3rd, 1997. Recurrent aphthous stomatitis: clinical characteristics and associated systemic disorders. Seminars in Cutaneous Medicine and Surgery 16, 278–283.)

manifestation in a range of systemic conditions, and a detailed medical history should be carefully taken.

Diagnosis

- History and clinical features.
- Blood tests for full blood count (FBC) and differential white cell count (WCC), iron studies (including serum ferritin), serum vitamin B_{12} levels, and folate and red cell folate in particular (if anaemia or latent anaemia suspected).

Management

- Symptomatic care with mouth rinses:
  - Chlorhexidine gluconate 0.2%, 10 mL three times daily.
  - Minocycline mouthwash, 50 mg in 10 mL water three times daily for 4 days for children over 8 years of age.
  - Benzydamine hydrochloride 0.15% and chlorhexidine 0.12% (Difflam C®).
- Topical corticosteroids:
  - Triamcinolone in Orabase® (although this may be difficult to apply in children).
  - Beclomethasone dipropionate or fluticasone propionate asthma inhalers sprayed onto the ulcers.
  - Betamethasone dipropionate 0.05% (Diprosone OV) ointment.
- Systemic corticosteroids only in most severe cases of major aphthous ulceration with consideration of steroid-sparing agents in recalcitrant cases managed by medical physician.
- Herpetiform ulceration seems to respond best to minocycline mouthwashes.

Biopsy should only be considered if there is any doubt about the clinical diagnosis. Haematological investigations should be carried out to exclude anaemia or haematinic deficiency states (when appropriate, replacement can improve the ulceration or bring about resolution). As with all oral ulceration, symptomatic care with appropriate analgesics and antiseptic mouthwashes is appropriate. In those cases of severe recurrent oral ulceration, systemic corticosteroids may be used, although their use is best avoided in children. Minocycline mouthwashes should not be used in children under the age of 8 years to avoid tooth discolouration. Major aphthae tend to occur in older children.

> **CLINICAL HINT**
>
> Minor aphthae occur in recurrent crops of two to five ulcers, sparing the palate and dorsum of the tongue.

BEHÇET SYNDROME

This condition is characterized by recurrent aphthous ulceration together with genital and ocular lesions, although the skin and other systems can also be involved. Lesions may affect other parts of the body. Behçet syndrome can be subdivided into four main types:

- Mucocutaneous form: classical form with involvement of oral and genital mucosa and conjunctiva.
- Arthritic form with arthritis in association with mucocutaneous lesions.
- Neurological form with central nervous system involvement.
- Ocular form with uveitis in addition to oral and genital lesions.

Diagnosis

- History and clinical presentation.

Management

> **CLINICAL HINT: BLOOD TESTS FOR RECURRENT ULCERATION**
>
> - Full blood count including differential white cell count.
> - Erythrocyte sedimentation rate (suggestive of inflammatory diseases).
> - Vitamin B_{12} and folate.
> - Iron studies
>   - Total iron-binding capacity.
>   - Serum iron.
>   - Ferritin.
> - Antinuclear antibodies (associated with systemic lupus erythematosus, Sjögren syndrome, scleroderma, rheumatoid arthritis).
> - C-reactive protein (suggestive of inflammatory bowel disease).
> - Angiotensin converting enzyme (test for sarcoid disease).
> - Immunoglobulin (IgA/IgG) antigliadin antibodies (test for coeliac disease).

As for recurrent aphthous ulceration, systemic treatment is usually required. Referral to appropriate specialist team for management of extra-oral manifestations is needed.

ERYTHEMA MULTIFORME, STEVENS–JOHNSON SYNDROME AND TOXIC EPIDERMAL NECROLYSIS

Three conditions exist that present with similar clinical signs and histopathological appearances. Like many conditions, varied nomenclature and misdiagnosis have clouded and confused the diagnosis/es. There is now a view that these are distinct pathological entities and, perhaps importantly, might be initiated by quite distinct aetiological agents. The alternative view is that these disorders represent different presentations of the same basic disorder, distinguished by the severity and extent of the lesions.

Erythema multiforme (von Hebra) (Figure 10.9A–D)

The original description of erythema multiforme was that of a self-limiting but often recurrent and seasonal skin disease with mucosal involvement limited to the oral cavity. The lips are typically ulcerated with blood staining and crusting. The characteristic macules ('target lesions') occur on the limbs but with less involvement of the trunk or head and neck. These lesions are concentric

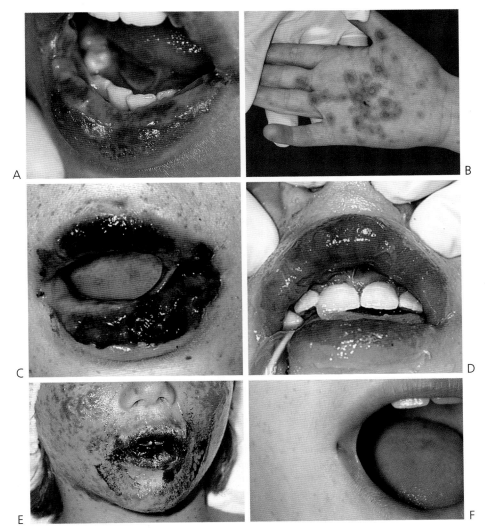

Figure 10.9 (A) Erythema multiforme presenting with pan-stomatitis and severe dehydration. Treatment included rehydration and symptomatic care of the ulceration. (B) Typical target lesions seen in erythema multiforme. (C) Ulceration of the lips may be severe and in this case resulted in the lips becoming fused together by the slough and crusting. (D) The mouth was debrided under general anaesthesia. (E) Stevens–Johnson syndrome with severe mucocutaneous involvement. This child required admission to the intensive care unit for 3 days. (F) Stricture of the lateral commissure of the lips because of scarring following an episode of Stevens–Johnson syndrome.

with an erythematous halo and a central blister. Although the lesions are extremely painful, the course of the illness is self-limiting, and healing is uneventful.

Stevens–Johnson syndrome (Figure 10.9E, F)

The condition presents with acute febrile illness, generalized exanthema, lesions involving the oral cavity and a severe purulent conjunctivitis. The skin lesions are more extensive than those of erythema multiforme. Stevens–Johnson syndrome is characterized by vesiculobullous eruptions over the body, in particular the trunk, and severe involvement of multiple mucous membranes including the vulva or penis and conjunctiva. The course of the condition is longer, and scarring may occur. Some authors have used the term 'erythema multiforme major' for Stevens–Johnson syndrome, defining the condition as a severe form of erythema multiforme, but this is disputed by others. Although Stevens–Johnson syndrome patients are acutely ill, death is rare.

Toxic epidermal necrolysis

Similar to the clinical presentation of Stevens–Johnson syndrome, toxic epidermal necrolysis (TEN), or Lyell syndrome, is a severe, sometimes fatal, bullous drug-induced eruption where sheets of skin are lost. It resembles third-degree burns or staphylococcal scalded skin syndrome. Oral involvement is similar to Stevens–Johnson syndrome. TEN may be misdiagnosed as a severe form of Stevens–Johnson syndrome (given the controversy over nomenclature), but the use of steroids is controversial, given an increase in mortality with their use in this disease.

Aetiology

Erythema multiforme is often initiated by herpes simplex reactivation. There is some evidence that Stevens–Johnson syndrome is initiated by a *Mycoplasma pneumoniae* respiratory infection or drug reaction. TEN is drug induced.

Clinical presentation

A summary of the three conditions is shown in Table 10.3. There is an acute onset of fever, cough, sore throat and malaise, followed by the appearance of the lesions on the body and oral cavity ranging from 2 days to 2 weeks after the onset of symptoms. These break down quickly in the mouth to form ulcers. The most striking feature is the degree of oral mucosal involvement that may lead in all three cases to a pan-stomatitis and sloughing of the whole oral mucosa. There is extensive ulceration and crusting around the lips, oral haemorrhage and necrosis of skin and mucosa leading to secondary infection. There may be difficulty in eating and drinking, which complicates the clinical course, and there is usually extreme discomfort from both the skin and oral lesions that may necessitate narcotic analgesics.

Management

If there is a known precipitating factor such as herpes simplex infection, then antivirals such as topical acyclovir can be used in an attempt at prophylaxis. Management is generally symptomatic and supportive. A major problem during the course of the illness is fluid balance and pain, much of which arises from secondary infection of the oral lesions. Debridement of the oral cavity with 0.2% chlorhexidine gluconate or benzydamine hydrochloride and chlorhexidine (Difflam C®) is effective in removing much of the necrotic debris from the mouth. Extensive areas of ulceration tend to be less responsive to chlorhexidine, and a minocycline mouthwash may prove more effective. The role of systemic corticosteroids is controversial, but they may be necessary in severe cases. Their use in recurrences may obviate the need for hospital admission.

Management also includes:
- Adequate fluid replacement and total parenteral nutrition if required.
- Pain control, which may necessitate the use of narcotics and sedation.

TABLE 10.3 ■ Differential diagnosis of erythema multiforme, Stevens–Johnson syndrome and toxic epidermal necrolysis

Signs	Erythema multiforme (EM minor)	Stevens–Johnson syndrome (EM major)	Toxic epidermal necrolysis (Lyell syndrome)
Aetiology	HSV reactivation in some cases	HSV reactivation? *Mycoplasma*? Drug-related	Drug-related – trimethoprim and sulfamethoxazole (Bactrim), carbamazepine lamotrigine
Recurrence	75% have multiple recurrences – two to three per year	Usually single but may recur	May recur in response to initiating agent
Target lesions	Yes, typical concentric target lesions on extremities	No, or atypical vesiculobullous eruptions on trunk, head and neck	Skin involvement is so severe that no separate lesions are ever seen
Skin	Raised papules acrally distributed	Multiple tissue involvement usually severe	Severe skin involvement, similar to burns. Confluent sloughing of the skin
Mucosa	Crusting and bleeding of lips	Crusting and bleeding of lips. Severe multiple mucosal involvement – oral, ocular and genital	Severe multiple mucosal involvement
Course	Within 2 weeks	>2 weeks: oral lesions may take months	Healing phase will take many months
Management	Short course of high-dose systemic steroids. Fluid maintenance	Fluid maintenance. Debridement of oral lesions. Narcotic analgesics/ sedation? Antibiotics for *Mycoplasma pneumoniae*? Short course of high dose systemic steroids	Similar to burns management. Resuscitation and fluid maintenance. Narcotic analgesics. Intubation and intensive care unit admission
Sequelae	Healing without scarring	May be scarring and oral stricture	Blindness may occur and there is a high mortality
Histopathology	Similar in all three conditions: subepidermal vesicles and bullae		

HSV, Herpes simplex virus.

PEMPHIGUS

Pemphigus vulgaris is an important vesiculo-bullous disease mainly affecting adults; however, children can be also affected. The lesions are intraepithelial and rapidly break down, so that affected individuals are often unaware of blistering, complaining instead of ulceration, mainly affecting the buccal mucosa, palate and lips.

Diagnosis

There may be a positive Nikolsky sign (separation of the superficial epithelial layers from the basal layer produced by rubbing or gentle pressure), and cytological examination can reveal the presence of Tzanck cells. Direct immunofluorescence using frozen sections from an oral biopsy will reveal intercellular immunoglobulin (IgG) deposits in the epithelium that are diagnostic for this disease. Indirect immunofluorescence on blood samples is used to complement diagnosis.

Management

- Systemic corticosteroid therapy in conjunction with steroid-sparing agents.
- Topical corticosteroids are used for oral lesions.
- Antiseptic or minocycline mouthwashes and analgesia as necessary.

> **CLINICAL HINT**
>
> Crusted, blood-stained lips are typical of erythema multiforme. Examine the palms of the hands for the characteristic target lesions.

All of these mucocutaneous conditions in children heal with scarring and are managed similarly.

EPIDERMOLYSIS BULLOSA (Figure 10.10)

Epidermolysis bullosa is a term used to describe several hereditary blistering disorders of the skin and mucosa. EB is described by increased skin/mucosa fragility to minimal mechanical trauma, with disturbances at the dermoepidermal junction. This results in blistering, peeling, erosions, ulcerations, wounds or scars. Within the hereditary variants, there are four major classical types, depending on the location of the structural defect within the skin:

- EB simplex: the most common type of EB, transmitted as an autosomal dominant or autosomal recessive.
- Junctional EB: with demidesmosome defect, transmitted as an autosomal recessive trait.

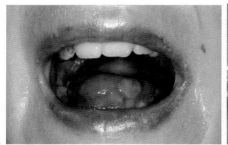

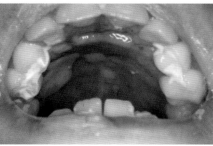

A   B

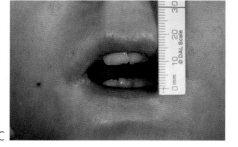

C

Figure 10.10 Vesiculobullous diseases often present with ulceration attributed to fragility and breakdown of the preceding vesicles or bullae. Epidermolysis bullosa is a severely debilitating disease presenting with multiple large ulcers that heal with scarring (A, B), loss of tissue and stricture. Limitation of opening severely complicates the provision of oral care and dental treatment (C). (Courtesy Dr. Joana Monteiro, London.)

- EB, autosomal recessive or dominant, characterized by scarring following blistering.
- Kindler EB, a rare type of EB, more common in consanguineous populations.

Other related skin fragility disorders include conditions with superficial skin cleavage, such as keratinopathic ichthyoses.

Blisters may form from birth or appear in the first few weeks of life, depending on the form of the disease. Growth may lead to improvement or worsening of the clinical features. Depending on the type and severity, several co-morbidities may develop, including anaemia, oesophageal stricture, corneal ulceration, progressive skin contractures, mitten deformities of hands and development of squamous cell carcinoma. Oral features include enamel hypoplasia related to junctional EB, microstomia following scarring in severe forms of dystrophic EB and reported absence of tongue papillae in severe forms of dystrophic EB.

Management

Management is often extremely difficult because of oral strictures and fragility of the skin and oral mucosa. Restricted mouth opening and limitation of tongue movement as a result of scarring can make oral hygiene challenging. Children with EB often require a highly caloric, soft diet which contributes to their increased caries risk. Intensive preventive dental care is essential to prevent dental caries, combined with treatment of early decay. In severe forms, orthodontic treatment may involve early interventions such as serial extractions. Supportive care for mucositis may be required with the use of chlorhexidine gluconate mouthwashes and benzydamine hydrochloride (Difflam™). Dental treatment under general anaesthesia may be challenging as a result of difficulties intubating and oral strictures. Mouth stretching exercises and surgical release of the commissures may be necessary. It is important to cover instruments with copious lubricant; the use of rubber dam is essential to protect the oral mucosa from trauma resulting from suction tips. Lancing of blisters may be necessary following dental treatment.

SYSTEMIC LUPUS ERYTHEMATOSUS

Systemic lupus erythematosus is a chronic inflammatory multisystem disease occurring predominantly in young women. The hallmark of systemic lupus erythematosus is the presence of antinuclear antibodies which form circulating immune complexes with DNA. Oral ulceration often occurs in systemic lupus erythematosus, and treatment of the condition usually involves the use of systemic corticosteroids.

OROFACIAL GRANULOMATOSIS AND CROHN DISEASE (Figure 10.11)

Although not primarily an ulcerative condition, oral ulceration may be the presenting sign in orofacial granulomatosis. Orofacial granulomatosis may be confined to the orofacial region and precede or be a manifestation of Crohn disease, an inflammatory condition of the gastrointestinal tract, or of sarcoidosis.

Presentation

- Diffuse, painless swelling of the lips and cheeks, often initially recurrent and then becoming persistent.
- Diffusely swollen gingivae (Figure 10.11B).
- Linear ulceration or fissuring of the buccal and labial sulcus. A characteristic 'cobblestone' appearance of the buccal mucosa (Figure 10.11A) with aphthous-like ulceration.
- Polypoid tags of vestibular and retromolar mucosa.
- Children may also present with diarrhoea, failure to thrive, weakness, fatigue, anorexia and perianal fissuring or skin tags as manifestation of Crohn disease.

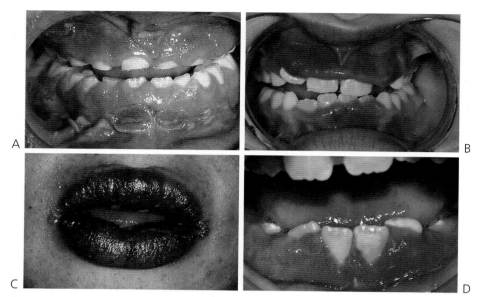

Figure 10.11 Presentations of orofacial granulomatosis/Crohn disease. (A) The intraoral appearance is pathognomonic with swelling of the gingivae; the patient also had a cobblestone appearance of the buccal mucosa and ulceration of the labial and buccal sulci. (B) A different presentation with bright red swollen gingivae. (C) The patient initially presented with a painless swelling of the lips and had evidence of malabsorption, perianal fissuring and bowel problems and was diagnosed with Crohn disease. Management was with systemic corticosteroids. (D) Crohn disease. This child has recurrent flare-ups of his disease that is characterized by concurrent deterioration of his oral disease.

- Oral changes have been found in between 10% and 25% of patients with Crohn disease and, importantly, their appearance may precede other systemic symptoms.

Diagnosis

- Biopsy of oral lesions. The granulomas may be quite deep within the submucosa, and if possible, a minor salivary gland should be included in the specimen.
- Blood tests, including:
  - FBC, differential WCC (to exclude leukaemia), erythrocyte sedimentation rate and C-reactive protein.
  - Serum angiotensin-converting enzyme level to identify or exclude sarcoidosis.
  - Antisaccaromyces cerevisiae antibodies (ASCAs) often associated with Crohn disease whereas antineutrophil cytoplasm antibodies (p-ANCA) recognized as marker for ulcerative colitis and can be useful to distinguish between inflammatory bowel conditions.
- Barium studies, endoscopy and biopsy of the lower bowel if Crohn disease is suspected.

Management

- Some cases of orofacial granulomatosis have been shown to be a response to topical medicaments or dietary components. An exclusion diet can be considered to identify food intolerance, in particular cinnamon and benzoates.

Crohn disease

- Prednisolone. Corticosteroids are usually commenced at a high dosage (2–3 mg/kg daily for 6–8 weeks) to gain control of the disease and are then reduced. Clinicians should be

aware of the significant adverse effects of high-dose and long-term use of corticosteroids in children.
- Dietary management for malabsorption.
- Metronidazole for perianal disease.
- Immunomodulators:
  - Methotrexate, azathioprine.
  - γ-interferon/α-interferon.
  - Infliximab, adalimumab and certolizumab pegol (tumour necrosis factor alpha [TNF] inhibitors)

More recently, methotrexate, budesonide and infliximab (a monoclonal antibody that neutralizes TNF-α) and ustekinumab (an anti-interleukin) have also been used in the management of Crohn disease. Research continues into the use of paratuberculosis therapy (rifabutin, clarithromycin and clofazimine).

MELKERSSON–ROSENTHAL SYNDROME

Melkersson–Rosenthal syndrome is regarded by some as a form of orofacial granulomatosis.

Presentation

- Recurrent/persistent orofacial swelling.
- Facial nerve paralysis.
- Fissured (plicated) tongue.

Melkersson–Rosenthal syndrome is a diagnosis sometimes made without this triad – there is controversy regarding its existence or place within the disorders characterized by orofacial granulomata.

Pigmented, vascular and red lesions

If a lesion is red or bluish in colour, there should be the suspicion of a vascular lesion. These lesions will blanch on pressure with a glass slide (or end of a test tube if access is difficult) (Figure 10.12) as the blood is pushed from the vessels. Melanotic lesions are rare in children (other than physiological pigmentation). A characteristic melanin-pigmented oral lesion in young children is the melanotic neuroectodermal tumour of infancy.

DIFFERENTIAL DIAGNOSIS

- Physiologic pigmentation (Figure 10.13).
- Vascular lesions:
  - Haemangioma.
  - Other vascular malformations.

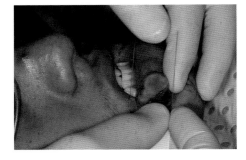

Figure 10.12 Compressing a lesion on the lower lip with a glass slide. Blanching indicates the presence of a vascular lesion caused by emptying of blood from the lesion.

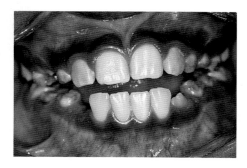

Figure 10.13 Racial pigmentation of the attached gingiva. This should not be confused with heavy metal toxicity, which is limited to the marginal gingivae.

- Haematoma.
- Petechiae and purpura.
- Hereditary haemorrhagic telangiectasia.
- Sturge–Weber syndrome.
- Pigmented lesions (containing melanin):
  - Melanotic neuroectodermal tumour of infancy.
  - Peutz–Jeghers syndrome.
  - Addison disease.
- Other red/blue/purple lesions:
  - Juvenile spongiotic gingival hyperplasia.
  - Giant cell granuloma: peripheral (epulis) or central.
  - Eruption cyst.
  - Langerhans cell histiocytosis.
  - Geographic tongue.
  - Median rhomboid glossitis.
  - Hereditary mucoepithelial dysplasia.
  - Cyanosis.
  - Heavy metal toxicity.

LESIONS OF VASCULAR ORIGIN

Haemangioma/localized vascular anomaly (Figure 10.14A, B)

Haemangiomas are endothelial hamartomas. Typically present at birth, they may grow with the infant but then may regress with time to disappear by adolescence. As such, they require no treatment other than observation, excepting cosmetic concerns.

OTHER VASCULAR MALFORMATIONS

Arteriovenous malformations include birthmarks, blood vessel and lymphatic anomalies. These may be life-threatening conditions, which can occasionally present with profound haemorrhage. Arteriovenous malformations have been classified by Kaban and Mulliken (1986) according to their flow characteristics. They are either:

- Low-flow lesions: capillary, venous, lymphatic or combined port-wine stains, Sturge–Weber syndrome.
  Or
- High-flow lesions: arterial with arteriovenous fistulae (Figures 10.14C and 10.15). Present with mobile and sometimes painful teeth, a bruit and palpable pulses, bleeding from gingivae and bony involvement.
- Combined lesions: extensive combined venous and arteriovenous malformations.

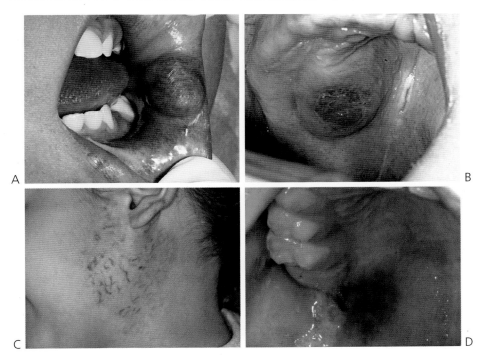

Figure 10.14 (A, B) Different presentations of haemangiomas in infants. (C) A high-flow vascular malformation that is warm to touch, and a bruit is palpable. (D) It is essential that the correct diagnosis of a vascular malformation is made, as there is a potential for life-threatening haemorrhage.

Diagnosis

- Presentation may be subtle, such as prolonged bleeding from the gingivae after toothbrushing, or alternatively a torrential single episode of haemorrhage.
- Vascular lesions are often warm to touch (although this can be difficult to determine if wearing latex gloves).
- Radiographically, there may be enlargement of the periodontal ligament space and a diffuse abnormal trabeculation of the bone.
- A bruit or pulse may be felt over high-flow lesions.
- Teeth may be hypermobile and may have pulsatile movements.
- Facial asymmetry may become apparent as lesions expand.
- Digital subtraction angiography (Figure 10.15C) is required for definitive diagnosis of feeder vessels and the distribution of the lesion.
- Magnetic resonance angiography can be used to aid diagnosis; however, digital subtraction angiography has the advantage that embolization can be performed at the same time.

Management

- Low-flow lesions can be removed by careful surgery with identification and ligation of feeder vessels. Larger lesions can be managed with cryotherapy, laser ablation or injection of sclerosing solutions.
- High-flow lesions require selective embolization of vessels, but these will generally recur after embolization owing to revascularization from contralateral supply and recanalization

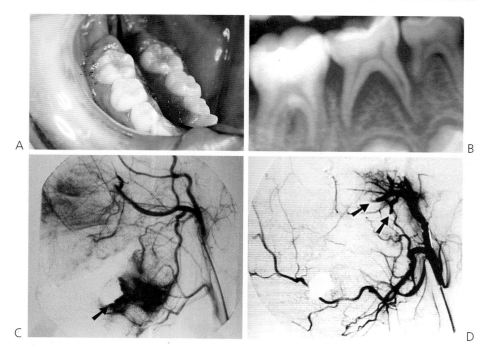

Figure 10.15 A high-flow arteriovenous malformation in the mandible. (A) This child presented with an unusual erythematous enlargement of the gingivae around the mandibular right first permanent molar in addition to mobile second primary molar. (B) Periapical radiograph shows widening of the periodontal ligament space, but there are no indicative changes in the trabecular pattern of the bone. During the biopsy, 350 mL (20% of total volume) of blood was lost after extraction of the second primary molar. The haemorrhage was controlled with an iodoform pack (arrowed). (C) Subsequently, an angiogram was ordered. The extent of the lesion inferior and posterior to the pack is seen. (D) The lesion was managed by embolizing the inferior alveolar and maxillary arteries (*arrows*) and the mandible was resected later.

of the embolized artery. Repeat embolization and resection of the entire lesion are often necessary involving jaw reconstruction.

- If a tooth is accidentally removed and a torrential haemorrhage results, some clinicians suggest that the extracted tooth should be immediately replaced and additional measures used to control the haemorrhage. These rare but potential life-threatening events call for urgent assistance and response.

CLINICAL HINT

Vascular lesions blanch on pressure.

LYMPHANGIOMA (Figure 10.16)

- Diagnosis of developmental lymph vessel abnormalities must exclude vascular involvement. Surgical excision is only necessary if of functional or aesthetic concern.
- Cystic hygroma (Figure 10.16C) is a term used to describe a large lymphangioma involving the tongue, floor of mouth and neck. Expansion of the lesion may cause respiratory obstruction, and treatment usually involves multiple resections over time, management with laser ablation or cryosurgery.

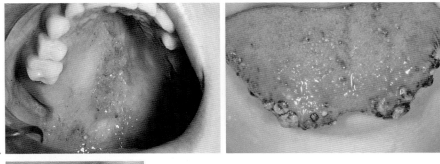

A   B

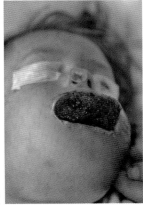

Figure 10.16 (A) Lymphangioma in the palate. (B) A lesion involving the tongue. (C) A large cystic hygroma that was managed with cryosurgery.

C

PETECHIAE AND PURPURA

Petechiae are small pinpoint submucosal or subcutaneous haemorrhages. Purpura or ecchymoses present as larger collections of blood. These lesions are usually present in patients with severe bleeding disorders or coagulopathies, leukaemia and other conditions such as infective endocarditis. Initially bright red in colour, they will change to a bluish-brown hue with time as the extravasated blood is metabolized.

HEREDITARY HAEMORRHAGIC TELANGIECTASIA (RENDU–OSLER–WEBER DISEASE)

An autosomal dominant disorder presenting as a developmental anomaly of capillaries. Lesions may be small, flat or raised haemorrhagic nodules or spider naevi. Bleeding as a result of involvement of the gastrointestinal tract and respiratory tract can lead to chronic anaemia.

STURGE–WEBER SYNDROME (Figure 10.17)

This syndrome that typically presents with:
- Encephalotrigeminal angiomatoses.
- Epilepsy.
- Intellectual disability.
- Calcification of the falx cerebri.

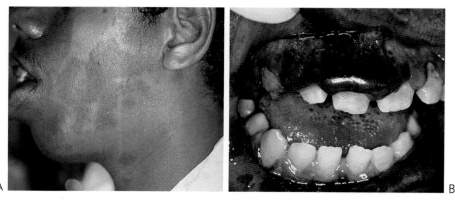

Figure 10.17   (A, B) Sturge–Weber syndrome showing the extent of the capillary vascular malformation in the face which is contiguous with intraoral involvement.

- Vascular lesions involve the leptomeninges, and peripheral lesions appear along the distribution of the 5th nerve.

Extraction of teeth within regions of the affected jaws should be performed with caution and only after thorough investigation of the extent of the anomaly, although it has been reported that they are usually uncomplicated (see other vascular malformations earlier).

MAFFUCCI SYNDROME

Presents with multiple haemangiomas and enchondromas of the small bones in the hands and feet. Only a small number of cases will manifest with oral lesions, mainly haemangiomas.

MELANIN-CONTAINING LESIONS

Peutz–Jeghers syndrome

An autosomal dominant disorder manifesting as multiple small, pigmented lesions of oral mucosa and circum-oral skin appearing almost like dark freckles. There is an important association with intestinal polyposis coli which requires gastrointestinal investigation.

RED LESIONS

Eruption cyst or haematoma

Follicular enlargement appearing just before eruption of teeth. These lesions tend to be blue-black, as they may contain blood. They usually require no treatment unless infected. The parents and child should be reassured and the follicle allowed to rupture spontaneously, or it may be surgically opened if infected (Figure 10.18).

Localized juvenile spongiotic gingival hyperplasia (Figure 10.19)

This lesion is reasonably common but poorly identified. The usual presentation is a florid, bright-red, sessile lesion appearing on the attached gingiva, usually in the anterior maxilla. It is more common in children in the mixed dentition and predominately in girls. It is more accurately a gingival (epithelial) hyperplasia rather than a lesion originating from an inflammatory process. It does not respond to changes in oral hygiene. There is a lack of consensus as to how localized

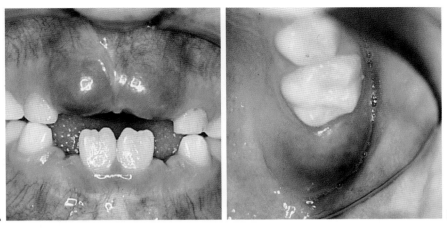

A   B

Figure 10.18 Eruption cysts may be associated with any tooth. (A) Two eruption cysts associated with the maxillary central incisors. (B) Eruption cyst of the maxillary first permanent molar.

juvenile spongiotic gingival hyperplasia should be managed, ranging from conservative excision to cryotherapy and photodynamic therapy with diode lasers.

Hereditary mucoepithelial dysplasia

A rare disorder where there is a reduced number of desmosomes attaching the epithelial cells to each other. Lens cataracts, corneal lesions leading to blindness, skin keratosis and alopecia are associated with a fiery red mucosa involving both keratinized and nonkeratinized mucosa. Diagnosis is confirmed by gingival and/or mucosal biopsy. Transmission electron microscopy is necessary to demonstrate the reduced number of desmosomes and amorphous intracellular inclusions. The oral lesions are usually asymptomatic. Loss of sight is progressive because of corneal vascularization. Corneal grafts are unsuccessful, as they too undergo vascularization.

Geographic tongue (Figure 10.20A)

This condition is also termed 'glossitis migrans', 'benign migratory glossitis', 'erythema migrans' or 'wandering rash of the tongue'. It presents as areas of depapillation and erythema with a heaped 'serpentine-like', keratinized margin on the lateral margins and dorsal surface of the tongue. It can be associated with a fissured tongue. The lesions appear as map-like areas (hence the 'geographic') and may change in their distribution over a period of time (hence the 'migratory'). The areas affected may return to normal and new lesions appear at different sites on the tongue. Sometimes, symptomatic, topical corticosteroids may be beneficial for those children in pain.

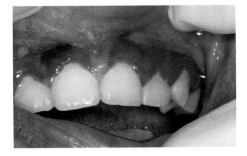

Figure 10.19 Localized juvenile spongiotic gingival hyperplasia showing the florid bright-red gingival inflammation and hyperplasia seen around the labial gingivae.

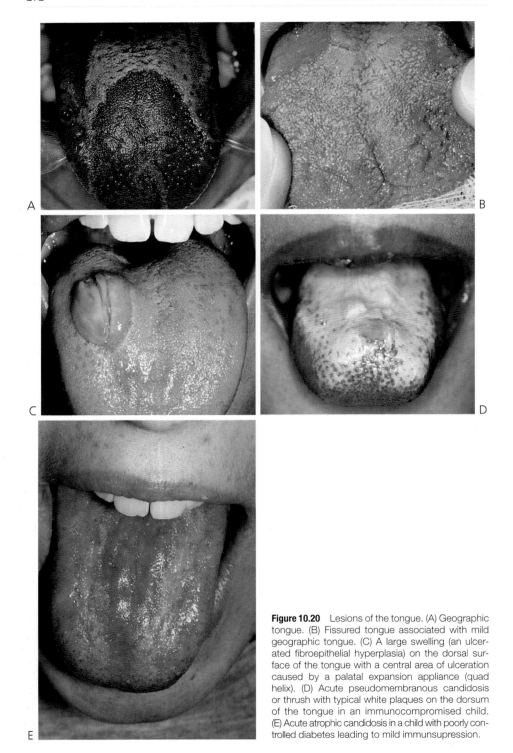

Figure 10.20 Lesions of the tongue. (A) Geographic tongue. (B) Fissured tongue associated with mild geographic tongue. (C) A large swelling (an ulcerated fibroepithelial hyperplasia) on the dorsal surface of the tongue with a central area of ulceration caused by a palatal expansion appliance (quad helix). (D) Acute pseudomembranous candidosis or thrush with typical white plaques on the dorsum of the tongue in an immunocompromised child. (E) Acute atrophic candidosis in a child with poorly controlled diabetes leading to mild immunsupression.

Fissured tongue (Figure 10.20B)

Also termed 'plicated tongue', 'scrotal tongue', 'fissured tongue' or 'lingua secta'. The tongue in these patients is fissured, the fissures being perpendicular to the lateral border. Although this is usually considered a variation of normal, it is a commonly found condition in children with Down syndrome. Some patients with a fissured tongue will also have geographic tongue. Fissuring of the tongue is also a feature of Melkersson–Rosenthal syndrome.

Epulides and exophytic lesions

An epulis is a nonspecific term to merely describe a lump on the gingiva or the alveolar mucosa. These are exophytic lesions growing outwards from the epithelial surface and may be pedunculated (arising from a stalk) or sessile (flattened and raised with a broad base).

DIFFERENTIAL DIAGNOSIS

- Inflammatory hyperplasias:
  Pyogenic granuloma.
  Fibrous epulis.
  Giant cell granuloma: central or peripheral (epulis).
- Congenital epulis of the newborn.
- Squamous papilloma/viral wart.
- Focal epithelial hyperplasia/Heck disease.
- Condyloma acuminatum.
- Eruption cyst/haematoma.
- Melanotic neuro-ectodermal tumour of infancy.
- Tuberous sclerosis.
- Mucocoele.
- Lymphangioma.

PYOGENIC GRANULOMA (Figure 10.21A)

This misnamed lesion (i.e., no pus and no granulomas) is actually an (ulcerated) lobulated capillary haemangioma. Hence, these lesions tend to bleed easily and are covered with a thin fibrin membrane and may recur if not fully excised. They are often pedunculated, and considering their size and, hence, the amount of vasculature needed to support this growth, it is understandable why bleeding might be an issue during removal. Excisional biopsy is recommended.

FIBROUS EPULIS (Figure 10.21B)

One of the most common epulides that is seen in children resulting from an exuberant fibro-epithelial reaction to plaque. Commonly arising from the interdental papillae and covered by epithelium, they range in colour from pink to red to yellow. Those appearing yellow are ulcerated.

Management

Oral hygiene and surgical excision. Lesions may recur, particularly if good oral hygiene is not maintained.

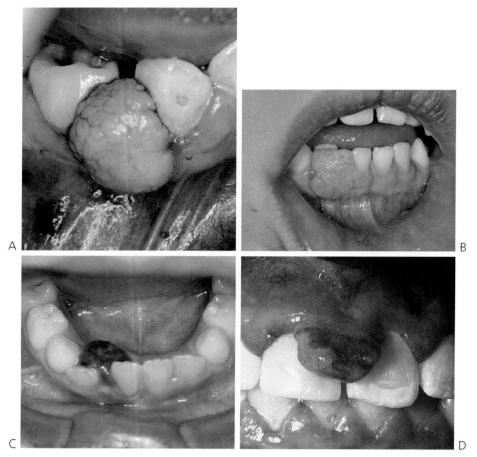

Figure 10.21 Gingival swellings. (A) Pyogenic granuloma; note the slow growth of the lesion as shown with the migration and separation of the teeth. (B) Fibrous epulis. (C) Peripheral giant cell granuloma/giant cell epulis. (D) Epulis associated with angiomata in a child with tuberous sclerosis.

GIANT CELL GRANULOMA: CENTRAL OR PERIPHERAL (EPULIS) (Figure 10.21C)

These lesions usually occur in the region of the primary dentition. The colour of these lesions tends to be dark purple. Bone loss of the alveolar crest can sometimes be observed as 'radiographic cupping'. It is important to ensure that there is no intraosseous component radiographically, as in this case the diagnosis would be a central giant cell granuloma. As with all giant cell lesions of the jaws, hyperparathyroidism should be considered in the differential diagnosis. True central lesions are typically aggressive, and local resection may be required.

Management

- Surgical excision.
- Haematological investigations for calcium, phosphate, alkaline phosphatase and parathyroid hormone.
- Lesions may regrow if not totally excised.

TUBEROUS SCLEROSIS (Figure 10.21D)

Tuberous sclerosis is an autosomal dominant disorder characterized by seizures, mental retardation and adenoma sebaceum of the skin. Epulides or generalized nodular gingival enlargement may be present. Some of these may result from vascular malformations and may bleed profusely when excised. Hypoplasia of the enamel is often observed as surface pitting; this can be demonstrated particularly effectively by the use of disclosing solution.

SQUAMOUS PAPILLOMA (Figure 10.22A)

A squamous papilloma is a benign neoplasm caused by the human papilloma virus (HPV), presenting as a cauliflower-like growth on the mucosa. The colour of the lesion depends on the degree of keratinization.

Management

Surgical excision, including the stalk and a border of normal tissue.

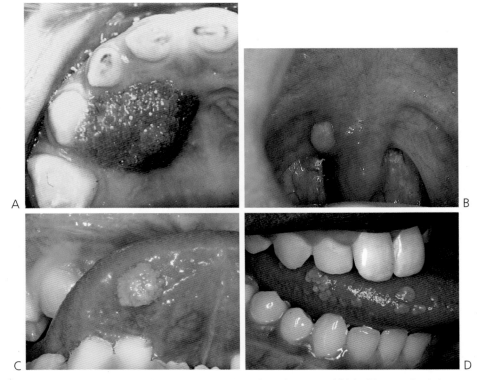

Figure 10.22 Infective epulides. (A) A papilloma in the palate of a young child. In this case, the lesion was associated with viral warts on the extremities; hence, this is assumed to be a viral papilloma. (B) A small viral wart on the uvula. (C) A good example of the exophytic nature of viral warts, present on the dorsal surface of the tongue. (D) Focal epithelial hyperplasia with the characteristic lesions on the slide of the tongue. (Courtesy Dr. Charmaine Hall, Royal Children's Hospital, Melbourne.)

VIRAL WARTS (VERRUCA VULGARIS) (Figure 10.22B, C)

This is the cutaneous form of the HPV infection. Lesions may be single or multiple and may appear similar to the papilloma or as the common wart seen on the hands and fingers.

Management

Surgical excision. If multiple lesions are present extraorally, dermatological management may also be required.

HECK DISEASE (FOCAL EPITHELIAL HYPERPLASIA) (Figure 10.22D)

These pale white multiple exophytic lesions, commonly appearing on the side of the tongue or lips, are also associated with HPV infection. In some children, there is a genetic predisposition to those who may be affected (types 13 and 32).

Gingival enlargements (overgrowth)
DIFFERENTIAL DIAGNOSIS

- Drug-induced hyperplasia:
  - Phenytoin.
  - Cyclosporin A.
  - Nifedipine.
  - Verapamil.
- Syndromes with gingival enlargement as a presenting feature:
  - Hereditary gingival fibromatosis.
  - Zimmerman–Laband syndrome and other rare, usually autosomal recessive, syndromes.
  - Other systemic conditions such as metastatic spread of neoplasms (see Figure 10.23)

PHENYTOIN ENLARGEMENT (Figure 10.24A, B)

Not all patients taking phenytoin have gingival enlargement. Principally, there is enlargement of the interdental papillae. There may be delayed eruption of teeth because of the bulk of fibrous tissue present and ectopic eruption. Overgrowth has been suggested to result from decreased collagen degradation and phagocytosis, as well as increased collagen synthesis. Withdrawal of the drug

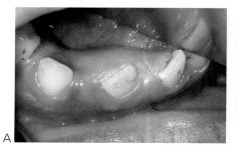
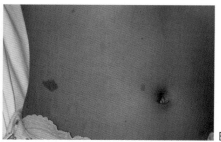

A   B

Figure 10.23   Gingival enlargement may present because of neoplasia or other growths (A) Enlargement of the lower jaw caused by neurofibromatosis type 1. The bone was unaffected and the only the soft tissue in the anterior mandible was affected. (B) Characteristic café-au-lait hyperpigmentation on the torso in the same child.

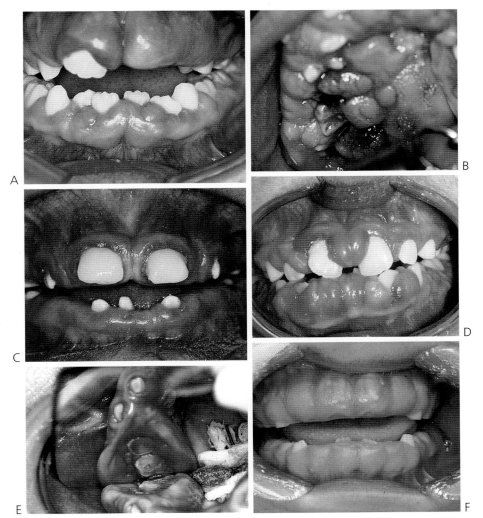

Figure 10.24 (A) Phenytoin-associated gingival enlargement. This initially involves the interdental papillae and then adjacent tissues. (B) The phenytoin-associated gingival enlargement can become so extensive as to cover the whole palate. An acute periodontal abscess was associated with this case. (C) Cyclosporin A-associated gingival enlargement in a child following end-stage renal failure and kidney transplantation. The enamel is malformed because of the effects of the renal disease. (D) Cyclosporin A-associated gingival enlargement in a child following heart transplantation. (E) Hereditary gingival fibromatosis. (F) Gingival enlargement and delayed eruption of teeth associated with Zimmermann-Laband syndrome.

will bring about resolution in all but severe cases. Oral hygiene is most important in controlling overgrowth, as there is always a component of plaque-induced gingival enlargement.

Management

- Maintenance of oral hygiene.
- Use of chlorhexidine 0.2% mouthwashes.
- Gingivectomy may be required to allow eruption of teeth or for aesthetics.

Vitamin B supplementation has been found to lessen gingival overgrowth in those children on anticonvulsant medication.

CYCLOSPORINE A-ASSOCIATED ENLARGEMENT (Figure 10.24C, D)

A significant number of children now undergo kidney, liver, heart or combined heart/lung transplantation. The mainstay of immunosuppressive antirejection chemotherapy is cyclosporin A. Gingival overgrowth occurs in between 30% and 70% of patients and is not strictly dose related but may be more severe if the drug is administered at an early age. Individual patients appear to have a threshold below which gingival overgrowth will not occur. Overgrowth appears to be higher in those human leukocyte antigen (HLA) B37-positive patients and lower in HLA DR1-positive patients.

NIFEDIPINE AND VERAPAMIL ENLARGEMENT

Both these drugs are calcium-channel blockers used to control coronary insufficiency and hypertension in adults; their main use in children is to control cyclosporin-induced hypertension after transplantation. An increase in the extracellular compartment volume is responsible for enlargement that occurs in addition to the enlargement caused by cyclosporin A, which is invariably used in these patients.

Management

- As with phenytoin enlargement, maintenance of oral hygiene is mandatory.
- Gingivectomy if required.
- In children with severe enlargement, a full mouth procedure may be required. In these cases, periodontal flap procedures are preferable as primary closure can be achieved.

HEREDITARY GINGIVAL FIBROMATOSIS (Figure 10.24E)

Gingival enlargement may be a feature of several syndromes, some of which include learning disabilities. These syndromes may occur sporadically or as an autosomal dominant or an autosomal recessive trait.

Management

Gingivectomy or periodontal flap procedures as required to allow tooth eruption and maintain aesthetics. Histopathological examination of the excised tissue may assist in diagnosis of some of the rarer causes of syndromic gingival enlargement (e.g., juvenile hyaline fibromatosis).

ZIMMERMANN–LABAND SYNDROME (Figure 10.24F)

This is a rare autosomal dominant disorder associated with course facial appearance, hypertrichosis, mild intellectual disability, joint hyperflexibility and delayed eruption of teeth because of gingival fibromatosis.

Premature exfoliation of primary teeth

Premature loss of primary teeth is a significant diagnostic event. Most conditions that present with early loss are serious, and a child presenting with unexplained tooth loss warrants immediate investigation. Teeth may be lost because of metabolic disturbances, severe periodontal disease, connective tissue disorders, neoplasia, loss of alveolar bone support or self-inflicted trauma.

DIFFERENTIAL DIAGNOSIS

- Neutropenias:
  - Cyclic neutropenia.
  - Congenital agranulocytosis.
- Qualitative neutrophil defects:
  - Prepubertal periodontitis.
  - Juvenile periodontitis.
  - Leucocyte adhesion defect.
  - Papillon–Lefèvre syndrome.
  - Chédiak–Higashi disease.
  - Acatalasia.
- Metabolic disorders:
  - Hypophosphatasia.
- Connective tissue disorders
  - Ehlers–Danlos syndrome (types IV and VIII).
  - Erythromelalgia.
  - Acrodynia.
  - Scurvy.
- Neoplasia:
  - Langerhans cell histiocytosis.
  - Acute myeloid leukaemia.
- Self-injury (see Chapter 13):
  - Hereditary sensory neuropathies.
  - Lesch–Nyhan syndrome.
  - Psychotic disorders.

PERIODONTAL DISEASE IN CHILDREN (Figure 10.25D)

Although gingivitis is not uncommon in children, periodontitis with alveolar bone loss is usually a manifestation of a serious underlying immunological deficiency. Two forms of periodontal disease in children, prepubertal periodontitis and juvenile periodontitis, are associated with characteristic bacterial flora including *Actinobacillus actinomycetemcomitans*, *Prevotella intermedia*, *Eikenella corrodens* and *Capnocytophaga sputigena*. The presence of these bacteria is thought to be related to decreased host resistance, specifically neutropenia or neutrophil function defects. Although B-cell defects show few oral changes, altered T-cell function will manifest with severe gingivitis, periodontitis and candidosis.

CLASSIFICATION OF PERIODONTAL DISEASES

Table 10.4 details the new terminology used to describe the different periodontal diseases. The new terminology for prepubertal periodontitis is now generalized aggressive periodontitis or periodontitis associated with systemic disease. However, in children, it is important to understand that any periodontal disease in a young child is associated with some form of immune dysfunction. Although any classifications should aid in the description of a particular disease entity, it is essential for clinicians to understand the different presentations and the pathogenesis of the disease.

NEUTROPENIAS AND QUALITATIVE NEUTROPHIL DEFECTS

Neutropenia

- Peripheral blood levels lower than 1500/mL.
- Acute forms usually fatal.

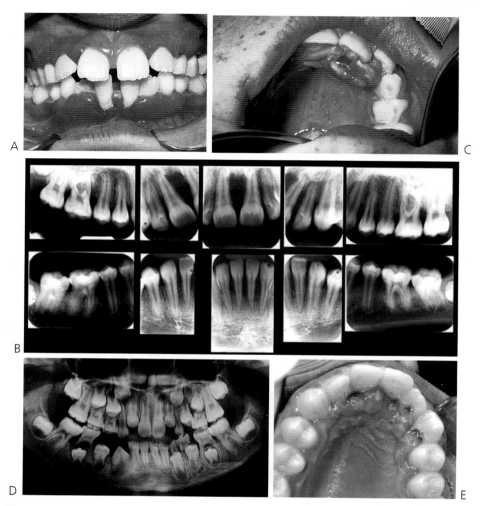

Figure 10.25 (A) Gross gingival inflammation in an adolescent with cyclic neutropenia. This girl lost most of her primary teeth by the age of 7 years. (B) Periapical radiographic survey showing the extent of bone loss and angular defects in another child with cyclic neutropenia. (C) Severe unexplained palatal ulceration in a child with a leucocyte adhesion defect. The maxillary left incisor exfoliated a short time later. (D) Prepubertal periodontitis, also associated with a leucocyte adhesion defect. It is important to assess normal eruption patterns and to be suspicious of loss of teeth in the absence of caries or other pathology. (E) Acute necrotizing ulcerative gingivitis (ANUG) in a 15-year-old boy, showing the characteristic destruction of the interdental papilla. ANUG is rare in children and is seen only in those who are immunocompromised to debilitated.

- Chronic forms have indolent progression.
- Cyclic (see later in the chapter) characterized by recurrent episodes.
- Intermittent as part of Shwachman–Diamond syndrome.

CYCLIC NEUTROPENIA (Figure 10.25A, B)

In this condition, there is an episodic decrease in the number of neutrophils every 3 to 4 weeks. Peripheral neutrophil counts usually drop to zero, and during this time the child is extremely

TABLE 10.4 ■ **Terminology used to classify periodontal diseases**

Old terminology	Current terminology
Prepubertal periodontitis	Generalized aggressive periodontitis
	Periodontitis associated with systemic disease
Localized juvenile periodontitis	Localized aggressive periodontitis
Acute necrotizing ulcerative gingivitis (ANUG)	Necrotizing periodontal disease

(From Research, Science and Therapy Committee, 2003. Periodontal diseases of children and adolescents. American Academy of Periodontology. Journal of Periodontology 74, 1696–1704.)

susceptible to infection. Recurrent oral ulceration often occurs when cell counts are low. Gingival and periodontal involvement occurs with the emergence of teeth and is progressive.

Management

- Early preventive involvement.
- Dental care through all stages of cycle.
- Chlorhexidine 0.2% mouthwashes or gel.
- Elective extraction of primary teeth may be considered in severe cases.
- In some familial cases, the condition appears to totally regress during adolescence.

LEUCOCYTE ADHESION DEFECT (Figure 10.25C, D)

A rare autosomal recessive condition associated with a reduced level of adhesion molecules on peripheral leucocytes resulting in severely reduced resistance to infection. The CD11/CD18 molecules are necessary for effective phagocytosis. Children present with delayed wound healing, persistent severe oral ulceration, cellulitis without pus formation, severe gingival inflammation, periodontitis and premature loss of primary teeth. Also present is a persistently high leucocytosis and reactive marrow, without evidence of leukaemia. One important indicator of this condition is late separation of the umbilical cord after birth.

Diagnosis

Diagnosis is confirmed by examining leucocytes for surface expression of CD11/CD18 markers using immunofluorescence techniques and cytofluorographic analysis.

Management

- Many children succumb to overwhelming infection.
- Granulocyte transfusion and bone marrow transplantation may be effective in some cases.

PAPILLON–LEFÈVRE SYNDROME (Figure 10.26)

An autosomal recessive condition manifesting as hyperkeratosis of the palms and feet and progressive exfoliation of all teeth from periodontal disease. *A. actinomycetemcomitans* has been implicated in the periodontal disease, which is associated with a qualitative neutrophil defect and mutations in the lysosomal protease cathepsin C gene on 11q14–21. Primary teeth commence shedding from the time of eruption, with no evidence of root resorption. All primary teeth are usually lost before the permanent teeth erupt, when they in turn are exfoliated.

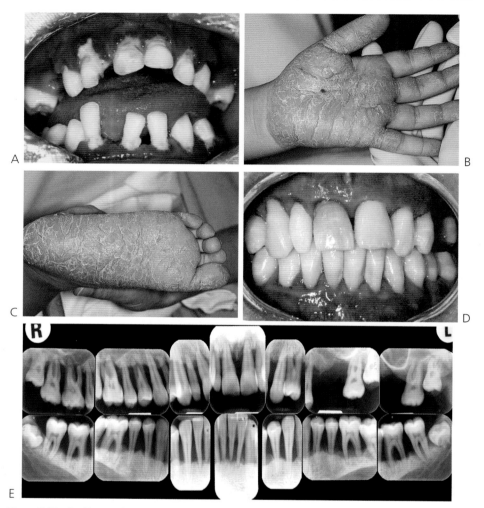

Figure 10.26 Papillon–Lefèvre syndrome. (A) The initial presentation of the child with severe periodontal disease–associated tooth mobility. Many of these teeth exfoliated within 6 months. (B, C) The characteristic appearance of the hands and feet in the same child. (D, E) The permanent dentition in a boy of 17 years, following long-term antibiotic treatment that has failed to improve the prognosis of the dentition.

Diagnosis

- The oral changes and skin lesions are pathognomonic for this condition.
- Selective anaerobic culturing for *A. actinomycetemcomitans* is difficult, and a more reliable alternative is to use an enzyme-linked immunosorbent assay to detect IgG antibodies against this organism.

Management

No treatment is particularly successful. Extraction of any remaining primary teeth before eruption of the permanent teeth has been advocated. Intensive periodontal therapy with metronidazole and chlorhexidine to eliminate or reduce *A. actinomycetemcomitans* may be successful in delaying the inevitable exfoliation of teeth, although the basic neutrophil function defect remains. Treatment of other family members has also been recommended, including pets (especially dogs), if they are found to harbour the bacteria. Several papers have reported the use of vitamin A derivatives in management that may improve the prognosis. All patients require planned full clearances and dentures to avoid pain and disfigurement. It is important to consider proceeding with extractions soon after the eruption of the permanent dentition to minimize excessive bone loss.

CHÉDIAK–HIGASHI DISEASE

This is a rare autosomal recessive disorder affecting lysosomal storage and causing a qualitative neutrophil defect. There is defective neutrophil chemotaxis and abnormal degranulation that result in poor intracellular killing. Abnormal B-cell and T-cell function and thrombocytopenia have also been reported. Most children die by 10 years of age because of overwhelming sepsis. Teeth are shed because of severe periodontal disease with rapid alveolar bone loss.

HUMAN IMMUNODEFICIENCY VIRUS–ASSOCIATED PERIODONTAL DISEASE IN CHILDREN

There are few cases documenting periodontal disease in young children. In adolescents, there are reports of acute necrotizing ulcerative gingivitis and a characteristic linear marginal gingival erythema. Excellent oral hygiene and plaque control are essential, combined with supportive therapy including chlorhexidine and metronidazole as required.

LANGERHANS CELL HISTIOCYTOSIS (Figure 10.27)

This condition was previously termed 'histiocytosis X' and included the conditions eosinophilic granuloma, Hand–Schüller–Christian disease and Letterer–Siwe disease. The abnormality in common is a proliferation of histiocytes. Oral lesions characteristically occur in all four quadrants and characteristically affect the tissues overlying or supporting the primary molar teeth. The lesions typically extend forward to the canines but rarely involve the incisors.

Presentation

- Malaise, irritability.
- Anogenital and postauricular rash.
- Diabetes insipidus.
- Premature exposure by alveolar resorption and subsequent loss of primary teeth, especially molars.
- Radiographically, teeth appear to be 'floating in air'.
- Typically, all four quadrants are involved.

Diagnosis

- Biopsy of oral or skin lesions; cells positive for S100 and CD1a.
- Transmission electron microscopy of Langerhans cells shows characteristic Birbeck granules.

Management

- Excision and curettage of oral lesions and extraction of involved teeth are required to control oral lesions.
- Multiagent chemotherapy is required for disseminated disease and is most effective if commenced early.

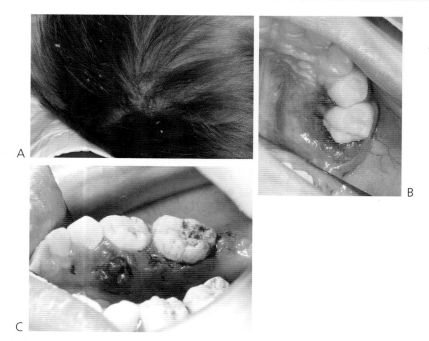

Figure 10.27   (A) Cradle cap–like rash on the head and severe ano-vulval or ano-perineal rash are common presentations of disseminated Langerhans cell histiocytosis (LCH). LCH characteristically presents intraorally with lesions in all four quadrants (B) and (C). All the posterior teeth were excessively mobile and retained only by soft tissue. Note the perforation of the lesions through the lingual alveolus (C).

Metabolic disorders

HYPOPHOSPHATASIA (Figure 10.28)

A decrease in serum alkaline phosphatase and an increase in the urinary excretion of phosphoenolamine (PEA) are pathognomonic for hypophosphatasia. The more usual form is transmitted as an autosomal dominant trait, whereas the autosomal recessive form is invariably lethal. Loss of at least some of the incisor teeth usually occurs before 18 months. Several authors have identified groups of children who manifest only dental changes, namely the early loss of teeth without any rachitic bone changes; the term 'odontohypophosphatasia' has been suggested for these patients, but this is inappropriate because the presentation of loss of teeth alone is only one end of the spectrum in the variable expression of this disease. In these children, there are less severe changes, and we have observed that the permanent dentition can be unaffected.

Diagnosis

- Serum alkaline phosphatase level under 90 U/L. The normal range is 80 to 350 U/L; however, growing children often have levels well in excess of these values (>400 U/L).
- Urinary PEA and serum pyridoxal-5-phosphate (vitamin B_6) tests are required to confirm the diagnosis. A skeletal survey of the long bones is necessary, as rachitic changes may be present in severe cases.
- Sections of the exfoliated teeth show abnormal or absent cementum.

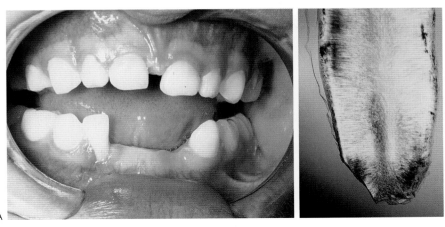

Figure 10.28   (A) Hypophosphatasia presenting with exfoliation of the maxillary and mandibular anterior teeth around 2 years of age. There is minimal gingival inflammation, and hard tissue sections (B) show absence of cementum.

EHLERS–DANLOS TYPE IV AND TYPE VIII

These inborn errors of metabolism present as disorders of collagen formation. Typically, there is hyperextensibility of skin with capillary fragility, bruising of the skin and hypermobility of the joints. Types IV and VIII may present with dental complications, mainly progressive periodontal disease leading to the loss of teeth.

ERYTHROMELALGIA

A very rare condition, characterized by sympathetic overactivity, causing an endarteritis and the extremities feeling hot. One case has been reported with loss of primary and permanent teeth at 4 years of age. The child had extreme hypermobility of the joints and slept on a tiled floor in the middle of winter because of the heat in her legs. She also had an unexplained tachycardia of 200 beats per minute and presented a diagnostic dilemma for many months. The teeth exfoliated because of necrosis of alveolar bone.

ACRODYNIA (PINK DISEASE)

Mercury toxicity causes alveolar destruction and sequestration. This is extremely rare now, although in the past it was not uncommon with the use of teething powders containing mercury.

ACATALASIA

Autosomal recessive catalase deficiency in neutrophils leading to periodontal destruction. Extremely rare outside Japan.

SCURVY (Figure 10.29)

Almost unknown today, this nutritional deficiency of vitamin C results in a connective tissue disorder. Tooth loss is attributed to a failure of proline hydroxylation and consequent reduced collagen synthesis. Children with special needs, who have extremely restricted diets and, hence,

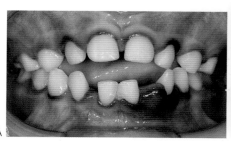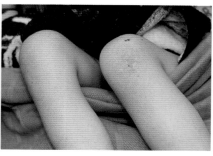

A　　　　　　　　　　　　　　　　　　　　　　　　　　　　　　　　　　　　　　B

Figure 10.29 (A) Scurvy. This disease is almost unheard of now; however, children present with mobile teeth and marked gingival inflammation. (B) Characteristic petechial haemorrhages on the extremities because of capillary fragility.

nutritional deficiencies, have presented with this rare disorder. They have difficulties and refusing to walk, often presenting in pain during dressing because of microsubperiosteal haemorrhages. Skin lesions may also present (Figure 10.29B).

Oral pathology in the newborn infant

DIFFERENTIAL DIAGNOSIS

- Keratin cysts of the newborn:
  - Epstein pearls.
  - Bohn nodules.
- Congenital epulis of the newborn.
- Granular cell tumour (granular cell myoblastoma).
- Melanotic neuro-ectodermal tumour of infancy.
- Natal/neonatal teeth.

CYSTS IN THE NEWBORN

Epstein pearls (Figure 10.30A)

These hard, raised nodules are small keratinizing cysts arising in epithelial remnants trapped along lines of fusion of embryological processes. They appear in the midline of the hard palate, most commonly posteriorly.

Bohn nodules (Figure 10.30B)

These are remnants of the dental lamina and usually occur on the labial or buccal aspect of the maxillary alveolar ridges.

Management

No treatment is required other than reassurance of the parents.

CONGENITAL EPULIS (Figure 10.31B)

The congenital epulis is a rare benign lesion of unknown origin found only in neonates. Lesions are equally distributed between maxillary and mandibular arches and may be multiple in about 10% of reported cases; they are 10 times more common in girls than in boys. It arises from the

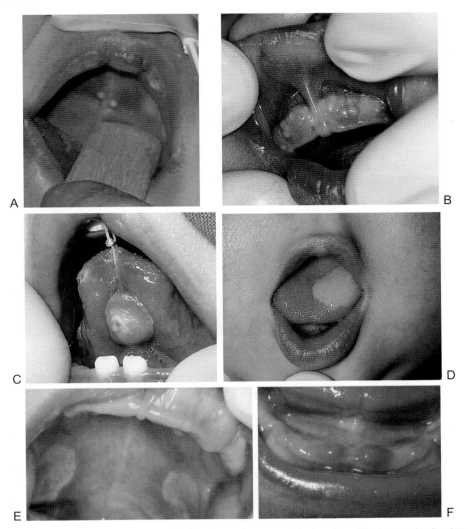

Figure 10.30 Oral pathology in infants. (A) Epstein pearls appear at the junction of the hard and soft palate while Bohn nodules (B) occur on the dental alveolus in newborns. (C) Fibroepithelial hyperplasia on the ventral surface of the tongue caused by trauma from the erupting mandibular incisors. (D) White sponge naevus of the tongue. (E) Bednar ulceration. This peculiar ulceration of the palate may occur in infants because of trauma from breast or bottle feeding. (F) Bilateral eruption cysts in a newborn.

gingival crest but is thought not to be odontogenic in origin. The swelling is characterized by a proliferation of mesenchymal cells with a granular cytoplasm and is usually pedunculated. There is controversy over the histogenesis of this lesion. The congenital epulis is histologically indistinguishable from the extra-gingival granular cell tumour, which is usually seen on the tongue. Immunohistochemically, the congenital epulis is S100 negative, whereas the granular cell tumour is positive for both CD68 and S100. It has been suggested that the congenital epulis is a non-neoplastic, perhaps reactive, lesion arising from primitive gingival perivascular mesenchymal cells with the potential for smooth muscle cytodifferentiation.

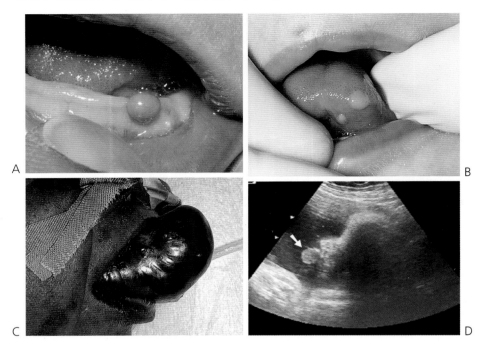

Figure 10.31 Granular cell tumours in children. (A) Multiple granular cell myoblastomas of the tongue lip. They are yellowish in appearance and are sessile. (B) The most common presentation of a congenital epulis, which is a true granular cell tumour. Usually pedunculated, they occur on the alveolus and usually regress and exfoliate over a few months. (C) This extremely large congenital epulis is measuring 4 cm in length. (D) The lesion was diagnosed prenatally on ultrasound (*arrow*).

Alternative terminology

Congenital granular cell tumour, Neumann tumour, granular cell epulis, gingival granular cell tumour.

Management

Lesions often regress with time, although large lesions which interfere with feeding may require surgical excision. Large lesions are sometimes present at birth and may be life-threatening because of respiratory obstruction. The eruption of the primary dentition is unaffected by either surgical or conservative management, and recurrence is uncommon.

MELANOTIC NEUROECTODERMAL TUMOUR OF INFANCY

A rare but important paediatric tumour derived from neural crest cells, this occurs predominantly in the maxilla. The condition may be present at birth, and all recorded cases have been diagnosed by 4 months of age. Similar to a neuroblastoma, there may be high levels of vanillylmandelic acid (a catecholamine end-product) in the urine. Lesions may be multicentric with close approximation to, but not involving, dental tissues, reflecting their ectomesenchymal origin. Intraorally, lesions appear as circumscribed swellings that may have the appearance of normal mucosa or have a blue-black hue and may be associated with premature eruption of the primary incisors.

Diagnosis

Computed tomography followed by excisional biopsy because of the extremely rapid growth of the lesion. This condition is usually so unique, at this age and at this site, that diagnosis is not difficult.

Management

- Enucleation of the tumour and involved primary teeth.
- Curettage of the bony floor of the multiple cavities.
- Radiotherapy is contraindicated.
- Recurrences are extremely rare.

Diseases of salivary glands

DIFFERENTIAL DIAGNOSIS

- Mucocoele.
- Ranula.
- Sialoliths.
- Mumps.
- Autoimmune parotitis.
- Bilateral parotitis associated with bulimia (sialosis).
- Aplasia (or hypoplasia) of major salivary glands.

MUCOCOELE (Figure 10.32A–C)

Mucous extravasation cyst

The most common mucous cyst in the oral cavity, the mucous extravasation cyst arises from damage to the duct of one of the minor salivary glands in the (lower) lip or cheek. Often caused by lip biting or other minor injuries, mucus builds up in the connective tissue to become surrounded by fibrous tissue. Most mucocoeles are well-circumscribed bluish swellings, although traumatized lesions may have a keratinized surface.

Management

- Some cysts regress spontaneously.
- Surgical excision, ideally together with the associated minor salivary glands.

Mucous retention cyst

Less common than the mucous extravasation cyst, the retention cyst has a similar or identical clinical appearance but is lined by epithelium. It is more common in the upper lip and palate, whereas the extravasation cyst is more typical of the lower lip.

RANULA (Figure 10.32D, E)

A mucous (extravasation) cyst of the floor of the mouth caused by damage to the duct of either the sublingual or submandibular glands. A soft, bluish swelling presents on one side of the floor of the mouth. A plunging ranula occurs when the lesion herniates through the mylohyoid muscle to involve the neck.

Management

- Surgical excision.
- Large lesions may require marsupialization in the first instance.

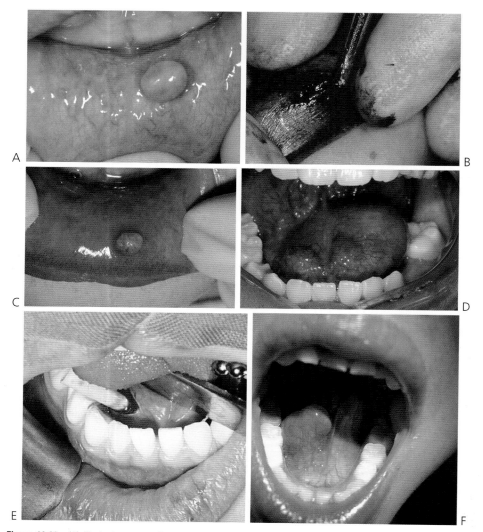

Figure 10.32 (A) Typical presentation of a mucocoele on the lower lip. Most lesions require removal. (B) Semilunar incision with exposure of cyst which may be removed with blunt dissection. (C) Over time, the appearance of these lesions may change with fibrosis and keratinization. (D) A mucous cyst of the floor of the mouth; a ranula. (E) Insertion of a drain lateral to Wharton duct to marsupialize the cyst. (F) Swelling of the submandibular duct because of a siaolith.

SIALADENITIS

Inflammation of the major salivary glands may result from:

- Viral infection:
  - Mumps or cytomegalovirus infection. Present with bilateral nonsuppurative parotitis, usually epidemic.
  - Human immunodeficiency virus (HIV) infection and AIDS; 10% to 15% of children with AIDS will manifest bilateral parotitis.

- Bacterial infections:
  - Suppurative, usually retrograde infection.
- Autoimmune:
  - Sjögren syndrome (usually seen in older patients).
  - Bilateral autoimmune parotitis. Punctate sialectasis appearance on sialogram.
- Chronic sialadenitis:
  - Usually caused by unilateral obstruction of a major salivary gland, either by stricture, epithelial plugging or a sialolith (calculus) causing obstruction and inflammation (Figure 10.31F). Pain occurs during eating and if there is acute exacerbation of infection.
- Bulimia:
  - This can present with a nontender bilateral salivary gland enlargement which is often thought to be a sialadenitis but reflects sialosis, a noninfective, noninflammatory hyperplasia of the salivary glands.

CLINICAL HINT

A periodontal probe is useful for gently exploring the terminal part of a major salivary gland duct. This can identify a small calculus or dislodge an epithelial plug. This should not be attempted in younger and/or anxious patients.

Management

- Massage of the gland/milking of the duct for cases of recurrent epithelial plugging.
- Antibiotics to control infection in the acute phase.
- Removal of sialolith. Note: a suture should be passed under the duct behind the sialolith to prevent it being displaced backwards.
- In long-standing cases of obstructive sialadenitis, removal of the gland may be necessary.

SALIVARY GLAND TUMOURS

Most tumours of the salivary glands in children are vascular malformations. Pleomorphic adenomas are uncommon. Malignant neoplasms such as mucoepidermoid carcinoma, adenocarcinoma and sarcoma are extremely uncommon and affect mainly older children and adolescents. The parotid is the most common site for such tumours.

DIAGNOSTIC IMAGING OF THE SALIVARY GLANDS

Radiology

Mandibular occlusal films are useful for imaging salivary calculi in the submandibular duct. These may also be seen on panoramic radiographs, albeit with the mandible superimposed.

Sialography. Used to demonstrate a stricture of the duct and gland architecture.

Computed tomography, magnetic resonance imaging, ultrasound. If neoplasms are suspected. Can be combined with sialography.

Nuclear medicine

Demonstrates salivary gland function. A technetium-99m tracer seeks major protein-secreting exocrine and endocrine glands. The isotope is readily taken up by the major salivary glands. Lemon juice is then administered orally to assess function and clearance of the glands.

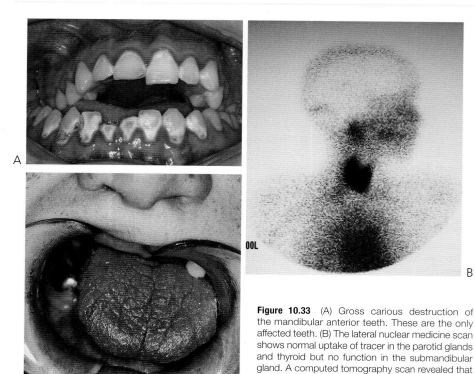

Figure 10.33 (A) Gross carious destruction of the mandibular anterior teeth. These are the only affected teeth. (B) The lateral nuclear medicine scan shows normal uptake of tracer in the parotid glands and thyroid but no function in the submandibular gland. A computed tomography scan revealed that only rudimentary glands were present. (C) A 4-year-old boy who, after three procedures under general anaesthesia to treat gross caries in his primary dentition, was subsequently diagnosed with aplasia of his major salivary glands.

APLASIA OF SALIVARY GLANDS (Figure 10.33)

A number of cases of congenital salivary gland agenesis have been reported. Major salivary gland hypoplasia is an uncommon presentation of a child with gross caries in unusual sites. Caries of the lower anterior teeth should be regarded with suspicion in a young child, as it may indicate aplasia of the submandibular glands. It is uncommon for children to be on medication that will cause severe xerostomia, and so aplasia/hypoplasia should always be considered.

Diagnosis

Reduced uptake of technetium pertechnetate.

Radiographic pathology in children

The location, size and distribution of radiographic anomalies are important in determining a differential diagnosis. Slowly growing lesions will displace teeth within the jaws, whereas more aggressive or rapidly growing lesions may resorb teeth. It is also important to have due regard for adjacent structures and the anatomy of where a lesion might derive from and ultimately spread. Space-occupying lesions in children are predominately sarcomas rather than carcinomas that are seen in adults.

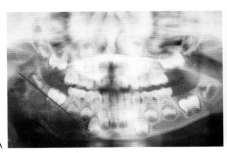 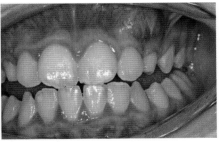

A   B

Figure 10.34   (A) *Line* drawn through the cemento–enamel junction of teeth associated with pathology in the jaws. Lesions apical to this line tend to be nonodontogenic in origin, with the body of the lesion extending away from the teeth. Those lesions coronal to this line are usually odontogenic in origin. (B) A bluish-coloured swelling of a cyst associated with an unerupted upper left permanent canine. When managing lesions presenting with this colour, it is important to eliminate a lesion of vascular origin.

The position of the lesion and the direction of the displacement of the tooth are important. Observing the radiograph, a line can be drawn through the cemento–enamel junction of the associated teeth. Lesions that arise coronal to this line are generally odontogenic in origin (see Figure 10.34). The tooth tends to be displaced away from the occlusal plane towards the cortical plates. Lesions apical to this line tend to be nonodontogenic. The body of the lesion tends to extend away from the teeth. Some lesions may have different presentations that change over time.

Descriptions of some of the following lesions have been covered in this section, while others will be discussed in other chapters of this book, as referred (Table 10.5).

PERIAPICAL RADIOLUCENCIES

Radiolucencies in the periapical region are usually associated with pulpal necrosis. All of these lesions tend to be inflammatory in origin, but remember that healing lesions may appear similar to those that are active, and sequential radiographs may be required to properly assess progression or healing. It is important to determine the integrity of the lamina dura around the apex of the tooth. Disruption or expansion of the periodontal ligament space indicates pathology.

Inflammatory lesions

- Periapical granuloma, abscess, surgical defect, scar.
- Radicular cyst.
- Transient apical breakdown postluxation of an incisor tooth (see Chapter 9).

RADIOLUCENCIES ASSOCIATED WITH THE CROWNS OF TEETH

Radiolucencies that are associated with the crowns of unerupted teeth are generally odontogenic.
- Dentigerous cyst (Figure 10.35).
  The dentigerous or follicular cyst is the most common pathological entity associated with unerupted teeth. Some 75% are located in the mandible and usually present as a painless bony expansion and failure of eruption of the associated tooth that may be displaced a significant distance. The cyst enlarges by expansion from the increased hydrostatic pressure within the cavity. In early stages, it may be difficult to distinguish between an expanded follicle and a hyperplastic dental follicle. In some cases, the cyst lining becomes contiguous with the oral epithelium, forming an eruption cyst. The cyst is usually covered

TABLE 10.5 ■ Differential diagnosis of radiographic pathology in the jaws

Radiolucencies

Periapical	Periapical granuloma, abscess, surgical defect, scar
	Radicular cyst
	Transient apical breakdown postluxation of an incisor tooth
	Traumatic bone cyst
Associated with crown of unerupted tooth	Dentigerous (follicular) cyst
	Inflammatory follicular cyst
	Eruption cyst
	Paradental cyst
	Keratocystic odontogenic tumour
	Adenomatoid odontogenic tumour
	Ossifying fibroma
Separate isolated	Nonepithelial lined bony cavities
	Primordial cyst
	Solitary bone cyst/traumatic bone cyst/haemorrhagic bone cyst
	Stafne bone cyst
	Aneurysmal bone cyst
	Nonodontogenic fissural or developmental cysts
	Fissural cysts
	Median palatine cyst
	Incisive canal cyst
	Nasolabial cyst
	Odontogenic cysts and tumours
	Keratocystic odontogenic tumour
	Ameloblastic fibroma
	Others
	Central giant cell granuloma
	Hyperparathyroidism
	Ossifying fibroma
Multiple or multilocular	Keratocystic odontogenic tumour
	Central giant cell tumour
	Cherubism
	Giant cell lesion of hyperpararthyroidism
	Langerhans cell histiocytosis
	Central haemangioma of bone
	Odontogenic myxoma
	Ewing sarcoma
	Vascular malformations of the jaws
	Desmoplastic fibroma
	Metastatic tumours
Generalized bony rarefactions	Hyperparathyroidism
	Thalassaemia
	Langerhans cell histiocytosis
	Fibrous dysplasia
	Renal osteodystrophy
	Metastatic tumours

TABLE 10.5 ■ **Differential diagnosis of radiographic pathology in the jaws** (Continued)

Radiolucencies	
Mixed radio-opaque and radiolucent lesions	Odontoma, compound or complex
	Ameloblastic fibro-odontoma
	Calcifying odontogenic cyst (Gorlin cyst)
	Calcifying epithelial odontogenic tumour (Pindborg tumour)
	Adenomatoid odontogenic tumour
	Odontogenic fibroma
	Fibrous dysplasia
	Garre osteomyelitis
	Osteosarcoma
Radio-opacities	Retained roots
	Odontomas and supernumerary teeth
	Bony exostoses, torus palatinus, torus mandibularis
	Osteoma
	Foreign bodies
	Focal sclerosing osteomyelitis
	Condensing osteitis
	Gardner's syndrome
	Cleidocranial dysplasia

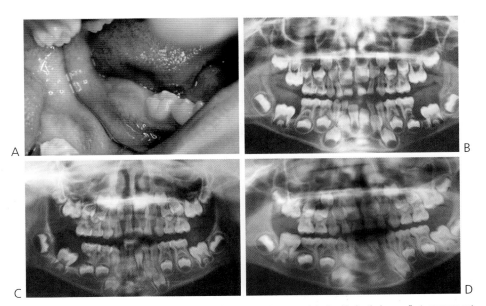

Figure 10.35 An unusual case of bilateral dentigerous cysts associated with both lower first permanent molars. (A) Uninflamed swelling distal to the second primary molar. (B) Radiographic changes showing expansion of the follicle and resorption of the root of the lower left second primary molar. (C) A large dentigerous cyst around the crown of the tooth 46. This was managed by marsupialization. (D) The appearance 6 months postsurgery showing bony infill and eruption of the tooth.

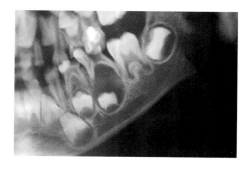

Figure 10.36 Inflammatory follicular cyst. The necrotic lower left second primary molar has caused inflammatory changes in the follicle of the premolar with displacement of this tooth.

by a very thin wall of bone, but the cortical plate invariably remains intact. Aspiration typically reveals a straw-coloured fluid containing cholesterol crystals.

The cyst lining represents a metaplastic change in the reduced enamel epithelium and histologically is seen as thin, nonkeratinized, stratified squamous epithelium, but flattened or low cuboidal cells typical of the reduced enamel epithelium may be seen along with islands of odontogenic epithelial rests. Some cysts show inflammatory changes, and when there is communication with the oral cavity, the cyst cavity may be infected. The epithelium of a dentigerous cyst may undergo neoplastic transformation. Treatment is by enucleation of marsupialization (Figure 10.35C, D).

- Inflammatory follicular cyst (Figure 10.36) (see Chapter 11).
- Eruption cyst (see Chapter 11).
- Paradental cyst (Figure 10.37).

    The paradental cyst is an inflammatory odontogenic cyst usually seen on the buccal aspect of the lower molars. It is thought to arise from the cell rests of Malassez. When there is a communication with the oral environment because of partial eruption or pericoronitis, the cyst becomes infected, and actinomyces species and other anaerobic microorganisms are found frequently. However, this is not classified as 'actinomycosis', which is a soft tissue lesion with characteristic yellow sulphur granules.

- Keratocystic odontogenic tumour (previously known as odontogenic keratocyst).

    The keratocystic odontogenic tumour (KCOT) was re-categorized as a true neoplasm by the World Health Organization in 2005. It is locally aggressive and has a very high risk of recurrence reported to be between 3% and 60%. Approximately 70% of these lesions occur in the mandible with the typical presentation similar to a dentigerous cyst with

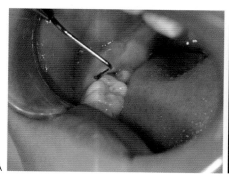
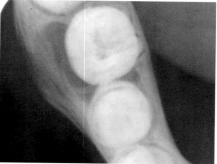

A

B

Figure 10.37 Paradental cyst. (A) A deep pocket on the buccal of a newly erupted lower right first permanent molar. (B) The true mandibular occlusal film shows the expansion of the buccal cortical plate and the associated bone loss with this cyst.

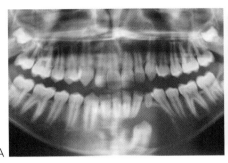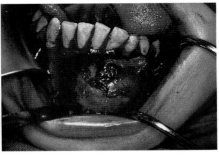

A   B

Figure 10.38 Adenomatoid odontogenic tumour. (A) This large cyst associated with the crown of the unerupted tooth 33 has caused displacement of the adjacent incisors and premolars, but there is no resorption of the roots. Hence, the lesion is slowly growing. (B) The appearance at surgery.

painless expansion; however, it may appear in association with the crown of an unerupted tooth, as an isolated radiolucency, as a multilocular lesion or as multiple isolated lesions. Radiographically, they have smooth well-demarcated borders but are locally invasive, and the cortical plate may be perforated or in the maxilla; the lesion may extend into the antrum. Histologically, there is a parakeratinized stratified squamous epithelial lining with a relatively flat epithelial–mesenchymal junction. The contents of the cyst have been described as caseous or having a yellow, cheese-like consistency, and hence aspiration is essential before surgical intervention.

Because of the aggressive nature of the KCOT, a more radical treatment approach is advised. Recurrence is caused by the budding of daughter cysts from the basal layer, an increased mitotic activity of the epithelium and local invasion of surrounding bone. Although marsupialization and enucleation with curettage have similar rates of recurrence, there is no surgical morbidity associated with resection. More recently, application of the fixative Carnoy solution (60% ethanol, 30% chloroform and 10% glacial acetic acid) has shown some promise in reducing recurrence with these lesions.

■ Adenomatoid odontogenic tumour (Figure 10.38).

The adenomatoid odontogenic tumour is a benign, slowly growing unilocular lesion that presents as a well-circumscribed radiolucency in maxilla or mandible. There may be islands of calcification within the lesion accounting for either a radiolucent or mixed radiographic presentation. There is contention as to whether this is a true tumour or a hamartoma, as they never recur. Management is by enucleation.

SEPARATE ISOLATED RADIOLUCENCIES

Odontogenic cysts and tumours

■ Ameloblastic fibroma (Figure 10.39) (see also Chapter 11).

The ameloblastic fibroma is a slowly growing, mixed odontogenic tumour containing both epithelial and mesenchymal tissues. If dentine is identified in the specimen, then the lesion is classified as an ameloblastic fibrodentinoma and tends to occur in young children.

There is discussion as to whether there is a continuum of perturbed differentiation from the ameloblastic fibroma, through the ameloblastic fibrodentinoma, to the ameloblastic fibroodontoma (see later in the chapter) and the odontomas. The former two lesions tend to occur at a later age than the latter two and, although all share similar histological features, are considered to form from different mechanisms. This means that although

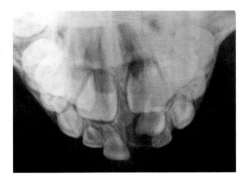

Figure 10.39 Ameloblastic fibroma associated with a maxillary supernumerary tooth. There is enlargement of the follicle surrounding the supernumerary that should arouse suspicion that there is other pathology associated with this tooth, as a dentigerous cyst is uncommonly found with supernumerary teeth in a child of this age.

conservative management is appropriate initially, revision may be required, as malignant transformation to the ameloblastic fibrosarcoma is commonly seen requiring wide surgical resection.
- KCOT (see p. 296).

Nonepithelial lined bony cavities

- Solitary bone cyst/traumatic bone cyst/haemorrhagic bone cyst (Figure 10.40).
  These pseudocysts are unlined cavities usually in the mandible; however, there is little evidence that these anomalies form following bleeding in the medullary spaces after trauma. These are asymptomatic and are usually found during routine radiographic surveys. The lamina dura of adjacent teeth is intact and there is no expansion of the bone, and without treatment, they probably resolve spontaneously; however, without a definitive diagnosis, the finding of a large radiolucency in the mandible warrants investigation.
- Stafne bone cyst (cavity).
  Although this may have the radiographic appearance of a cyst, this is merely a depression in the lingual aspect of the mandibular ramus and is occupied by the submandibular salivary gland.
- Aneurysmal bone cyst.
  The aneurysmal bone cyst is a rare expansile lesion seen in long bones as well as in the jaws. Of unknown aetiology, it is comprised of fibrous connective tissue interposed between blood-filled spaces. Aspiration yields fresh blood. The cortical plate is expanded but infrequently perforated and may present as a single or multilocular radiolucency.

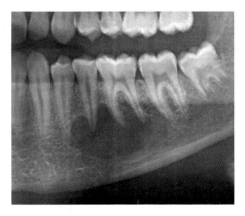

Figure 10.40 Solitary bone cyst. There is no expansion of the cortical plate, and the lamina dura of the teeth is intact.

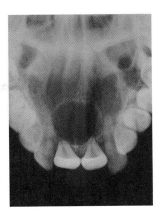

Figure 10.41 Incisive canal cyst. This cyst appears as a well-circumscribed radiolucency in the midline of the anterior palate. Notice the displacement of the central incisors.

Nonodontogenic fissural or developmental cysts

This group of cysts arises possibly from remnants of embryonic epithelial tissue; nasopalatine cysts will be lined with stratified squamous epithelium or pseudostratified ciliated columnar epithelium and are commonly observed as heart-shaped radiolucencies posterior to the upper central incisors.

- Incisive canal/nasopalatine duct cyst (Figure 10.41).
- Nasolabial cyst.
- Median palatine cyst.

Others

- Central giant cell granuloma.
  Previously thought to be a reparative process, the central giant cell granuloma is seen much more frequently in females and mainly in the mandible. It is clinically and radiographically identical to the appearance of hyperparathyroidism except that the latter is polyostotic and serum calcium and parathyroid hormone levels are elevated, while phosphorus levels are decreased. Histologically, there is a mass of connective tissue with multiple multinucleated osteoclast-like giant cells. More recently, central giant cell lesions have been managed with interferon-α and calcitonin.
- Hyperparathyroidism (see earlier and Chapter 12).
- Ossifying fibroma.
  This fibroosseous disease presents as a uni- or polyostotic lesion in either jaw, the radiographic appearance of which is either a radiolucency or mixed depending on the degree of calcification within the lesion. Previously termed the 'cemento-ossifying fibroma', the lesion is well encapsulated but is more locally aggressive in younger patients. Trabecular juvenile ossifying fibroma affects children and young adolescents, more commonly females, where there is rapid expansion of bone that may involve the cortex.

MULTIPLE OR MULTILOCULAR RADIOLUCENCIES

These are often termed soap-bubble lesions. Concern should also arise by the presence of any multilocular radiolucency, as this represents areas of pathological expansion, bone lysis and invasion.

- KCOT (Figure 10.42A).
- Nevoid basal cell carcinoma syndrome (NBCCS); OMIM No. 109400 (Figure 10.42B).
  Also known as Gorlin–Goltz syndrome, NBCCS is transmitted as an autosomal dominant mutation of the PTCH1 gene at 9q22.3–q31 but may be associated also with a 9q deletion. Similar to many autosomal dominant conditions, there is variable expressivity but complete

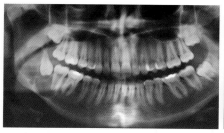
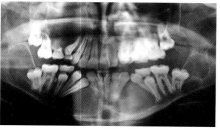

A

B

Figure 10.42 (A) Keratocystic odontogenic tumour of the right ramus of mandible in a 16-year-old patient. The presentation of these lesions may be quite variable. They are commonly associated with the crown of an unerupted tooth but may appear as multiloculated lesions or as a single radiolucency. (B) Gorlin syndrome. Panoramic radiograph of a 15-year-old girl presenting with multiple keratocystic odontogenic tumours and basal cell carcinomas on her face.

penetrance. The major criteria for a diagnosis of NBCCS include multiple KCOTs, basal cell carcinomas, palmar–plantar pits and calcification of the falx cerebri. Other features include rib and vertebral anomalies, medulloblastoma and ophthalmic anomalies. Patients have characteristic facies with frontal and parietal bossing and increased head circumference, hypertelorism and a broad nasal bridge. Patients need to be regularly monitored for the appearance of basal cell carcinomas. The jaw cysts are managed as for other KCOTs.

- Central giant cell granuloma/tumour.
- Cherubism (see Chapter 11).
- Hyperparathyroidism (see Chapter 12).
- Langerhans cell histiocytosis (see p. 283).
- Vascular malformation of jaws (arteriovenous malformation) (see p. 266).
- Odontogenic myxoma.

  Similar in radiographic appearance to the ameloblastoma, the myxoma is a mixed tumour of mesenchymal and odontogenic origin. Occurring mainly from 10 years of age onwards, it presents as a painless swelling; however, adjacent teeth may become loose or exfoliate. Histologically, there is a mass of fibroblast-like cells in a myxoid stroma. Although benign, these lesions display local aggressive infiltration requiring wide surgical resection.

- Rare tumours of bone.
  - Ewing sarcoma.
  - Desmoplastic fibroma (Figure 10.43A).
- Metastatic tumours (especially rhabdomyosarcoma Figures 10.43B, C and 10.44).

GENERALIZED BONY RAREFACTIONS

- Hyperparathyroidism.
- Thalassaemia (see Chapter 12).
- Langerhans cell histiocytosis.
- Fibrous dysplasia (Figure 10.45).

  Fibrous dysplasia presents as a monostotic or polyostotic lesion where there is abnormal growth and replacement of medullary bone by fibro-osseous tissue. The polyostotic form is more common in childhood. The areas affected are often painful, especially the limbs. Radiographically, the bone appears to have a ground-glass appearance.

  McCune–Albright syndrome (OMIM No. 174800) is described as the triad of polyostotic fibrous dysplasia, unilateral skin hyperpigmentation (café-au-lait spots) and precocious puberty. There may be generalized endocrine hyperfunction resulting in increased growth

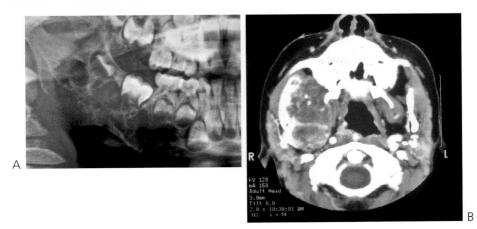

Figure 10.43 The diagnosis of a multilocular or soap-bubble lesion must always be treated with concern. These are invasive lesions and prompt referral is necessary. (A) Desmoplastic fibroma of the right mandible. (B) A large rhabdomyosarcoma involving the ramus of the right mandible and infratemporal fossa the extent of which is visible on the computed tomography scan.

hormone, catecholamines (Cushing syndrome), hyperthyroidism and hyperparathyroidism in addition to increased sex hormones. It is caused by a mutation of the GNAS1 gene at 20q13.32. There is no treatment other than bony recontouring in cases of severe disfigurement. Bisphosphonates are often prescribed to relieve pain experienced in the long bones.

- Renal osteodystrophy (see Chapter 12).

MIXED LESIONS WITH RADIOPACITIES AND RADIOLUCENCIES

- Odontoma (see Chapter 11).
- Ameloblastic fibro-odontoma (Figure 10.46; see also Chapter 11).

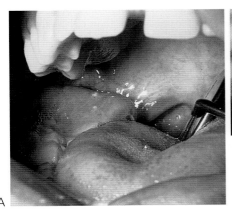

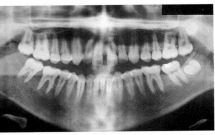

Figure 10.44 (A) A large gingival swelling in the retromolar triangle was associated with a metastatic fibrosarcoma from the abdomen in a 17-year-old boy. Not all such tumours present with multilocular radiolucencies. This patient presented with mobile right lower molars caused by metastatic infiltration of the tumour. (B) The panoramic radiograph shows only diffuse changes in the trabecular pattern of bone in the right body and ramus.

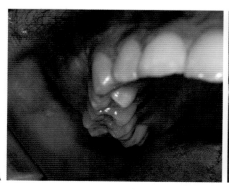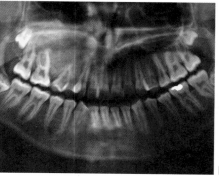

Figure 10.45 (A) This 16-year-old boy presented unable to fit his sports mouth guard properly because of the painless expansion of bone in his right maxilla. (B) Panoramic radiograph of the bone with the characteristic 'ground glass' appearance.

Similar to the ameloblastic fibroma (see earlier), this benign odontogenic tumour is distinguished by ameloblast-like cells with elements of enamel and dentine present in the lesion. It has been suggested that the ameloblastic fibro-odontoma is an early stage in the development of an odontoma and may be classified as a hamartoma, and so conservative management with enucleation is indicated.

- Calcifying epithelial odontogenic tumour (Pindborg tumour).

First described in 1955 by Jens Pindborg, this uncommon, benign odontogenic tumour has been termed the Pindborg tumour. It is believed to arise from cells of the stratum intermedium. It is usually unilocular and may be associated with an unerupted tooth. Radiographically, the lesion is well circumscribed with islands of varying degrees of radio-opacity. Histologically, the lesion is comprised of polygonal epithelial cells, interspersed with islands of calcification, and deposits of amyloid-like material. It has a high rate of recurrence.

- Calcifying odontogenic cyst (Gorlin cyst).

The Gorlin cyst presents as a single mixed radiolucency in either arch, although it may be associated with an odontome, an ameloblastic fibroma or fibro-odontome or even an ameloblastoma. Characteristic of this lesion is the presence of 'ghost cells' in the lining.

- Adenomatoid odontogenic tumour.
- Odontogenic fibroma.
- Ossifying fibroma.

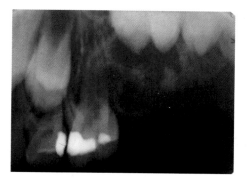

Figure 10.46 Ameloblastic fibro-odontoma. Similar in presentation to the ameloblastic fibroma, this less aggressive lesion typically presents with a mixed radiographic appearance with radiolucencies and opacities.

- Fibrous dysplasia (Figure 10.45).
- Garré osteomyelitis (periostitis ossificans).
- Osteosarcoma.

  Although the average age for the appearance of osteosarcoma is in the fourth decade of life, this rapidly growing, malignant tumour of the bone may affect children. It is primarily an osteolytic lesion displaying a characteristic 'sunray' pattern seen radiographically. It may present with pain and swelling over the area and is managed with chemotherapy and surgery.

RADIOPACITIES IN THE JAWS

- Retained roots.
- Odontomas and supernumerary teeth (see Chapter 11).
- Focal sclerosing osteomyelitis (condensing osteitis).
- Cleidocranial dysplasia (see Chapter 11).
- Gardner syndrome (see Chapter 11).
- Bony exostoses; torus mandibularis or torus palatinus.
- Osteoma.
- Foreign bodies.

Further reading

Infections

Doson, T.B., Perrott, D.H., Kaban, L.B., 1989. Pediatric maxillofacial infections: a retrospective study of 113 patients. Journal of Oral and Maxillofacial Surgery 47, 327–330.

Flaitz, C.M., Baker, K.A., 2000. Treatment approaches to common symptomatic oral lesions in children. Dental Clinics of North America 44, 671–696.

Heggie, A.A., Shand, J.M., Aldred, M.J., et al., 2003. Juvenile mandibular chronic osteomyelitis: a distinct clinical entity. International Journal of Oral and Maxillofacial Surgery 32, 459–468.

King, D.L., Steinhauer, W., Garcia-Godoy, F., et al., 1992. Herpetic gingivostomatitis and teething difficulty in infants. Pediatric Dentistry 14, 82–85.

Oral ulceration

Challacombe, S.J., 1997. Oro-facial granulomatosis and oral Crohn disease: are they specific diseases and do they predict systemic Crohn disease? Oral Diseases 3, 127–129.

Field, E.A., Brooks, V., Tyldesley, W.R., 1992. Recurrent aphthous ulceration in children: a review. International Journal of Paediatric Dentistry 2, 1–10.

Flaitz, C.M., Baker, K.A., 2000. Treatment approaches to common symptomatic oral lesions in children. Dental Clinics of North America 44, 671–696.

Harris, J.C., Bryan, R.A., Lucas, V.S., et al., 2001. Dental disease and caries related microflora in children with dystrophic epidermolysis bullosa. Pediatric Dentistry 23, 438–443.

Has, C., Bauer, J.W., Bodemer, C., et al., 2020. Consensus reclassification of inherited epidermolysis bullosa and other disorders with skin fragility. British Journal of Dermatology 183, 614–627.

Krämer, S.M., Serrano, M.C., Zillmann, G., et al., 2012. Oral health care for patients with epidermolysis bullosa – best clinical practice guidelines. DEBRA International. International Journal of Paediatric Dentistry 22, 1–35.

Léauté-Labrèze, C., Lamireau, T., Chawki, D., et al., 2000. Diagnosis, classification and management of erythema multiforme and Stevens–Johnson syndrome. Archives of Disease in Childhood 83, 347–352.

Letsinger, J.A., McCarthy, M.A., Jorozzo, J.L., 2005. Complex aphthosis: a large case series evaluation algorithm and therapeutic ladder from topicals to thalidomide. Journal of the American Academy of Dermatology 52, 500–508.

Natah, S.S., Konttinen, Y.T., Enattah, N.S., et al., 2004. Recurrent aphthous ulcers today: a review of the growing knowledge. International Journal of Oral and Maxillofacial Surgery 33, 221–234.

Rogers, R.S., 3rd, 2003. Complex aphthosis. Advances in Experimental Medicine and Biology 528, 311–316.

Scully, C., 1981. Orofacial manifestations of chronic granulomatous disease of childhood. Oral Surgery, Oral Medicine and Oral Pathology 57, 148–157.

Sedano, H.O., Gorlin, R.J., 1989. Epidermolysis bullosa. Oral Surgery, Oral Medicine and Oral Pathology 67, 555–563.

Tay, Y.-K., Huff, J.C., Weston, W.L., 1996. *Mycoplasma pneumoniae* infection is associated with Stevens–Johnson syndrome, not erythema multiforme (von Hebra). Journal of the American Academy of Dermatology 35, 757–760.

Weston, W.L., Morelli, J.G., Rogers, M., 1997. Target lesions on the lips: childhood herpes simplex associated with erythema multiforme mimics Stevens–Johnson syndrome. Journal of the American Academy of Dermatology 37, 848–850.

Vascular lesions

Kaban, L.B., Mulliken, J.B., 1986. Vascular anomalies of the maxillofacial region. Journal of Oral and Maxillofacial Surgery 44, 203–213.

Epulides

Kaiserling, E., Ruck, P., Xiao, J.C., 1995. Congenital epulis and granular cell tumour: a histologic and immunohistochemical study. Oral Surgery, Oral Medicine and Oral Pathology 80, 687–697.

Gingival overgrowth

Miranda, J., Brunet, L., Roset, P., et al., 2001. Prevalence and risk of gingival enlargement in patients treated with nifedipine. Journal of Periodontology 72, 605–611.

Pernu, H.E., Pernu, L.M.H., Huttunen, K.E., et al., 1992. Gingival overgrowth among renal transplant recipients related to immunosuppressive medication and possible local background factors. Journal of Periodontology 63, 548–553.

Ross, P.J., Nazif, M.M., Zullo, T., et al., 1989. Effects of cyclosporin A on gingival status following liver transplantation. Journal of Dentistry for Children 56, 56–59.

Premature exfoliation of teeth

Erturk, N., Dogan, S., 1991. Distribution of *Actinobacillus actinomycetemcomitans* and *Porphyromonas gingivalis* by subject age. Journal of Periodontology 62, 490–494.

Frisken, K.W., Higgins, T., Palmer, J.M., 1990. The incidence of periodontopathic micro-organisms in young children. Oral Microbiology and Immunology 5, 43–45.

Hartman, K.S., 1980. Histiocytosis X: a review of 114 cases with oral involvement. Oral Surgery, Oral Medicine, and Oral Pathology 49, 38–54.

Littlewood, S.J., Mitchell, L., 1998. The dental problems and management of a patient suffering from congenital insensitivity to pain. International Journal of Pediatric Dentistry 8, 47–50.

Macfarlane, J.D., Swart, J.G.N., 1989. Dental aspects of hypophosphatasia: a case report, family study, and literature review. Oral Surgery, Oral Medicine, and Oral Pathology 67, 521–526.

Meyle, J., Gonzales, J.R., 2000. Influences of systemic diseases on periodontitis in children and adolescents. Periodontology 26, 92–112.

Prabhu, N., McDonald, J., Cass, D., et al., 2015. Congenital granular cell tumour: an unusual antenatal presentation with a 12-year follow-up. South African Dental Journal 70, 50–52.

Preus, H.R., 1988. Treatment of rapidly destructive periodontitis in Papillon–Lefèvre syndrome. Laboratory and clinical observations. Journal of Clinical Periodontology 15, 639–643.

Rasmussen, P., 1989. Cyclic neutropenia in an 8-year-old child. Journal of Pediatric Dentistry 5, 121–126.

Research, Science, Committee, Therapy, 2003. Periodontal diseases of children and adolescents. American Academy of Periodontology. Journal of Periodontology 74, 1696–1704.

Slayton, R.L., 2000. Treatment alternatives for sublingual traumatic ulceration (Riga–Fedé disease). Pediatric Dentistry 22, 413–414.

Toomes, C., James, J., Wood, A.J., et al., 1999. Loss-of-function mutations in the cathepsin C gene result in periodontal disease and palmoplantar keratosis. Nature Genetics 23, 421–424.

Watanabe, K., 1990. Prepubertal periodontitis: a review of diagnostic criteria, pathogenesis and differential diagnosis. Journal of Periodontal Research 25, 31–48.

Salivary gland agenesis

Whyte, A.M., Hayward, M.W.J., 1989. Agenesis of the salivary glands: a report of two cases. British Journal of Radiology 62, 1023–1028.

Radiographic pathology

Kaczmarzyk, T., Mojsa, I., Stypulkowska, J., 2012. A systematic review of the recurrence rate for keratocystic odontogenic tumour in relation to treatment modalities. International Journal of Oral Maxillofacial Surgery 41, 756–767.

Sharif, F.N.J., Oliver, R., Sweet, C., et al., 2010. Interventions for the treatment of keratocystic odontogenic tumours (KCOT, odontogenic keratocysts, OKC). Cochrane Database of Systematic Reviews (9), CD008464.

General

Hall, R.K., 1994. Pediatric orofacial medicine and pathology. Chapman and Hall Medical, London.

World Wide Web Database

Online Mendelian Inheritance in Man, OMIM (TM), 2000. McKusick-Nathans Institute for Genetic Medicine. Johns Hopkins University, Baltimore, MD. National Center for Biotechnology Information, National Library of Medicine (Bethesda, MD). Online. Available: www.ncbi.nlm.nih.gov/omim/.

Dental anomalies

Mike Harrison   ■   Angus C. Cameron   ■   Richard P. Widmer

...whilst many practitioners strive rightly to delay the first 'tooth-cutting' restoration, conversations with a substantial number of adults with [amelogenesis imperfecta] suggest that this professional restraint may be unwelcome and paternalistic. Some of these same adults will recount that, if they had realised that restored teeth must eventually fail, they would have chosen tooth-tissue destructive, but aesthetically more attractive restorations earlier in their adolescence, in order to appear most 'ordinary' to their peers at an important time in social development.

Crawford PJM, Aldred M, and Bloch-Zupan, 2007

Introduction

The diagnosis and management of dental anomalies are important areas of paediatric dentistry. Although most dental anomalies present in childhood, many are misdiagnosed or left untreated, perhaps because of lack of experience or because the case is perceived to be 'too difficult'.

In this chapter, reference to particular inherited conditions is made to entries in the Online Mendelian Inheritance in Man (OMIM). This online database is a catalogue of genetic disorders developed by Dr Victor McKusick of the Johns Hopkins University and the National Center for Biotechnology Information (see References and further reading). When a dentist is trying to reach a diagnosis or formulate a treatment plan for rare dental anomalies, case reports published online can be a good source of information but must be read with caution. Discussion with colleagues or an experienced paediatric dentist is always recommended. Genetic investigation for dental anomalies is rarely indicated, but a small number of conditions with oral manifestations do require referral to specialist paediatric services.

Considerations in the management of dental anomalies

- Informing and supporting the child and parent.
- Establishing a diagnosis.
- Consider if medical referral required.
- Interdisciplinary formulation of a definitive treatment plan.
- Elimination of pain.
- Restoration of aesthetics.
- Provision of adequate function.
- Maintenance of occlusal vertical dimension.

- Use of intermediate restorations in childhood and adolescence.
- Planning for definitive treatment at an optimal age.

TREATMENT PLANNING FOR CHILDREN WITH DENTAL ANOMALIES

Treatment planning should be multidisciplinary. Decision making must involve the child and the parents and should consider the present and future needs and development of the child. Although children will cope with a range of appliances and treatments during childhood, early adolescence represents a period of social adjustment, as well as the transitional changes in the dentition. It is perhaps the most difficult time in which to formulate a long-term plan. Teenagers are most concerned about aesthetics, yet it may be too early to provide definitive restorations; extensive orthodontic treatment may be required or later orthognathic surgery. In hospital dental services, various teams exist to carry out a treatment plan and/or manage these cases and a list of specialists is suggested here. Note the involvement of the child's family dental practitioner.

The team approach

- Paediatric dentist.
- Orthodontist.
- Prosthodontist.
- Surgeon.
- Speech pathologist.
- Clinical psychologist.
- Family dental practitioner.

It is essential to seek advice from colleagues in the management of children with uncommon dental conditions. Local and international collaboration provides the best opportunities to increase our knowledge and improve the outcomes for these children.

Dental anomalies at different stages of dental development

It is convenient to consider dental anomalies by the development stage at which they arise.

DENTAL LAMINA FORMATION STAGE

Induction and proliferation

- Hypodontia (isolated or syndromic).
- Supernumerary teeth.
- Double teeth (geminated or fused teeth).
- Odontomes (complex and compound).
- Odontogenic tumours, particularly the spectrum of ameloblastic fibroma/fibrodentinoma/fibro-odontome (dependent on differentiation and the presence and type of calcification within the lesion).
- Keratocystic odontogenic tumours (KCOTs).

HISTODIFFERENTIATION

Developmental defects of multiple dental tissues

- Regional odontodysplasia.
- Segmental odontomaxillary dysplasia (SOD).

MORPHODIFFERENTIATION

Abnormalities of size and shape

- Macrodontia.
- Microdontia (isolated or syndromic).
- Invaginated odontome (dens invaginatus).
- Evaginated odontome (dens evaginatus).
- Carabelli trait.
- Taurodontism.
- Talon cusp.
- Hutchinson incisors and mulberry molars in congenital syphilis.

MATRIX DEPOSITION

Organic matrix deposition and mineralization

- Enamel:
  - Fluorosis.
  - Chronological enamel hypoplasia.
  - Molar–incisor hypomineralization.
  - Amelogenesis imperfecta.
- Dentine:
  - Dentinogenesis imperfecta.
  - Dentinal dysplasia.
  - Vitamin D-resistant rickets.
  - Preeruptive intracoronal resorptive lesions.

ERUPTION AND ROOT DEVELOPMENT

- Premature eruption.
- Natal and neonatal teeth.
- Eruption cyst.
- Delayed eruption.
- Primary failure of eruption (PFE).
- Ectopic eruption.
- Impactions.
- Transposition of teeth.
- Arrested root development from systemic illness (or treatment of systemic illness).
- Failure of eruption associated with inflammatory follicular cysts.
- Failure of eruption in amelogenesis imperfecta.
- Failure of eruption in cleidocranial dysplasia (CCD).
- Failure of eruption in cherubism.

Formation of dental lamina

HYPODONTIA

Alternative terminology: hypodontia, oligodontia, anodontia.

Hypodontia, oligodontia and anodontia are terms that can be interpreted to refer to progressive degrees of missing teeth, although the term 'hypodontia' is preferred because it is inclusive of any number of missing teeth (Figure 11.1A). 'Oligodontia' refers to six or more missing teeth,

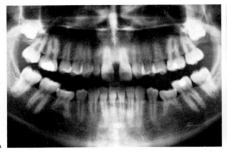
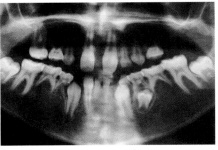

A   B

Figure 11.1   (A) The teeth most commonly missing are the last teeth in each series, namely the upper lateral incisors, the second premolars and the third molars. (B) Panoramic radiograph of a boy with autosomal dominant ectodermal dysplasia with absence of both primary and permanent teeth.

and 'anodontia' to the complete absence of teeth. It is implicit in all cases that the teeth are missing because of failure of development. The term 'congenitally missing teeth' is a misnomer when applied to the permanent dentition because these teeth do not commence development until after birth (and with regard to the primary dentition, one cannot usually determine this clinically at birth); 'partial anodontia' is a nonsense term. Some degree of hypodontia is relatively common, occurring sporadically or with a hereditary component. The teeth most commonly absent are the last teeth in each series (i.e., the lateral incisor, the second premolar and the third molar). Clinically, it is less important to know how many but rather which types of tooth are absent. It is particularly unusual for a patient to be missing central incisors, canines or first permanent molars. Multiple missing teeth in a child should lead to investigations to determine if there are other affected family members. The presence of a rudimentary or conical maxillary lateral incisor may be associated with the absence of the same tooth on the opposite side of the arch. This anomaly may be a familial trait or sometimes the mildest manifestation of an underlying genetic disorder.

Frequency

Primary teeth	~0.1%–0.7%	Male : female	Ratio unknown
Permanent teeth	~2%–9%	Male : female	1 : 1.4

Third molars > maxillary lateral incisors > second premolars > mandibular central incisors.

Major conditions manifesting hypodontia

Hypodontia is a major clinical feature of over 50 syndromes. These include:
- Ectodermal dysplasias.
- Cleft lip and/or palate.
- Trisomy 21 (Down syndrome).
- Chondroectodermal dysplasia (Ellis–van Creveld syndrome).
- Rieger syndrome.
- Incontinentia pigmenti.
- Oro-facial-digital syndrome.
- William syndrome.
- Craniosynostosis syndromes.

Ectodermal dysplasias.   Ectodermal dysplasia describes a group of developmental, often inherited disorders involving structures derived from ectoderm, that is, hair, teeth, nails, sweat glands and salivary glands. The most common is the X-linked hypohidrotic form (OMIM 305100,

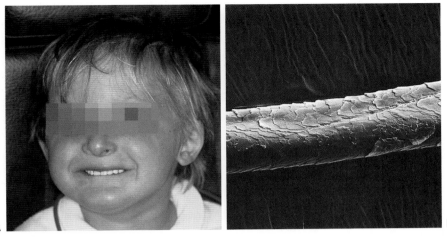

A   B

Figure 11.2 (A) Typical appearance of a boy with X-linked hypohidrotic ectodermal dysplasia (wearing a denture). The skin around the eyes is dry and wrinkled and may be pigmented (not shown here). (B) The hair is fine and sparse and often displays longitudinal grooves on the surface under the scanning electron microscopy.

EDA1, Xq12–q13.1; short arm of X chromosome). In this condition, the usual presentation is a male child with:

- Multiple missing teeth (Figure 11.1B).
- Fine, sparse hair (Figure 11.2A, B).
- Dry skin (Figure 11.2A).
- Maxillary hypoplasia.
- Eversion of the lips.
- Peri-orbital skin pigmentation with creases.

Teeth are small and conical, often with a large anterior diastema (Figure 11.3). Heterozygous females are often identified by dental examination, and their manifestations may be limited to a single missing tooth or to a peg lateral incisor (see the Lyon hypothesis, later in the chapter).

In the group of ectodermal dysplasias, autosomal dominant and recessive modes of inheritance are also seen. In such families, there will not be such a striking difference in the degree of the disorder between males and females compared with X-linked hypohidrotic ectodermal dysplasia (Figures 11.2A and 11.4).

Changes in the gene *WNT10A* have been implicated in many cases of nonsyndromic hypodontia, often with a severe dental phenotype and very mild disturbances of extraoral structures of ectodermal origin.

Mutations in the *MSX1* gene (4p16.1) have been identified in families with missing third molars and second premolars with or without clefting, as well as in families with tooth-nail (Witkop) syndrome. *PAX9* (14q12–q13) gene mutations have been found in other families with autosomal dominant missing teeth, particularly multiple molar agenesis. More genes implicated in missing teeth and other anomalies continue to be identified.

In some countries, dental care (including prevention, orthodontics and prosthetics) for affected children may be provided under government-funded schemes.

Management

The aim of treatment is to provide adequate function, maintain the vertical dimension and restore aesthetic appearance. Ideally, for social reasons, treatment should begin at around 2 to 3 years of age. There is often considerable parental pressure to 'normalize' the appearance, and this needs to

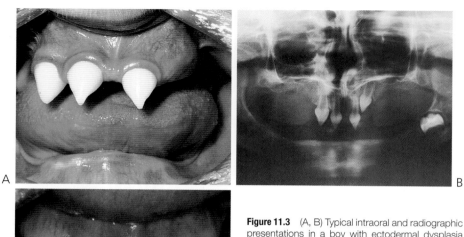

Figure 11.3 (A, B) Typical intraoral and radiographic presentations in a boy with ectodermal dysplasia with multiple missing teeth; the teeth that are present are small and conical in shape. In the regions where teeth are absent, alveolar bone does not develop. (C) Composite resin build-ups of the conical teeth have provided improvement in the aesthetics; however, the problem of the diastema remains, given that there are only a few teeth for orthodontic anchorage.

be balanced against the needs of the child. A first step is often the placement of composite restorations to mask the 'fang-like' appearance of any conical anterior teeth (Figure 11.3A). Provision of partial dentures (or, in severe cases, full dentures) can start at any age, often around the time the child starts school, as soon as the child allows adequate impressions to be taken. Often, however, the first denture is initially worn in the pocket(!), but as the child grows, there is often a desire to have a more ordinary appearance. With encouragement and positive reinforcement, most children will soon try their new appliances.

Treatment planning for children with hypodontia

Treatment planning should be multidisciplinary and should consider the present and future needs and development of the child, while also considering the concerns of the parents (Figure 11.5).

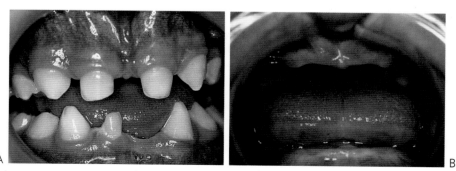

Figure 11.4 (A) This child is a heterozygous female with the X-linked form of ectodermal dysplasia and is less severely affected than her brother who has anodontia (B).

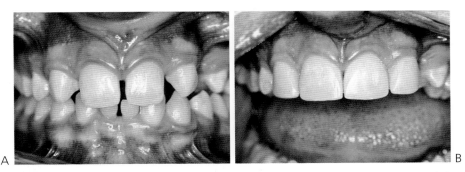

Figure 11.5 (A, B) Closure of an anterior diastema and reshaping of the canines with composite resin in a child with absence of the upper lateral incisors. The successful masking of upper canines to appear like lateral incisors is dependent very much on their size.

Treatment options

- Acid-etch retained, composite resin build-ups of conical teeth (Figure 11.6).
- Composite resin or bonded orthodontic buttons can also be added to provide undercuts for denture clasps and retainers.
- Partial dentures: conventional or overdentures (Figure 11.7).
- Surgical exposure of ectopic or impacted teeth.
- Orthodontic management of spaces.

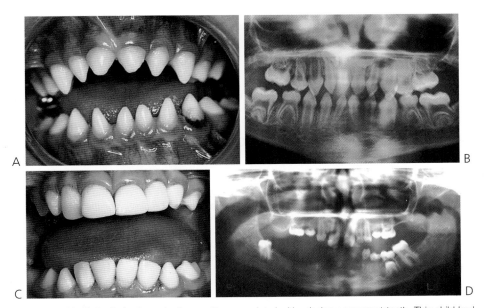

Figure 11.6 (A, B) Conical primary teeth are often associated with missing permanent teeth. This child had an autosomal recessive form of ectodermal dysplasia and was missing almost all of the permanent teeth. (C) These teeth have been built up with composite resin strip crowns. (D) Radiographic appearance of the same child at 15 years of age. Most of the primary teeth have exfoliated even in the absence of a permanent successor. There has also been loss of bone in the region of the tuberosity as a result of pneumatization of the sinus that will complicate implant placement.

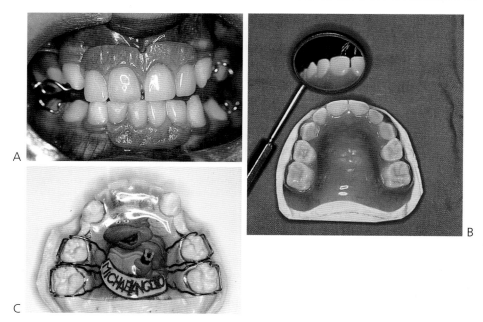

Figure 11.7 (A–C) Dentures for young children with ectodermal dysplasia. (A) Young children tolerate dentures extremely well, and Adams cribs and ball retainers provide retention around primary molars. In this case, an overdenture covers two conical, widely spaced incisors. (B) A full upper denture for a child of 30 months will require periodic relining and re-making as the child grows. (C) Stock prosthetic teeth are sometimes difficult to obtain, but paediatric denture teeth may be made freehand from acrylic and the palate can be customized.

- Laboratory-fabricated composite resin veneers, crowns and bridges.
- Osseointegrated implants (usually after the cessation of growth).

THE LYON HYPOTHESIS (X CHROMOSOME INACTIVATION)

CLINICAL HINTS: PROVISION OF DENTURES FOR YOUNG CHILDREN

Generally, children can tolerate dentures well; nevertheless, provision of the upper denture before the lower may be one way of increasing acceptance. The aim is for these children to be wearing appliances that give them a dentition similar to their peers, to enhance their self-esteem and to promote normal speech development and masticatory function by the time they are at kindergarten or primary school. Dentures need to be re-made at regular intervals, and a same-age model from an unaffected child should be used as a template for the occlusion.

- Use fast-setting alginate impression material or a bite-registration elastomeric material and sit the child upright with the head forwards.
- Use Adam clasps on molars and ball retainers between upper canines and first molars.
- Use overdentures when there are multiple missing teeth and/or irregular spacing.
- Fluoride supplementation should be used with overdentures.
- Resilient or soft liners aid retention.
- Make dentures with irregular, or partly erupted, teeth during the mixed dentition stage.
- Long school holidays are often a good time for the provision of new dentures.

During cellular differentiation, one of the two X chromosomes in each female somatic cell is inactivated. This means that in families with X-linked disorders, approximately 50% of the cells of heterozygous females will express the mutant gene disorder, whereas the remainder will express the normal gene. In the tissues affected by the condition, such females have a mosaic of affected and normal cells. This is of particular importance in X-linked forms of conditions such as haemophilia, hypohidrotic ectodermal dysplasia, vitamin D-resistant rickets and amelogenesis imperfecta. Thus, heterozygous females with X-linked hypohidrotic ectodermal dysplasia may have missing teeth, although they are invariably less severely affected than males. Similarly, in haemophilia A, heterozygous females do not usually have a clinical bleeding abnormality, but this can occur if lyonization is severely skewed so that there is a preponderance of cells producing factor VIII under control of the mutant gene.

DENTOALVEOLAR CLEFTING

In patients affected by dentoalveolar clefting, disruption of the dental lamina at that site, there may be abnormal cellular induction or proliferation. This may give rise to either missing teeth, usually the maxillary lateral incisor, and/or supernumerary teeth adjacent to the cleft. In children with nonsyndromic orofacial clefting, hypodontia has been shown to be more common away from the cleft site, in both maxilla and mandible.

SOLITARY MEDIAN MAXILLARY CENTRAL INCISOR SYNDROME (OMIM 147250)

Solitary median maxillary central incisor syndrome (Figure 11.8) is very rare. It presents with a midline symmetrical maxillary central incisor. The condition may also be associated with other midline disturbances such as cleft palate, choanal stenosis or atresia, imperforate anus

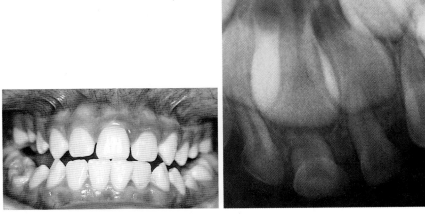

Figure 11.8 (A) Solitary median maxillary central incisor syndrome presenting with a symmetrical incisor in the midline. This child had a mild growth hormone deficiency, with his height on the 10th centile. (B) Periapical radiograph of the same patient in the primary dentition showing the single primary and permanent central incisors.

or umbilical hernia and is probably the mildest part of the spectrum of the holoprosencephaly malformation complex. Of importance in some cases is the association with hypoplasia of the sella turcica, pituitary dysfunction, growth hormone deficiency and subsequent short stature. The syndrome is usually diagnosed based on the dental manifestations, and the dentist should always refer to specialist paediatric services for further investigation. A mutation in the *SHH* gene (7q36) has been identified in one family, but it is probable that there is genetic heterogeneity in the condition.

Ultimately, management of the dental anomaly is by orthodontic and prosthodontic therapy, determined by space considerations. In most cases, the single central incisor is moved to one side of the midline with either creation of space for a prosthodontic replacement or the adjacent lateral incisors are recontoured.

OSSEOINTEGRATED IMPLANTS IN CHILDREN

There has been much controversy about the timing of placement of osseointegrated implants in children. To date, there has been only limited published material about early placement and any long-term consequences. It is generally understood that implants act similarly to anky-losed teeth and do not move occlusally with the growing bone around adjacent natural teeth. Animal research has confirmed that most fixtures do become osseointegrated in growing jaws; however, there was no evidence from this research that the fixtures behaved like normal teeth during development. In the mandible, the fixtures came to lie lingual to the natural teeth; in the maxilla, they came to lie palatal and superior to the adjacent teeth and did not follow the normal downwards and forwards growth of this bone. This latter point is important when considering the placement of implants in the anterior maxilla. Furthermore, placement of fix-tures retarded alveolar growth locally and changed the eruptive path of distally positioned tooth buds. Implants should, in most cases, not be considered before the cessation of growth. It should be noted, however, that in children with conditions such as ectodermal dysplasia, alveolar bone does not develop where teeth are not present. Consequently, it may be considered appropriate, particularly where there are multiple missing teeth, to place implants much earlier in these children than in those with a normal alveolus. Recent research suggests that in cases of anodontia, implants are best placed in the mandibular canine region at around 8 to 10 years of age (which is after the period of maximal mandibular transverse growth) to facilitate lower denture retention.

Disorders of proliferation

SUPERNUMERARY TEETH (Figure 11.9)

- Supernumerary teeth arising as a result of budding of the dental lamina are usually an iso-lated anomaly.
- Multiple supernumerary teeth are a feature of CCD, skeletal dysplasia and Gardner syn-drome, a form of familial adenomatous polyposis.
- The shape of the supernumerary may resemble a tooth of the normal series (a supplemental tooth), in which case it can be incisiform, caniniform or molariform; otherwise it may be conical or tuberculate.
- Most often present as a result of failure of eruption of one or more permanent teeth. Usually appear as conical or tuberculate forms.
- Supernumerary teeth have been considered to be manifestations of a separate dentition (occurring between the primary and permanent dentitions), and consequently, it may be possible to predict when and where supernumeraries may form (Jensen & Kreiborg, 1990).

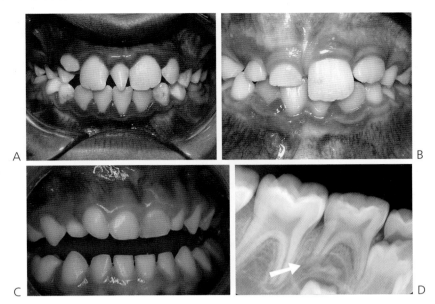

Figure 11.9 Common presentation of supernumerary teeth. (A) Conical teeth often erupt, except when inverted. (B) The late eruption of a permanent central incisor is most commonly caused by a supernumerary tooth. (C) Supplemental upper primary lateral incisor. (D) Supernumerary teeth may occur in any part of the jaws. In the lower premolar region they are usually found lingual and slightly superior to the normal premolar tooth.

Alternative terminology

Mesiodens (a term restricted to supernumerary teeth in the midline of the maxilla), paramolar, distomolar, hyperdontia, supplemental teeth.

Frequency

Primary teeth	~0.3%–0.8%	Male:female	Ratio unknown
Permanent teeth	~1.0%–3.5%	Male:female	1:0.4

- 98% occur in the maxilla, 75% of which are mesiodens.

Diagnosis

- Failed or eruption disturbance of permanent tooth (Figure 11.9B).
- Unexpected radiographic finding.
- As part of a syndrome such as CCD (Figure 11.10).

Management

- If a supernumerary tooth is obstructing the eruption path of an adjacent tooth, or has any associated pathology, it should be removed as soon as convenient. However, with all dento-alveolar surgery, there are risks that need to be considered, such as nerve injury or damage to adjacent teeth and anaesthetic risk. In some cases, the risks will outweigh the benefits, and it may be better to leave the supernumerary tooth in situ (i.e., if the supernumerary is in the posterior hard palate).

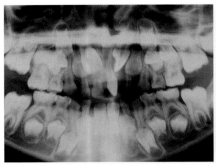
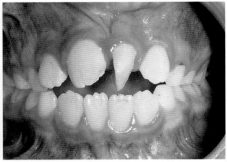

A   B

Figure 11.10 (A, B) Dependent on the degree of displacement, given adequate space, most central incisors will erupt normally once an obstruction such as a supernumerary tooth is removed. The rotation can be corrected later.

- A supernumerary primary incisor may be retained if there is sufficient room for it. The tooth should be extracted when the permanent lateral incisor is ready to erupt if it is not expected to exfoliate normally.
- Supplemental permanent lateral incisors usually present with the primary supernumerary tooth. Usually, the more distal of the two permanent teeth is the supernumerary tooth.
- Identification of a supernumerary tooth that is similar in form and size to the adjacent tooth can be made by comparing the teeth with those on the opposite side of the dental arch. The tooth that more closely resembles the size and shape of the normal lateral incisor should be retained unless there are orthodontic reasons otherwise.
- Conical teeth often erupt and are easily extracted (Figures 11.9A and 10).
- Tuberculate and/or inverted conical teeth require surgical removal as early as possible to allow uninhibited eruption of the permanent teeth (Figure 11.11).
- It is essential to localize the position of the tooth to be removed before surgery. Periapical films using a tube-shift technique can be used to locate the tooth; however, this is always open to errors and misinterpretation. Panoramic and standard maxillary occlusal films may be used in the same way.
- Digital imaging techniques using cone-beam computed tomography (CBCT) provide high-definition, three-dimensional (3D) imaging of the head and neck with much reduced radiation exposure than traditional computed tomography (Figure 11.11). However, plane radiographs remain the standard views for children, except in very complex cases where CBCT images may change the planned intervention.
- During surgical removal, care should be taken to avoid disturbing the developing permanent teeth.
- Before 10 years of age: if the unerupted central incisor is correctly aligned, the treatment of choice is to remove the supernumerary surgically and allow normal eruption of the permanent tooth. Gingival exposure may be required later because of surgical scar formation that can inhibit final soft-tissue emergence. Some authorities recommend the simultaneous removal of primary canines to counteract this tendency. Inverted supernumeraries can be removed less traumatically if surgery is performed early; however, this needs to be done with caution to avoid damage to the adjacent teeth.
- After 10 years of age, or if the central incisor is malaligned: surgical exposure with or without bonding of orthodontic brackets or chains and subsequent traction may be required (Figure 11.12).

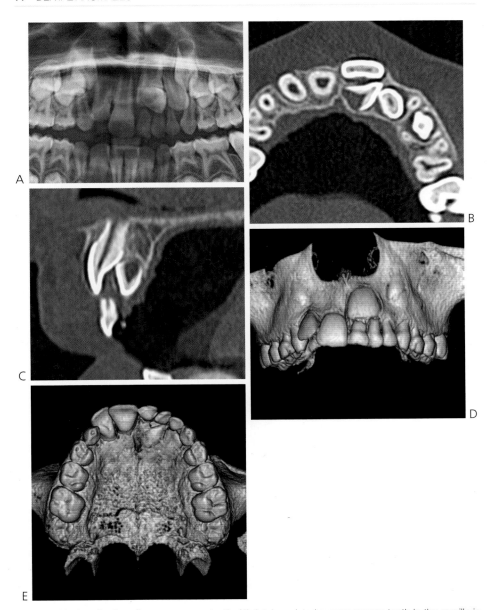

Figure 11.11 Localization of supernumerary tooth. (A) A tuberculated supernumerary tooth in the maxilla is impacting the upper left central incisor. A panoramic film is useful in determining the vertical and horizontal angulation of the permanent tooth. It is important to know if there will be enough room for the tooth to erupt spontaneously. (B, C) This can be correlated with images from a cone-beam tomography. Axial and sagittal sections show that the 21 tooth is labial positioned with little impediment to its eruptive path. (D, E) This can be confirmed using the three-dimensional reconstructions that can also provide a visual aid during surgery. Note the presence of a supplemental primary lateral incisor.

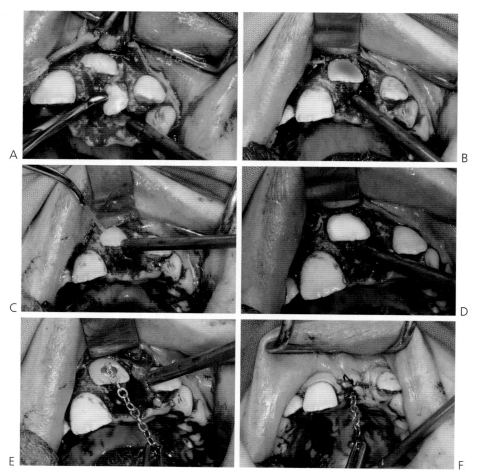

Figure 11.12 Surgical exposure and bonding of a gold chain to a central incisor which was impacted by a supernumerary tooth. (A) Elevation of the labial and palatal flaps and removal of the supernumerary. (B) Acid-etch applied to the labial surface of the upper left central incisor. (C) Rinsing the acid etch gel from the tooth. (D) The appearance of the etch pattern on the prepared tooth. (E) Bonding of a gold chain attachment to the labial surface of the incisor. (F) The flap is closed, and the chain is sutured to the gingiva with surgical nylon. The chain will be attached to an archwire and orthodontic traction will be applied to orthodontically align the tooth.

CLINICAL HINT: REMOVAL OF SUPERNUMERARY TEETH

- Most maxillary supernumerary teeth are best removed surgically via a palatal approach. The only exceptions are those that are inverted, conical in shape and positioned between the roots of the central incisors. Usually the crown is found lying adjacent to the anterior nasal spine and is best approached via a labial flap.

CLEIDOCRANIAL DYSPLASIA (OMIM 119600) (Figure 11.13)

CCD is a skeletal dysplasia with significant dental manifestations. The majority of cases of CCD are caused by mutations of the gene *RUNX2*, and there may be an autosomal dominant mode of inheritance, although sporadic cases are frequent.

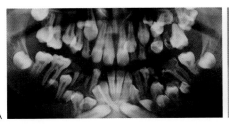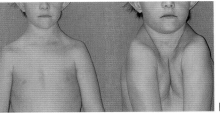

A   B

Figure 11.13 (A) Case of cleidocranial dysplasia with 18 supernumerary teeth. (B) A boy with cleidocranial dysplasia showing the characteristic absence of the clavicles.

Manifestations

- Short stature.
- Aplasia or hypoplasia of one or both clavicles (Figure 11.13B).
- Delayed ossification of fontanelles and sutures.
- Frontal bossing.
- Hypertelorism and maxillary hypoplasia.
- Wormian bones in cranial sutures.
- Multiple supernumerary teeth (Figure 11.13A).
- Delayed eruption of teeth, even in those regions without supernumerary teeth.
- Dentigerous cyst formation.

Management

- Early diagnosis and documentation.
- Early planned removal of nonresorbing primary teeth.
- Surgical removal of supernumerary teeth.
- Surgical exposure (uncovering) of permanent teeth.
- Orthodontic traction, when required, and alignment and consideration of orthognathic surgery when growth is complete.

The mechanism of delayed eruption remains contentious. Recent research has demonstrated that there is no difference in the amount of either cellular or acellular cementum in patients with CCD. The formation of the primary teeth is usually normal; however, the delay in permanent tooth eruption is most probably attributed to a combination of the presence of supernumerary teeth and decreased bone resorption because of insufficient osteoclast activity.

Note that the simple extraction of a primary tooth will not guarantee the eruption of the impacted permanent tooth. A two-stage surgical procedure is usually required with an attachment placed on the permanent tooth followed by orthodontic traction. The first procedure involves exposure of the anterior segments with removal of the anterior primary teeth and any supernumeraries that may be present. The permanent teeth are surgically exposed, and bonded gold chains are attached for orthodontic traction. The anterior teeth are then aligned orthodontically. The second stage involves extraction of the primary molars, surgical removal of remaining supernumerary teeth and exposure of the premolars and molars in the buccal segments. Definitive orthodontic therapy follows; orthognathic surgery may be required in cases with severe skeletal Class III malocclusion. Treatment extends over many years, often with the need for multiple surgical procedures, so clinicians should be aware of the child's ability to cope and the family's willingness bring the child for frequent appointments. Support from clinical psychiatry may be useful, particularly with respect to other aspects of CCD such as short stature and painful joint hypermobility.

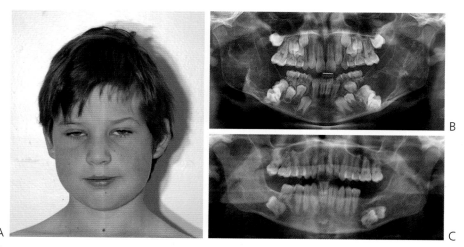

Figure 11.14 Cherubism. (A) An 8-year-old boy with characteristic facies of cherubism. (B) The panoramic radiograph shows almost symmetrical multilocular radiolucencies in the angles of the mandible of an 8-year-old boy. The displacement of developing molars and delayed eruption of teeth are typical. (C) These cases should be managed conservatively. With no treatment, the condition burns out, and 13 years later, there has been almost complete resolution of the condition. Several of the lower molars remain impacted with no prospect of them being functional teeth; however, the patient has a bilateral stable and functional occlusion.

CHERUBISM (OMIM 118400) (Figure 11.14)

Cherubism is a self-limiting fibro-osseous disorder caused by mutations in the *SH3BP2* gene at 4p16.3.

Patients may present in childhood with facial swelling and/or failure of eruption of teeth, typically the mandibular molars. Radiographs will reveal multilocular radiolucencies, typically involving the angles of the mandible. A biopsy will reveal multinucleate giant cells in a fibrous tissue stroma. Developing teeth in the affected area tend to be displaced and fail to erupt at the normal time. Both jaws can also be affected, as can the ribs. The facial swelling reflects the involvement of the underlying bone. In some patients, the sclera in the lower part of the eyes may be exposed to give the cherubic or heavenward gaze that gives the condition its name. In some cases, there is no discernible facial swelling, and the condition is identified as a result of routine radiographic studies such as for orthodontic treatment planning, or because of delayed eruption of teeth.

The condition progresses into adolescence and then tends to resolve, so that by the third or fourth decade, radiographic changes may no longer be found. In some families, more affected males than females may be identified; this is a result of reduced penetrance in females and needs to be taken into account in genetic counselling. A subset of patients with cherubism is more severely affected, with the multilocular radiolucencies affecting the whole of the mandible and maxillae. In mildly affected cases regular review may be all that is necessary; in more severely affected cases surgical reduction may be considered if the patient is distressed by their appearance.

INFLAMMATORY FOLLICULAR CYSTS (see Chapter 10)

Some children may present with failure of eruption of a mandibular premolar associated with a radiolucency involving the roots of the primary molar and crown of the unerupted premolar (see Figure 7.2B and Figure 10.36). There is controversy as to whether such cases are as a result of radicular cyst formation associated with the roots of the primary tooth (which is considered by some to be a rare occurrence) or dentigerous cyst formation around the crown of the premolar. The common characteristics of such cases tend to be:

- Prior endodontic treatment of the primary molar.
- A radiolucency involving the roots of the primary molar and crown of the permanent successor.
- Displacement of the permanent successor away from the alveolar crest.

Histopathological examination tends to show intense acute and chronic inflammation of the curetted tissue which is lined by hyperplastic stratified squamous epithelium. Such cases have been designated 'inflammatory follicular cysts', with persistent inflammation from the endodontically treated primary molar leading to an inflammatory enlargement of the follicle of the underlying permanent tooth.

Similar cystic changes can occur in the follicles of unerupted permanent incisors when pulp necrosis of the overlying primary incisor is left untreated. Delayed eruption of the permanent incisor when compared with the ipsilateral tooth should always be investigated, particularly if the retained primary incisor is discoloured or carious.

ODONTOMES (Figure 11.15)

Odontomes occur because of disordered differentiation and often present because of failure of eruption of a permanent tooth. In compound odontomes, a multiplex of irregular denticles are

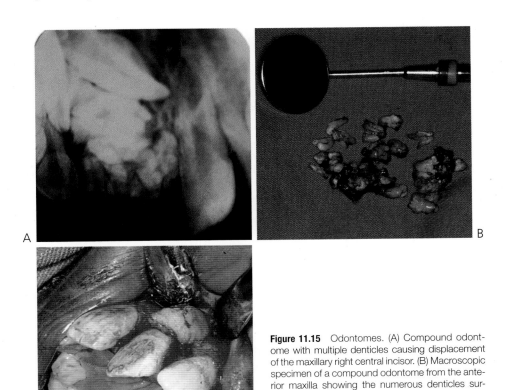

A

B

C

Figure 11.15 Odontomes. (A) Compound odontome with multiple denticles causing displacement of the maxillary right central incisor. (B) Macroscopic specimen of a compound odontome from the anterior maxilla showing the numerous denticles surrounded by a well-defined capsule. (C) Complex odontome following elevation of a labial flap.

found in a circumscribed soft tissue stroma. Complex odontomes are disordered lesions with a discrete, haphazard mass of calcified tissue containing all dental elements. There is either a normal complement of teeth or the odontome replaces a tooth of the normal series.

Management

- Surgical enucleation.
- Depending on the time of diagnosis, permanent teeth may be ectopically positioned and may require surgical exposure and orthodontic alignment.

ODONTOGENIC TUMOURS (see also Chapter 10)

The ameloblastic fibroma, fibrodentinoma and fibro-odontome are uncommon benign odontogenic mixed tumours. All are seen as altered differentiation of the tooth bud: in an ameloblastic fibroma no hard tissue is formed, in an ameloblastic fibrodentinoma only dentine-like tissue is recognizable, and in an ameloblastic fibro-odontome enamel is also formed. The lesions tend to be well demarcated.

Management

- Surgical enucleation.
- Follow-up of erupting permanent dentition if teeth are displaced by the lesion.

KERATOCYSTIC ODONTOGENIC TUMOURS (see Chapter 10)

KCOTs may arise in place of a tooth of the normal series or from the dental lamina in addition to a normal complement of teeth. They constitute 5% to 15% of odontogenic cysts.

REGIONAL ODONTODYSPLASIA (Figure 11.16)

Regional odontodysplasia is a sporadic defect in tooth formation with segmental involvement, usually localized to one, or part of one, quadrant, but it may cross the midline to affect the contralateral central incisor. All dental tissues are involved in a bizarre dysplasia with severely hypoplastic teeth which are slow to erupt and which typically radiographically show a ghost-like appearance. The aetiology of the condition is unclear.

- Usually presents initially with abscessed primary teeth before or soon after eruption.
- Some cases are associated with superficial vascular anomalies.

Alternative terminology

Ghost teeth.

Management

- In spite of attempts to restore teeth with preformed metal crowns or composite resin, most affected teeth require extraction. Permanent successors of affected primary teeth are invariably affected, although sometimes to a lesser degree. There is no justification for bony excision at the time of tooth removal. If the affected permanent teeth fail to erupt and are completely covered by bone, then it is reasonable for these teeth to be left in situ, which will preserve bone and the height of the alveolus. There is no suggestion that there is a higher rate of cystic degeneration in such teeth. Successful autologous tooth transplantations into the sites of removal of affected teeth have been reported.

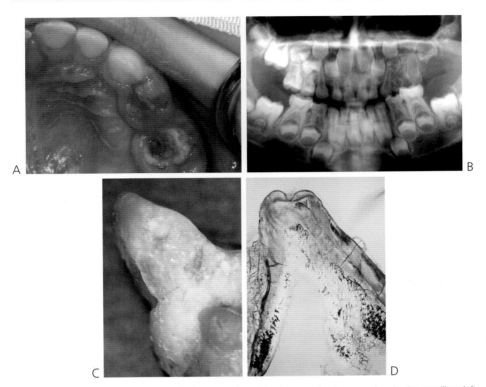

Figure 11.16 (A) Regional odontodysplasia presenting with abscessed primary molars in the maxillary left quadrant, soon after eruption. (B) The panoramic radiograph shows involvement of all the teeth in this quadrant, including the permanent teeth. (C) Grossly abnormal enamel in an affected tooth and (D) the hard tissue section demonstrates the disruption of odontogenesis. (Courtesy Dr. N. Pai, Sydney, Australia.)

- Partial dentures are required to restore the lost teeth.
- Implants may be appropriate.

SEGMENTAL ODONTOMAXILLARY DYSPLASIA (Figure 11.17)

This condition affects the teeth and the adjacent bone, distinguishing it from regional odontodysplasia and fibrous dysplasia. Typically, SOD presents as a unilateral expansion of the maxilla in a segment of the dental arch. The teeth in the affected segment are dysplastic, with hypoplastic or hypomineralized enamel, or developmental absence of permanent teeth may be seen. The gingivae are often enlarged in the affected segment, and there is an associated expansion of the alveolar ridge similar to that seen in monostotic fibrous dysplasia of the maxilla. This bony expansion can sometimes cause facial asymmetry, and the overlying facial skin can be hyperpigmented or exhibit hypertrichosis.

Management

- Although preservation of affected teeth is important, the priority may be to establish diagnosis by extraction of the worst-affected teeth along with a bone biopsy.
- SOD is a benign condition and does not require resection of the affected bone.
- Aesthetic considerations are needed for very rare occurrences in the anterior maxilla.

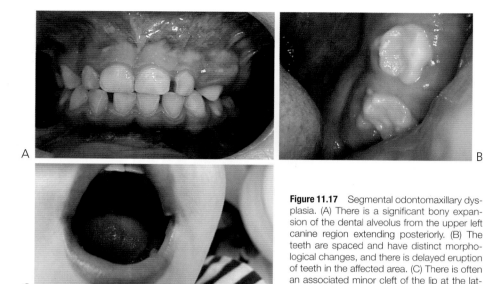

Figure 11.17 Segmental odontomaxillary dysplasia. (A) There is a significant bony expansion of the dental alveolus from the upper left canine region extending posteriorly. (B) The teeth are spaced and have distinct morphological changes, and there is delayed eruption of teeth in the affected area. (C) There is often an associated minor cleft of the lip at the lateral commissure.

Abnormalities of morphology

MACRODONTIA (Figure 11.18)

- Any tooth larger than normal for that particular tooth type.
- True macrodontia involving the whole dentition is extremely rare. More commonly, single teeth are abnormally large because of an isolated disturbance of development.

Aetiology

- Unknown for a single tooth, but generalized macrodontia may be caused by a hormonal imbalance, as this has been described in pituitary gigantism. It should be remembered that an illusion of generalized macrodontia will occur if the jaws are small relative to the size of the teeth.

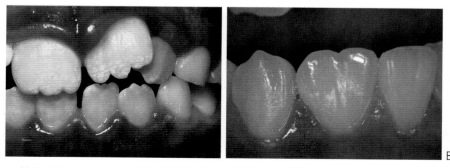

Figure 11.18 Morphological anomalies. (A) Mamelons, which are variations of normal anatomy. (B) Double tooth involving the right mandibular incisor, probably caused by fusion of the lateral and central incisor tooth germs.

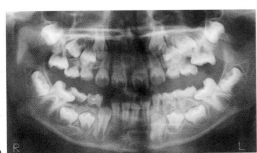 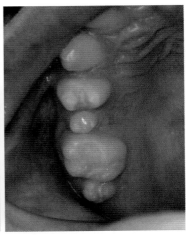

A   R   L   B

Figure 11.19 Macrodontia. (A) Generalized macrodontia associated with KBG syndrome. These children present with intellectual disabilities, broad facies, short stature and skeletal abnormalities. (B) Syndromic microdontia affecting multiple teeth as opposed to isolated microdontia that usually affects only a single tooth.

- May also be associated with hemifacial hyperplasia.
- True macrodontia should not be confused with the fusion or gemination of adjacent tooth units or a supernumerary to form a single tooth.
- Macrodontia is associated with KBG syndrome (the initials are taken from the surnames of the families first reported with the condition). These children present usually with a triad of short stature, intellectual disability and macrodont upper incisors. However, one of the authors has described a family with generalized macrodontia affecting all primary and permanent teeth. Other abnormalities may include microcephaly and a typical facial appearance with bushy eyebrows, anteverted nostrils and hypertelorism (Figure 11.19B).

Alternative terminology

Megadontia

Frequency

Primary dentition	Unknown
Permanent dentition	~1.1%

More common in males.

Management

- Stripping to reduce tooth size is ineffective and should be done with great caution, as the enamel is usually of normal thickness.
- Can be combined with composite resin build-up of the antimere if only one tooth is affected.
- Extraction and replacement by a prosthesis.
- Aesthetic adjustment of an isolated macrodont tooth by incisal edge 'notching' and the generation of a labial groove to break up light reflections may be helpful in some cases.

MICRODONTIA (Figure 11.19B)

- One or more teeth are smaller than normal for the tooth type.
- The most common form of microdontia affects only one or possibly two teeth; it is much rarer in the primary than in the permanent dentition.
- This anomaly most often affects the maxillary lateral incisors and third molars. It is noteworthy that the affected teeth are usually the ones that are also most often missing.
- Supernumerary teeth are frequently microdont.
- Patients with ectodermal dysplasia often present with microdontia.

True generalized microdontia

All of the teeth are of a normal morphological form, but they are smaller than normal teeth. This condition is exceedingly rare but can occur in pituitary dwarfism and some other skeletal dysplasias.

Generalized relative microdontia

The teeth are of normal size but appear relatively small with respect to the jaws that are larger than normal.

Alternative terminology

Peg-shaped laterals.

Frequency

Most data are available only for maxillary lateral incisors.

Primary dentition	<0.5%
Permanent dentition	~2.0% (maxillary lateral incisors)

More common in females.

Management

- Composite resin additions to improve shape.
- The profile of the tooth is narrower at the gingival margin than a normal-sized tooth (emergence profile), and there is therefore a limit to how large the tooth can be enlarged with a restoration without producing an overhang at the gingival margin or an unsightly interdental shadow.
- Orthodontic alignment of the upper labial segment and extraction of the tooth may be required, and prosthetic replacement with nonpreparation adhesive bridges (or implants in adulthood) should also be considered.

CLINICAL HINT: ACID-ETCH COMPOSITE RESIN BUILD-UPS

In patients with missing teeth, the central incisors can be conical in form. When closing an anterior diastema, it is often preferable to add composite to the distal aspect of the crown rather than the mesial. The diastema can be closed orthodontically to avoid a 'flared' appearance of the tooth crown that tends to look artificial. A more vertical mesial proximal surface and the addition of composite to the distal surface give a better appearance with a more normal distal angle and arch form.

DOUBLE TOOTH (Figure 11.20)

This anomaly is manifest as a structure resembling two teeth that have been joined together. In the anterior region, the anomalous tooth usually has a groove on (at least) the labial surface and

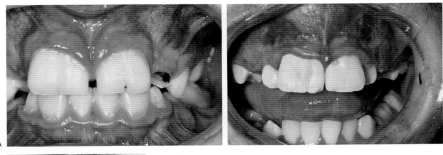

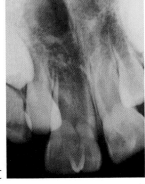

Figure 11.20 (A) Two double teeth formed by the fusion of each of the maxillary central incisors with supernumerary teeth. Two root canals were present in each tooth. (B) Bilateral double teeth caused by gemination. A single root canal was present in each tooth (C).

a notch in the incisal edge. Although rarer in the posterior region, the cuspal morphology can be suggestive of two teeth that are joined together. Radiographs are necessary to determine if there is a union of the pulp chambers, and even then it may be speculative. If the 'double tooth' is present together with a normal complement of teeth in the same quadrant, then it is presumed to have arisen as a result of gemination; if the number of teeth is reduced, then fusion of tooth germs is assumed. If teeth have been extracted or exfoliated, the use of the neutral term 'double tooth' avoids the need to arbitrarily decide if this is as a result of gemination or fusion.

Alternative terminology

Fusion, gemination, connation, schizodontia, dichotomy.

Frequency

Primary dentition	~2.5%
Permanent dentition	~0.2%

Fusion, gemination or a 'double tooth' in the primary dentition should alert the clinician to the possibility of disturbances in the permanent dentition. These can range from an absent tooth, an extra tooth, a microdont tooth or no disturbance at all.

Fusion

Joining of two teeth of the normal series or a normal tooth and a supernumerary tooth by pulp and dentine. Two canals are usually present. The tooth has arisen from two tooth germs, and so the number of teeth in the dentition is normally reduced by one unit. If, however, the normal tooth is fused to a supernumerary, the number of teeth in the arch will be normal. This fusion is assumed to occur between normal and supernumerary teeth because of the close proximity of the tooth buds.

Gemination

Budding of a second tooth from a single tooth germ. Usually one root canal is present.

Management

- The central groove on the labial and palatal surfaces of a double tooth is prone to dental caries; therefore early application of a fissure sealant is recommended.
- Very rarely, surgical separation of fused teeth may be possible. The roots should be completely separate, and a pulp-capping technique planned if the coronal pulp is shared. The lack of cementum on the cut surface of the root may result in external resorption or a periodontal defect. Subsequent orthodontic alignment and restorative treatment may be needed to reshape the remaining crown.
- Reshaping or reduction of a double tooth with a single canal (geminated tooth) may be attempted by modifying the appearance of the labial groove and the use of composite resin, but is often impossible and extraction may be the only alternative. Orthodontic treatment and/or prosthetic replacement are/is then required. Implants may be an option for adolescents.
- Planned extraction and surgical separation outside the mouth with replantation might also be considered, although this is not always successful because of resorption subsequent to replantation.

CLINICAL HINT: FUSED AND GEMINATED TEETH

Large geminated teeth present difficult management issues. It is essential to diagnose whether a single canal or separate canals are present. Plain radiographs are often of little benefit, especially when the abnormal tooth is in the central incisor region and there is superimposition of the lateral incisor which erupts palatal to the double tooth because of a lack of space. Cone-beam tomography can be helpful to determine the pulp and root morphology (Figure 11.21).

Concrescence

Joining of two teeth, one of which may be a supernumerary, by cementum. Concrescence most commonly affects the maxillary second and third permanent molars in older adults. Apart from when involving supernumeraries, this condition is rarely seen in children.

DENS INVAGINATUS (Figures 11.22 and 11.23)

The maxillary lateral incisors may have a developmental invagination of the cingulum pit with often only a thin hard tissue barrier between the oral cavity and the pulp. Pulp necrosis often occurs soon after eruption of the affected tooth and may lead to a canine fossa abscess or cellulitis. This anomaly may occur in other teeth such as the maxillary central incisors and canines.

Alternative terminology

Invaginated odontome, dens in dente (if an enamel structure is present within the canal), dilated odontome.

Frequency

Primary dentition	~0.1%
Permanent dentition	~4%

More common in males.

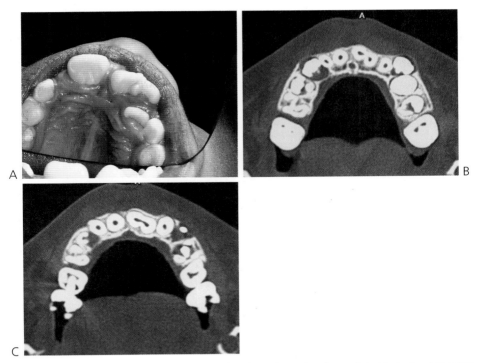

Figure 11.21 (A) It is often very difficult to determine the root canal anatomy of double teeth when using periapical films because of superimposition of the lateral incisor that has usually erupted palatally. Computed tomography can be used to determine the true internal anatomy of the root canal. (B) Apically, it appears that there are two distinct canals; however, a more coronal section shows that there is communication between the canals. (C) This contraindicates surgical separation of the roots. The diagnostic value of this radiography must be weighed against the radiation exposure.

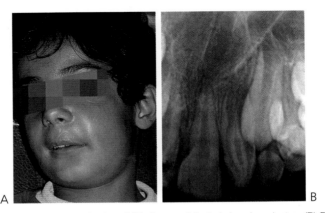

Figure 11.22 (A, B) Maxillary canine fossa cellulitis from an infected dens invaginatus. (B) Because of root canal morphology and the severity of the infection, the tooth was removed. The patient required hospital admission, with high-dose intravenous antibiotics and surgical drainage of the abscess under general anaesthesia.

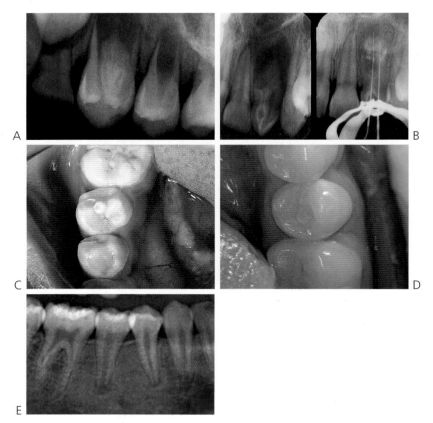

Figure 11.23 (A) Dens invaginatus in a maxillary first premolar tooth. (B) Ultimately, the prognosis is related to the ability to adequately instrument and obturate the canals of these teeth. Temporary endodontic dressings can be placed in such teeth to relieve symptoms and treat infection, but it is almost impossible to obturate such canals. (C) Dens evaginatus. (D) Dens evaginatus where the tubercle has fractured off and the tooth has become necrotic. This child presented in acute pain with a facial cellulitis. The radiograph (E) shows the periapical area.

Management

- If newly erupted, palatal pits and fissures should be sealed as a preventive measure.
- If caries is evident, then place an acid-etched retained composite resin restoration with minimal preparation.
- If symptomatic and the root canal morphology is favourable, endodontic treatment can be attempted.
- If the internal anatomy is complex and the root canal is not negotiable, then, in the event of infection, extraction is necessary. The presence of this anomaly should be carefully considered during orthodontic treatment planning.
- The same tooth on the opposite side should be carefully assessed for the same problem.

DENS EVAGINATUS (Figure 11.23C, D)

- An enamel-covered tubercle usually projecting from the occlusal surface of a premolar tooth.
- Usually bilateral and more common in the mandible.

- There is evidence of pulp tissue within the tubercle in around 50% of cases.
- Radiographs may show occlusal extension of the pulp chamber.

Alternative terminology

Leung cusp, dens evaginatus, tuberculated premolar, axial core type odontome, occlusal enamel pearl, composite dilated odontome, interstitial cusp.

Frequency

Primary dentition	Almost unknown
Permanent dentition	~4% (almost exclusively in people of Asian extraction)

More common in females.

Management

- The tubercle can easily fracture because of occlusal interference, leaving the internal pulp extension exposed. Thus reduction of the cusp and composite coverage is advisable, presuming that a minimal pulpotomy is being performed even if not clinically evident. An alternative prophylactic measure is to support the sides of the tubercle with composite resin and then to recontour the occlusal surface to produce a central ridge. Ideally, both options should be performed before the tooth comes into complete occlusion.
- If fractured or subject to attrition, pulp exposure occurs frequently. Because this exposure occurs soon after eruption, the apex of the tooth is often open, and the long-term prognosis is less certain. Extraction of the tooth may be considered after orthodontic consultation. If the tooth is to be retained, a calcium hydroxide dressing is appropriate with an apexification procedure (see Chapter 9) to stabilize the tooth if orthodontic therapy is to commence later (and subsequent definitive endodontic treatment). More recently, revascularization has been proposed in the management of these teeth.
- If diagnosed early, an elective (Cvek) pulpotomy can be performed in an attempt to allow normal root formation.

TALON CUSP (Figure 11.24)

This is a horn-like projection of the cingulum of the maxillary incisor teeth. It may reach the incisal edge of the tooth.

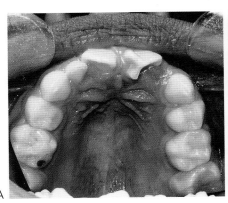
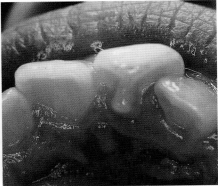

A   B

Figure 11.24   (A) Talon cusp. (B) T-cingulum. The cingulum cusp has pulp horns, and removal of the cusp will often result in an exposure of the pulp.

Alternative terminology

T-cingulum, Y-shaped cingulum.

Frequency

Primary dentition	Almost unknown
Permanent dentition	~1%–2%

Management

- If there is no interference with the occlusion, no treatment is required.
- Fissure sealants to prevent caries in the grooves between the various parts of the tooth.
- If occlusal interference is present, small progressive reduction of enamel only to avoid pulp exposure, or elective pulpotomy, to allow root completion.

TAURODONTISM

Used to describe a molar tooth with a pulp chamber that is vertically enlarged at the expense of the roots. The distance from the cemento–enamel junction to the furcation of the root may be greater than the distance from the furcation to the apices. The tooth, therefore, has a long body and short roots, with a tendency towards a single root or apical displacement of the furcation. The anomaly appears to be caused by delay or failure of invagination of Hertwig epithelial root sheath. Taurodontism may have a genetic basis. Several syndromes and conditions such as ectodermal dysplasias, X-chromosome aneuploidies and some families with (autosomal dominant) amelogenesis imperfecta have this anomaly. The latter is interesting, as the pulp chamber is, of course, determined by the surrounding dentine. Taurodontism may also be reflected in single-rooted teeth, with the pulp canals being wider than usual.

Frequency

Uncommon rather than rare. Enlarged pulp chambers may also be seen in:
- X-linked hypophosphataemic rickets (vitamin D–resistant rickets).
- Vitamin D–dependent rickets.
- Hypophosphatasia.
- Dentinogenesis imperfecta (some cases).
- Regional odontodysplasia.
- Klinefelter syndrome.
- Shell teeth.

CONGENITAL SYPHILIS

Although now very rare in most parts of the world, congenital syphilis presents with several important diagnostic dental manifestations. Both primary and permanent incisors have tapering crowns and central notching of the incisal edge. This tapering or screwdriver-like appearance is important in the differential diagnosis, as there are other causes of nonsyphilitic notching of the incisal edge (e.g., trauma). This screwdriver morphology is also seen in Nance–Horan syndrome. The crowns of the molar teeth have a 'cobbled' or 'mulberry' appearance in congenital syphilis.

Developmental defects of enamel

Developmental defects of enamel can be acquired or inherited.

CHRONOLOGICAL DISTURBANCES

Any severe systemic event during the development of the teeth (i.e., from 3 months in utero to 20 years of age) may result in some dental abnormality. Many of these anomalies are subclinical and can only be observed in hard-tissue sections as changes in the incremental deposition lines. The neonatal line is manifest in all primary teeth, but unless there is a severe physiological disturbance or foetal distress, the disturbance may not be clinically evident. Different teeth will show defects at different levels of the crown depending on the stage of crown formation at the time the disturbance occurred. The resulting enamel may be reduced in quality (usually hypomineralization) and/or quantity (hypoplasia). A hypomineralization enamel defect that has undergone posteruptive breakdown should not be described as 'hypoplastic'.

More than 100 aetiological agents have been reported to cause developmental defects of enamel. Those causing localized defects are listed in Table 11.1 and those causing generalized defects are listed in Table 11.2.

Developmental defects of enamel can be considered according to their clinical appearance:

- Discolouration.
- Opacity.
- Opacity with posteruptive breakdown.
- Hypoplasia.

In general, the aims of management are to treat associated pathology and pain, provide adequate aesthetic appeal, maintain occlusal function and maintain the vertical dimension.

TOOTH DISCOLOURATION

Tooth discolouration may be extrinsic or intrinsic in nature. Extrinsic staining is superficial and occurs after tooth eruption. Intrinsic discolouration may result from a developmental defect of enamel or internal staining of the tooth (Figure 11.25). Although such internal staining is manifest as a change in tooth colour, the intrinsic defect may affect the dentine primarily or exclusively. See Table 11.3 for the differential diagnosis of tooth discolouration.

OPACITY

Opacities result from a defect in the quality of the enamel, affecting the translucency of the tissue. Hypomineralization results in a change in the porosity of the enamel, altering the refractive index to light compared with normally mineralized enamel. This may be located below the enamel surface, which otherwise remains intact.

TABLE 11.1 ■ **Aetiological agents shown to produce developmental defects of enamel with a localized distribution**

Acute osteomyelitis	Gunshot wounds to jaws
Acute trauma to primary teeth	Irradiation
Ankylosis	Jaw fracture
Cleft palate	Laryngoscopy
Congenital epulis	Periapical infection of primary teeth
Electrical burn to mouth	Periodontal ligament injection
Extraction of primary teeth	

TABLE 11.2 ■ **Environmental aetiological agents shown to produce developmental defects of enamel and discolouration with a generalized distribution**

Prenatal	Perinatal	Postnatal	
Anaemia	Bile duct defects	Adrenal hyperfunction	Lead intoxication
Cardiac disease	Breech presentation	Cytotoxic medications	Measles
Congenital allergies	Caesarean section	Bulbar poliomyelitis	Mumps
Congenital syphilis	Erythroblastosis fetalis	Candida-endocrinopathy syndrome	Nephrotic syndrome
Cytomegalovirus	Haemolytic disorder	Chickenpox (varicella)	Neurological disorders
Diabetes	Hepatitis	Cholera	Otitis media
Fluoride	Intrapartum haemorrhage	Congenital cardiac disease	Pneumonia
Hypoxia	Low birth weight	Diphtheria	Pseudohypothyroidism
Pregnancy toxaemia	Neonatal asphyxia	Encephalitis	Renal dysfunction
Malnutrition	Neonatal hypocalcaemia	Fluoride	Scarlet fever
Renal disease	Placenta praevia	Gastrointestinal disturbances	Sickle cell anaemia
Rubella	Prematurity	Hyperpituitarism	Smallpox
Stress	Prolonged labour	Hyperthyroidism	Stress
Thalidomide	Respiratory distress syndrome	Hypogonadism	Tetracyclines
Urinary tract infection	Tetanus	Hypoparathyroidism	Tuberculosis
Vitamin A deficiency	Tetracyclines	Hypothyroidism	Typhus
Vitamin D deficiency	Traumatic birth injuries	Intestinal lymphangiectasia	Vitamin A deficiency
	Twinning		Vitamin C deficiency
			Vitamin D deficiency
			Vitamin D intoxication

FLUOROSIS (Figure 11.26, Table 11.4)

Dental fluorosis is a qualitative defect of enamel resulting from a chronic increase in fluoride concentration within the micro-environment of the ameloblasts during the mineralization of enamel (Aoba & Fejerskov, 2002). Therefore, children aged 1 to 3 years are the most susceptible to develop fluorosis in the most visible maxillary anterior areas. One important factor in recognizing fluorosis is that it primarily affects permanent teeth and is bilateral, appearing similarly on equivalent teeth that developed at the same time on each side of the mouth. This distinguishes fluorosis from other types of hypomineralization. Because it is a dose-related condition, a diagnosis of dental fluorosis requires a detailed history of fluoride exposure. At 1 parts per million (ppm) of fluoride in public water supplies, up to 10% of the population will show very mild opacities attributable to fluorosis (although this may depend on individual water consumption); interestingly, this seems to be a

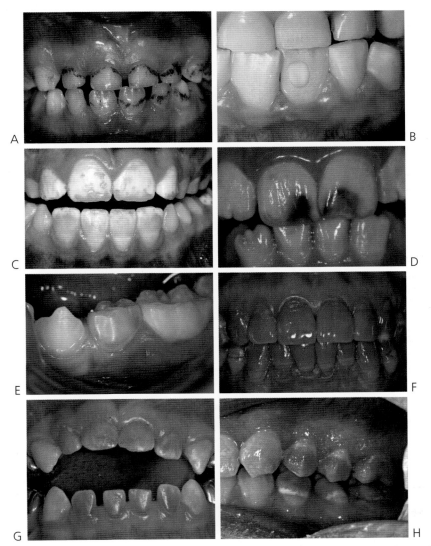

Figure 11.25 Tooth discolouration. (A) Brown-black superficial staining from chromogenic bacteria. (B) Localized enamel opacity caused by the root apex of a traumatized primary incisor. (C) Superficial extrinsic staining from the use of iron supplementation. (D) Brown discolouration caused by incorporation of blood pigments into the enamel following trauma to the primary dentition. (E) Pink discolouration caused internal resorption of the tooth 74. (F) Tetracycline staining in a child from South-east Asia. Tetracycline-containing liquid preparations are no longer routinely prescribed for children; however, tetracyclines may be included in some homoeopathic preparations in some countries. (G) Blue-brown appearance of dentinogenesis imperfecta. (H) Chronological discolouration of an unknown aetiology. There is a precise pattern to the hypomineralization and appearance of the posterior teeth; however, the anterior teeth, in particular the canines that are developing at the same age, are unaffected.

TABLE 11.3 ■ Causes of tooth discolouration

Colour	Aetiology	Comments
Extrinsic discolouration		
Green	Chromogenic bacteria	Usually cervical and gingival areas
Yellow	Bile pigments from gingival crevicular fluid	Biliary atresia and jaundice
Black-brown	Ferrous sulphate	Iron supplementation
	Chromogenic bacteria	Arrested caries
Intrinsic discolouration with localized staining on one or several teeth		
Yellow/brown	Developmental defects	Usually after trauma or infection
White	Developmental defects	Subsurface decalcification in permanent teeth, after trauma or infection
Pink	Internal resorption	Seen before exfoliation or after trauma
Grey/Black	Amalgam staining	Leakage of old amalgam restorations causing discolouration at the periphery
Chronological staining of dentition		
Bright yellow	Tetracycline	Unoxidized fluorophore, seen in newly erupted teeth
Yellow/grey-brown	Tetracycline	Erupted teeth, oxidized fluorophore (ultraviolet light)
Yellow-brown	Systemic illness	Developmental defect of enamel affecting all teeth forming during illness
Generalized intrinsic staining of teeth, either single or complete dentition		
Grey-brown	Necrotic tooth	Usually after trauma
Yellow-brown to dark yellow	Amelogenesis imperfecta	Both dentitions are affected
Green-blue	Hyperbilirubinaemia	Seen in children with end-stage liver disease and premature infants
Blue-brown (opalescent)	Dentinogenesis imperfecta	Uniformly affected teeth, may be associated with osteogenesis imperfecta
Red-brown	Congenital porphyria	All teeth affected
White	Fluorosis/nonfluorotic	Usually only permanent dentition

minimum value and the proportion of opacities increases as fluoride levels either fall below 1 ppm or rise above ppm.

Severe forms of dental fluorosis are usually seen in areas where the natural concentration of fluoride in the water is very high. Mild forms of fluorosis are less frequently seen worldwide since the reduction or elimination of systemic fluoride supplements and the raised awareness of careful evaluation of all fluoride sources before additional fluoride sources are prescribed. However, the dental profession must consider very carefully their fluoride regimes for children younger than 6 years of age, weighing carefully their risks and benefits. It is interesting to note that most studies show that people do not notice mild fluorosis.

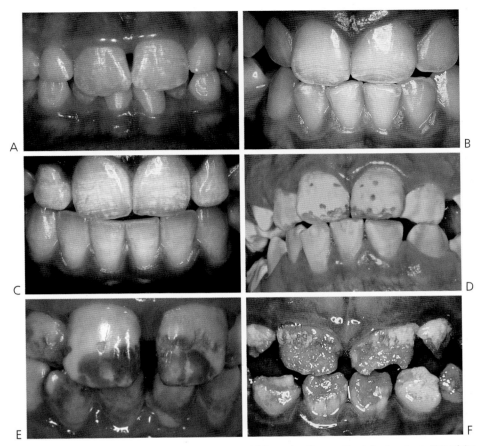

Figure 11.26 Different severities of fluorosis. (A) Very mild fluorosis with opacities following the outline of the perikymata. The primary teeth are unaffected. In younger children, the enamel is generally more opaque. (B) In an older child, the translucency of the incisal edge is evident, but the opacities follow the same horizontal lines of the perikymata. (C) Mild fluorosis with white flecking through the crowns of the incisors. Note that the lower incisors are only minimally affected. This is still a surface opacity that will improve over time or may be conducive to treatment with microabrasion. (D) Moderate opacity affecting the whole crown. Note that the pits and brown mottling is secondary to tooth-surface wear and the acquisition of stains. (E) Score 6, staining of intact enamel and discrete pitting. (F) Score 6, a more severe appearance with significant loss of enamel.

To reduce the risk of mild fluorosis, parents of children under 6 years of age should:

- Supervise brushing to check on fluoride toothpaste usage.
- Place a smear or pea size of paste on the brush depending on the age of the child.
- Store the toothpaste out of reach, so that a child will be unable to eat or suck the toothpaste.
- Avoid giving children 1 mg fluoride supplements.
- Not give baby vitamin drops containing a fluoride supplement.

The appearance of fluorotic enamel changes over time with natural abrasion of the outer surface of the teeth, especially in cases of mild fluorosis. In its mildest forms, fluorosis is manifest as hypomineralization of the enamel, leading to opacities. These can range from tiny white flecks to confluent opacities throughout the enamel, making the crown totally lacking in translucency. Mild fluorosis is characterized by opaque lines following the perikymata. With increasing

TABLE 11.4 ■ **Tooth surface index of fluorosis**

Score	Description (teeth not dried)
Score 0	No evidence of fluorosis
Score 1	Less than one-third of visible enamel as areas showing a parchment white colour. Tips of incisors and posterior teeth showing snowcapping
Score 2	Parchment white fluorosis totals at least one-third but less than two-thirds of visible enamel surface
Score 3	Parchment white fluorosis totals at least two-thirds of visible surface
Score 4	Any of preceding levels of fluorosis plus staining from light to brown
Score 5	Discrete pitting which is usually discoloured when compared with surrounding enamel
Score 6	Discrete pitting, plus staining of intact enamel
Score 7	Confluent pitting, plus large areas of enamel may be missing. Dark brown stain is usually present

(From R.G. Rozier (1994). Epidemiologic indices for measuring the clinical manifestations of dental fluorosis: Overview and Critique. Advances in Dental Research 8(1), 1994. https://doi.org/10.1177/08959374940080010901.)

severity, the opaque lines merge and more irregular cloudy areas become visible. More severe cases will have a totally opaque, chalky appearance. In a small number of cases, there will be punched-out pits and the outermost enamel will be gradually lost (Figure 11.26D). Hypoplasia (Figure 11.26F) occurs at higher concentrations of fluoride. When the tooth first erupts, the surface of even the most severely affected enamel may be intact; however, with wear, areas of enamel are lost and stains are taken up into the porosities. Severely affected cases may require microabrasion or restoration with composite resin, either in a localized or a more generalized manner. Many opacities are incorrectly labelled as fluorosis without adequate justification or investigation of the patient's fluoride history.

Management of stains and opacities

- Extrinsic stains can be removed with abrasives.
- Mild discolouration may be improved using peroxide-based bleaching agents.
- Intrinsic stains, if superficial, may be removed with microabrasion techniques.

Microabrasion. It must be understood that microabrasion techniques involve removal of the surface opaque layer of enamel. The opaque but often bright white layer of enamel is removed, and children and parents are often disappointed at the appearance of the normal 'yellow' colour of the permanent crown. It is important to make an initial decision whether to attempt to alter the entire dentition to this darker colour or to continue with the piecemeal adjustment of darker areas to match the overall 'paper-white' appearance. In present-day society, the latter decision may prove to be satisfactory or even desirable. Acid-based techniques may create more porosity in the enamel, which may accumulate more stains over time.

Hydrochloric acid: 18% (with or without the use of pumice). Rubber dam should always be used and must be secured by ligation around individual teeth and sealing with copal-ether varnish or a proprietary sealer. Orabase® paste applied to the gingival margin before dam placement can be used to protect the soft tissues from any acid leakage. An aqueous slurry of sodium bicarbonate may be laid on the dam around the teeth to neutralize any inadvertent excess acid. A hydrochloric acid/pumice slurry is applied to the affected area using a slowly rotating rubber cup for 10 seconds only, and then rinsed thoroughly with water. Application is repeated a maximum of 10 times. This technique is potentially destructive to enamel and soft tissues and must be used with caution.

Alternatives

- Abrasion with a mixture of pumice and 37% phosphoric acid (etchant).
- Polishing labial surfaces with a multi-fluted tungsten-carbide bur.
- Application of a 2% neutral sodium fluoride.
- Recent research has shown that mild fluorosis can also be remineralized and the opacity reduced by casein phosphopeptide-amorphous calcium phosphate (CPP-ACP) or CPP-amorphous calcium phosphate fluoride. The enamel should be pretreated with sodium hypochlorite to denature any residual protein.
- It is suggested that after any abrasion procedure the enamel be polished with a fine polishing paste (non coloured toothpaste is suitable) using a rubber cup.

Deep intrinsic stains require removal of the affected enamel and rebuilding, usually with composite resin. Although localized marks may be dealt with by this method, treatment using composite resin or porcelain as full-face veneers, or crowns, should ideally be delayed in adolescents until the gingival attachment is established at the cemento-enamel junction. The longevity of hybrid composite resins has improved substantially, along with their colour stability, strength and translucency. These materials may be placed quickly and more cost-effectively than porcelain and other complex restorations such as crowns. Modern materials generally provide for densely white shades that make matching possible. Always keep treatment options open. Involvement in contact sports may be another reason for delaying placement of complex restorations.

ENAMEL HYPOPLASIA (Figure 11.27)

A defect in quantity that causes an altered contour of the surface of the enamel. This is caused by initial failure of the deposition of enamel protein, but the same clinical effect could also result if there is a mineralization defect that leads to loss of enamel substance after eruption. In the former case, the enamel is often hard and glassy; in the latter, it will usually pit on probing. In some trauma cases, tissue may be lost after formation and is not regarded as a true hypoplasia. Examples of hypoplastic defects following trauma are shown in Figure 9.20.

Management

- Localized hypoplastic defects may be restored with composite resin. Pitting defects may need initial localized debris or stain removal with either rotary instruments or amine peroxide bleaching systems.
- Maintain posterior support, and preformed metal crowns may be required to restore grossly hypoplastic molars. These teeth may be exquisitely sensitive to thermal and osmotic stimuli, and treatment is made difficult by an inability to achieve good isolation of teeth that are only partially erupted. Glass ionomers may be used temporarily to restore hypoplastic occlusal defects and prevent caries.
- A realistic assessment of the likely longevity of affected first molars is important from an early age. Consideration should be given to the elective loss of these teeth as part of an occlusal developmental plan for the child. A preassessment accompanied by orthodontic advice not later than 8 years of age is recommended.
- Complex restorative treatment involving onlays, veneers and crowns should generally be delayed until late adolescence, but the selective use of metal, adhesively retained onlays may provide a long-term solution in some molar cases.

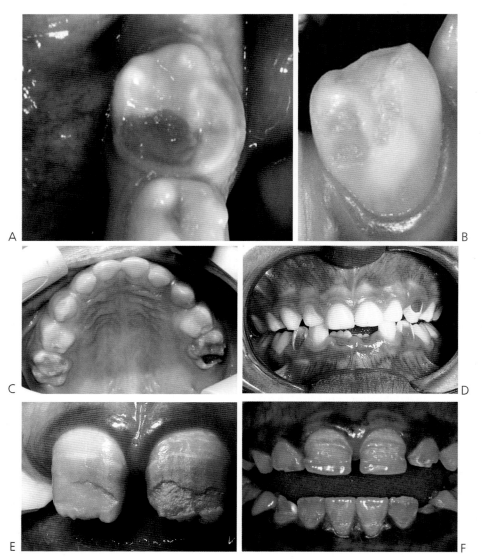

Figure 11.27 (A, B) Enamel hypoplasia associated with preterm delivery, foetal distress and neonatal hypoxia. All second primary molars and canines were affected, but the first primary molars were normal, indicating a chronological event. (C) Chronological hypoplasia may affect the primary dentition; this child suffered foetal distress and meconium aspiration at delivery. It is possible that the tips of the cusps of the first permanent molars are similarly affected. (D) Localized hypoplasia of primary canines. These anomalies present as small pit defects on the labial surface of primary canine teeth and often become carious. A minute area of hypoplasia is visible on the maxillary right canine, and all the other canine teeth are carious, while the remainder of the teeth are caries free. (E) Another form of chronological hypoplasia with hypomineralization of the permanent incisors. Note that there is normal enamel at the cervical region and the primary teeth are unaffected. (F) Chronological enamel hypoplasia after a childhood illness from 11 months up to around 18 months of age. The incisal edges of the maxillary lateral incisors are affected. Fortunately, there is little hypomineralization of the teeth, making the dentition more easily restored with composite resin.

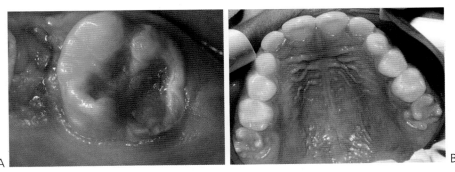

Figure 11.28 Molar incisor hypomineralization. Teeth may be variably affected in the one mouth. (A) Severely affected upper first permanent molar with loss of enamel and hypomineralization. (B) An otherwise intact dentition shows typical molar–incisor hypomineralization. The incisors (palatal surface) are less severely affected than the molars.

Molar–incisor hypomineralization (Figure 11.28)

Molar–incisor hypomineralization (MIH) is a condition that, although recognized as a clinical entity for some time, is still a subject of considerable study. It presents as a qualitative change in enamel that, initially, is of normal thickness, ranging from localized opacity through opacity with discolouration and obvious poor quality to posteruptive enamel breakdown. The cervical enamel appears to be normal in most affected first permanent molars. One or more first permanent molars may be affected in a quasi-chronological but inconsistent manner, together with (usually lesser) effects on one or more incisors. The presentation is puzzling because as few as one molar or as many as all four may be affected. Often affected teeth are extremely sensitive, and this can be an indicator of poor ability to gain complete anaesthesia of the affected teeth. Use of either low-viscosity glass isonomer cement sealants soon after eruption or remineralizing agents such as CPP-ACP toothpastes can help decrease sensitivity and reduce posteruptive breakdown.

Many possible aetiological factors, especially those related to childhood disease and maternal illness during the third trimester, have been suggested. Research is under way in many international centres to define the aetiological factors, because knowledge of these would permit early preventive and restorative interventions. The prevalence ranges widely; however, it is between 10% and 15% in many communities worldwide, with around 5% of the population being severely affected. It is believed that MIH may account for a large proportion of the restorative needs of children in many communities and therefore is an important public health issue.

A familial tendency to the condition has been recognized by some authors. Irrespective of the exact aetiology of MIH, it is important to recognize that this condition represents a chronological disturbance in tooth formation between birth and 24 months of age. Enamel hypomineralization can affect any teeth in the permanent dentition; however, there is a very low prevalence compared with the first molars.

Enamel hypomineralization also affects second primary molars, with a prevalence of approximately 6%. The atypical location of caries can alert the dentist to the true nature of the defect, even when carious destruction of coronal tissue has removed clinical signs of defective enamel. Caries on the distal aspects of second primary molars and caries in these teeth when the rest of the primary dentition is disease-free are both important signs. It is important to tell the parents that there is a positive predictive value of similar defects occurring in the permanent molars, and that these must be checked frequently as they are erupting.

MANAGEMENT

- The ideal restorative approach for these cases has yet to be determined; however, if intracoronal restorations are planned, composite resin should be used. Some research indicates that pretreating the enamel with 5% sodium hypochlorite after etching increases bond strength significantly. Preformed metal crowns are an option for severely affected teeth; however, it needs to be explained to the child and parents that this is an intermediate phase of treatment, and further restorative work will be required at maturity. Trimming the length of the preformed metal crown for partly erupted first permanent molars so as to obtain a fit just apical to the maximum convexity of the crown makes such placement easier in many cases.
- There is a clear association between repeated, well-meaning attempts by practitioners to place 'minimal', adhesive or other treatments for these molars, without adequate local anaesthesia, and a real antipathy to dental treatment on the part of the affected children. Local analgesia should be used for the treatment of these cases, but it should be noted that even under these conditions pain control will not always be adequate, and treatment may be compromised. General anaesthesia is often required to provide high-quality dental care for these children.

Amelogenesis imperfecta

The term 'amelogenesis imperfecta' is usually applied to inherited defects of the enamel of both primary and permanent teeth (Figures 11.29–11.32). Although the definition implies a family history, for practical purposes it seems reasonable to extend this to include sporadic cases and also

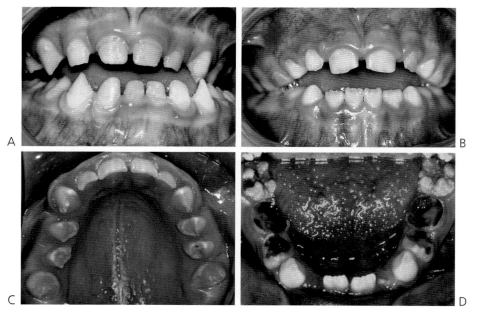

Figure 11.29 Different forms of predominately hypoplastic amelogenesis imperfect (AI). (A) Autosomal recessive with a rough hypoplastic phenotype. (B) Autosomal dominant with smooth hypoplasia with a marked anterior open bite. Note the open contact points in these two cases. (C) Hypoplastic AI teeth are yellow-brown with spacing between the teeth. (D) Rough or grossly pitted forms may be susceptible to caries as they are extremely difficult to keep clean.

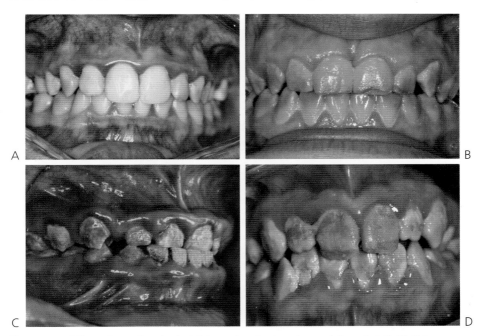

Figure 11.30 Different forms of predominately hypomineralized amelogenesis imperfect. (A–D) All these cases are characterized by varying degrees of hypomineralization. The enamel is so soft that it can be removed with an excavator. Note the discolouration and gross build-up of calculus on all tooth surfaces.

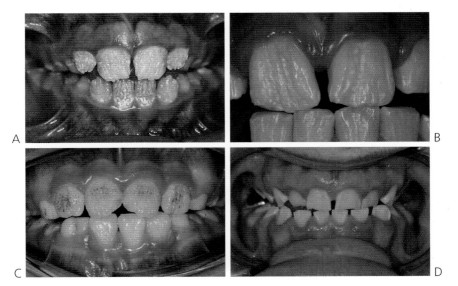

Figure 11.31 Different forms of amelogenesis imperfect (AI) with X-linked inheritance. (A, B) Typical appearance of vertical hypoplastic grooves in females. These represent enamel derived from different clones of ameloblasts that have undergone lyonization (X chromosome inactivation). (C) Pitting hypoplastic AI represents another clinical variety of X-linked AI. (D) X-linked AI in a male. All the enamel is affected uniformly.

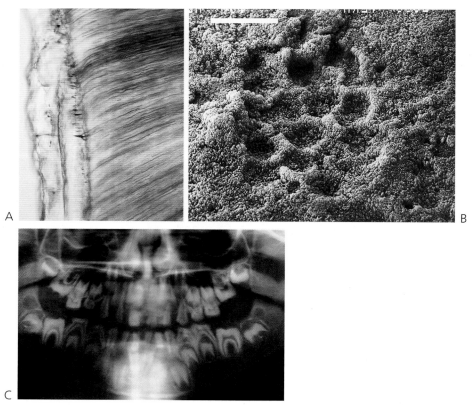

Figure 11.32 (A) Hard tissue section of autosomal dominant amelogenesis imperfecta showing extremely thin enamel in this particular patient. (B) Scanning electron micrograph of a similar patient with abnormal etching pattern of enamel. (C) Panoramic radiograph showing absent or very thin enamel in this form of amelogenesis imperfecta.

to those cases where the enamel defects are associated with extraoral features, as found in some syndromes (i.e., focal dermal hypoplasia or the trichodento-osseous syndrome).

CLINICAL HINT: QUESTIONS CONCERNING SEVERELY HYPOMINERALIZED FIRST PERMANENT MOLARS

Always consider the long-term implications of your treatment.
- Is it preferable to extract the first molar at 8 to 9 years of age and allow the second molar to migrate mesially?
- What impact will the treatment plan have on the future behaviour of the child?
- Many of these teeth are extremely sensitive; will local anaesthesia be effective?
- Once a preformed metal crown has been placed, what are the treatment options at age 20 years? A clear record of the state of the underlying tooth at crown placement is essential for the later restorative dentist.
- Does it matter if a third molar is not present; does this affect your decision?
- Is it preferable to leave a child free of disease, but also free of any restoration that will require multiple replacements throughout life?

FREQUENCY EXAMPLES

- Estimated 1 : 14 000 in the United States.
- Up to 1 : 800 in northern Sweden.

Few studies of prevalence have been carried out, and there may be marked differences according to the population studied.

DIAGNOSIS

- Based on a combination of the mode of inheritance and clinical and radiographic appearances.

AMELOGENESIS IMPERFECTA VARIANTS WITH MENDELIAN INHERITANCE

- X-linked (Xp22.3–p22.1) (OMIM 301200): The AMELX gene on the short arm of the X chromosome which codes for amelogenin, the major enamel matrix protein, has been shown to be mutated in several families with X-linked amelogenesis imperfecta.
- X-linked (Xq22–q28) (OMIM 301201): Another locus for X-linked amelogenesis imperfecta has been identified on the long arm of the X chromosome.
- Autosomal dominant (OMIM 104500): A number of genes in the 4q11–q21 region appear to be implicated in causing autosomal dominant amelogenesis imperfecta in some families. Mutations in the enamelin gene, which maps to the same region, have been identified. Families with autosomal dominant amelogenesis imperfecta with taurodontism (ADAIT) as part of the trichodentoosseous (TDO) syndrome have mutations in the DLX3 gene; one family with ADAIT without other features of TDO syndrome has also been found to have a mutation in the same gene, whereas in other ADAIT families, mutations in the DLX3 gene have been excluded. With time, it is expected that this area will be better understood, as it is probable that as yet unknown genes are involved in the disorder in some families.
- Autosomal recessive (OMIM 204650): Mutations in the matrix metalloproteinase-20 (MMP-20) or kallikrein-4 (KLK-4) gene appear to cause autosomal recessive amelogenesis imperfecta.
- Sporadic cases.

PHENOTYPES

Phenotypes range from markedly hypoplastic (thin) enamel (Figure 11.29) (either uniformly with spacing between adjacent teeth or irregularly giving rise to pits or grooves) to varying degrees of hypomineralization (poorly formed enamel) with altered colour and translucency (Figure 11.30). In many cases, both hypoplasia and hypomineralization are seen together. The colour of the teeth is presumed to reflect the degree of hypomineralization of the enamel; the darker the colour, the more severe the degree of hypomineralization.

In X-linked amelogenesis imperfecta (Figure 11.31), females exhibit vertical bands of altered enamel (manifesting lyonization; see Lyon hypothesis, earlier in the chapter). There may be vertical grooves (because of hypoplasia) and/or vertical bands of enamel of altered colour or lucency (because of hypomineralization) or a combination of the two. In such families, there will be no male-to-male transmission, whereas the heterozygous females may pass on the trait to children of either sex.

In some patients affected by amelogenesis imperfecta, one or more teeth fail to erupt, presumably because of a more severe disturbance of the enamel organ, and may undergo resorption of their crowns. In some cases (up to 50%), a skeletal anterior open bite or lateral open bite is seen.

CLASSIFICATION OF AMELOGENESIS IMPERFECTA

There has been great controversy and confusion created with different nomenclature and classifications. Indeed, up to 14 different forms of the condition are described in some texts. It should be noted that all of these different manifestations are based on the clinical and radiographic appearance. It is essential that diagnosis and classification be based on the mode of inheritance and phenotype. Understanding the mode of inheritance is essential for genetic counselling. However, setting aside questions of inheritance for our present purposes, from a clinical treatment planning perspective, two clinically distinct basic forms are considered here.

PREDOMINANTLY/EXCLUSIVELY HYPOPLASTIC FORMS (Figure 11.29)

- Thin enamel.
- Lack of contact points between teeth.
- Enamel may be rough, smooth or randomly pitted.
- Heterozygous females with X-linked amelogenesis imperfecta manifest lyonization (see p. 347) with vertical banding of normal and abnormal enamel.
- Teeth may be delayed in eruption.
- Unerupted teeth may undergo resorption.
- Anterior or lateral open bite associated with about 50% of cases.
- Radiographically, it may be difficult to distinguish enamel from dentine if the former is extremely thin.

PREDOMINANTLY/EXCLUSIVELY HYPOMINERALIZED FORMS (Figure 11.30)

- May be normal thickness of enamel, at least initially.
- Yellow to brown in colour.
- Enamel may be softer than normal, tends to chip and can be penetrated with an explorer. In severely hypomineralized cases, the enamel may be scraped away with a scaler.
- Teeth may erupt with enamel of normal thickness, but it can be quickly lost, exposing highly sensitive dentine.
- Large masses of supragingival calculus may be present.
- Radiographically, it can be difficult to distinguish between enamel and dentine because of a decreased degree of mineralization of enamel.
- Unerupted teeth may undergo resorption; radiographic review is needed to monitor this.

Management (Figures 11.33 and 11.34)

- Appropriate diagnosis, taking into account the mode of inheritance and phenotype.
- Continued commitment to and support of both children and families. These are disfiguring, painful conditions, and children may be badly teased by their peers.
- Preservation of molar teeth with full coverage restorations to maintain vertical dimension.
- Early orthodontic assessment.
- Composite resin veneers over anterior teeth for aesthetics. It is possible to bond composite resin successfully to hypoplastic and hypomineralized enamel. Adequate margins may be difficult to achieve because of the poor quality of the enamel.
- Preformed paediatric zirconia crowns offer new treatment options.
- Preformed metal crowns or gold onlays on molars or laboratory-made composite resin crowns may be useful.
- Care is required when trial-fitting crowns, because defective enamel can be easily scraped or flaked off the tooth in some cases.

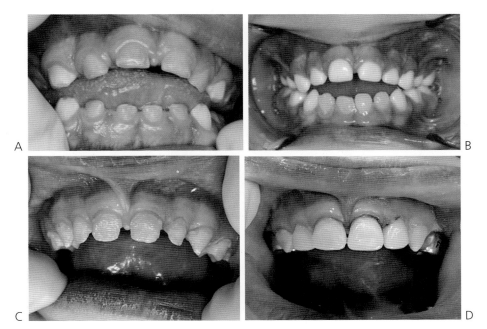

Figure 11.33 Two different restorative options for amelogenesis imperfecta (AI). (A, B) Full mouth rehabilitation with zirconia paediatric crowns. Placement is facilitated by the spacing between the teeth in this hypoplastic form. (Courtesy A/Prof. James Lucas, AM, Melbourne). (C, D) Restoration of a hypoplastic AI case with composite resin strip crowns on the anterior teeth and stainless steel crowns on molars.

- Ideally, delay definitive treatment with porcelain and precious metals until late adolescence. However, some middle-aged patients have commented that, had they known that their dentition was going to 'fail' at that stage, they would have preferred their practitioner to have been less 'conservative' in their teenage years and to have provided more conventional restorative care. Two points arise:
  - Modern composite resins have improved greatly, and 'adolescent' treatment now is hopefully more aesthetic and longer lasting than previously.

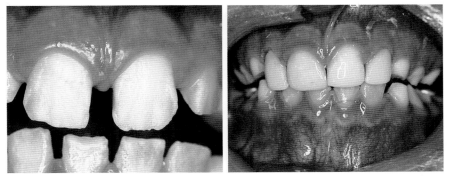

Figure 11.34 Different management options for amelogenesis imperfect in the permanent dentition. Composite bonding in a case with rough hypoplasia of the enamel. Etching times should be slightly longer than usual; however, the roughness of the enamel surface aids in mechanical retention.

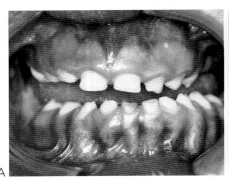
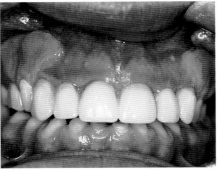

A   B

Figure 11.35 A patient with autosomal recessive dystrophic epidermolysis bullosa and amelogenesis imperfecta. The posterior teeth failed to erupt and underwent spontaneous replacement resorption within the alveolus. Because of the small crown length and the prominent alveolus, an overdenture without a labial flange was constructed.

- There is evidence of a clear association between these conditions and lack of self-esteem. It is as important here as anywhere in dentistry to treat the whole patient, and not only the teeth.
- Overdentures may be an option in children with small, hypoplastic teeth (Figure 11.35).
- Orthodontic, prosthodontic and possible orthognathic/periodontal surgery to correct anterior open bite in hypoplastic forms (Figures 11.36 and 11.37).

Genetic counselling for enamel disorders

Although many causative genes have now been identified in the amelogenesis imperfectas, there is significant clinical variability and overlap within and between types. Genetic testing may be

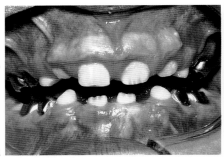
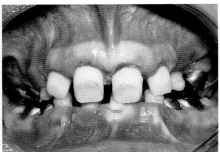

A   B

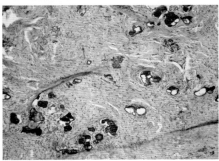

C

Figure 11.36 (A, B) A case of autosomal dominant amelogenesis imperfecta with failure of eruption of the anterior teeth. Many of the posterior teeth were unerupted and undergoing resorption. Initial surgical exposure of the anterior segments did not aid their complete eruption. The gingivae contained small islands of calcification, which may be a significant factor in the failure of eruption (C). Periodontal surgery with apically repositioned flaps was used to fully expose the crowns.

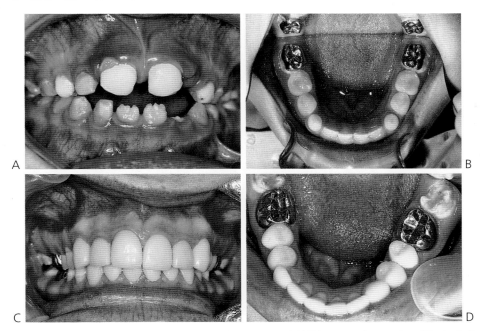

Figure 11.37 (A) Not all cases using composite resin are successful. With progressive eruption of the teeth, it is difficult for the patient to keep the gingival margins clean and the restoration may therefore fail. (B) Cast gold onlays are useful to protect the occlusal surfaces. No preparation of the crown was performed. (C, D) Onlays, veneers and composite crowns were cemented with composite luting cement.

possible, but it is difficult to predict how useful this information would be to an affected individual or family. Counselling may be helpful in some circumstances, provided it is given by someone with the appropriate training.

CLINICAL HINTS: BONDING TO ABNORMAL ENAMEL

- Acid-etch composite resin seems to bond more successfully to hypoplastic enamel than to hypomineralized enamel.
- In severely affected dentitions, it is preferable to place preformed metal crowns on primary molar teeth very early (e.g., at around 3–4 years of age) to preserve the vertical dimension and allow maximal eruption of the first permanent molar.
- Cast metal (precious or base-metal) onlays on suitable permanent posterior teeth have the best long-term clinical success.
- Regular radiographic examination is required to detect early caries.

Disorders of dentine

DENTINOGENESIS IMPERFECTA (OMIM 125490) (Figure 11.38)

Dentinogenesis imperfecta is an inherited disorder of dentine, which may or may not be associated with osteogenesis imperfecta. The term 'hereditary opalescent dentine' is sometimes used for the isolated condition. Both osteogenesis imperfecta and dentinogenesis imperfecta are transmitted as autosomal dominant traits and are clinically indistinguishable dentally, although they have a different genetic basis. Osteogenesis imperfecta is caused by mutations in the type I collagen

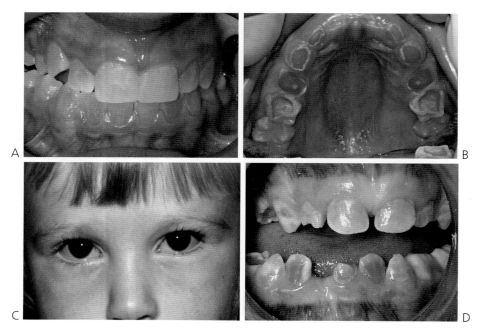

Figure 11.38 Manifestations of dentinogenesis imperfecta. (A) Dentinogenesis imperfecta. Dark discoloura-tion of the crowns which appear normal in size and shape. (B) Severe attrition in the primary dentition in a case of dentinogenesis imperfecta. (C) Blue sclera associated with osteogenesis imperfecta. (D) Primary dentition in a child with osteogenesis imperfecta.

genes (e.g., *COL1A1*, *COL1A2*) and dentinogenesis imperfecta to mutations in the dentine sialo-phosphoprotein I gene (*DSPP*). Some individuals and families with osteogenesis imperfecta may have clinical evidence of dentinogenesis imperfecta, but in other families there may be variable expression of the trait. Within these families, some individuals may have abnormal dentine, while others are clinically unaffected as far as the teeth are concerned. However, because of the same collagen defect, all such children with osteogenesis imperfecta may have abnormal dentine, albeit at a subclinical level. The possibility of osteogenesis imperfecta should be considered in children presenting with dentinogenesis imperfecta and investigated by measurement of bone density if necessary. The presence of blue sclera or a history of bone fractures should alert the clinician to osteogenesis imperfecta.

Dental manifestations

- Amber, grey to purple-bluish discolouration or opalescence (Figure 11.38).
- Pulpal obliteration (Figure 11.39).
- Relatively bulbous crowns.
- Short, narrow roots.
- Enamel may be lost after tooth eruption, exposing the soft dentine, which rapidly wears. This is probably because of inherent weakness in the dentine rather than because of an enamel defect or abnormality at the dentinoenamel junction.
- Mantle dentine appears normal.
- Circumpulpal dentine is poorly formed with abnormal direction of tubules. Small soft tissue inclusions represent remnants of pulpal tissue.

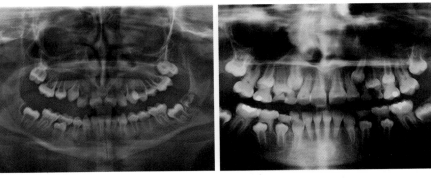

A   B

Figure 11.39   (A) Radiographic manifestations of dentinogenesis imperfecta showing short, bulbous crowns with wide-open root canals. (B) With further development, these teeth undergo pulpal canal obliteration; however, periapical pathology is fortunately rare.

Management

- Preservation of the vertical dimension of the occlusion.
- Continued commitment to and support of both children and families, providing adequate aesthetics and function through childhood and adolescence.
- Protection of posterior teeth from attrition using full coverage restorations.
- Provision of aesthetic appeal.
- Preformed metal crowns for posterior teeth.
- Initially composite resin to build up anterior teeth, possibly followed later by porcelain crowns. (These teeth will remain or even become increasingly brittle throughout life. Conventional crowns requiring tooth preparation may never be the treatment of choice, but see earlier, under 'Amelogenesis imperfecta'.)
- Overdentures or even full dentures may be required in severe cases.

We have followed cases over many years into adulthood. The initial optimism over retaining these teeth for a lifetime has been tempered by the eventual failure of complex restorative work and the loss of teeth in early adulthood. Clinicians must be sensitive to the implications of long-term failure and the aesthetic, functional and indeed financial legacy with which the patient is left.

OSTEOGENESIS IMPERFECTA (OMIM 166200)

Most cases of autosomal dominant osteogenesis imperfecta are caused by mutations in the genes that encode Type 1 collagen (COL1A1 and COL2A2), with some rare dominant or recessive forms being caused by other recently identified novel genes.

The essential features are:
- Bone fragility.
- Blue sclera (Figure 11.38C).
- Progressive hearing loss.
- Dentine changes (Figure 11.39).

DENTINAL DYSPLASIA: RADICULAR DENTINE DYSPLASIA (SHIELDS TYPE I DD) (OMIM 125400)

- Also described as 'short root anomaly', this appears to be a distinct entity from dentinogenesis imperfecta. Both dentitions can be equally affected. The teeth may be lost early because of periapical infection or spontaneous exfoliation caused by the short roots.

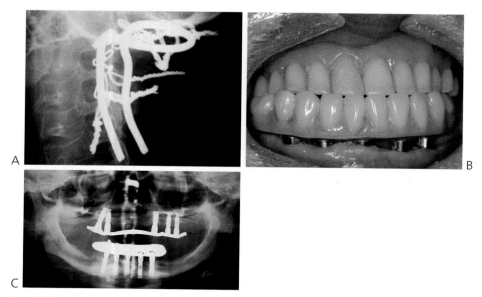

Figure 11.40 (A) The 'Ransford Loop' used to stabilize the vertebral column in a child with type IV osteogenesis imperfecta and basilar compression. This life-saving procedure is performed by an anterior approach through the pharynx, splitting the palate and sectioning the odontoid process of C2. The vertebral column is then wired to the occipital bone. This child initially presented with trigeminal neuralgia caused by pressure from C2 on the pons. (B) In spite of the bone pathology, osseointegrated implants can be successfully placed in patients with osteogenesis imperfecta. The same patient was rehabilitated with implant-supported dentures following his surgery. (C) The panoramic radiograph shows the survival of the implants at 9-year follow-up.

- Autosomal dominant transmission.
- Teeth with very short or absent roots but clinically normal crowns (Figure 11.41).
- Total or partial obliteration of radicular pulp before eruption but with demilune of coronal pulp shown on the radiographs of molar teeth.
- Mantle and coronal dentine are histologically normal.

Management

- In spite of excellent preventive care, these affected teeth are commonly lost because of loss of enamel, pulp necrosis or periodontal disease.

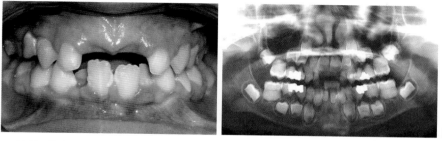

Figure 11.41 Radicular dentinal dysplasia. (A) The general appearance of the teeth is relatively normal. (B) Although radiographically it appears that there is complete absence of the pulp chamber, a small horizontal band of pulp is evident at the beginning of root formation that is quite abnormal in appearance. (Courtesy Prof. M.-C. Maniere, Strasbourg, France.)

- Prophylactic preformed metal crowns.
- Endodontic therapy may be successful if there is minimal pulpal obliteration.
- Long-term prognosis for the dentition is poor.

DENTINAL DYSPLASIA: CORONAL DENTINAL DYSPLASIA (SHIELDS TYPE II DD) (OMIM 125420)

- The consensus now is that this is a variant of dentinogenesis imperfecta rather than a distinct entity. The primary teeth have a typical amber discolouration and undergo tooth wear associated with loss of the enamel and appearance of 'shell teeth' radiographically.
- Normal crown and root form.
- Varying degrees of pulp canal obliteration.
- Altered pulp morphology resembling a 'thistle-shaped' pulp chamber.
- Intrapulpal calcifications (pulp stones).

Management

Similar to the management of dentinogenesis imperfecta, however, some authors suggest that no treatment is required, as there are few sequelae. If there is enamel loss in the primary dentition, then full coverage restorations should be placed (preformed metal crowns). If the permanent dentition is clinically normal, then no special care may be needed.

DIFFERENT CLASSIFICATION OF DENTINE ANOMALIES

Many texts describe up to four different forms of dentinogenesis imperfecta. All these dentine anomalies are autosomal dominant in inheritance. Dentinogenesis imperfecta has been mapped to 4q13–21. Linkage studies of families with coronal dentine dysplasia (Shields type II DD) have shown that the candidate mutation occurs in a region on 4q that overlaps the most likely location of the dentinogenesis imperfecta locus. Further, a similar locus has been determined to that of dentinogenesis imperfecta Shields type III (Brandywine isolate – OMIM 125500). These results suggest that dentinogenesis imperfecta (Shields type II) Shields type III and DD type II (coronal dentinal dysplasia) are allelic or the result of mutations in tightly linked genes. Subsequent studies have identified that the mutated gene in all of these phenotypes is the *DSPP* gene. Radicular dentinal dysplasia may be a separate entity.

X-LINKED HYPOPHOSPHATAEMIC RICKETS (OMIM 307800) (Figure 11.42)

- Also termed X-linked vitamin D-resistant rickets, it is caused by a defect in the *PHEX* gene located at Xp22.
- X-linked disorder with rachitic changes in long bones associated with a failure of distal tubular reabsorption of phosphate in the kidneys. The rickets is unresponsive to vitamin D and traditionally treated with daily oral phosphate supplements.
- Short stature.
- Bowing of the legs.
- Scaphocephaly: an elongated skull as a result of premature fusion of the sagittal suture.
- Males severely affected; females may show milder features (typically short stature with bowing of legs), often not affecting the teeth.
- Low serum phosphate.
- Elevated alkaline phosphatase.

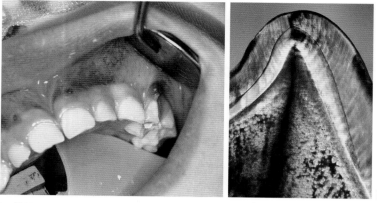

Figure 11.42   (A) X-linked vitamin D–resistant rickets presenting with multiple abscessed teeth in the absence of caries. (B) Under polarized light, the hard tissue section demonstrates globular dentine and a pulp horn that extends to the dentinoenamel junction, resulting in early exposure caused by attrition and, subsequently, pulpal necrosis.

Dental manifestations

- Multiple spontaneous abscesses in the absence of dental caries or trauma.
- Elongated pulp horns, which often extend up to the dentinoenamel junction, can be exposed with minimal attrition of the overlying enamel. An abscess can develop many months after silent pulp death.
- Large pulp chambers and delayed apical root closure.
- Enamel occasionally has hypomineralization or hypoplastic defects.
- Possibly reduced radiodensity of dentine on radiographs.
- Patients may have repeated orthopaedic procedures and indwelling mechanics to promote bone straightening or lengthening. The avoidance of sepsis is essential. Treatment planning should include collaboration with orthopaedic colleagues and may demand the regrettable removal of infected teeth at times of particular infection risk.
- Novel therapies to treat the skeletal defect in X-linked hypophosphatemia may not correct the dental defects. Bone is a metabolic tissue which is constantly remodelled, whereas the mineralized tissues of the dentition have no metabolic maintenance once formed.

PREERUPTIVE INTRACORONAL RESORPTIVE DEFECTS (Figure 11.43)

These defects are dentine lesions found on unerupted teeth, usually detected on routine dental radiographs. They have often erroneously been referred to as 'preeruptive caries' or 'dentine cysts'. They are often located adjacent to the dentine–enamel junction in the occlusal aspect of the crown. There is evidence that these defects develop as a result of coronal resorption. On opening into the lesion, it is often empty or filled with an amorphous tissue comprising small particles of tubular dentine and crystalline material. Resorptive cells such as osteoclasts and macrophages may be found. When the tooth erupts, the lesion is likely to be rapidly colonized by oral flora, and the lesion becomes similar to a carious lesion.

Management

The cavity should be restored conservatively. It has been proposed that these lesions may be responsible for many of the lesions that are clinically undetected in molar teeth that progress to rapid carious breakdown and, ultimately, loss of the tooth.

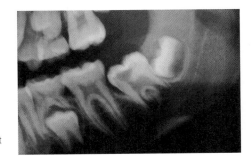

Figure 11.43 Preeruptive intracoronal resorptive defect in an unerupted mandibular second molar.

Dental effects of prematurity and low birth weight

Normal birth weight for gestational age	>2500 g
Low birth weight	>1500–2500 g
Very low birth weight	<1500 g
Extremely low birth weight	<1000 g

PROBLEMS IN EXTREME PREMATURITY

- Hyaline membrane disease and respiratory insufficiency.
- Hyperbilirubinaemia (Figure 11.46D).
- Necrotizing enterocolitis.
- Cerebral intraventricular haemorrhage.
- Oxygen retinopathy.

The limiting factor in survival is based on lung development, and infants weighing less than 400 g at birth or those born before 24 weeks rarely survive. Hyaline membrane disease is now treated with synthetic surfactant, although very young babies often develop pneumothoraces caused by the prematurity and fragility of the alveoli. Cerebral intraventricular bleeding and necrotizing enterocolitis with the resulting sepsis are common causes of mortality and morbidity.

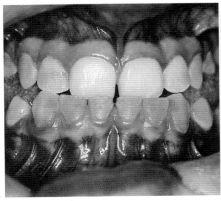
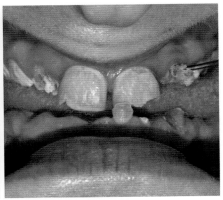

A   B

Figure 11.44 (A) It appears initially that the permanent dentition may not be as severely affected as the primary dentition in osteogenesis imperfecta. In this child, the severe skeletal Class III malocclusion and the posterior open bite required a surgical solution. (B) Clinical photograph of the same case at 30 years of age shows the destruction of the dentition over time resulting in the eventual loss of all of her teeth.

Surviving children may be left with problems of growth retardation, delayed cognitive development and a range of other abnormalities.

DENTAL IMPLICATIONS

- Hypoglycaemia.
- Hypocalcaemia with reactive pseudohyperparathyroidism.
- Hyperbilirubinaemia, causing intrinsic staining of the teeth.
- Intubation trauma, causing enamel hypoplasia/hypocalcification. The maxillary central incisors are most often affected (Figure 11.46E). If the baby is intubated orally, palatal grooving may occur. Tooth eruption may be delayed, although it is often normal for the 'corrected' age after adjustment for prematurity.
- Chronological opacities or hypoplasia.

Disorders of tooth eruption

Eruption of teeth is not always correlated with somatic development. Children with growth disturbances may exhibit delayed eruption or the delay may be resulting from other causes such as gingival overgrowth owing to medication such as phenytoin. More importantly, premature exfoliation of teeth is invariably associated with severe systemic disease (see Chapter 10) and requires investigation (Figures 10.28, 11.45).

Delayed eruption of the primary dentition requires no treatment other than determining that all teeth are present. It is uncommon for children to require surgical exposure of the teeth in infancy. Parents should be reassured that there is considerable variability in the eruption of teeth (plus or minus 6 months for primary teeth, plus or minus 1 year for permanent teeth). In the permanent dentition, delayed eruption beyond this range should be investigated for the presence of supernumeraries and other pathology. Although the actual timing of tooth eruption is variable, evidence of progress in tooth crown and root development and the eruption sequence are of much more relevance. In contrast, the failure of eruption of a contralateral tooth more than 6 months after the appearance of its partner requires investigation.

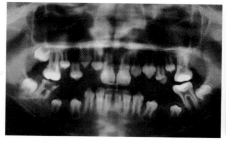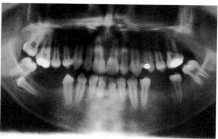

A   B

Figure 11.45   Teeth require guidance for normal eruption. (A) In this case, several primary teeth and the mandibular right first permanent molar were removed because of gross caries and pulpal necrosis. (B) While the second molar has drifted slightly mesially, the second premolar has rotated and drifted distally and impacted against the second molar. Had the second primary molar not been removed, it is unlikely that this premolar would have drifted.

NATAL AND NEONATAL TEETH (Figure 11.46)

A natal tooth is present at birth, whereas a neonatal tooth is one that erupts within 30 days of birth. In almost all cases, this is simply the early eruption of a normal primary incisor tooth. The development of this tooth is consistent with the expected stage of development of a primary

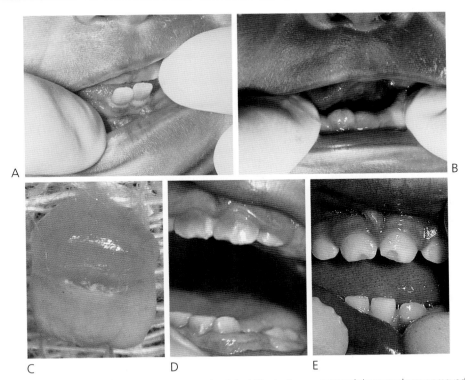

Figure 11.46 (A) Natal teeth in a 36-week premature infant. The teeth were extremely loose and were removed. (B) A newborn infant with two mandibular incisors soon to erupt. The reduced enamel epithelium has fused with the gingivae, and teeth will probably erupt within a few days. (C) A neonatal tooth from a 27-week premature infant. Note the extent of the crown formation is consistent with the chronological age. If a natal tooth is extracted without removing the dental papilla, then a root may develop from the odontoblasts and Hertwig epithelial root sheath. (D, E) Dental effects of prematurity: hyperbilirubinaemia staining of the enamel (D) and hypoplastic defects on the incisal edges of the central incisors caused by laryngoscopy (E).

incisor at birth (i.e., only five-sixths of the crown is formed without any root being present). This lack of root development accounts for the mobility of the tooth. Babies with posterior natal teeth should be carefully investigated for other systemic conditions that may be associated with syndromes or other diseases.

Management

- The most important point to consider is whether the nursing mother can adequately establish breast-feeding. If either the nipples or the ventral surface of the infant's tongue is being traumatized, the tooth should be removed.
- If the tooth is not excessively mobile, it should be retained, as it can become firm with time as the root continues to develop.
- If the tooth is excessively mobile, then it may spontaneously exfoliate; however, because of the theoretical risk of aspiration or ingestion, it should be electively removed.
- If tooth removal is indicated, care should be taken to extract the entire tooth, as the crown only may be removed leaving behind the pulpal tissue. If this is the case, the dentine and a root will form subsequently; the root will then require removal at a later date.
- The permanent teeth should be unaffected by extraction of the primary tooth.

CLINICAL HINT: EXTRACTING NATAL AND NEONATAL TEETH

- Always protect the airway when removing these teeth by placing a gauze in the back of the mouth. The teeth are easily dislodged or dropped. A pair of haemostats or similar will provide a firm grip on the tooth to be removed.
- Check the medical history for significant jaundice, which may predispose to postoperative bleeding.

INFRAOCCLUDED (SUBMERGED) PRIMARY MOLARS (Figure 11.47)

It is quite common for primary molars to become infraoccluded; however, it is controversial as to whether all teeth are truly ankylosed. The mechanism by which this occurs is unknown, but it has been suggested that a cessation of normal primary root resorption may stimulate healing and then ankylosis as the bone remodels. Some teeth never appear in the mouth, and this infraocclusion may result from a failure or partial failure of teeth eruption, particularly secondary primary molars. If ankylosis occurs posteruption, the tooth will appear to submerge into the alveolus (in fact, the tooth remains stationary while the alveolar bone grows around it and adjacent teeth erupt). The timing of the removal of an ankylosed tooth is based on the position of the first permanent molar and the extent of the resorption of the primary tooth.

Management

- If there is radiographic evidence of resorption of the roots, then removal should be delayed, as the vast majority of these teeth will exfoliate normally, because the tooth is probably not ankylosed.
- Orthodontic consultation.
- If the premolar is congenitally absent, early removal of the submerging primary molar might be indicated.
- Surgical removal of the ankylosed tooth is to be avoided before eruption of the first permanent molar as this latter tooth will migrate mesially and space loss is likely to occur together

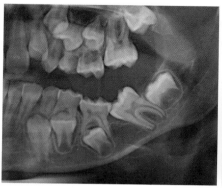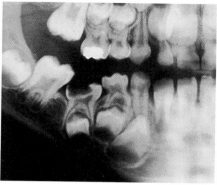

A   B

Figure 11.47 Failure of eruption of the mandibular left second primary molar. It is questionable whether these teeth are truly ankylosed. It is important to wait until the first permanent molar has erupted before surgical removal to avoid impaction of the second premolar. (A) In this case, the 36 tooth was also impacted underneath the 75 tooth. (B) Some unerupted primary molars also become carious, as they are difficult to clean. Infraoccluded teeth are difficult to remove, especially if there is space loss and they should therefore be sectioned and elevated to minimize excessive bone loss. In some cases, surgical removal may be needed.

with impaction of the second premolar. Once the permanent tooth has erupted, the primary tooth may be removed and a space maintainer inserted.

■ Retain space and use orthodontic treatment to align the permanent molar as required.

CLINICAL HINTS: SUBMERGED TEETH

- Submerged primary molars are difficult to remove intact surgically, and there may be significant comorbidity associated with surgery.
- Where space has been lost because of migration or tipping of the first permanent molar, consider orthodontic uprighting in the first instance. Space can be maintained to await normal root resorption or facilitate more conservative surgical removal later.

ECTOPIC ERUPTION OF PERMANENT CANINES

The incidence of impacted canines in the maxilla is 2%, and the majority lie in a palatal position. The anomaly can be associated with small or absent lateral incisors. In about 12% of cases with impacted canines, the lateral incisor root will undergo some resorption.

The normal age of eruption is 11 ± 2 years and the crown should certainly be palpable in the labial sulcus at 9 to 10 years of age. If the canine is not palpable, further investigation is indicated to check for impaction or ectopic eruption. Intraoral radiographs taken at right angles to each other and the technique of parallax can be used to localize their position or, alternatively, a panoramic radiograph. CBCTs are the best for localizing ectopic or impacted permanent canines because these provide a 3D position of the tooth.

Interceptive extraction of the deciduous canines can improve the position of the permanent teeth, and the maximum improvement will be seen within 12 months (Ericson & Kurol, 1988). The success of this approach is reduced, however, if the arch is already crowded (Power & Short, 1993).

ECTOPIC ERUPTION OF FIRST PERMANENT MOLARS (Figure 11.48)

This can be an indication of an inadequate arch length, and a radiographic survey is required to confirm the presence of premolar teeth. The permanent teeth may resorb the distal margins of the second primary molars; this is more common in the maxilla.

Management

■ Where there is impaction of the permanent molar against the distal of the second primary molar, slicing or discing of the distal surface of the primary molar will allow the spontaneous eruption of the permanent molar.

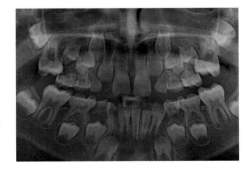

Figure 11.48 Bilateral ectopic eruption of the first permanent molars, causing resorption of the second primary molars. In these positions, it is unlikely that the first permanent molars will erupt, and space loss has already occurred. The primary molars were extracted, and a space-regaining appliance constructed.

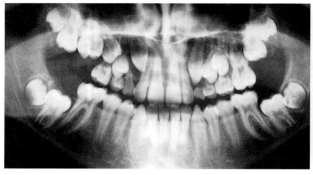
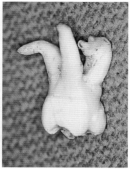

A   B

Figure 11.49 (A, B) Failure of eruption of the first permanent molars is not uncommon. Surgical exposure of the crown may be sufficient to allow these teeth to erupt. Note that root development will continue in spite of a failure of tooth eruption, and deviation of the roots will occur when the roots reach the cortical bone, in this case the antral floor. This root deviation may not be evident on radiographs, especially in the maxilla, and extraction of these teeth may prove extremely difficult.

- Placement of orthodontic separators or brass ligature wire is usually difficult and uncomfortable and has mixed success.
- Where the resorption of the primary molar is advanced, the loss of this tooth is indicated, and space-regaining mechanics should be considered once the permanent molar has erupted (see Fig. 11.48).
- Parents should be warned that further orthodontic treatment is usually required because of arch length deficiencies.
- PFE is a rare condition that is characterized by nonsyndromic eruption failure of permanent teeth in the absence of mechanical obstruction. It typically affects the first molars and/or second molars. The molars do not erupt and also do not respond to orthodontic traction; rather, efforts to pull them leads to ankylosis. This condition can be familial.

FAILURE OF ERUPTION OF FIRST PERMANENT MOLARS (Figure 11.49)

Failure of eruption of a first permanent molar is an uncommon finding; however, no one has yet been able to explain the mechanism as to why these teeth do not erupt. During surgical intervention it is invariably noted that these teeth are not ankylosed. Because of this, eruption could be encouraged by surgical exposure and bonding an orthodontic device for traction – however, the treatment is lengthy and unpredictable.

PRIMARY FAILURE OF ERUPTION IN MULTIPLE QUADRANTS

In some nonsyndromic patients, PFE in the absence of mechanical obstruction can be seen in multiple quadrants. This is known to be associated with mutations in parathyroid hormone receptor 1 (*PTHR1*) and can be inherited as an autosomal dominant trait. Some rare skeletal dysplasias are also associated with *PTHR1* mutations, but the dental condition appears to be unrelated.

ROOT DEVELOPMENT (Figure 11.50)

Just as enamel can be affected by systemic illness, so too can root development be delayed, altered or arrested by systemic disease. This is most commonly seen when radiotherapy causes shortening and tapering of the roots of premolars (see Chapter 10). Excessive orthodontic forces may also cause root resorption.

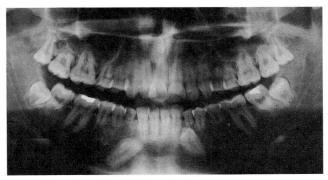

Figure 11.50 Arrested root development in a child who developed Stevens–Johnson syndrome at 10 years of age. Root development ceased at that time (probably as a result of the treatment as much as the disorder itself), and all teeth except the third molars were affected. It is interesting that these molars, which were not undergoing calcification, were unaffected.

DENTAL AGE (MATURITY) DETERMINATION

The paediatric dentist can be asked to help in age assessment, for example, when migrant children have lost their parents. It is important to take into consideration ethnicity and variation in somatic growth potential.

Tooth eruption may not be as important as tooth crown calcification and root development. The most widely used and accepted method is that developed by Demirjian (1978), based on the panoramic radiographic appearance of tooth calcification at different ages.

Although there remains little doubt that peak height velocity, skeletal development and sexual maturation are associated, dental development seems to be independent of general somatic development.

Even a specialist in paediatric dentistry should be cautious about offering an accurate dental age assessment, and these queries should be referred to a specialist in the subject, such as a forensic odontologist.

Loss of tooth structure

- Attrition:
    - From wear of one or more teeth in one arch against one or more teeth in the opposing arch.
- Erosion:
    - Exogenous from diet, habits or environment.
    - Gastro-oesophageal reflux.
    - Bulimia.
- Abrasion.
- Exogenous tooth substance loss from diet, habits or environment.

ENAMEL EROSION

The prevalence of erosion in children and adolescents has been reported recently as very high, with over half of 14-year-olds in a UK population having moderate erosion, with an increased prevalence seen in lower socio-economic groups. The aetiology of erosion in children and adolescents is varied, and it has been suggested that the increased consumption of fruit juices and carbonated drinks is the most important factor, with the sale of soft drinks increasing by 56% over the past decade.

The erosive potential of acidic drinks is related to:

- Titratable acidity.
- pKa.
- Type of acid.
- Calcium chelation ability.
- Method and temperature of consumption.

Carbonated soft drinks contain carbonic acid, and often organic acids (commonly citric acid) are added to improve taste and 'mouth feel'. Citrate ions strongly chelate calcium in both acidic and basic environments, decreasing the amount of free ionic calcium available in both saliva and at the enamel surface and thereby enhancing demineralization. The erosive potential of 'diet' soft drinks is similar to that of sugared drinks; however, their potential to increase caries risk is decreased markedly. The method of drinking can also affect the extent of erosion, with the decrease in intraoral pH becoming greater as the beverage is held in the mouth or is drunk by 'long sipping'; when the beverage is gulped, intraoral pH does not decrease significantly.

The long-term and short-term consequences of dental erosion are marked, with the need for extensive and costly dental care and potential loss of teeth. The concomitant dental sensitivity can be severe and debilitating. It has been shown that even a few intakes of acidic drinks on a regular basis may be associated with considerable dental erosion. It is important to question the child and parent(s) carefully as to the total family usage of such drinks (fruit squashes, fresh fruit juices, particularly citrus juices, carbonated drinks and colas) in the first instance. The taking of study models and the institution of an exclusion diet for 3 months may show a diagnostic 'tide mark' of unattacked tooth substance at a later review.

PREVENTION OF EROSION

- Cessation or restriction of exposure to the aetiological factor.
- Modification of beverage erosivity seems to have the greatest future potential for reducing tooth structure loss. Recent research has concentrated on the addition of calcium and/or phosphate and pH alteration of soft drinks.
- Families are bombarded with advice on healthy eating. They may find advice to limit intake of fruit juices confusing, and careful explanation is required.

GASTRO-OESOPHAGEAL REFLUX (Figure 11.51A)

When loss of enamel by erosion cannot be explained by dietary factors, reflux must be considered. Children with reflux will show enamel erosion, which is a smooth loss of tooth structure, characteristically with any restorations standing proud. Some children have undiagnosed, asymptomatic reflux that presents first with enamel erosion.

Diagnosis

- Barium swallows may not demonstrate reflux.
- 24-h pH manometry is required to assess the extent of reflux.

Management

- Diagnosis and treatment of reflux condition before definitive restoration of the teeth.
- Histamine blockers (H_2 antagonists) such as ranitidine and cimetidine.
- Antiemetics (prokinetic agents) such as metoclopramide.

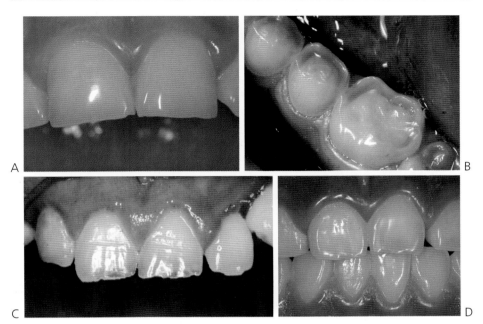

Figure 11.51 (A) Enamel erosion with asymptomatic gastro-oesophageal reflux. The first presentation of this child to a dentist was because of the erosion. Note the smooth, almost glassy appearance of the incisors. (B) Severe erosion in a 12-year-old boy showing the outline of enamel with exposed dentine. (C) Erosion can be seen in the chipping and translucency of the incisal edges. (D) Tooth substance loss from sucking on lemons.

- Composite resin, preformed metal crowns, glass ionomer cement coverings or onlays over the posterior teeth.
- Onlays on posterior teeth to protect occlusion and maintain vertical height.
- Professional application of fluorides. Nocturnal mouthguards with fluoride toothpaste as mechanical barriers against acid attack and fluoride to promote remineralization.

Further reading

Hypodontia

Fleming, P., Nelson, J., Gorlin, R.J., 1990. Single maxillary central incisor in association with mid-line anomalies. British Dental Journal 168, 476–479.

Freire-Maia, N., Pinheiro, M. (Eds.), 1984. Ectodermal dysplasias: a clinical and genetic study. Alan R Liss, New York.

Hall, R.K., 1983. Congenitally missing teeth – diagnostic feature in many syndromes of the head and neck. Journal of the International Association of Dentistry for Children 14, 69–75.

Hall, R.K., Bankier, A., Aldred, M.J., et al., 1997. Solitary median maxillary central incisor, short stature, choanal atresia/midnasal stenosis (SMMCI) syndrome. Oral Surgery, Oral Medicine, Oral Pathology, Oral Radiology, and Endodontics 84, 651–662.

Klineberg, I., Cameron, A., Hobkirk, J., et al., 2013. Rehabilitation of children with ectodermal dysplasia. Part 2: an international consensus meeting. International Journal of Oral & Maxillofacial Implants 28, 1101–1119.

Klineberg, I., Cameron, A., Whittle, T., et al., 2013. Rehabilitation of children with ectodermal dysplasia. Part 1: an international consensus meeting. International Journal of Oral & Maxillofacial Implants 28, 1090–1100.

van den Boogaard, M.J., Créton, M., Bronkhorst, Y., et al., 2012. Mutations in WNT10A are present in more than half of isolated hypodontia cases. 2012. Journal of Medical Genetics 49, 327–331.

Supernumerary teeth and other disorders

Hogstrom, A., Andersson, L., 1987. Complications related to surgical removal of anterior supernumerary teeth in children. Journal of Dentistry for Children 54, 341–343.

Jensen, B.L., Kreiborg, S., 1990. Development of the dentition in cleidocranial dysplasia. Journal of Oral Medicine and Pathology 19, 89–93.

Kreiborg, S., Jensen, B.L., 2018. Tooth formation and eruption – lessons learnt from cleidocranial dysplasia. European Journal of Oral Sciences 26 (Suppl 1), 72–80.

Omer, R.S.M., Anthonappa, R.P., King, N.M., 2010. Determination of the optimum time for surgical removal of unerupted anterior supernumerary teeth. Pediatric Dentistry 32, 14–20.

Papadaki, M.E., Lietman, S.A., Levine, M.A., et al., 2012. Cherubism: best clinical practice. Orphanet Journal of Rare Diseases 7 (Suppl. 1), S6.

Von Arx, T., 1992. Anterior maxillary supernumerary teeth. A clinical and radiographic study. Australian Dental Journal 37, 189–195.

Morphological anomalies

Nazif, M.M., Laughlin, D.F., 1990. Dens invaginatus in a geminated central incisor: case report. Journal of Pediatric Dentistry 12, 250–251.

Rakes, G.M., Aiello, A.S., Kuster, C.G., 1998. Complications occurring resultant to dens invaginatus: a case report. Pediatric Dentistry 10, 53–56.

Tsai, S.J.J., King, N.M., 1998. A catalogue of anomalies and traits of the permanent dentition of southern Chinese. Journal of Clinical Pediatric Dentistry 22, 185–194.

Regional odontodysplasia

Aldred, M.J., Crawford, P.J.M., 1989. Regional odontodysplasia: a bibliography. Oral Pathology and Medicine 18, 251–263.

Enamel hypomineralization

Cullen, C., 1990. Erythroblastosis fetalis produced by Kell immunization: dental findings. Journal of Pediatric Dentistry 12, 393–396.

Fleming, P., Witkop, C.J., Kuhlmann, W.H., 1987. Staining and hypoplasia caused by tetracycline. Journal of Pediatric Dentistry 9, 245–246.

Enamel hypoplasia

Aoba, T. , Fejerskov, O., 2002. Dental fluorosis: chemistry and biology.

Croll, T.P., 1990. Enamel microabrasion for removal of superficial dysmineralization and decalcification defects. Journal of the American Dental Association 129, 411–415.

Eli, H., Sarnat, H., Talmi, E., 1989. Effect of the birth process on the neonatal line in primary tooth enamel. Journal of Pediatric Dentistry 11, 220–223.

Pendrys, D.G., 1989. Dental fluorosis in perspective. Journal of the American Dental Association 122, 63–66.

Molar–incisor hypomineralization (MIH)

Beentjes, V.E., Weerheijm, K.L., Groen, H.J., 2002. Factors involved in the aetiology of molar–incisor hypomineralisation (MIH). European Journal of Paediatric Dentistry 3, 9–13.

Fayle, S.A., 2003. Molar–incisor hypomineralisation: restorative management. European Journal of Paediatric Dentistry 4, 121–126.

Silva, M.J., Scurrah, K.J., Craig, J.M., et al., 2016. Etiology of molar incisor hypomineralization – a systematic review. Community Dentistry and Oral Epidemiology 44, 342–353.

Weerheijm, K.L., 2003. Molar–incisor hypomineralisation (MIH). European Journal of Paediatric Dentistry 4, 114–120.

Weerheijm, K.L., Duggal, M., Mejare, I., et al., 2003. Judgement criteria for molar–incisor hypomineralisation (MIH) in epidemiologic studies: a summary of the European meeting on MIH held in Athens 2003. European Journal of Paediatric Dentistry 4, 110–113.

Amelogenesis imperfecta

Bäckman, B., Ammeroth, G., 1989. Microradiographic study of amelogenesis imperfecta. Scandinavian Journal of Dental Research 97, 316–329.

Crawford, P.J., Aldred, M., Bloch-Zupan, A., 2007. Amelogenesis imperfecta. Orphanet Journal of Rare Diseases 2, 17.

Dentine anomalies

Cole, D.E.C., Cohen, M.M., 1991. Osteogenesis imperfecta: an update. Journal of Pediatrics 115, 73–74.

Gage, J.P., Symons, A.L., Roumaniuk, K., et al., 1991. Hereditary opalescent dentine: variation in expression. Journal of Dentistry for Children 58, 134–139.

O'Carroll, M.K., Duncan, W.K., Perkins, T.M., 1991. Dentin dysplasia: review of the literature and a proposed sub-classification based on radiographic findings. Oral Surgery, Oral Medicine, and Oral Pathology 72, 119–125.

Seow, W.K., Brown, J.P., Tudehope, D.A., et al., 1984. Dental defects in the deciduous dentition of premature infants with low birth weight and neonatal rickets. Pediatric Dentistry 6, 88–92.

Seow, W.K., Latham, S.C., 1991. The spectrum of dental manifestations in vitamin D-resistant rickets: implication for management. Pediatric Dentistry 8, 245–250

Eruption disorders

Friend, G.W., Mincer, H.M., Carruth, K.R., et al., 1991. Natal primary molar: case report. Journal of Pediatric Dentistry 13, 173–175.

Masatomi, Y., Abe, K., Ooshima, T., 1991. Unusual multiple natal teeth: case report. Journal of Pediatric Dentistry 13, 170–172.

Sauk, J.J., 1988. Genetic disorders involving tooth eruption anomalies. In: Davidovitch, Z. (Ed.), The biological mechanisms of tooth eruption and root resorption. Birmingham, EBSCO Media, pp. 171–179.

Erosion

Jarvinen, V., Muerman, J.H., Hyvarinen, H., et al., 1988. Dental erosion and upper gastrointestinal disorders. Oral Surgery, Oral Medicine, and Oral Pathology 65, 298–303.

Taji, S., Seow, W.K., 2010. A literature review of dental erosion in children. Australian Dental Journal 55, 358–567.

General

Demirjian, A., 1978. Dental development: index of physiologic maturation. Medicine and Hygiene 36, 3154–3159.

Dure-Molla, M.de L., Fornier, B.P., Manzanares, M.C., et al., 2019. Elements of morphology: Standard terminology for the teeth and classifying genetic dental disorders. American Journal of Medical Genetics 179(10), 1913–1981.

Hall, R.K., 1994. Pediatric orofacial medicine and pathology. Chapman and Hall Medical, London.

World Wide Web Database

Online Mendelian Inheritance in Man, OMIM (TM), 2000. McKusick-Nathans Institute for Genetic Medicine, Johns Hopkins University (Baltimore, MD) and National Center for Biotechnology Information, National Library of Medicine (Bethesda, MD). Online. Available: http://www.ncbi.nlm.nih.gov/omim/.

CHAPTER 12

Management of medically compromised paediatric patients

Marcio A. da Fonseca ■ Evelina Kratunova

Introduction

Children and adolescents with disabilities and complex health problems are surviving longer because of advances in medical technologies and drug therapies, which may cause undesirable effects in the oral cavity and affect the delivery of dental care. In addition to that, oral and dental infections can compromise the patient's systemic health and delay medical treatment. The patient's caretakers may not make oral and dental care a priority owing to a lack of understanding of their importance or because they have many competing demands. Education of both the patient and the family as well as our medical colleagues about the importance of oral health is essential for the successful outcome of medical therapies and the child's quality of life. The dental professional must become acquainted with the patient's medical history and the therapies to deliver dental care in a safe manner.

This chapter discusses common paediatric medical conditions that require consideration in the provision of optimal dental treatment.

Congenital heart disease

Congenital heart disease (CHD) encompasses structural abnormalities of the heart or intrathoracic great vessels that occur in utero because of genetics, teratogens or maternal factors. It affects 9 : 1000 live births, or approximately 1% of births every year. CHD is the most common birth anomaly and the leading cause of death in children with congenital malformations. CHD that is suspected on a foetal ultrasound can be usually diagnosed by echocardiography at 18 to 22 weeks of gestation.

CHD can be divided in acyanotic and cyanotic ('critical CHD') lesions, which can be further classified into right heart obstructive lesions, left heart obstructive lesions and mixing lesions. Cyanotic defects comprise 25% of all CHD. Heart failure in children leads to poor growth, feeding difficulties, respiratory distress, exercise intolerance and fatigue.

Some children with CHD may present neurodevelopmental problems, such as adverse effects on language, memory, behaviour, fine and gross motor skills and social interactions, as well as psychological maladjustments because of low self-esteem.

ACYANOTIC CARDIAC DEFECTS (Figure 12.1)

These lesions involve shunting of blood from left to right, leading to increased pulmonary blood flow. The most common are:

- Atrial septal defect (ASD): an abnormal opening between the atria.
- Ventricular septal defect (VSD): an abnormal opening between the ventricles. It is the most common congenital cardiac lesion (30%).
- Patent ductus arteriosus (PDA): connection between the left pulmonary artery and the descending aorta.

Acyanotic cardiac anomalies

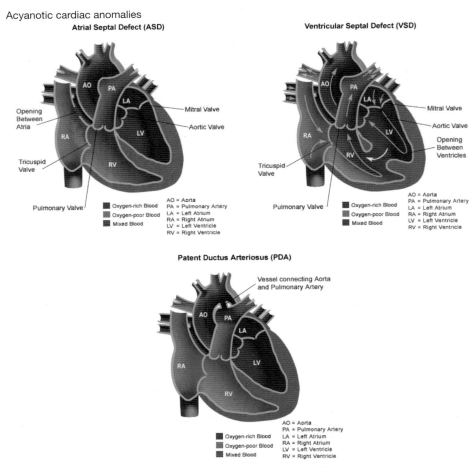

Figure 12.1 Structure of acyanotic anomalies of the heart.

CYANOTIC CARDIAC DEFECTS (Figures 12.2 and 12.3)

Right heart obstructive lesions

These defects cause significantly reduced blood flow through the lungs, thus the body does not get enough oxygenation:

- Tricuspid atresia: failure of development of the tricuspid valve, which controls blood flow from the right atrium to right ventricle.
- Pulmonary atresia: the pulmonary valve, which controls blood flow from the right ventricle to the pulmonary artery, does not form correctly.
- Tetralogy of Fallot: a combination of VSD, pulmonary stenosis, right ventricular hypertrophy and transposition of the aorta.
- Transposition of the great arteries: the aorta arises entirely from the right ventricle and the pulmonary artery from the left ventricle.

Cyanotic cardiac anomalies

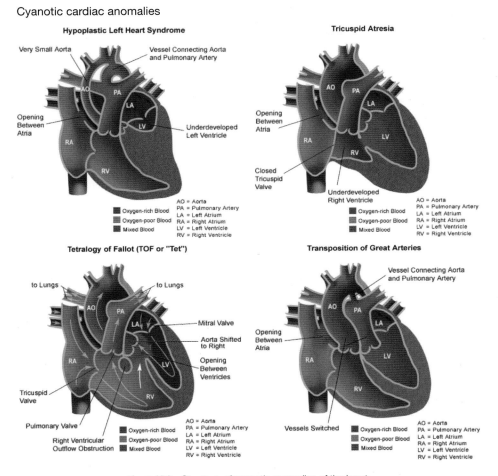

Figure 12.2   Structure of cyanotic anomalies of the heart.

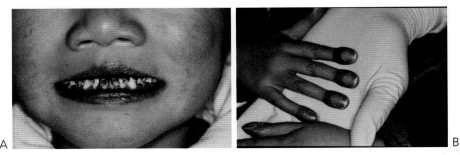

Figure 12.3   (A) Cyanosis of facial tissues and lips, as well as poor dentition in a 5 year-old boy with unrepaired Tetralogy of Fallot. (B) Clubbing of the fingers and cyanosis of the nail beds in the same patient. (Courtesy Prof. Marcio da Fonseca.)

Left heart obstructive lesions

These lesions prevent the proper amount of blood from traveling through the body.

- Coarctation of the aorta: narrowing of the aorta where the ductus arteriosus enters the aorta.
- Aortic stenosis: the aortic valve narrows, reducing or blocking blood flow from the left ventricle into the aorta.
- Pulmonary stenosis: caused by narrowing of the pulmonary valve, but may also involve the pulmonary arteries.

Complex defects

- Total anomalous pulmonary venous return: all pulmonary veins do not connect normally to the left atrium, but instead drain to the right atrium through an abnormal (anomalous) connection.
- Truncus arteriosus: an arterial trunk gives off the aortic arches and develops into the aorta and the pulmonary arteries.
- Hypoplastic left heart syndrome: the left side of the heart does not form correctly.

Oral and dental considerations

- Oral infections in childhood, such as caries and periodontal bleeding, appear to be associated with subclinical carotid atherosclerosis in adulthood. In addition to that, oral infections may be a risk factor for infective endocarditis (IE). Thus, excellent oral hygiene, aggressive caries prevention and elimination of all potential sources of odontogenic infection are essential for children with CHD.
- Children with certain cardiac conditions have limited cardiopulmonary reserve and may decompensate rapidly (Table 12.1). These conditions pose a challenge for the use of general anaesthesia (GA), conscious sedation and passive immobilization for uncooperative children in the dental practice. In such situations, the patient's cardiologist (and the anaesthesiologist in case of GA) must be consulted before the dental procedure.
- To gain weight, some children with CHD are prescribed highly caloric foods and drinks, which can lead to high caries risk, while others may need a nasogastric or gastrostomy tube, which may lead to increased calculus formation.
- The use of sonic or ultrasonic devices (e.g., scalers) or electrosurgery appliances in dental practice may interfere with implanted devices, such as pacemakers and ventricular assist devices. The cardiologist must be consulted before their use to determine whether the cardiac devices must be turned off.
- Adrenaline used with local anaesthesia is unlikely to create serious cardiovascular compromise because of its low volume, but the cardiologist must be consulted in cases of critical CHD and hypertrophic cardiomyopathy.

TABLE 12.1 ■ **Cardiac conditions at high risk for decompensation or sudden death during strenuous activity**

Coarctation of the aorta (depending on severity)	Congestive heart failure
Coronary insufficiency	Exercise-induced arrhythmias
Hypertrophic cardiomyopathy	Long QT syndrome
Marfan syndrome and aortic dilation	Pulmonary hypertension
Severe aortic stenosis	Severe untreated systemic hypertension
Severe ventricular outflow obstruction	Untreated cyanotic heart disease

- There is no contraindication for the use of nitrous oxide in patients with CHD.
- Some children with CHD may present neurodevelopmental problems, which, together with increased family stress and overprotection of the child, may create behaviour management concerns for the dental professional.
- Patients on anticoagulant agents (aspirin, warfarin) must have their international normalized ratio (INR) checked a few days before any oral or periodontal surgical procedure. Dental surgery can be safely performed, including mandibular block injections, even with an INR higher than 3.5 (ideal between 2 and 3).
- Anticoagulant therapy should not be interrupted before dental surgery; the risk of thromboembolism is more dangerous than prolonged bleeding caused by the dental procedure.
- Certain calcium channel blockers can cause gingival overgrowth.
- Patients with severe CHD may not tolerate prolonged periods lying in the supine position.
- Nonsteroidal antiinflammatory drugs (NSAIDs) should not be prescribed because they can exacerbate symptoms of heart failure and increase risk of bleeding. Paracetamol is the drug of choice.
- For information regarding prophylaxis against IE (see Appendix F).

Haematology

DISORDERS OF HAEMOSTASIS

Haemostasis is a complex process comprised of clot formation, followed by clot lysis and tissue remodelling. It depends on three main stages:

- Primary haemostasis: initiated at the site of a blood vessel injury and includes vascular response (vasoconstriction) and platelet aggregation.
- Secondary haemostasis: related to the assembly of the coagulation cascade and clot propagation.
  The tissue factor at the wound site is exposed and interacts with factor VIIa (extrinsic pathway), which leads to the generation of activated factor X. The activated factor X then activates prothrombin to thrombin in a reaction that requires factor V. The thrombin converts fibrinogen to fibrin. The components of the intrinsic pathway (factors VIII, IX, XI) amplify the same process.
- Tertiary haemostasis: fibrinolysis and breaking down of the clot.
  The termination of clotting phase involves antithrombin, tissue factor pathway inhibitor and the protein C pathway to regulate the extent of clot formation. Clot removal restores vessel patency – plasminogen binds fibrin and tissue plasminogen activator, resulting in active proteolytic plasmin that cleaves fibrin, fibrinogen and a variety of plasma proteins and clotting factors.

Main screening tests

Three tests are recommended for initial screening of bleeding disorders:

- Partial thromboplastin time (PTT): assesses the intrinsic coagulation system (factors VIII, IX, XI and XII) and common pathways (factors V and X, prothrombin and fibrinogen). This is the best single screening test for coagulation disorders.
- Activated PTT (APTT): a contact activator is added. APTT is prolonged in cases of mild to severe deficiency of factors VIII or IX.
- Prothrombin time (PT): measures the extrinsic (factor VII) and the common pathway.

Other investigations:

- INR is a method that standardizes PT assays and is used to assess the level of anticoagulation in patients on anticoagulant drugs.

- Platelet count: normal count is 150 000–450 000/10^9/L. However, this is ineffective in identifying disorders of platelet function, and if suspected, platelet function tests should be ordered.
- Thrombin time.
- Bleeding time is unreliable and no longer used as a screening test.
- Platelet function analyzer (PFA-100) measures platelet-dependent coagulation, but it is not sensitive enough to detect underlying mild bleeding issues.
- Patients with positive screening test results must be evaluated further and referred to a haematologist.

VASCULAR DISORDERS

Structural vascular abnormalities

Hereditary haemorrhagic telangiectasia. This is an autosomal dominant disorder associated with telangiectasias and arteriovenous malformations of the small vessels in the oropharynx, lungs, skin and gastrointestinal (GI) tract. Manifestations include epistaxis, telangiectasias on the lips and fingertips, GI bleeding and iron deficiency anaemia. Typical onset is in childhood, and most patients will show haemorrhagic symptoms by age 16 years.

Treatment: laser, surgery, oestrogen, oestrogen plus progesterone, thalidomide.

Acquired connective tissue disorders. Scurvy: vitamin C deficiency (<0.2 mg/dL or <11 μmol/L) causes impaired collagen synthesis and disturbances in vascular connective tissue leading to haemorrhagic symptoms.

Inherited disorders of connective tissue

Ehlers–Danlos syndrome. Ehlers–Danlos syndrome (EDS) represents a group of 13 syndromes manifesting deficiencies of vascular and perivascular collagen that can lead to blood vessel ruptures, manifested with easy bruising and haemorrhage. Classical EDS presents with joint hypermobility and hyperextensibility of the skin, which may lead to bruising (usually a mild bleeding tendency). Diagnosis is based on the genetic abnormality/abnormal type V collagen.

- Vascular type IV EDS (defects in COL3A1 gene) is associated with very extensive bruising and vascular ruptures can be fatal. Skin may be thin and wrinkled, but joint hyperextensibility is rare.

Osteogenesis imperfecta (see also Chapter 11). A connective tissue disorder that primarily affects bone; however, due to capillary fragility, bleeding tendencies may be present.

PLATELET DISORDERS

Thrombocytopenia

Thrombocytopenia is defined by a platelet count of less than 150 × 10^9/L. Thrombocytopenia can be acquired (immune or nonimmune cause) or congenital (very rare).

Clinical signs and symptoms associated with decreased platelet counts include:
- Spontaneous bleeding usually only develops with a platelet count less than 20 × 10^9/L.
- <15 × 10^9/L: Petechiae appear on the skin.
- <5 × 10^9/L: Oral petechiae, submucosal and mucosal bleeding.

Pathophysiological mechanism:
- Increased platelet destruction, including sequestration and pooling of platelets.

■ Decreased production of platelets due to bone marrow infiltration, suppression or failure or a defect in megakaryocyte development and differentiation.

Clinical manifestations:

■ Cutaneous bleeding: petechiae, nonpalpable purpura, ecchymoses.

■ Mucosal bleeding: epistaxis, gingival bleeding, bullous haemorrhage, menorrhagia.

■ Intracranial haemorrhage: rare and the most common cause of death in these patients.

Diagnosis relies on a detailed history, physical examination, laboratory testing (complete blood count, platelet count, peripheral blood smear) and determination of underlying aetiology.

Management depends on the aetiology and presence of an underlying disease.

Thrombocytosis

Thrombocytosis is an increased number of platelets $(450 \times 10^9/L)$ and may be associated with prolonged bleeding because of abnormal platelet function.

The aetiology includes reactive or autonomous processes:

■ Reactive thrombocytosis (secondary thrombocytosis): caused by pathophysiologic mechanisms that are extrinsic to the megakaryocyte. This is typically associated with anaemia, infection, noninfectious inflammation (i.e., reactions to medications, malignancy, trauma, rheumatologic conditions) and postsplenectomy.

■ Autonomous thrombocytosis results of cell-intrinsic mechanisms (within the megakaryocyte or its precursor cells) as seen in haematologic malignancies and familial thrombocytosis.

Diagnosis is based on history, physical examination and laboratory testing (repeat complete blood count, differential count, blood smear, serum ferritin). Management is dependent on the underlying cause.

Platelet function disorders

Inherited platelet function disorders

■ Glanzmann thrombasthaenia. This is an autosomal recessive disorder caused by qualitative or quantitative defects of the fibrinogen receptor (glycoprotein IIb/IIIa) that has an essential role in the adhesion and aggregation of platelets. The platelet count and morphology are normal; however, the platelets do not bind fibrinogen and aggregation does not occur. Management requires platelet transfusion, desmopressin (1-deamino-8-D-arginine vasopressin [DDAVP]) and/or activated coagulation factor concentrate (factor VIIa) before surgical treatment.

■ Bernard–Soulier syndrome. An autosomal recessive disorder in which the platelets are large and defective and unable to interact with von Willebrand factor (vWF). The genetic defects result in abnormal adhesive platelet receptor proteins (glycoprotein Ib). Symptoms include easy bruising and mucosal and postoperative bleeding.

Acquired platelet function disorders. These are caused typically by medications such as heparin, quinidine, trimethoprim sulfamethoxazole, aspirin (can irreversibly block thromboxane-induced platelet aggregation), NSAIDs (inhibit cyclooxygenase, but unlike aspirin, the inhibition is reversible), antihistamines, phenothiazines, valproic acid and guaifenesin.

INHERITED COAGULATION DISORDERS

Haemophilia

Haemophilia represents a group of inherited coagulation disorders with similar clinical manifestations caused by defects or deficiency in one of the clotting factors. The most common disorders are haemophilia A and von Willebrand disease (vWD), both manifesting a decrease in factor VIII

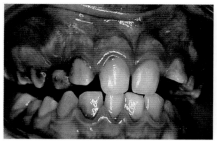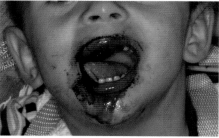

A B

Figure 12.4 (A) Gingival haemorrhage around an exfoliating maxillary right primary canine in a child with haemophilia B. Normally, exfoliation of primary teeth is not of major concern and bleeding is locally controllable. (B) A boy with haemophilia presenting following minor trauma to the labial frenum. Note the poorly formed clot in the mouth and continued oozing after several days.

levels. Factor VIII is produced by endothelial and liver sinusoidal cells. In its inactive form, factor VIII is bound to vW factor (vWF). At a blood vessel injury site, factor VIII separates from vWF and becomes activated. The factor VIII part of the molecule and factor IX are responsible for the activation of factor X in the intrinsic pathway of the coagulation cascade.

- Haemophilia A (X-linked recessive disorder): deficiency of factor VIII. It occurs in approximately 1 : 4000–5000 live male births; 75% of the cases are severe.
- Haemophilia B, also known as Christmas disease (sex-linked recessive disorder): deficiency of factor IX. The incidence is approximately 1 : 15 000–30 000 live male births; 30% to 50% of the cases are severe (Figure 12.4).
- Haemophilia C, also known as Rosenthal syndrome (autosomal recessive disorder): deficiency of factor XI; especially common in Ashkenazi Jews.

Classification of disease severity is based on factor activity level, which typically correlates with bleeding symptoms:

- Severe haemophilia: factor activity level less than 1% (<0.01 international units [IU]/mL).
- Moderate haemophilia: factor activity level between 1% and 5% of normal (0.01–0.05 IU/mL).
- Mild haemophilia: factor activity level between 5% and 40% of normal (0.05–0.40 IU/mL).

Clinical manifestations

- Severe haemophilia:
  - Spontaneous bleeding or bleeding in response to minor trauma.
  - The degree of bleeding is disproportionate to the injury.
  - Symptoms may begin from birth.
  - Delayed bleeding after trauma is common.
  - Bleeding can be substantial or persistent (oozing for days or weeks).
- Mild haemophilia may become apparent only with significant haemostatic challenge (trauma, surgery) and has been reported in about 25% of heterozygote female carriers.

Common bleeding sites include the oral mucosa, soft tissues, joints and brain. Late complications involve neurologic signs from intracranial haemorrhage and joint deformities from repetitive bleeding (haemarthroses).

Diagnosis

- Review of patient's and the family's bleeding history.
- Laboratory testing: screening tests of haemostasis, factor activity levels, and/or genetic testing. Prolonged APTT, normal PT, normal platelet count.

- Diagnostic criteria: confirmation of a factor activity level below 40% of normal (below 0.40 IU/mL) or a haemophilia gene mutation.

Management. Factor replacement therapy with plasma-derived proteins, recombinant proteins and recombinant proteins with modifications to extend half-life. A complication of factor replacement therapy is an immune response with development of alloantibodies (inhibitors), which is estimated to occur in 20% to 30% of cases of haemophilia A and 5% of cases of haemophilia B. The presence of inhibitors (usually immunoglobulin [Ig] G antibodies to factor VIII) requires bypassing agents, such as recombinant factor VIIa, or immune-modulating approaches with continuous factor exposure in conjunction with immunosuppressive drugs.

von Willebrand disease

Characterized by an impairment in the synthesis or the function of the vWF.

The vWF plays an important role in primary haemostasis by:
- Binding to both platelets and endothelial components
- Forming an adhesive bridge between platelets and vascular subendothelial structures
- Acting as a carrier protein for factor VIII

It is the most common inherited bleeding disorder; around 1% incidence in the general population. Clinical manifestations include bruising, mucocutaneous bleeding, heavy menstrual bleeding and postpartum bleeding. vWD is associated with mutations in the genes responsible for the production of vWF and is classified into three types:
- Type 1 (autosomal dominant disease): approximately 75% to 85% of all cases. It is associated with a partial quantitative deficiency of vWF.
- Type 2 (autosomal dominant disease) with four subtypes (2A, 2B, 2M and 2N): characterized by several qualitative abnormalities of vWF.
- Type 3 (autosomal recessive disorder): total deficiency of VWF.

Laboratory testing may show prolonged APTT, normal or slightly reduced platelet count, normal PT and normal thrombin time. Therapy is determined by the type and severity of vWD, level of haemostatic challenge, prior response to treatment and other existing haemostatic abnormalities. DDAVP is a synthetic analogue of vasopressin that promotes the release of vWF from storage pools in endothelial cells; plasma levels of vWF and factor VIII can be increased by three to fivefold for 8 to 12 hours. It is available for intravenous (IV), subcutaneous and intranasal routes of administration, with maximum levels reached in 30 to 60 minutes. Vasodilator side effects include tachycardia, hypotension, flushing and headaches. Patients with type 1 and most patients with type 2A respond to DDAVP.
- For minor bleeding or minor surgery: usually IV or intranasal DDAVP is recommended for patients who have shown a prior response to the medication.
- For major bleeding, major surgery or cases not responding to DDAVP: plasma-derived vWF concentrate or recombinant vWF (only in patients over 18 years of age) are indicated.
- Additional options include antifibrinolytic agents such as tranexamic acid (Cyklokapron), topical haemostatic agents, oestrogen and recombinant factor VIIa.

DENTAL MANAGEMENT

Dental management of children with suspected haemostasis disorders should begin with screening laboratory tests. If tests are abnormal, haematological consultation is required for a definitive diagnosis. Invasive dental procedures should be performed only after the extent of the problem has been determined. Extractions must never be performed without first consulting the haematologist. It is preferable to have platelet levels over 75×10^9/L before extractions. Endodontic procedures may be preferable to extractions to avoid the need for platelet transfusion.

DENTAL PROCEDURES

- Atraumatic technique is essential for all procedures.
- In the event that oral surgery is necessary, a sound surgical technique to minimize trauma and local measures to control bleeding, such as careful atraumatic suturing and socket dressings, are necessary.
- Maxillary infiltration anaesthesia can generally be administered slowly without pretreatment with platelet or factor replacement. However, if the infiltration injection is into loose connective tissue or a highly vascularized area, then factor replacement to achieve 40% activity level is recommended.
- Mandibular block injections should be avoided, as these may be complicated by a dissecting haematoma and airway obstruction. In the absence of suitable factor replacement, intraperiodontal ligament injections may be used.
- Nitrous oxide sedation can be an effective adjunct for restorative procedures.
- Use a rubber dam to protect the soft tissues.
- Endodontic treatment can be safely carried out without factor cover.
- Periodontal treatment with deep scaling and subgingival curettage requires factor replacement.
- Multiple extractions in severe haemophilia cases require hospital admission and haematological work-up.
- Postsurgical administration of antifibrinolytic agents such as tranexamic acid may be helpful in preventing clot lysis.

Characteristically, haemophilia bleeds are delayed by 12 to 24 hours because primary haemostasis is not impaired, and local pressure has little effect. It is worth noting that mild haemophilia may go undiagnosed. APTT is not sensitive to detect mild deficiencies of FVIIIc, and levels of FVIIIc 25 to 30 IU/dL can be associated with a normal APTT. In addition to that, FVIIIc values in mild haemophilia are temporarily increased (as occurs in unaffected persons) by stress, exercise and bleeding. If there is a convincing history of a bleeding tendency, always do a specific factor assay even if the initial screening tests are normal.

CLINICAL HINT

Questions commonly asked by parents are:
- Will my child's teeth erupt normally? Usually yes, but there is often more bleeding from a traumatized operculum that may require active intervention.
- Will my child's teeth fall out normally? Usually yes, unless continually traumatized, there is normally no abnormal bleeding associated with exfoliating primary teeth. However, if there is prolonged mobility and oozing occurs, then extraction may be necessary under appropriate factor cover to reduce the risk of persistent bleeding (Figure 12.4).
- Can a child with a bleeding disorder have orthodontic treatment? Yes, but if extractions are necessary, appropriate consultation with the haematologist is a must.

Red cell disorders

Mature red blood cells (RBCs) are released from the bone marrow into the circulation and typically survive for 100 to 120 days. About 1% of the circulating RBCs are destroyed daily and are replaced by new erythrocytes.

ANAEMIAS

Caused by decreased production of RBCs, increased loss of RBCs, premature destruction (haemolysis) of RBCs or a combination of these mechanisms. Anaemia is diagnosed when the haematocrit or haemoglobin (Hb) is at or below the 25th percentile for age, race and sex. Anaemia is considered to be present if the Hb level falls below 100 g/L. The cause of anaemia in children may be blood loss, iron, folate and vitamin B_{12} deficiency, bone marrow failure, haemolysis of RBCs or anaemia of chronic disorders.

Patient assessment for anaemia should include:

- History of symptoms: onset and severity, evidence of jaundice, blood loss (GI symptoms, menstrual history), medication/toxin exposure, associated chronic disease.
- Family history of anaemias or haemoglobinopathy.
- Signs of pallor, scleral icterus, jaundice, hepatomegaly and splenomegaly.
- Laboratory examination: complete blood count, including RBC indices, reticulocyte count and review of the peripheral blood smear.

Haemolytic anaemia

Results from premature destruction of RBCs. Bone marrow responds with a compensatory increase in RBC production. In severe haemolytic processes, the compensatory production of RBCs may cause an expansion of the medullary spaces, leading to bony deformities (skull and hands).

Haemolytic anaemias are classified as:

- Intrinsic haemolytic anaemias: caused by RBC abnormalities, such as in haemoglobinopathies (sickle cell disease [SCD], thalassemia), erythrocyte membrane defects and enzyme deficiencies (glucose-6-phosphate dehydrogenase, pyruvate kinase).
- Extrinsic haemolytic anaemias: caused by external pathologic processes that immunologically, chemically or physically damage normal RBCs, such as in autoimmune haemolytic anaemia, hypersplenism, systemic disease (including infections, liver and renal diseases), medication, toxins and microangiopathies (haemolytic uremic syndrome, thrombotic thrombocytopenic purpura, disseminated intravascular coagulation).

Aplastic anaemia

This is a rare disorder defined by pancytopenia and hypocellular bone marrow as a consequence of injury to or loss of haematopoietic stem cells. It may be either inherited or acquired:

- Inherited: bone marrow failure syndromes, such as Fanconi anaemia, dyskeratosis congenita, Shwachman–Diamond syndrome, amegakaryocytic thrombocytopenia and reticular dysgenesis.
- Acquired: medications, chemicals, radiation, infection, immune disorders.
  Symptoms and signs related to pancytopenia – bleeding, fatigue, neutropenia.
  Laboratory diagnosis: complete blood count (pancytopenia), confirmed by bone marrow aspiration and biopsy (hypocellularity of all three cell lines).

Treatment:

- Blood transfusions: chronic red cell transfusion therapy can lead to iron overload.
- Immunosuppressive therapy.
- In severe cases, haematopoietic stem cell transplant (HSCT).

HAEMOGLOBINOPATHIES

The Hb molecule is a soluble tetramer that does not polymerize. Normal RBCs contain three types of Hb:

- Hb A (composed of 2 α and 2 β globin chains): comprises 96% to 98% of the total Hb.
- Hb A2 (2 α and 2 δ chains): 1.5% to 3.2% of the total Hb.
- Foetal Hb (2 α and 2 γ chains): 0.5% to 0.8%. Newborns' blood consists of 60% to 80% foetal Hb, which is reduced to 10% to 20% within the first 6 months of life.

SICKLE CELL ANAEMIA

A point mutation in the β globin gene, causing substitution of valine for glutamic acid at the sixth amino acid of the β globin chain that results in the formation of defective (sickle) haemoglobin (HbS), which is poorly soluble when deoxygenated. The lifespan of the sickle RBC is reduced from 120 days to 12 to 17 days. Sickle cell anaemia is the most common genetic disorder of the blood (autosomal recessive).

Sickle cell trait

This is usually a benign carrier condition: one allele of the β globin gene carries the sickle Hb mutation and the other allele is normal (producing Hb AS with one normal β globin chain and one βS globin chain). Typically, HbS levels are below 40%. It is associated with a reduced risk of severe malaria and hospitalization in areas where *Plasmodium falciparum* malaria is endemic. It is also potentially protective against Burkitt lymphoma in Africa. Numerous reports have challenged its benign course because of a high incidence of morbidity and even mortality associated with the trait, including sudden deaths. Potential complications may include haematuria, renal disorders, diabetes, hypertension, stroke, preeclampsia, splenic infarction at high altitude, traumatic hyphaema and renal medullary carcinoma.

Sickle cell disease

SCD includes all cases with one βS globin mutation and a second β globin gene mutation, which can be also a sickle mutation or a different mutation (associated with β thalassemia, HbC disease).

Pathophysiology: Sickling occurs after a period of time necessary for sufficient intracellular polymerization to deform the cell. The polymer is a rope-like fibre that aligns with others, forming a bundle and distorting the RBC into a crescent (sickle) shape that interferes with its deformability. The polymer-containing sickled cells are trapped predominantly in the slow-flowing venular side of the microcirculation, which leads to more cells sticking together, resulting in local hypoxia, vasoconstriction, falling pH and low concentration of protective Hb types. Thus, HbS produces a problem of RBCs 'sticking' rather than 'sickling'.

The clinical picture is one of a chronic inflammatory vascular disease.

- SCD usually manifests in the first 6 months of life when foetal Hb is replaced by HbS.
- Hallmarks of SCD are anaemia and vasculopathy.
- Sickle cell crises can be vaso-occlusive, haemolytic (aplastic) and splenic sequestration, lasting between 5 and 7 days.
- Dactylitis (hand-foot syndrome) is seen in childhood and can lead to fusion and permanently shortened, deformed small bones.
- Growth disturbances are also common.

After 2 years of age, a typical manifestation is excruciating and symmetrical pain in the joints (hips, knees, elbows, shoulders, spine, sternum, pelvis and ribs), lasting from a few minutes to several days. Long-term RBC transfusions lead to iron overload. The chronic manifestations of SCD are multiple, including chronic organ ischaemia and infarction. Osteomyelitis is 200 times greater in SCD than in the normal population. There is an increased susceptibility to invasive bacterial infections under 5 years of age.

Patients present coagulation abnormalities because of increased platelet activation, depletion of anticoagulant proteins and abnormal activation of the fibrinolytic system. The leading cause of death and hospitalization is acute chest syndrome (pulmonary infiltrate obstructing different parts of the lungs).

Treatment:

- HSCT is the only curative therapy and must be performed before multiple organ dysfunction.
- Patients usually take folic acid daily.

- Children up to age 5 years receive daily penicillin V or an alternative antibiotic prophylaxis to prevent pneumococcal infection.
- Symptomatic cases may be treated with hydroxyurea, L-glutamine and iron-chelating agents.
- Vaso-occlusive pain episodes are managed with adequate hydration, pain control medication (including opioids) and nitrous oxide/oxygen therapy in the emergency room.

THALASSAEMIA

Thalassaemia is a group of inherited haemoglobinopathies characterized by reduced formation of α globin or β globin chains caused by mutations. It is the most common haemoglobinopathy, with approximately 5% of the world's population affected. The excessive globin chains precipitate and lead to damage of RBC precursors, deeming the erythropoiesis ineffective, and damaging the circulating RBCs, resulting in haemolytic anaemia.

α-Thalassaemia: caused by deletions or mutations of the four alpha globin genes on chromosome 16. One to four genes may be affected, resulting in a relative overproduction of β-chains. Homozygous α-zero thalassaemia (four alpha globin genes deleted) is incompatible with life, whereas carriers (1–2 gene deletions) have no clinical symptoms. Children with HbH disease (three alpha genes deleted/abnormal) may have mild anaemia or a transfusion dependent anaemia.

β-Thalassaemia: Of more clinical significance is homozygous β-thalassaemia major (Cooley anaemia). Because of the absence of the β-chain, there is a compensatory increased production of HbA_2 and HbF. As erythropoiesis is inadequate, the bone marrow is reactive and there is compensatory intermedullary haemopoiesis in the maxilla and diploe of the skull. There may be severe haemolytic anaemia with marked hepatosplenomegaly and failure to thrive. Those children with sickle/β-thalassaemia show evidence of vascular thrombosis with ischaemia to organs, especially bones.

Signs and symptoms may include:

- Variable degrees of anaemia
- Bone and skeletal changes, which lead to expansion of the medullary cavities
- Hepatosplenomegaly
- Impaired growth
- Iron overload, which can lead to cardiac, pulmonary and endocrine dysfunction
- Thrombosis
- Leg ulcers

Laboratory testing includes a complete blood count and blood smear, iron studies, Hb analysis and/or genetic testing.

Management:

- Allogeneic HSCT is a curative therapy.
- Transfusion therapy is used to reduce symptoms and morbidities.

Prognosis and survival: highly variable, continues to improve with advances in therapy.

ENZYME DEFICIENCIES

Glucose-6-phosphate dehydrogenase deficiency

Glucose-6-phosphate dehydrogenase deficiency (G6PD) is caused by a genetic defect in the RBC enzyme G6PD, which is important for the normal functioning of the RBC as it generates reduced nicotinamide adenine dinucleotide phosphate and protects erythrocytes from oxidative injury. It is the most common inherited RBC enzymatic defect, affecting approximately 400 million people worldwide. It is inherited in a sex-linked pattern, and heterozygous females are typically unaffected carriers.

Manifestations:

- Neonatal jaundice.
- Episodic or chronic Heinz body haemolytic anaemia.
- Increased susceptibility to infection in severe enzymatic deficiency.
- Possible protection against malaria.

Management depends on the severity of the deficiency and the clinical manifestations.

ORAL, DENTAL AND CRANIOFACIAL CONSIDERATIONS

Sickle cell and thalassemia

Review the medical history thoroughly, including the number of crises, transfusion complications (virus contamination, iron overload, etc.), medications, spleen function and hospitalizations.

- Craniofacial bones: There is decreased radiodensity with coarse trabecular pattern and increased marrow spaces due to erythroblastic hyperplasia and medullary hypertrophy that leads to frontal bossing, prominent zygomatic and parietal bones ('chipmunk facies') as well as malocclusion. The radiographic pattern adjacent to tooth roots has a 'stepladder' appearance. Radiographically, there is a widening of the diploic space, vertical trabeculations ('hair on end'), granular appearance and calvarial lesions ('doughnut lesions') in the skull. The inferior border of the mandible is thin, and there is loss of alveolar bone height with pronounced lamina dura and radiopaque lesions. Maxillary protrusion occurs with proclined incisors, possibly a result of cellular hyperplasia and circulatory factors. There is an increased risk of osteomyelitis, osteopenia and osteoporosis.
- Oral mucosa: Pallor, jaundice, glossitis, gingival enlargement and, in SCD, spontaneous facial swellings that may be confused with swelling caused by odontogenic infections.
- Malocclusion.
- Teeth: Delayed eruption, enamel defects, pulp calcifications, pulpal necrosis without dental pathology and interglobular dentin in periapical areas. Patients with SCD may present with facial and dental pain in the absence of odontogenic pathology, which is related to vaso-occlusive crises within the microcirculation of facial bones and dental pulps. Vaso-occlusive episodes near the mental foramen may result in persistent anaesthesia of the lower lip.
- There is a reduced dental caries experience in children with SCD until they stop taking penicillin prophylaxis between 5 and 7 years of age.
- Odontogenic infections, facial cellulitis and pain require a vigorous approach and may warrant hospitalization for IV antibiotics, hydration, pain management and close monitoring of the patient. Antibiotic prophylaxis before invasive dental procedures may be indicated to compensate for splenic dysfunction but should be discussed with the haematologist. All necessary dental interventions must be completed before the beginning of bisphosphonate therapy or HSCT conditioning.
- Elective surgery and dental procedures should be avoided during crises. GA is associated with a significant risk for postoperative complications, especially acute chest syndrome in SCD, and should be subjected to careful planning and interprofessional collaboration. The use of nitrous oxide sedation in dental surgery should be carefully monitored to reduce risk of hypoxia.

Bleeding disorders

- Consultation with the patient's haematologist before any dental intervention is essential.
- Typically, mild forms of platelet functional disorders and thrombocytopenia can be managed efficiently with adequate local measures or antifibrinolytic agents, but severe disorders may require systemic replacement therapy.

- Application of antifibrinolytic agents (ε-aminocaproic and tranexamic acid) can be used to prevent the lysis of clots after surgical interventions in the oral cavity. They inhibit the fibrinolysis by blocking the binding of plasminogen to fibrin and its subsequent activation to plasmin. They are administered orally pre- and postoperatively for a few days until the healing is adequate and may be provided as mouthrinses for patients on anticoagulation therapy.

Children on antithrombotic therapy

Anticoagulants are usually prescribed for children with valvular heart disease and prosthetic valves to reduce the risk of remobilization. If an extraction or surgery is required, it is necessary to decrease the clotting times to facilitate adequate coagulation but not to such an extent as to cause emboli or clotting around the valves. The dental management of these children is also complicated by their congenital cardiac defect and antibiotics may be required for prophylaxis against IE.

Therapeutic drugs used:

- Oral warfarin sodium (Coumadin): This is a vitamin K antagonist that depletes factors II, VII, IX and X. Usually 3–4 days are required for full anticoagulation onset, and its efficacy is assessed by PT level (factor VII levels).
- Heparin sodium (Heparin): Shorter acting and has an immediate onset (inhibits factors IX, X and XII). Can be administered either subcutaneously, using a low-molecular-weight derivative, or intravenously.
- Enoxaparin sodium (Clexane): Low-molecular-weight heparin which inhibits factor Xa and thrombin. Usually administered subcutaneously.

Dental management

- Alterations of the medication regimen are not indicated, as the risk of bleeding is lesser than the risk of thrombosis, and multiple dental extractions can be done even with an INR up to 3.5 (best between 2 and 3).
- Saliva ejectors should be used with care to avoid trauma of the mucosa, especially on the floor of the mouth.
- Soft tissues should be protected during treatment using rubber dam isolation.
- Elective orthodontic extractions should be replaced with alternative treatment strategies.
- Endodontic treatment is preferable to extractions (see Chapter 7).
- Pulpotomy procedures do not present a risk for prolonged bleeding.

Use of local haemostatic measures alone or in conjunction with systemic therapy depends on:

- Scale and the location of surgical intervention.
- Access to surgical site postoperatively (e.g., if postoperative bleeding causes airway obstruction, the intervention indicates systemic measures).

Local anaesthesia:

- For coagulation disorders: inferior alveolar nerve block administration requires systemic therapy because of a potential haematoma development that may present a risk of airway obstruction.
- For patients on anticoagulant medications: evidence shows that an inferior alveolar block is safe.
- Alternative techniques can be used (e.g., long buccal nerve infiltration with *Articaine*).
- Infiltration anaesthesia is usually safe.

Extractions:

- Ensure good wound closure and place sutures where feasible to achieve primary surgical closure.

- Effective removal of granulation tissue, as it can be a source of prolonged bleeding.
- Packing of extraction sockets with absorbable material (e.g., gelatin sponge) can be used to provide a stable scaffold for clot formation, except in cases of an odontogenic abscess, which needs an open wound to drain.
- Adequately placed pressure over time can be very effective; wet gauze is advised (to prevent sticking of the clot to it).
- Soft prefabricated splints can be placed over multiple extraction areas to provide sufficient pressure for haemostasis.
- Electrocautery can reduce intra- and postoperative bleeding; however, a large area of tissue necrosis may delay healing and present a source of delayed bleeding.

Management of postoperative haemorrhage

- Pressure pack application for a long time (30–60 minutes).
- Packing of the socket with a gelatin sponge or oxidized cellulose and pressure pack.
- Additional infiltration of local anaesthesia with vasoconstrictor (use with caution as it can result in delayed haemorrhage).
- Removal of large clots followed by pressure packs.
- Astringents can also be used (commercially available preparations with aluminium chloride are recommended). Postoperative restriction in physical activity, avoidance of hot food and drinks, soft diet, sleeping with raised head.
- Administration of coagulation factors may be necessary in severe cases.

Immunodeficiency

Immunodeficiency may be caused by quantitative or qualitative defects in neutrophils, primary immunodeficiencies involving T cells and B cells, complement or combined defects and secondary immunodeficiency or acquired disorders (Figure 12.5).

NEUTROPHIL DISORDERS

Neutropaenias (quantitative)

Neutrophils initiate response to invading bacteria and fungi and represent the first line of defence in the body. They are short-lived (6–8 hours circulating half-life) and then undergo apoptosis. Neutropenia is defined as an absolute neutrophil count (ANC) less than 1.5×10^9 L. Because neutropenia can be a presenting sign of immunodeficiency or a systemic autoimmune disorder, further screening is indicated.

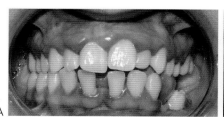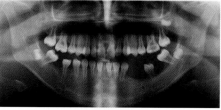

Figure 12.5 (A) 13-year-old girl with severe congenital neutropenia. Note poor oral hygiene and periodontal disease. (B) Panoramic radiograph shows dental caries, severe bone loss and missing permanent teeth due to extraction. (Courtesy Prof. Marcio da Fonseca.)

Severe chronic neutropenias

Congenital neutropenias. Cyclic neutropenia: This is an autosomal dominant disease caused by mutations in the ELA-2 or ELANE gene, which shorten the survival of neutrophil progenitors through accelerated apoptosis. There is a characteristic oscillation of blood neutrophil counts with periods of severe neutropenia every 18 to 28 days. This is the time it takes for a cohort of cells to pass through the bone marrow to their ultimate utilization and removal from the blood or tissues.

- Neutrophil levels can be near zero for 3 to 5 days when the bone marrow supply of neutrophils is exhausted, before recovering to near the lower limit of the normal count.
- During neutropenic periods, patients have painful oral ulcers, fevers, respiratory symptoms, cellulitis, abscesses and bacterial infections, which are potentially fatal.
- Regularly recurring oral ulcers are a useful sign that aid in the diagnosis.

Diagnosis: serial blood counts at least 3 days a week for 6 weeks or longer to see at least two nadirs, expecting the cycle to be approximately 21 days, concomitant with oral ulcers and other inflammatory features.

Responds well to granulocyte-colony stimulating factor (G-CSF).

Severe congenital neutropenia (Kostmann syndrome)

- Neutrophil counts are constantly extremely low: less than $0.2 \times 10^9/L$.
- Most cases are autosomal dominant caused by mutations in the ELA-2 or ELANE gene.
- Affected infants are chronically ill soon after birth, and 10% to 30% of patients develop acute myeloid leukaemia (AML) or myelodysplastic syndrome (MDS).
- Approximately 40% develop osteopenia and/or osteoporosis.

Diagnosis and management:

- Usually recognized in very young children because of fever and infections; neonates may present a severe acute umbilical infection.
- Gingivitis, oral ulcers and periodontal problems can develop within the first 2 years of life (Figure 12.5).
- HSCT is necessary if the patient does not respond well to high doses of G-CSF and for those who develop MDS or AML.

Metabolic diseases associated with neutropenia

Glycogen-storage disease type 1b

- Autosomal recessive defect in the glucose-6-phosphate transporter protein that prevents glycogen from being metabolized into glucose.
- 'Doll-like' facial appearance, stunted growth, hypoglycaemia, enlarged liver and spleen, failure to thrive, renal problems, recurrent infections.
- Bleeding tendencies resulting from splenomegaly due to platelet sequestration and destruction.
- Chronic neutropenia is caused by a defective function of cells responsible for killing bacteria.
- Patients present with oral ulcers, candidiasis, gingivitis, periodontitis and perioral infections
- Treatment: G-CSF.

Acquired neutropenias. Idiopathic neutropenia: May occur at any point in life for unknown reasons. Long-term treatment is with G-CSF.

Autoimmune benign chronic neutropenia: This is the most common form of neutropenia in infants and children. Generally, it presents in the first year of life (median age at diagnosis: 8–11 months), normalizing between 3 and 5 years of age. There is prolonged noncyclic neutropenia likely caused by antineutrophil antibodies, particularly IgG. The condition is usually not inherited, but a familial form (autosomal dominant) has been described. Patients present with recurrent infections, oral ulcers and oedematous fiery-red gingival tissues.

Treatment: not usually necessary, but antibiotics can be used for acute bacterial infections and G-CSF for serious infections only.

Other conditions associated with neutropenia

- Severe acquired aplastic anaemia.
- Viral illnesses: Almost any virus can cause transient neutropenia. More profound with infection by CMV, HIV, Epstein–Barr virus, influenza viruses and parvovirus B19.

Marrow failure syndromes

Fanconi anaemia is a chromosomal instability disorder caused by genetic defects in DNA repair. It results in bone marrow failure frequently in the first year of life and may affect almost any organ system.

- Short stature, skin abnormalities (café-au-lait spots, hypo/hyperpigmentation), upper limb abnormalities, renal anomalies, hypogonadism, microcephaly.
- 'Fanconi facies': micrognathia, mid-face hypoplasia, epicanthal folds.
- Increased risk of MDS, AML and solid tumours.
- HSCT is the only curative treatment for the haematologic manifestations of the disease.

Drug-induced neutropenias

Nonchemotherapeutic drug-induced neutropenia is relatively rare but potentially fatal with a mortality rate of approximately 5%.

- Most common drugs: amoxicillin, clotrimoxazole, ticlopidine, valganciclovir, matamizole, clozapine, sulfasalazine, thiamazole and carbimazole.
- Patients typically experience acute, severe neutropenia or agranulocytosis and symptoms of fever, chills, sore throat and joint and muscle pain within weeks or months after first exposure to a drug.
- Discontinuation of the drug usually solves the problem.

DISORDERS OF NEUTROPHIL FUNCTION (QUALITATIVE DISORDERS)

Result from impairment in neutrophil responses critical for host defence. Patients with defects in neutrophil function present in infancy with recurrent and/or difficult-to-treat bacterial infections involving the skin, mucosa, gingiva and lungs, draining lymph nodes, and/or tissue abscesses. Four key aspects should be considered in a patient with a history of infections: frequency, severity, location of infections and curative agent. Other factors to consider include the patient's age, medical condition and family history.

Disorders of adhesion and chemotaxis

The ability of neutrophils to adhere to endothelium, tissue matrix and invading microorganisms is essential for their migration from the bloodstream to infection sites, where they kill pathogens. Defects in these interactions and/or chemotaxis impair recruitment of neutrophils into sites of infection or inflammation, often with relative neutrophilia in peripheral blood but poor formation of pus. Individuals with defective chemotaxis develop rapidly advancing periodontal disease at a young age. Children and adolescents who present with periodontal disease without a clear aetiology must be evaluated for neutropenia or neutrophil dysfunction.

Leukocyte adhesion deficiency (LAD) type I – a rare autosomal recessive deficiency of γ-2 integrin, a leukocyte glycoprotein important for cell surface adhesion. Frequent skin and periodontal infections in both dentitions, delayed separation of the umbilical cord and deep tissue abscesses, typically with *Staphylococcus aureus* or Gram-negative enteric microbes, are observed.

- Patients with partial expression of LAD type I require good supportive care, including antibiotics and optimal oral care.
- Patients with severe LAD type I need allogeneic HSCT because of the severity of infections.
- LAD types II and III are very rare.

Localized aggressive periodontitis (see Chapter 10): Periodontal disease with atypical inflammation and usually absence of calculus affects typically the primary teeth, which may exfoliate because of bone loss.

Hyperimmunoglobulin E (Job) syndrome: Presents with a triad of elevated serum levels of IgE (>2000 IU/ml), *S. aureus* skin infections ('cold abscesses') and pneumonia. There are variable profound defects of neutrophil chemotaxis, which are independent of IgE serum fluctuations.

- Chronic candidiasis of mucosa and nail beds, hyperextensible joints, scoliosis, decreased bone density.
- Delayed or failure of exfoliation of primary teeth, oral ulcerations and gingivitis are present, but patients may not be prone to severe periodontitis.

Lazy leukocyte syndrome: Mutations in actin-interacting protein 1 (Aip1) that lead to recurrent infections, oral ulcers and periodontitis with early loss of teeth.

Papillon–Lefevre syndrome: An autosomal recessive condition with defects in chemotaxis, phagocytosis and intracellular killing because of deficiency in cathepsin C.

- Characteristic palmoplantar keratosis and severe aggressive periodontitis in both dentitions, sometimes without significant neutrophil abnormalities.

Trisomy 21 (Down) syndrome: These children have deficits in neutrophil chemotaxis, phagocytosis and intracellular killing and may present with periodontal disease from an early age.

Disorders of ingestion and degranulation

After phagocytosis, neutrophil granules fuse with phagosome membranes and release proteases, enzymes and antibacterial proteins into the phagosome lumen, which facilitates microbial killing.

Chediak–Higashi syndrome: This is an autosomal recessive condition caused by mutations in the CHS1 gene, a large protein thought to regulate lysosomal and granule trafficking. It is characterized by fusion of cytoplasmic granules that lead to the death of myeloid precursors. Surviving giant granules interfere with the diapedesis process.

- Ineffective granulopoiesis, moderate neutropenia and delayed and incomplete degranulation.
- Defective natural killer cells because of reduced content of hydrolytic enzymes.
- Partial oculocutaneous albinism, frequent *S. aureus* infections in skin and lungs, lymphadenopathy and neuropathies.
- Organelle abnormalities within platelets inhibit normal clot formation.

Patients present with gingivitis, periodontitis, tongue and buccal mucosa ulcers and premature loss of teeth in both dentitions. The majority of patients who survive childhood develop haemophagocytic histiocytosis. Treatment: allogeneic HSCT.

Disorders of oxidative metabolism

Reactive oxygen species play an important role in killing microbial pathogens. Defects in this metabolic pathway present with a number of conditions:

Chronic granulomatous disease: This is the most common clinically significant inherited disorder of neutrophil function, occurring in 1:200 000 live births. Patients present with recurrent, often life-threatening bacterial and fungal infections in the skin, lungs and lymph nodes; liver abscesses; osteomyelitis; and hypergammoglobulinemia. Splenomegaly, hepatomegaly and lymph node enlargement are present. Oral ulceration and gingivitis are present but usually not periodontitis.

Treatment: prophylactic trimethropim-sulfamethoxazole, itraconazole and γ-interferon or HSCT.

Myeloperoxidase deficiency (MPO): the most common inherited disorder of phagocytes with 1:4000 people presenting as an autosomal recessive condition with mutations in the MPO gene.

- Rarely associated with clinical symptoms, unless patients suffer from diabetes mellitus, which leads to disseminated candidiasis and other fungal infections.
- No prophylactic antibiotics needed because of lack of symptoms.

Disorders of defective clearance of neutrophils

Even healthy neutrophils can cause unwarranted collateral tissue damage if not cleared properly when they become apoptotic, which could lead to neutrophil necrosis and release of toxic content.

Associated with autoimmune inflammatory disorders (e.g., systemic lupus erythaematosus).

IMMUNE DISORDERS

Severe combined immunodeficiency

Severe combined immunodeficiency (SCID) represents a group of inherited immune deficiencies characterized by deficiency of T cells or T cell lymphoma caused by genetic mutations affecting T cells; most cases are X-linked. Patients present with frequent infections that often are fatal; thus SCID is considered a paediatric emergency.

Clinical features:

- Babies may present recurrent infections, chronic diarrhoea and failure to thrive.
- Lymphoid tissues, such as adenoids and tonsils, may be absent.
- Oral and genital candida and severe skin rash may occur.

Initial management: protection against infection – strict isolation, avoidance of live vaccines, use of IV immunoglobulin and antimicrobial prophylaxis. The most common treatment is HSCT, especially in the first 3.5 months of life (survival rate: 94%).

Wiskott–Aldrich syndrome is an X-linked recessive disease that causes impaired lymphoid development and maturation of lymphocytes. Presents with eczema, thrombocytopenia and immune deficiency.

22q11.2 deletion syndrome is the most common chromosomal microdeletion disorder (1:1000 live births). Several conditions have overlapping phenotypic features resulting from 22q11.2 deletion: DiGeorge syndrome, conotruncal anomaly facial syndrome, velocardiofacial syndrome and subsets of Opitz G/BBB and Cayler cardiofacial syndromes.

Oral and dental considerations

Neutrophil homeostasis and periodontal health: Neutrophils are the majority of cells recruited to the gingival crevice, forming a 'defence wall' against tooth-associated subgingival biofilm. Conditions associated with defects in mechanisms that regulate the production and life cycle of neutrophils lead to the development of periodontitis. The early forms of early-onset periodontitis are generally unresponsive to antibiotics and/or mechanical removal of the biofilm.

- Good oral hygiene and dental health are of paramount importance to prevent bacterial penetration into the periodontal tissues of affected patients. Once that happens, it is difficult to revert it.

TABLE 12.2 ■ **Most common types of childhood and adolescent cancers in the United States**

Children <14 years of age		Adolescents (15–19 years of age)	
Acute lymphoblastic leukaemia	26%	Hodgkin lymphoma	15%
Brain and central nervous system (CNS)	21%	Thyroid carcinoma	11%
Neuroblastoma	7%	Brain and CNS	10%

- Patients with severe congenital neutropenia may have osteoporosis and may be prescribed bisphosphonates.
- Treatment with G-CSF usually improves the periodontal condition, but patients may still show gingivitis and periodontal problems (Figure 12.5).
- Periodontal treatment in neutrophil disorders has been empirical and without consistent success. The outcome is usually tooth loss.

Childhood cancer

Childhood cancer accounts for about 1% of all cancer cases in the population and is the second leading cause of death in children between 1 and 14 years of age in the United States (Table 12.2). Internationally, the annual incidence of malignant tumours in children under 15 years is approximately 11 per 100 000 children. Approximately 600 to 700 children between birth and 15 years of age develop cancer each year in the United States. Whereas most adult cancers are carcinomas with strong aetiological associations, childhood cancers are a wide range of different histological types of tumour with less aetiological connection.

The incidence, either in childhood cancer as a whole or in individual types of cancer, varies little from one country to the next, and no racial group is exempt. Among more than 50 types of childhood cancers, the most common forms include leukaemias, lymphomas (Figure 12.6A), central nervous system (CNS) tumours, primary sarcomas of bone and soft tissues, Ewing sarcoma (Figure 12.6B), Wilms tumours, neuroblastomas and retinoblastomas. Acute leukaemias

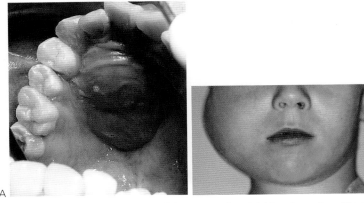

Figure 12.6 Examples of childhood cancer. (A) Asymptomatic palatal lymphoma in a 15 year-old girl. (B) 4 year-old boy with acute right facial swelling that appeared after a minor fall, subsequently diagnosed as Ewing's sarcoma. (Figure B, courtesy Prof. Marcio da Fonseca.)

and tumours of the CNS account for approximately one-half of all childhood malignancies. Multimodal therapy (chemotherapy, radiotherapy and surgery) has resulted in an overall 5-year survival rate of approximately 80% for childhood cancer. Signs and symptoms of childhood cancer can be nonspecific (Table 12.3 and Figures 12.7 and 12.8).

SOLID TUMOURS IN CHILDHOOD

Brain and spinal cord tumours

- Most common solid tumours in children.
- Some 40% located in the hemispheres (astrocytomas, gangliomas, primitive neuroectodermal tumour).
- Some 60% in the posterior fossa (medulloblastoma, ependymoma).
- Chemotherapy can be used to delay or avoid cranial radiotherapy in infants.
- The overall survival rate is approximately 60% at 10 years.

TABLE 12.3 ■ **Signs and symptoms of childhood cancer**

Frequent headaches, often accompanied by vomiting	Gingival enlargement (Figure 12.7)
Lymphadenopathy	Mediastinal or abdominal masses
Ongoing pain in an area of the body	Paleness or loss of energy
Persistent bone pain or limping	Rapid weight loss
Sudden eye or vision change	Sudden tendency to bruise and/or bleed
Testicular masses	Unexplained fever or illness
Unusual mass or swelling (chloroma) (Figure 12.8)	

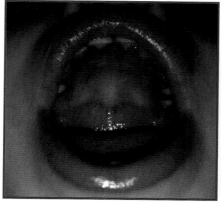
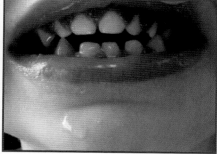

A   B

Figure 12.7   (A and B) Two-year-old boy with fever, loss of appetite, malaise, drooling, gingival erythema and swelling initially diagnosed with gingivo-herpetic stomatitis. As his clinical picture did not resolve after a few weeks, a complete blood count revealed acute lymphoblastic leukemia. (Courtesy Prof. Marcio da Fonseca.)

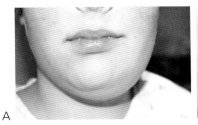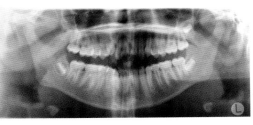

A   B

Figure 12.8 (A) Twelve-year old girl presented for a dental consult concerned about odontogenic infection causing left facial swelling. Patient had no dental disease and swelling was diagnosed as a chloroma caused by acute myelogenous leukemia. (B) Panoramic radiograph showing no dental disease or infection. (Couresy Prof. Marcio da Fonseca.)

Neuroblastoma

- Arises from neural crest derivatives in cells of the sympathetic nervous system found in the embryo or foetus.
- Develops in infants and children; rare after 10 years of age.
- Can occur anywhere in the body but most commonly in the abdomen.
- Diagnosis is confirmed by raised levels of urinary catecholamines and tissue biopsy.
- Prognosis depends on patient age at diagnosis, tumour stage and biological features of the tumour, especially presence of amplification of the n-myc gene. Children with high-risk disease (~50% of cases) have 25% survival rates even with aggressive chemotherapy, surgery, radiation and autologous HSCT.

Wilms tumour (nephroblastoma)

- Usually in one kidney only, presenting as an asymptomatic abdominal mass.
- Most often found in 3- to 4-year-old children.
- Often associated with aniridia and other congenital anomalies.
- Responds well to chemotherapy with or without radiotherapy to reduce the tumour mass and surgical removal depending on disease stage. Commonly lung, hepatic and skeletal metastases occur.

Rhabdomyosarcoma

- Most common type of soft tissue tumour and affects skeletal muscles anywhere in the body.
- Arises from embryonal mesenchymal tissue with potential for differentiation to skeletal (striated) muscle.
- Children often present with a painless, usually rapidly enlarging subcutaneous lump, almost anywhere in the body.
- Common sites include head and neck, genitourinary tract and extremities.
- Large lesions in the head and neck invade bone and jaw lesions are quite common in advanced cases.
- Treatment involves surgery with adjuvant chemotherapy and radiotherapy.
- Prognosis is influenced by site, subtype of rhabdomyosarcoma and stage at diagnosis.

Retinoblastoma

- Usually affects children around 2 years of age, rarely after 6 years.
- Strong hereditary component.
- Diagnosis is usually a white or yellow pupillary reflex (normally red reflex).
- Treatment often requires enucleation of the globe and postsurgical radiotherapy. Occasionally adjunct chemotherapy is also required.

Osteosarcoma

- Rare malignant tumour of bone, mostly in the metaphyseal region of long bones, with the distal femur being the most common site.
- Occurs in areas of rapid bone growth, usually in teenagers, causing bone pain and swelling of the area.
- Teenagers are the most common age group affected.
- Frequently metastasizes to the lung and requires wide resection of primary tumour plus multi-agent chemotherapy.

Ewing sarcoma

- Malignant tumour of bone in young teenagers, commonly involving the midshaft of long bones, pelvic bones and chest wall, although any bone may be involved, including facial bones (Figure 12.6B).
- Occurs most commonly in the proximal femur or pelvis and is characterized by densely packed small round cells.
- Treatment involves surgery, chemotherapy and local irradiation.
- The prognosis worsens with pelvic primary or metastatic disease.

Lymphomas

Lymphomas arise from the immune system (lymphocytes): lymph nodes, tonsils, thymus.
- Hodgkin lymphoma is a lymphoid malignancy characterized by the presence of Reed–Sternberg cells in the tumour. It is rare in children under 5 years of age, usually occurring in adolescents and young adults.
- Non-Hodgkin lymphoma is found in younger patients than Hodgkin lymphoma; rare under 3 years of age. It is characterized by rapid growth.

Langerhans cell histiocytosis

- This rare disorder is essentially a build-up of a subgroup of histiocytes called Langerhans cells, which initially present with an eczematous, purpuric rash on the hands, scalp and trunk. There is discussion as to whether this is a true neoplasm.
- Osteolytic lesions of the skull and mandible can occur, and premature exfoliation of primary teeth has been reported with eosinophilic granulomas.
- Prognosis depends on the extent of disease at diagnosis and the progression of lesions.

HAEMATOLOGICAL MALIGNANCIES IN CHILDHOOD

The leukaemias are a heterogeneous group of haematological malignancies caused by clonal proliferation of primitive white blood cells.

Abnormal profile of the blood count: neutropenia, anaemia, thrombocytopenia.

Acute lymphoblastic leukaemia (ALL): most common childhood malignancy, accounting for 80% to 85% of all childhood leukaemias. It has a peak incidence between 2 and 6 years of age. The head and neck manifestations include lymphadenopathy, sore throat, gingival bleeding and oral ulceration.

Management involves several phases of treatment with chemotherapy:
- Remission induction: to restore normal haematopoiesis.
- Consolidation: to prevent or treat CNS disease.
- Delayed intensification or reconsolidation: to reduce relapse probability.
- Maintenance: to suppress leukemic growth; lasts 2 to 3 years.

■ Intrathecal therapy (commonly methotrexate) has been used to replace cranial irradiation.

Cure rates for standard risk ALL are now over 90% on current protocols. If relapse occurs, 40% to 50% can be cured with chemotherapy and/or HSCT. Prognosis depends on age of onset, initial white cell count, cytogenetic abnormalities and other features. HSCT is reserved for very-high-risk patients or patients with relapse.

AML: The incidence of AML increases with age, thus it is primarily a disease of young adults and adults, accounting for 15% to 20% of acute childhood leukaemias.

■ AML with monocytic morphology (M4/M5) can manifest gingival infiltration and promyelocytic morphology (M3) is associated with disseminated intravascular coagulation.

■ Approximately 20% to 40% of patients cured with chemotherapy only; others will need HSCT.

DENTAL MANAGEMENT IN CHILDHOOD CANCER

Close collaboration between the child's oncologist and the paediatric dentist is essential when planning appropriate dental care. At the time of diagnosis and during the initial stages of chemotherapy, dental care may be provided even in private practices if guidelines are followed. Once the child has achieved remission, or has successfully completed treatment, routine dental care should be provided.

Elective dental treatment can be provided when between cycles of chemotherapy, in consultation with the oncology team, if blood levels are adequate. Children in maintenance can receive routine dental treatment, although a full blood count (FBC) is prudent if an invasive procedure is planned. Pulpal therapy of primary teeth during the induction and consolidation phase of chemotherapy is generally not recommended because of the possibility of failed treatment with subsequent dental abscess/infection developing in an immunodepressed child. When pulpal therapy of permanent teeth is needed, the risk of bacteraemia and potential septicaemia must be weighed against the potential benefits of maintaining the teeth.

Oral hygiene and care of acute effects of cancer treatment in the oral cavity:

■ Toothbrushing two to three times a day with a soft or medium brush should be done throughout the entire treatment, including for HSCT patients, regardless of the child's haematological and immunosuppressive status; toothbrushing does not increase the risk of bacteremia, fever or bleeding.

■ Foam brushes, sponges, swabs and super-soft brushes do not provide effective plaque removal and thus are not recommended.

■ Aqueous chlorhexidine rinses can be prescribed for patients with poor oral hygiene, periodontal disease or for those who cannot brush because of moderate or severe mucositis to reduce the bacterial and fungal load. However, chlorhexidine is not recommended to treat or prevent mucositis.

■ During periods of immunosuppression and thrombocytopenia, patients must avoid the use of dental floss, toothpicks and water irrigation devices because they may break the gingival tissues and create a port of entry for microorganisms.

■ Mouthwash mixtures of an antacid, topical anaesthetic and an antihistamine are not effective and are not recommended.

■ Patients should not swallow or gargle with solutions containing anaesthetics because they numb the gag reflex, which can lead to aspiration of foods, liquids, bacteria and oral tissues into the lungs.

■ For further information on oral hygiene and care of acute effects of cancer treatment in the oral cavity, consult the international guidelines published by the Multinational Association of Supportive Care in Cancer (https://www.mascc.org/mucositis-guidelines).

DENTAL TREATMENT

Dental care should be completed before cancer treatment starts:

- In non-HSCT cases, treatment can be prioritized and completed in between chemotherapy cycles when the blood counts are normal or close to normal, if dental treatment cannot be fully completed before cancer therapy starts.
- In HSCT cases, treatment must be completed before admission for the conditioning phase of the transplant because the patient may be immunosuppressed for months or years (in cases of chronic graft-versus-host disease [GVHD]).
- The patient's physician must be consulted before any dental procedure to check the haematological and immunosuppressive status.
- The ANC should be above 0.5 cells × 10^9/L (500 cells/mm^3) for dental procedures. If the ANC is below that level, avoid elective procedures. In emergency cases, discuss the approach to dental care with physician.
- Platelet levels should be greater than 75 cells × 10^9/L (75 000/mm^3) for invasive dental procedures. Between 40 and 75 cells × 10^9/L, platelet transfusions may be considered because of potential for prolonged bleeding. When platelets are under 40 cells × 10^9/L, consider deferring care. If that is not possible, discuss the approach with the physician. The need for treatment must be balanced around the risks and complications of the procedure and the possible sequelae if treatment is not performed.
- Patients may also present prolonged bleeding because of poor quality of platelets, liver disorders, coagulations issues etc. In that case, additional blood tests must be ordered to check for coagulation factors and platelet disorder.
- Antibiotic prophylaxis before invasive dental procedures for patients who have a central line (Figure 12.9) is a controversial issue. There is no evidence to support the use of antibiotic prophylaxis to prevent catheter-related infections after a dental procedure. However, the catheter may indirectly interfere with a valve function or may rub against the endocardium, creating a wound which could potentially lead to IE. Discuss antibiotic coverage with the physician.
- The vinca alkaloid class of chemotherapeutic agents (e.g., vincristine, vinblastine) can cause neuropathic pain in the jaws. The pain is constant and deep, often bilateral, usually in the mandible. The pain may resemble a toothache, but patients cannot isolate the 'offending' tooth.
- Patients at high risk for dental caries and prolonged xerostomia (e.g., in cases of localized radiation to the salivary glands or oral chronic GVHD) should receive supplemental fluoride (rinses, gels, varnish or toothpastes with fluoride content) and be monitored closely by a dental professional.

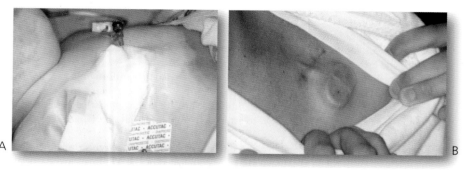

A   B

Figure 12.9 (A) Partially implanted central venous catheter. (B) Subcutaneously implanted central venous catheter (port). (Courtesy Prof. Marcio da Fonseca.)

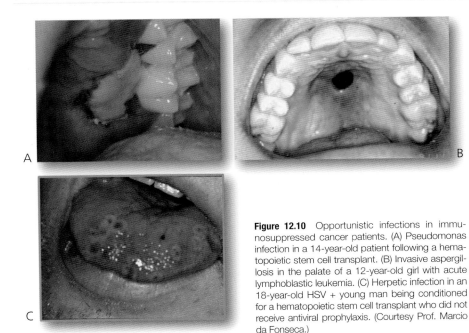

Figure 12.10 Opportunistic infections in immunosuppressed cancer patients. (A) Pseudomonas infection in a 14-year-old patient following a hematopoietic stem cell transplant. (B) Invasive aspergillosis in the palate of a 12-year-old girl with acute lymphoblastic leukemia. (C) Herpetic infection in an 18-year-old HSV + young man being conditioned for a hematopoietic stem cell transplant who did not receive antiviral prophylaxis. (Courtesy Prof. Marcio da Fonseca.)

- Immunosuppressed patients are at a high risk for opportunistic oral infections (Figure 12.10).

Patients who were immunosuppressed and those who experienced mucosal changes (e.g., mucositis, oral chronic GVHD) are at high risk of developing oral and pharyngeal cancer later – because of DNA changes in cells as well as infections by oncogenic microorganisms (e.g., human papilloma virus, Epstein–Barr virus, etc.)

CHEMOTHERAPY

The cytotoxic drugs used during chemotherapy can cause immediate and long-term damage to several organs:

- Liver.
- Kidney.
- Intestine.
- Germ cells of the testes and ovaries.
- Lung.
- Heart.
- Brain.

Direct stomato-toxicity is caused by the cytotoxic action of the chemotherapeutic agents on oral mucosal cells leading to inflammation, thinning and ulceration of the mucosa (mucositis Figure 12.11). Mucositis usually starts between 5 and 7 days after chemotherapy is administered, lasting about 14 to 21 days. Saliva function may also be diminished, although this response has not been reported as common in children. These problems are commonly encountered in the induction and consolidation phases of chemotherapy when relatively high doses of multi-agent therapy are employed.

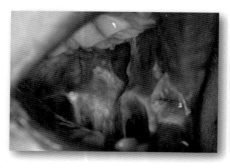
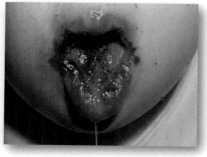

A   B

Figure 12.11   (A) Moderate mucositis caused by chemotherapy in a 14 year-old male patient. Note tissue atrophy, erythema, lichenoid changes and ulceration. (B) Severe mucositis in a 6-year-old female with Down syndrome. Note the thick saliva, erythema, ulceration of lips and tongue, and bleeding. (Courtesy Prof. Marcio da Fonseca.)

RADIOTHERAPY

Radiotherapy may be used:
- Before surgery to shrink tumour bulk.
- Alone as the only treatment.
- In combination with other therapies such as chemotherapy.
- Following other modalities to eliminate residual neoplastic cells.

Previously, cranial irradiation was used widely to manage and prevent leukaemic infiltration in the CNS (CNS prophylaxis) in children with ALL and other haemopoietic cancer. More commonly, intrathecal chemotherapy is now used. Radiotherapy is also used for primary solid tumours and in total body irradiation (TBI) as part of conditioning before HSCT. TBI and radiotherapy to the face produce mucositis, which is usually seen between 5 and 7 days after radiotherapy, lasting from 14 to 21 days. The severity of mucositis depends on the dosage of radiotherapy and whether fractionated versus whole-dose radiation is used. Mucositis may cause oral pain and difficulty in performing oral hygiene, speaking, eating and drinking.

When radiotherapy involves the major salivary glands, xerostomia occurs frequently within a few days, producing a viscous, acidic saliva. Loss or alteration of taste (hypo- or dysgeusia) may also occur, prompting the patient to change to a softer, more cariogenic diet to alleviate soreness and dryness of the oral cavity. This is a factor in the aetiology of rapid dental caries that has been reported in these patients if they are not given adequate preventive therapy. Radiation-induced dental caries has a distinctive generalized cervical pattern, and sometimes the complete dentition can be destroyed in a relatively short period.

LATE SYSTEMIC EFFECTS OF CHILDHOOD NEOPLASIA AND TREATMENT

Dramatic advances in the treatment of childhood cancer in the past three decades have led to the long-term cure of 70% of the children diagnosed today. Because about 1 in 600 children develop cancer before the age of 15 years, almost 1 young adult in every 1000 will be a long-term survivor of childhood cancer. As the number of survivors of a variety of paediatric cancers increases, the oro-dental sequelae of effective medical treatment in these patients are emerging. Many children for whom oncology treatment results in a stable remission can expect to follow a healthy life. Recurrence of the original malignancy or another cancer may occur a few years later, although the likelihood of this becomes increasingly remote as time passes.

Consequently, successfully treated paediatric oncology patients are never 'discharged', their health being regularly monitored throughout their life. Late effects following paediatric cancer treatment may include:

- Growth retardation, unequal or reduced growth
- Cognitive impairments and behavioural issues.
- Deficiencies in vision and hearing.
- Endocrine imbalances and altered function, especially thyroid and pituitary glands.
- Infertility.
- Cardiac and lung damage.
- Secondary malignancy.
- Other, less common effects include epidermal and mucosal changes such as skin hyperpigmentation, cutaneous telangiectasia, subcutaneous tissue atrophy and permanent thinning or loss of hair.

Postcancer surgery effects

Surgical removal of a solid tumour in the oral cavity can cause:

- Disfigurement (temporary or permanent) (see Figure 12.12A–C).
- Loss of teeth and function.
- Stenosis and paraesthesia.

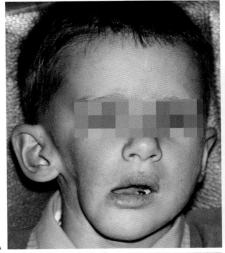

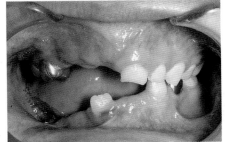

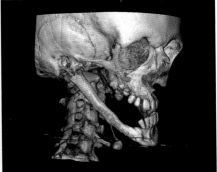

Figure 12.12 (A) Late effects of surgery and radiotherapy for a rhabdomyosarcoma of the right mandible involving the parotid, neck and infratemporal fossa. This child underwent a hemimandibulectomy and radical neck dissection, followed by reconstruction with a free vascular rib graft (B). Note the limited oral opening and the facial deformity (C).

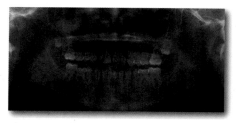

Figure 12.13   13-year-old patient diagnosed at 3 years of age with stage IV neuroblastoma on the adrenal gland that metastasized to the eye. Received 6 cycles of Cytoxan, doxorubicin and vincristine prior to an autologous hematopoietic stem cell transplant conditioned with melphalan, carboplatin and etoposide. He also received human anti-murine antibody therapy, rituxan and cyclophosphamide, as well as radiation to the eye and abdomen. Note several congenitally missing teeth, small mandibular premolars and short, V-shaped roots with early apical closure. (Courtesy Prof. Marcio da Fonseca.)

Craniofacial and dental development following chemo- and radiotherapy

Chronic problems involving target tissues lead to impairment of growth and development of hard and soft tissues, and the effects of chemotherapy and radiotherapy appear to be synergistic.

Generally, the nature and degree of these complications vary widely and depend on several factors including:

- The type and location of malignancy.
- The age of the patient. Children younger than 6 years of age are affected more severely than older patients, as their primary and permanent teeth are actively developing.
- Total dosage and timing of chemotherapeutic agents and radiotherapy.
- The initial oral health status and the level of dental care before, during and after therapy.

Other factors and considerations:

- Long-term dental developmental effects may include agenesis, microdontia, crown disturbances of size, shape, enamel and pulp chamber, and root abnormalities in shape, length and early apical closure (Figure 12.13).
- Chemotherapy causes ameloblast and odontoblast death, but they are not affected during nonproliferative or germinal stages.
- When chemotherapy is used alone, the craniofacial growth may not be affected significantly.
- Radiotherapy also causes ameloblast and odontoblast death, including presecretory odontoblasts.
- The mandible is four times more radiosensitive than the maxilla because of the radiosensitivity of dividing cells in the condylar cartilage. An altered craniofacial growth pattern with diminished mandibular growth is often associated with a field of irradiation that includes a portion of ascending ramus and the mandibular condyle.
- Progressive endarteritis is a complication that can occur in irradiated bone and can lead to postradiation osteonecrosis. The mandible is particularly prone to this complication; however, this is less common in children. If an area of necrotic or hypovascular bone becomes infected following a dental extraction or surgery, refractory osteomyelitis may ensue. Endarteritis may also cause fibrosis in the masticatory muscles and subsequent trismus.
- TBI used for HSCT conditioning may lead to reduced mandibular and maxillary growth.

Xerostomia and oral health

Generally, there is a lower incidence of radiation-induced dental caries in children compared with adults. Facial irradiation and chemotherapy can also damage irreversibly the acini cells of the major salivary glands, resulting in xerostomia. This condition may be transient because of the lower dosage of radiation used in children and the greater regenerative capacity of the exocrine cells. With the exception of children who have received irradiation involving the salivary glands, many long-term survivors of childhood cancer have no worse oral health or dental disease than the well child. Others, however, can be significantly more prone to dental caries because of enamel defects, xerostomia, oral GVHD and parental overindulgence.

HEMATOPOIETIC STEM CELL TRANSPLANTATION

HSCT is used to replace hematopoietic cells in the management of certain lymphomas, some brain tumours, neuroblastoma and following a relapse in leukaemias. It may also be used in certain haemoglobinopathies, bone marrow failure, immune disorders and congenital metabolic diseases. Stem cells may be derived from the bone marrow, peripheral blood or umbilical cord/placental blood, and may be classified according to the donor as:

- Autologous: from the patient's own cells.
- Allogeneic: from a sibling or unrelated donor.
- Syngeneic: from an identical twin.

Children undergoing HSCT conditioned with myeloablative regimens develop the typical oral mucosal changes of ulceration, atrophy, lichenoid changes, hyperkeratosis, keratinization and erythema (i.e., mucositis), which start 5 to 7 days after the beginning of conditioning and last up to 21 days posttransplantation. During this period, oral pain may be severe and require narcotic analgesia. The use of keratinocyte growth factor (palifermin) has been demonstrated to reduce this complication in adults undergoing autologous transplantation, and paediatric studies of this promising treatment are in progress. However, its cost is prohibitive at this time.

Oral infections with *Candida albicans*, *herpes simplex*, *cytomegalovirus* and *varicella zoster* are the major infective agents seen in children undergoing HSCT, if inadequate prophylaxis is given. These conditions can be life-threatening if not treated aggressively at diagnosis. Bleeding or crusting of the lips and gingival oozing are seen commonly but are seldom serious.

Graft-versus-host disease

This condition occurs when transplanted T cells recognize the host tissues as foreign. GVHD is a major problem following HSCT, with clinical manifestations in up to half of patients. The acute form of GVHD tends to occur within days of HSCT, with signs of fever, rash, diarrhoea and abnormal liver function leading to jaundice. Chronic GVHD may start at 80 days posttransplant and is characterized by lichenoid or scleroderma-like changes of the skin (Figure 12.14),

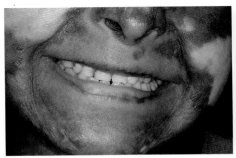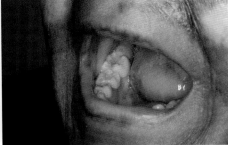

Figure 12.14 An 8-year-old male with severe oral chronic graft-versus-host disease following an autologous haematopoietic stem cell transplant at age 3 years for chronic granulomatous disease. Note the loss of the vermillion border, perioral fibrosis, dental caries, loss of tongue papillae, thickened saliva, lichenoid changes on buccal mucosa, gingivitis, and hypo- and hyperpigmentation of skin. (Courtesy Prof. Marcio da Fonseca.)

keratogingivitis, abnormal liver function, pulmonary insufficiency and intestinal problems. Oral manifestations of GVHD vary with the severity of the conditions but often include:

- Oral mucosal erythema, ulcers and lichenoid changes.
- Oral sensitivity (to spicy and acidic foods, carbonated beverages, acidic drinks, toothpaste).
- Salivary gland dysfunction.
- Atrophic glossitis, microstomia and perioral and soft tissue fibrosis in severe cases (Figure 12.14).
- Palatal mucoceles and sometimes marked icteric coloration of the oral tissues.
- Pyogenic granulomas.
- Oral infections.
- Loss of lingual papillae.

Management of chronic GVHD necessitates a multidisciplinary approach. The goal of treatment entails effective care as well as minimizing toxicity and relapse. Long-term systemic immunosuppression with prednisone and other agents is often needed. Extracorporeal photopheresis may lead to disease remission. Topical treatments can be effective to help with symptoms, such as steroid mouthwashes, creams and gels, steroid injections into large ulcerations, Biotene® oral products and sodium bicarbonate diluted in water to help with disturbances in taste (dysgeusia) and thick saliva. Careful attention to oral health with close communication with the treating medical team is needed to give the best outcomes.

- The oral cavity may be the first or only site of chronic GVHD following an HSCT.
- Patients who develop oral chronic GVHD tend to be deeply immunosuppressed for a long period of time, thus the physician must authorize any dental procedures, including supragingival dental cleanings.

Medication-related osteonecrosis of the jaw

The old term 'bisphosphonate-related osteonecrosis of the jaw' (BRONJ) is now part of a larger umbrella called 'medication-related osteonecrosis of the jaw' (MRONJ) to accommodate the growing number of jaw osteonecrosis cases caused by other antiresorptive medications (denosumab) and antiangiogenic therapies. Osteonecrosis of the jaws is a well-described complication of these medications in adults but has not yet manifested as a disorder in children. Although there have been no reported cases of MRONJ in children, there has been a significant increase in the use of these drugs in the management of children with connective tissue disorders and decreased bone density, including:

- Congenital osteoporosis: osteogenesis imperfecta.
- Secondary osteoporosis: immobility, chronic use of steroid medications.
- Focal orthopaedic conditions: avascular necrosis, Perthes disease; fracture nonunion; Ilizarov limb lengthening; bone cysts.
- Other bone disorders: fibrous dysplasia, idiopathic juvenile osteoporosis.

There is an increased association of MRONJ with invasive dental procedures such as extractions. Although the risks for children are unknown, clinicians should be aware of this potentially destructive condition. There is no concurrence regarding the optimal bisphosphonate drug in children, dosage or duration of treatment. The more serious side effects linked to bisphosphonates in adults, such as uveitis, thrombocytopenia or oesophageal or oral ulcerations, are rare in children. Potent bisphosphonates have established therapeutic half-lives of over 8 years, so there may be long-term, low to very low, residual risk of MRONJ in these patients.

Adolescents and young adults requiring bisphosphonate therapy, particularly in the setting of malignancy, may also be at increased risk of MRONJ, and caution needs to be applied in the undertaking of extractions and oral and periodontal surgery in this patient group. Currently there is no cure for MRONJ.

Nephrology

ACUTE KIDNEY INJURY

Acute kidney injury (AKI) is currently the preferred term instead of acute renal failure, as it reflects better on the continuum of renal dysfunction rather than the end stage of failed kidney function. AKI is the sudden loss of kidney function caused by decreased glomerular filtration rate (GFR), retention of urea and other nitrogenous waste products, and dysregulation of extracellular volume and electrolytes. AKI has a multifactorial aetiology and is commonly classified by anatomical location:

- Prenal AKI: associated with reduced renal perfusion because of hypovolemia, or decreased effective arterial volume (in heart failure, sepsis, or cirrhosis).
- Intrinsic AKI: caused by injury to the renal parenchyma (in prolonged hypoperfusion, sepsis, nephrotoxins, or severe glomerular diseases).
- Postrenal AKI: develops from anatomic obstructions to the lower urinary tract.

Clinical manifestations of paediatric AKI range from a minimal elevation in serum creatinine to renal failure. Signs and symptoms owing to impaired renal function include oedema, reduced urine output, gross haematuria and/or hypertension. Laboratory findings indicative for AKI include elevated serum creatinine, hyperkalaemia, serum sodium abnormalities, metabolic acidosis, hypocalcaemia and hyperphosphatemia. The diagnosis is based on history, signs and symptoms of renal impairment, laboratory findings, renal imaging and rarely a kidney biopsy.

Acute exacerbation of chronic kidney disease (CKD) is typically the differential diagnosis of AKI.

CHRONIC KIDNEY DISEASE

Irreversible renal damage and/or reduced kidney function that continuously decreases over time. The aetiology is associated with a heterogeneous group of conditions:

- Congenital renal disease (60% of cases): obstructive uropathy, renal hypoplasia and renal dysplasia.
- Glomerular disorders: more common in children over 12 years of age.
- CKD clinical presentation varies depending on severity of kidney impairment and type of underlying disorder:

In early CKD stages, patients are asymptomatic. Cases are identified by elevated serum creatinine for age, abnormal urinalysis or image detection of kidney disease.

- Moderate to severe CKD cases may manifest with poor growth.
- Severe CKD cases may present with signs and symptoms of uremia (weakness, fatigue, anorexia, or vomiting).
- CKD is classified with regard to the level of kidney function.

Complications of CKD include abnormal fluid and electrolyte levels, mineral and bone disorders, anaemia, cardiovascular risk factors (e.g., hypertension), endocrine disorders, growth impairment, hyperuricemia and uremia.

Diagnosis is based on patient history (age at onset of symptoms, duration of symptoms, clinical features), risk factors (family history, congenital kidney and/or urinary tract anomalies) and physical examination (measurement of growth parameters, blood pressure, cardiovascular assessment, examination of the extremities for bony deformities and oedema).

Laboratory testing (serum creatinine, electrolytes, complete blood count, urinalysis and quantification of urinary protein by a urine protein to creatinine ratio) can determine the stage of renal impairment and detect the development of potential complications. Ultrasonography is used to assess the growth and structure of the kidneys. CKD is typically progressive and can lead to end-stage renal disease.

Renal osteodystrophy

Childhood CKD is associated with early development of abnormalities in bone metabolism. Failure of timely management will lead to renal osteodystrophy and CKD-mineral and bone disorder. Renal osteodystrophy has several pathologic manifestations including osteitis fibrosa cystica, adynamic bone disease, osteomalacia and mixed osteodystrophy.

Management depends on the child's level of kidney function and focuses on prevention of phosphate retention and hypovitaminosis D, as they are main contributors to secondary hyperparathyroidism.

End-stage renal failure and renal replacement therapy

End-stage renal disease (ESRD) in children is defined when their glomerular filtration rate (GFR) falls under 15 mL/min per 1.73 m² and persists for more than 3 months. Causes of paediatric ESRF include congenital kidney and urinary tract malformations (40%), glomerular disorders (25%) and genetic renal diseases (15%). Acquired glomerular disease is the predominant aetiology in later age. Renal replacement therapy involves kidney transplantation, haemodialysis (HD) and peritoneal dialysis. Management decisions vary with respect to the patient's age and available resources.

- Paediatric patients on HD require easy and reliable vascular access and often have an arteriovenous fistula placed.
- For very small children (weight <15 kg), a central venous catheter is provided for HD.
- Complications of chronic dialysis include malnutrition, poor growth, mineral and bone disorders, anaemia, increased risk of neurodevelopmental and psychosocial impairment, IE and cardiovascular disease.
- Renal transplantation is the treatment of choice for children, as it is associated with superior patient survival rates and better growth and developmental outcomes compared with chronic dialysis.
- Children frequently undergo preemptive transplantation (CKD stage 4, avoiding dialysis) from a living related donor.
- With living donors, graft survival is reported to be greater compared with deceased donor allografts.
- Paediatric renal transplant recipients have better survival rates than adults. The major causes of death are infection and cardiopulmonary disease.
- After successful renal transplantation, most children have improved growth, and a catch-up growth is also observed. Factors limiting growth are poor renal allograft function and corticosteroid therapy.
- Transplant recipients have a long-term risk of complications (hypertension, cardiovascular disease, recurrent infection, malignancy, type 2 diabetes, mineral-bone disorders, surgical sequelae and recurrence of the primary disease).

Oral and dental considerations

Soft tissues

- Oral mucosa may appear pale because of reduced erythropoietin (anaemia).
- Ecchymosis, petechiae and haemorrhages may be observed owing to:
  - Alteration in platelet aggregations (consequence of uremia).
  - Patients on HD may be receiving anticoagulants (heparin).
  - The HD machine destroys platelets.
- Uremic stomatitis is common in advanced renal failure patients with blood urea nitrogen levels over 300 mg/mL.
- Mucositis and glossitis can be present.

- 'Uremic frost' may present intraorally (otherwise appears on skin); white patches from urea crystal perspiration on epithelial surfaces (can be seen with dry mouth).
- Bacterial and candida infections (uremia may lead to suppression of lymphocytic responses and cell-mediated immunity).
- Gingival overgrowth is a drug-induced response in patients taking immunosuppressants (post renal transplantation) and/or calcium channel blockers to control blood pressure.
- Periodontal health may be affected by the high level of calculus accumulation, common in renal patients.
- Calculus is a product of precipitation of calcium-phosphorus and calcium oxalate; facilitated by the elevated pH, decreased salivary magnesium and high levels of salivary urea and phosphorus.

Patients may complain of:

- Pain, infection/inflammation.
- Altered (dysgeusia) or metallic taste (uremic fetor).
- Dry mouth: caused by the adverse effects of medication, reduced fluid intake and low salivary flow rate.
- Bad breath (uremic breath): consequence of the high salivary concentration of urea (converted to ammonia) and changes in the phosphate, protein concentrations and in the salivary pH.

Hard tissues

- Developmental dental hard tissue defects are associated with systemic disturbances because of disruptions of calcium, phosphorus or vitamin D metabolism in early life (Figure 12.15).
- Pulp canal narrowing/calcifications (pulp stones).
- Delayed eruption of the permanent teeth.
- Caries experience appears to be lower in this patient population because of the highly buffered and alkaline saliva (elevated urea and phosphate concentrations).

Renal osteodystrophy and compensatory hyperparathyroidism. Lytic lesions of the mandible or maxilla, known as brown tumours, can also occur in severe renal failure because of secondary hyperparathyroidism. Histologically, these lesions are similar to giant cell tumours and usually resolve following correction of hypocalcaemia and hyperphosphataemia with vitamin D metabolites. Hypocalcaemia occurs because of increased phosphate retention and decreased calcium absorption. Active calcium absorption from the gut depends on the presence of the active metabolite, 25-hydroxy-cholecalciferol (vitamin D_3). However, vitamin D metabolism is impaired because of failure of the hydroxylation of 25-hydroxy-cholecalciferol to 1,25-dihydroxy-cholecalciferol in the diseased kidney. In an attempt to raise serum calcium, there is a secondary hyperparathyroidism, and calcium is removed from bone stores, giving rise to the characteristic radiographic appearance of renal osteodystrophy.

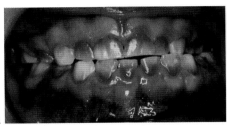 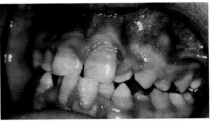

A   B

Figure 12.15 Effects of renal disease on teeth. (A) Yellow-brown discoloration of primary teeth. (B) Yellow discoloration and enamel hypoplasia in an adolescent. (Courtesy Prof. Marcio da Fonseca.)

Other dental changes include:

- Decreased trabeculation, demineralization, 'ground-glass' bone appearance.
- Decreased cortical bone thickness.
- Loss of lamina dura.
- Radiolucent giant cell lesions.
- Brown tumours (commonly in the maxilla).
- Skeletal base enlargement.
- Metastatic soft tissue calcifications.
- Increased risk of jaw fracture.
- Increased tooth mobility.
- Abnormal bone healing of extraction sockets (deposition of sclerotic bone around the socket).

Dental management

- Consultation with the medical provider to determine:
  - Immune status, susceptibility to infection, management of bacteremia from dental interventions (need for antibiotic prophylaxis).
  - Risk of excessive bleeding, especially in patients undergoing HD (anticoagulant therapy and maintained vascular access).
- Rigorous prevention, early diagnosis and prompt treatment of oral conditions.
- For patients on HD, elective dental procedures should be performed on the day after dialysis (having eliminated circulating toxins, high intravascular volume, less patient fatigue, less heparin circulating).
- Nephrotoxic medication should be avoided, and therapeutic agents that metabolize through the kidneys should be prescribed with dose reduction.
- Patients on long-term corticosteroids (nephrotic syndrome) may require supplemental corticosteroid cover to avoid adrenal crisis.

Dialysis

Children receiving dialysis often exhibit somatic growth retardation and have bleeding tendencies because of increased capillary fragility and mechanical destruction of platelets by the dialysis machine, which leads to thrombocytopenia. In addition, children on HD receive anticoagulation with IV heparin and can experience other complications such as infection of the port site and increased risk of hepatitis. In children receiving peritoneal dialysis, complications can occur with catheter placement, including peritonitis and exit-site infections. However, peritoneal dialysis is easier to manage in children, requiring less time for the fluid exchange, less restriction of food and fluid intake, and fewer haemodynamic problems compared with HD.

- Children on HD and anticoagulant therapy can be successfully managed with pretreatment DDAVP and antibiotic prophylaxis to prevent infection of the access device.
- Any dental treatment, especially extractions, should be performed the day after dialysis when the heparin is no longer active (heparin half-life is 4 hours, but residual effects can occur for 24 hours).
- Sockets should be packed with a haemostatic agent and sutured well. Platelet transfusions are to be avoided if possible.
- Children on continuous ambulatory peritoneal dialysis can be managed more conservatively.

Drug interactions

Drug interactions can occur in children with ESRF who are managed with long-term antihypertensives and steroids. Medications that are metabolized in the kidney or nephrotoxic should be avoided in children with renal insufficiency. These include:

- Cefalotin (cephalothin).
- Paracetamol (acetaminophen).
- Nonsteroidal antiinflammatory agents.
- Tetracycline.

Dentists should also be aware that renal excretion of drugs is also impaired and their half-life may be extended. However, if children are adequately haemodialysed, it may be necessary to increase dosage of drugs to obtain the necessary pharmacological effect. Adjustment of a drug dosage as well as timing of intake should be made in consultation with the child's nephrologist.

Gastroenterology

BILIARY ATRESIA

Two congenital conditions are responsible for the majority of children requiring liver transplantation, namely biliary atresia and α_1-antitrypsin deficiency. Biliary atresia is a progressive, idiopathic, fibro-obliterative disorder with obstructed extrahepatic biliary tree, manifested exclusively in the neonatal period. The overall incidence is low; approximately 1 : 10 000 to 20 000 live births. It is the most common cause of neonatal jaundice and the most common indication for liver transplantation in children (60%–80% of patients with biliary atresia will eventually require a transplant). Typically, infants are born full-term, healthy. By 8 weeks of age, signs of generalized jaundice (scleral icterus, acholic stools, dark urine, firm liver and splenomegaly) develop. Ideally, surgical intervention (hepatoportoenterostomy or Kasai procedure) should be done before 60 days of age.

- Associated with risk for fat-soluble vitamin deficiencies.
- Affected infants are typically given high-calorie formula and nutritional supplements to sustain normal rates of growth. Nasogastric feed may also be required.
- Cases with persistent jaundice 3 months after the Kasai procedure, failure to thrive, complications of portal hypertension and progressive liver dysfunction are indicated for liver transplantation.

α_1-Antitrypsin deficiency

- Deficiency in hepatic secretion of α_1-globulin.
- Leads to progressive hepatomegaly and cirrhosis.
- Treated by liver transplantation.

Liver function tests

- These include serum aminotransferases, bilirubin, alkaline phosphatase, albumin and PT.
- Serum aminotransferases are nonspecific and are elevated in most liver diseases.
- FBC and coagulation profile should be routinely checked.
- Albumin (a decrease may reflect impaired protein synthesis).

HEPATITIS

Hepatitis A virus infection

Hepatitis A virus (HAV) spreads via the faecal–oral route and has an incubation period of 15 to 50 days. This is seen in children as an acute, self-limited illness manifested with:

- Nonspecific symptoms: fever, malaise, anorexia, vomiting, nausea, abdominal pain/discomfort and diarrhoea.
- Jaundice (conjugated hyperbilirubinemia): usually occurs 1 week after onset of symptoms.
- Mild hepatomegaly.

- Choluria (bilirubin in the urine) and aminotransferases are also elevated in the prodromal period.
- Only 30% of children under 6 years of age develop symptomatic hepatitis, which often lasts less than 2 weeks.

Acute liver failure is rare, affecting less than 1% of all cases. The diagnosis is made by the detection of serum anti-HAV IgM (positive at the onset of symptoms, peaks during the acute phase and remains for approximately 4 to 6 months). Hepatitis A vaccine is part of the recommended childhood and adolescent immunization schedule and is also recommended for international travellers and patients with chronic liver disease. Postexposure prophylaxis may be done with the HAV vaccine or immune globulin.

Hepatitis B virus infection

There are around 250 million hepatitis B virus (HBV) chronic carriers (positive for hepatitis B surface antigen) in the world, and almost 600 000 of them die of related liver disease yearly. Effective vaccination programs have led to a significant decrease in the incidence of new HBV.

Clinical manifestations of HBV infection:
- Acute phase: ranging from subclinical or anicteric hepatitis to icteric hepatitis and, in some cases, fulminant hepatitis.
- Chronic phase: manifestations vary from an asymptomatic carrier state to chronic hepatitis, cirrhosis, and hepatocellular carcinoma.
- Extrahepatic manifestations also can occur with both acute and chronic infection.

HBV is carried in blood and other body fluids (saliva, tears, semen and vaginal secretions). Ways of transmission include parenteral contact, sexual intercourse or infection of the baby at birth from an infected mother. Vaccination against HBV before an exposure is the best prevention and it is recommended for newborns in most countries.

Interpretation of hepatitis B test results
- If the HBsAg test is positive the blood is automatically tested for the 'e' antigen. If 'e' is negative, the patient is a chronic healthy carrier.
- If the 'e' antigen is positive, the patient is a chronic active carrier.

Chronic healthy carrier (HBsAg +ve, e −ve)
- The degree of infectivity of these patients, although significant, is thought to be less than that of chronic active carriers. The liver function test for this patient should be normal.

Chronic active carrier (HBsAg +ve, e +ve)
- The chronic active carrier has active viral replication and is very infective. These patients have active liver disease, and their liver function may be abnormal.
- It is important to liaise directly with the patient's doctor in the first instance when planning dental treatment and to do so again at regular intervals.

Hepatitis C virus infection

- There is a lower prevalence in children than in adults, and perinatal transmission is by far the most common source of hepatitis C virus (HCV) in children.
- HCV generally progresses slowly in children, and serious consequences (cirrhosis or hepatocellular carcinoma) are rare during childhood.
- Infant HCV (acquired by transfusion or perinatal transmission) may clear spontaneously (20–45%).

- Acute HCV infection in children may be under-recognized, as fulminant disease course is rare. Generally, patients are observed for 6 to 8 weeks to determine for spontaneous clearance. Treatment is considered only for those with persistent viremia.
- In adults, direct-acting antiviral agents have been successfully used and are expected to transform treatment in children in near future.

PAEDIATRIC ACUTE LIVER FAILURE

Paediatric acute liver failure is a complex, rapidly progressive clinical syndrome. Manifestations include nonspecific prodromal period (abdominal discomfort, malaise with or without fever) and symptoms of jaundice, encephalopathy and hepatomegaly. Aetiology is variable depending on the age group and includes:

- Unknown/idiopathic.
- Dose-related medications: paracetamol (acetaminophen), isoniazid, halothane, propylthio-uracil and anticonvulsant drugs including valproate.
- Infectious diseases (e.g., hepatitis A, herpes simplex virus).
- Autoimmune hepatitis.
- Wilson disease: most common metabolic condition associated with PALF in children over 5 years of age.

GASTROEOSOPHAGEAL REFLUX DISEASE

Gastroeosophageal reflux (GOR) associated with regurgitation is common in infants and typically resolves by 18 months of age. Gastroeosophageal reflux disease (GORD) is GOR with pathological complications. Signs and symptoms of GORD include:

- Recurrent regurgitation that continues beyond 2 years of age.
- Refusal of food (solids).
- Frequent complaints of heartburn.
- Dysphagia.
- Progressive asthma (not responsive to standard therapy).
- Recurrent pneumonia.
- Chronic hoarseness or stridor.

It is important to recognize that many children may have quite asymptomatic but severe GORD.

Diagnosis can be done empirically based on history and physical examination, using barium contrast radiography to exclude anatomical abnormalities, endoscopy and histology.

- Oesophageal pH monitoring, bronchoalveolar lavage, nuclear scintigraphy or oesophageal manometry is useful in specific clinical situations.
- Endoscopic evaluation identifies esophagitis, which is typically caused by GORD. Eosinophilic esophagitis should be ruled out.
- The relationship of GORD with asthma is not clear.

Management is case specific and may include:

- Antacids or histamine type 2 receptor antagonists for short-term relief of symptoms.
- Lifestyle changes including weight management in overweight patients, elevation of the head at night and avoidance of food that exacerbate symptoms (chocolate, caffeine, spicy foods).
- Prokinetic agents improving gastric emptying.
- Antireflux surgery (Nissen fundoplication).

COELIAC DISEASE

Coeliac disease (CD) is a genetically determined sensitivity to dietary gluten and related proteins contained in wheat, barley and rye associated with immune-mediated inflammatory changes of the small intestinal mucosa. The estimated prevalence is less than 1% of the general population. Morphological improvement of the small intestinal mucosa occurs with a gluten-free diet usually within a few weeks to months. CD reoccurs if gluten is reintroduced. The prevalence of CD is higher in patients with Down syndrome, type 1 diabetes mellitus (T1DM), selective IgA deficiency, autoimmune thyroid disease and Turner and Williams syndromes. Signs and symptoms include:

- Malabsorption: diarrhoea, steatorrhea, weight loss.
- Nutrient, vitamin and iron deficiency.
- Histologic changes (including villous atrophy) on small intestinal biopsy.
- Resolution of symptoms and mucosal lesions with gluten-free diet.
- Non-GI manifestations: dermatitis herpetiformis, delayed growth and pubertal development, neurologic disease, behavioural symptoms, arthritis, dental enamel defects, liver disease.
- CD is associated with hyposplenism.

Diagnosis is confirmed with serologic testing (positive transglutaminase-IgA antibodies and antiendomysial antibodies), endoscopy and biopsy.

Treatment: most cases respond well to strict gluten-free diet, including avoidance of any wheat, rye and barley products. Compliance is very important for successful outcomes.

INFLAMMATORY BOWEL DISEASE

Inflammatory bowel disease is comprised of two distinct disorders: Crohn's disease and ulcerative colitis (UC). It has a peak incidence between the ages of 15 and 30 years.

Crohn's disease

Crohn's disease is an immune-mediated inflammatory disease that causes transmural inflammation of any portion of the intestinal tract but typically involves the ileum, ileum and cecum, or ileum and entire colon. The incidence is approximately 5 to 10 new cases per 100 000 individuals per year, and up to 25% of the cases are in children under 18 years of age. The aetiology and pathophysiology are poorly understood; however, both genetic and environmental factors may be implicated. Signs and symptoms include:

- Intestinal manifestations: abdominal pain, weight loss, diarrhoea and haematochezia
- Extraintestinal manifestations:
  - Skin, eyes, joints, hepatobiliary and respiratory systems.
  - Oral lesions (Table 12.4) occur in up to 40% of children: muco-gingivitis, aphthous ulcers, swelling, fissures and oral Crohn's disease (oral chronic granulomatous disease).
  - Nutritional deficiency.
  - Growth failure affects 30% of children and adolescents.
  - Significant perianal disease (fistulae, skin tags, abscesses).

Treatment decisions require assessment and monitoring of disease location and activity.

- Magnetic resonance imaging, upper endoscopy and colonoscopy with biopsies for treat-to-target approach.
- Radiolabelled white cell count.
- Therapeutic medication: different regiments depending on disease severity including glucocorticoids, aminosalicylates, immunomodulators (azathioprine, 6-mercaptopurine, methotrexate), antitumour necrosis factor drugs or combination therapy.

TABLE 12.4 ■ **Oral manifestations of Crohn's disease and inflammatory bowel disease**

Specific findings	Nonspecific findings
• Indurated tag-like lesions	• Aphthous stomatitis
• Cobblestoning of mucosa	• Pyostomatitis vegetans
• Mucogingivitis	• Angular cheilitis
• Linear ulcerations	• Persistent submandibular lymphadenopathy
• Mucosal polyps	• Recurrent buccal abscesses
	• Perioral erythema with scaling
	• Glossitis

Management:
- Oral lesions: topical prednisolone syrup may be helpful.
- Lip lesions: 0.1% triamcinolone application.
- Comprehensive health care: monitoring growth and nutritional status, infection risk, psychological issues and cancer surveillance.

Ulcerative colitis

This is an immune mediated inflammatory disease that affects the mucosal layer of the colon and rectum that mainly affects teenagers but can also occur earlier in life. Clinical presentation may vary:
- Mild to moderate UC: diarrhoea (frequently containing blood), weakness, anaemia, abdominal pain and sometimes weight loss.
- Acute severe UC: severe abdominal pain, haematochezia, tenesmus, fever, leukocytosis and hypoalbuminemia.

Treatment: similar to Crohn disease.

Oral and dental considerations

Liver disease
- Intrinsic green discoloration of teeth, alveolar bone and oral mucosa owing to biliverdin, the oxidation product of the bilirubin molecule (Figure 12.16).
- Hard tooth structures and/or groups of teeth forming after liver graft or postjaundice resolution develop normally (i.e., are not discoloured).
- Treatment of discoloured teeth depends on the patient's aesthetic concern. Incisors can be managed with vital bleaching (limited results if dentin is pigmented), direct or indirect composite resin restorations/veneers and porcelain veneers/crowns after full skeletal growth is achieved.

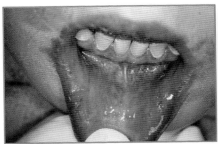 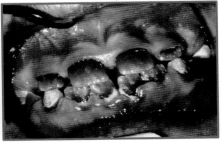

A   B

Figure 12.16   Effects of liver disease in the oral cavity. (A) Jaundiced oral tissues in a child with history of biliary atresia. (B) Green tooth pigmentation and poor periodontal health in a 12 year-old girl with history of severe liver disease. (Courtesy Prof. Marcio da Fonseca.)

- Developmental enamel defects (hypoplasia/hypomineralization) are not specific for liver disease and can present as a feature to any other severe systemic disturbances.
- Dental treatment aims to address aesthetic concerns in incisors (composite resin restorations/veneers) and rehabilitate structural defects of the affected teeth (resin restorations, stainless steel crowns).

Dental caries risk may be increased in children with liver disease because of:

- A diet high in calories and sugar, especially in patients with biliary atresia.
- Frequent administration of sweetened liquid medicines.
- Overwhelming demand for medical care may prevent families from following rigorous dental prevention.

Dental management:

- Always consult with the patient's physician before doing dental procedures.
- Coagulation disorders may be associated with liver disease and lead to prolonged bleeding.
- Therapy with antifibrinolytic medication, vitamin K and fresh frozen plasma.
- Effective local measures after tooth extractions should be implemented, including socket packing with clot-inducing materials (e.g., oxidized cellulose polymer, gelatin sponge).
- Ingestion of blood during dental care may increase the risk for hepatic coma; thus, using high-speed suction should be prevented.
- Amide local anaesthetic solutions (e.g., xylocaine) that metabolize in the liver should have dose reduction.

LIVER AND OTHER SOLID ORGAN TRANSPLANTATION

A pretransplant dental assessment is essential to reduce the risk of oral complications following organ transplant and immunosuppression. The presence of dental caries and oral infections will necessitate delay in transplantation until all potential foci of infection are eliminated. Comprehensive dental treatment and institution of a rigorous preventive program are recommended before transplant to reduce the risk of subsequent oral diseases. Antibiotic prophylaxis as per the protocol for prevention of IE may be used before invasive surgical procedures in patients who are immunodepressed.

Delayed eruption:

- Immunosuppressive therapy: corticosteroid therapy may contribute to slow growth and skeletal maturation, as well as delayed eruption of permanent teeth.
- Gingival overgrowth (medication and plaque-induced) may occur, leading to tooth emergence issues.

Gingival overgrowth:

- Immunosuppressants (e.g., cyclosporine) and calcium channel blockers (e.g., nifedipine) are known to cause medication-induced gingival overgrowth.
- Gingival irritants, including dental plaque, calculus, orthodontic appliances, dental restoration defects and mouth breathing can increase its severity.
- The severity of manifestation is greater in adolescents possibly because of the added effects of estrogenic, progesterone and growth hormone (GH).

Management:

- Achieving and maintaining excellent oral hygiene.
- Chemical plaque control with chlorhexidine.
- Metronidazole and azithromycin are known to reduce gingival overgrowth.
- Surgical excision (gingivectomy) or gingival recontouring (gingivoplasty) may be indicated in severe cases.
- If possible, change to immunosuppressive medications (mycophenolate mofetil, tacrolimus) that have fewer effects on gingival tissues.

Dental management considerations

Before liver transplantation:
- Intensive oral hygiene therapy and preventive care to reduce the risk of infection.
- Comprehensive dental care.

After liver transplantation:
- Regular and routine dental care after physician authorizes (usually 6 months posttransplant), with rigorous caries prevention.
- Head and neck cancer surveillance: long-term use of immunosuppressive drugs is associated with risk of cancer.

Inflammatory bowel disease and coeliac disease

The role of the paediatric dentist is potential recognition of oral manifestations in undiagnosed asymptomatic patients and early medical referral for evaluation.

Oral manifestations in CD include:
- Developmental enamel defects.
- Recurrent aphthous ulceration/stomatitis.
- Angular cheilitis.
- Atrophic glossitis.

Endocrinology

TYPE 1 DIABETES MELLITUS

T1DM or insulin-dependent diabetes mellitus is the most common form of diabetes in children It is an insulin deficiency caused by destruction of the pancreatic beta cells. It comprises approximately 75% of all cases of diabetes in patients under 19 years of age.
- The incidence varies worldwide from 0.1 to 65 per 100 000 children under 15 years of age.
- Two age peaks of T1DM: 4 to 6 years and 10 to 14 years.
- Although no exact triggers have been identified, it is suggested that exposure to environmental factors may cause the disease in genetically susceptible individuals.
- Classic signs and symptoms result from hyperglycaemia:
  Polyuria, polydipsia, weight loss and lethargy.
  Diabetic ketoacidosis: often an initial presentation in children under 6 years of age.

The diagnosis is based upon detected abnormalities of glucose metabolism:
- Fasting plasma glucose of 126 mg/dL or higher (7 mmol/L) on at least two occasions.
- Symptoms of hyperglycaemia and a plasma glucose of 200 mg/dL or higher (11.1 mmol/L).
- Plasma glucose of 200 mg/dL or higher (11.1 mmol/L) measured 2 hours after a standard glucose load in an oral glucose tolerance test.
- History or presence of prolonged candida infection should prompt screening for T1DM with blood and urine glucose concentrations.

Insulin therapy is the mainstay of treatment:
- Rapid-acting and/or short-acting insulins: administered 5 to 15 minutes before meals for the rapid-acting type and 20 to 30 minutes before meals for the short-acting type.
- Intermediate-acting Neutral Protamine Hagedorn insulin: given in a targeted manner in combination with long-acting insulins (given before breakfast will cover lunch).
- Long-acting insulin: given once or twice a day.
- Intensive insulin therapy combines a basal level of insulin together with premeal boluses of a rapid-acting insulin. This regimen can be delivered by two methods:
  - Injections of a long-acting insulin analogue once or twice daily and rapid- or short-acting insulin before each eating.

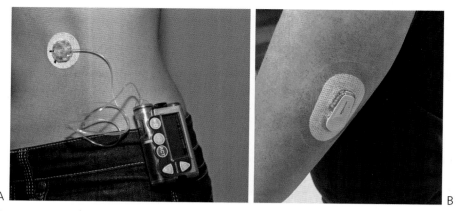

Figure 12.17 (A) An insulin pump showing the position of the subcutaneous canula, usually sited in the abdomen. The pump can be programmed to deliver a basal level of insulin and bolus doses as required with meals mimicking the function of the pancreas. (B) A wireless glucose sensor that provides continuous monitoring of blood glucose level, the data linking to a smart phone.

- Insulin pump to deliver a continuous subcutaneous infusion of a rapid- or short-acting insulin, supplemented by boluses before eating.
- Blood glucose monitoring is required for optimal glycaemic control:
  Fingersticks (at least four times daily)
  Devices for continuous glucose monitoring (Figure 12.17).

Dental implications

Patients with diabetes and their families are at increased risk for psychological disorders, such as depression and anxiety, which result in poor glycaemic control. Addressing these psychosocial issues improves glycaemic control.

Well-controlled diabetic children. Patients with well-controlled diabetes need no or minimal modifications to dental care and can receive dental treatment in the usual way, except when a general anaesthetic is required. The best measure of control is the level of glycosylated haemoglobin (HbA_{1c}). The target for most children is a value of less than 6.5% (≤53 mmol/mol).

- For routine dental appointments, the child should eat a normal meal before the dental procedure, although a glucose source should always be available to treat hypoglycaemia.
- Fasting before a general anaesthetic requires careful blood glucose monitoring and adjustment of insulin doses during the fasting period. This is to prevent extremes of hyper- and hypoglycaemia. Insulin doses and the possibility of IV fluid therapy should be discussed with the child's treating paediatrician/endocrinologist.
- Postsurgical healing can be delayed, particularly if blood glucose control is suboptimal and oral sepsis can be an additional risk.
- It is often possible to manage many T1DM children requiring GA in day-stay facilities, provided that children can begin taking fluids shortly after their procedure. Other children may require admission to a paediatric hospital, with a dextrose and insulin infusion set-up to maintain blood sugar levels (BSLs) and avoid complications during the fasting and postoperative periods. It is obviously essential to liaise with the treating endocrinologist.

Poorly controlled diabetic children. Severe and poorly controlled disease may present with xerostomia, burning mouth and/or tongue, candida infection, altered taste, dental caries, progressive periodontal disease, oral neuropathies, parotid enlargement, sialosis and delayed wound healing. Periodontal disease is a consequence of impaired leukocyte function, microvascular changes (gingiva and alveolar mucosa) and abnormal collagen metabolism.

Dental management

- Pain and infection can increase insulin resistance; hence, prompt management of orofacial infections is important.
- Dental anxiety and stress can cause rapid metabolic changes leading to blood glucose elevation; monitoring of blood glucose levels before and after invasive dental treatment is required for adequate insulin supplementation.
- Short dental visits with appropriate timing (should not interfere with diet and insulin control) are preferable.

Diabetic emergencies

Hypoglycaemia (levels of blood glucose <2.2 mmol/L): triggered by reduced glucose supply to the brain.
- Initial presentation: anxiety, pallor, nausea, sweating, tremor, tachycardia, palpitations, visual disturbance and perioral tingling.
- Further progression: confusion, irrational and/or aggressive behaviour, slurred speech, coma.
- Conscious patient: prompt oral administration of glucose is advised (50 g drink, tablets or gel).
- Uncooperative or unconscious patients require administration of 1 mg (1 unit) intramuscular (IM) glucagon.
- Vital signs should be monitored.
- Typically, full recovery is achieved within 15 minutes. Emergency services should be called if the recovery is delayed.

Hyperglycaemia: caused by insulin deficiency, usually develops slowly over several hours.
- Signs and symptoms include thirst, drowsiness, weak pulse, blurred vision, hypotension.
- Acidosis may develop additionally, leading to deep breathing.
- Ketosis (breath smell of acetone).
- Requires medical attention and administration of insulin and correction of the respiratory and metabolic acidosis.

Important points

- Administration of insulin in hypoglycaemia can lead to brain damage and death.
- If glucose is given to a hyperglycaemic patient, the condition will not improve and can be used as a diagnostic test (if blood glucose cannot be measured).
- The accuracy of glucometers may not be accurate at high BSLs (>20 mmol/L).

TYPE 2 DIABETES MELLITUS

Characterized by hyperglycemia, insulin resistance and relative impairment in insulin secretion. The incidence has increased in younger patients, linked to the rise in childhood obesity. Management of type 2 diabetes mellitus includes maintenance of glycaemic control and treatment of comorbidities.

PITUITARY DISORDERS

Hypopituitarism

Hypopituitarism (complete or partial) may be either congenital or secondary to pituitary or hypothalamic disease (tumours, infections, trauma or after exposure to ionizing radiation). These children need to be managed in conjunction with a paediatric endocrinologist to prevent potentially serious complications of pituitary hormone deficiency.

Deficiency of the hormones of the anterior pituitary:

- Adrenocorticotropic hormone (ACTH) deficiency results in cortisol deficiency.
- Thyroid-stimulating hormone (TSH) deficiency (secondary/central hypothyroidism) has similar manifestations as those of primary hypothyroidism.
- Deficient secretion of the gonadotropins follicle-stimulating hormone and luteinizing hormone results in hypogonadotropic (secondary) hypogonadism.
- GH deficiency in children typically presents as short stature.

Pituitary hormone excess

Overproduction of GH in childhood before the fusion of the epiphyseal growth plates leads to elevated levels of serum GH and insulin-like growth factor 1 and causes accelerated and excessive linear growth (pituitary gigantism). The same process in adulthood (acromegaly) has no effect on height. It can present as a feature in genetic syndromes, such as McCune–Albright syndrome, multiple endocrine neoplasia types 1 and 4, the paraganglioma-pheochromocytoma-pituitary adenoma association and Carney complex. Diagnosis is based on clinical findings, bone radiographs, thyroid function tests, sex steroid hormone concentrations and a karyotype.

Dental implications

- Precocious and accelerated development of the craniofacial skeleton.
- Prognathism.
- Accelerated dental development and eruption.

Dental management

Dental management of patients with pituitary disorders focuses mainly on the management of the associated craniofacial malformations. Treatment needs to be planned carefully and coordinated in a multidisciplinary setting. No contraindications exist for comprehensive dental healthcare, but the treating endocrinologist must be consulted before any invasive treatment or GA.

THYROID DISORDERS

Hypothyroidism

Congenital primary hypothyroidism. One of the most common preventable causes of intellectual disability worldwide (1:2000 to 1:4000 newborns). Untreated congenital hypothyroidism leading to severe developmental delay (cretinism) is rare in those countries where neonatal testing is performed (TSH with or without fT4) and treatment with synthetic thyroxine started in the first 1 to 2 weeks of life. Almost 85% of the cases are sporadic, typically caused by thyroid dysgenesis. Timing of diagnosis and treatment are critical because delayed treatment results in lower intelligence. Newborn screening programs occur in most countries.

Central hypothyroidism. Caused by defects in the production of TSH in the CNS because of hypothalamic or pituitary dysfunction.

Acquired hypothyroidism. This is the most common disturbance of thyroid function in children typically caused by autoimmune thyroiditis. It leads to short stature, poor pubertal and intellectual development and goitre.

Diagnosis is based on physical examination, laboratory findings (serum free T4 and TSH) and testing for antithyroid peroxidase antibodies and antithyroglobulin antibodies (autoimmune aetiology).

Treatment objective is to restore normal growth and development:

- Symptomatic cases: replacement therapy with levothyroxine.
- Subclinical cases: T4 therapy.

Once growth and pubertal development are complete, thyroid hormone treatment can be discontinued and thyroid function re-evaluated. Side effects of therapy include temporary behaviour symptoms and poor school achievement. Delayed therapy may not restore full growth potential in children.

Dental implications of untreated or suboptimally treated hypothyroidism

- Decreased vertical facial growth.
- Decreased cranial base length and flexure, maxillary protrusion and open bite with typical immature facial patterns.
- Delayed eruption of teeth and increased spacing between both primary and permanent teeth.
- Developmental anomalies such as enamel hypoplasia have been reported.
- Mouth breathing and dysgeusia (altered taste).

Hyperthyroidism

Hyperthyroidism can occur because of:

- Autoimmune hyperstimulation of the gland (Graves disease or Hashimoto thyroiditis).
- Inflammatory disorders (subacute thyroiditis).
- Iodine excess.
- Rarely neoplasm.

In children, the most common causes are Graves disease and thyroiditis. Thyrotoxicosis is more common in females and is most likely to appear between 8 and 16 years of age, usually associated with a goitre. Graves disease is caused by autoantibodies that bind to the thyrotropin receptor (TSHR-Ab), stimulating growth of the thyroid and overproduction of thyroid hormone. It is relatively rare, with a frequency of 1 : 10 000 children.

Clinical manifestations. Diffuse goitre, weight loss/failure to gain weight, tachycardia and increased cardiac output, increased GI motility, proximal muscle weakness, tremor, hyperreflexia, sleep disturbance, distractibility with unexplained poor school performance and emotional lability. In children, the disease is associated with modest acceleration of linear growth and epiphyseal maturation.

Management includes antithyroid drug therapy (thionamides), radioactive iodine or thyroidectomy. Lifelong monitoring of thyroid function is recommended, regardless of treatment choice and outcome.

Dental implications

- Accelerated growth and development of the craniofacial complex and skeleton.
- Precocious eruption of teeth.
- Increased susceptibility to caries and periodontal disease, burning mouth syndrome.
- Osteopenia or poor bone mass accrual.

Typical orofacial changes are increased vertical facial height with anterior open bite and mild mandibular prognathism.

Dental management

- In general, a child with well-controlled thyroid disease can undergo dental management similar to any other child. Where possible, thyroid function should be normalized before dental intervention. In the unusual situation where this is not possible, close collaboration with a paediatric endocrinologist is recommended.
- The principal concern in children with thyroid disorders is the increased risk associated with GA. The hypothyroid patient is at risk of extreme delay in emergence from GA.
- If a child with inadequately controlled hyperthyroidism is anaesthetized, there is a risk of precipitating a thyroid storm, a very dangerous condition of tachycardia and acute onset of fever, with possible cardiac failure and death. The untreated patient is also at risk from oral infection or surgical procedures, as a thyroid crisis may be precipitated.
- Rarely, intercurrent infections may precipitate significant worsening of hyperthyroidism. As such, oral infections should be treated aggressively and thyroid function (TSH and fT4) monitored. Rare side effects of antithyroid drugs include parotitis and agranulocytosis, which predispose the patient to bleeding episodes, ulcero-necrotic lesions and chronic oral infections.
- In patients with a poorly controlled condition, severe oral infection, CNS depressants and extensive surgical challenge can precipitate a myxedematous coma (bradycardia, hypothermia, severe hypotension and seizures).

PARATHYROID DISORDERS

Hypoparathyroidism

Parathyroid hormone (PTH), along with vitamin D, regulates serum calcium through direct effects on bone and kidneys and indirect effects on the GI tract. Hypoparathyroidism results from structural or functional deficiencies in the parathyroid glands. In children, it most commonly presents as hypocalcaemia in the neonatal period in association with complex disorders, such as Di George sequence and CATCH22 disorders.

The aetiology of hypoparathyroidism includes:

- Destruction of the parathyroid glands: autoimmune, surgical.
- Abnormal development of the parathyroid gland.
- Altered regulation of PTH production.
- Impaired PTH function.

Hypoparathyroidism results in hypocalcaemia, ranging from mild (perioral numbness, paraesthesia of the hands and feet, muscle cramps) to life-threatening seizures, refractory heart failure and laryngospasm.

Diagnosis is based on history, physical examination and laboratory testing (serum calcium and PTH).

Emergency IV administration of calcium gluconate is indicated for patients with tetany, seizures or markedly prolonged QT intervals on electrocardiogram.

Therapy for chronic hypoparathyroidism includes calcium and vitamin D supplementation.

Pseudohypoparathyroidism

A group of heterogeneous disorders associated with unresponsiveness to PTH in the proximal renal tubules, as well as hypocalcaemia and hyperphosphatemia with elevated PTH concentrations.

Hyperparathyroidism

Primary hyperparathyroididsm is defined as elevated PTH concentration, leading to hypercalcaemia. In majority of cases, the hypercalcaemia is an incidental finding of biochemical screening tests.

Dental implications of untreated hypoparathyroidism

- Circumoral paraesthesia and spasm of the facial muscles have been reported in severe hypocalcaemia.
- Hypoplasia of enamel, wide pulp chambers and pulp calcifications.
- Hypodontia and root anomalies are common clinical findings.
- Tooth eruption can be markedly delayed or arrested.
- Soft tissue calcifications.
- Increased risk of acute and chronic oral candidiasis attributed to associated immune dysfunction.

Dental management

- Because of the increased risk of jaw fractures, atraumatic surgery/extraction techniques should be implemented.
- The possibility of the presence of brown tumours should be considered for correct differential diagnosis.

ADRENAL GLAND DISORDERS

The adrenal cortex produces three major classes of steroid hormones: glucocorticoids, mineralocorticoids and sex hormones. Glucocorticoids (cortisol) have an important role in carbohydrate, fat and protein metabolism; assist in the maintenance of normal blood pressure; and protect the body against stresses of various types. Mineralocorticoids (aldosterone) help maintain salt and water balance through their action on the kidney. Adrenal sex hormones help complement the actions of the gonadal steroids in the development of sexual characteristics and reproductive capability.

Adrenal insufficiency (Addison disease) is an impaired synthesis and release of adrenocortical hormones.

- Primary: intrinsic disease to the adrenal cortex. Patients have deficiencies of one or more hormones produced in the adrenal cortex (glucocorticoids, mineralocorticoids and adrenal androgens). In infants, the most common cause is classic congenital adrenal hyperplasia.
- Central: related to impaired production of ACTH as a result of:
  - Pituitary disease (secondary adrenal insufficiency).
  - Interference with corticotropin-releasing hormone release from the hypothalamus (tertiary adrenal insufficiency).

Clinical symptoms of adrenal insufficiency

- Fatigue, nausea and vomiting, weight loss.
- Anorexia with salt craving.
- Skin hyperpigmentation.
- Mineralocorticoid deficiency, leading to hypotension, dehydration and electrolyte abnormalities.
  - Adrenal crisis with vomiting and diarrhoea, sometimes with severe abdominal pain or unexplained fever, weight loss and anorexia. Low blood cortisol levels may result in an acute adrenal crisis (hypotension and collapse, electrolyte disturbance and hypoglycaemia), which can be precipitated by a relatively minor stress.
- Serum electrolyte abnormalities, such as hyponatremia with or without hyperkalaemia, metabolic acidosis and hypoglycaemia (especially in young children).
- Hypotension or shock, particularly if disproportionate to apparent underlying illness.

Dental management of adrenal insufficiency

- All patients with adrenal insufficiency require glucocorticoid replacement during stressful times: consult with the physician. Glucocorticoid doses must be increased during physiologic stress, using doses ranging from two to four times the replacement dose, depending on the stressor.
- GA sharply increases glucocorticoid requirements, in addition to the stress of surgery itself. Typically, an IV bolus is given at the beginning of surgery, followed by a postoperative regimen.
- Adrenal crisis is a medical emergency that is managed with immediate steroid supplementation. Secondary adrenal insufficiency is caused either by prolonged administration of steroids, resulting in the suppression of endogenous cortisol, or by a central lack of ACTH. Children do not usually present with obvious clinical signs, unless stressed. An adrenal crisis can occur without warning.
- It is important to confirm the diagnosis and medical management with the endocrinologist before commencement of dental treatment. Children with adrenal insufficiency must have a plan for stress glucocorticoid therapy before undertaking dental treatment. Failure to do so may result in serious medical complications for the child. Always consult the patient's specialist endocrine consultant.
- Patients with primary adrenal insufficiency also require mineralocorticoid replacement.

CONGENITAL ADRENAL HYPERPLASIA

One of the most commonly known autosomal recessive disorders, congenital adrenal hyperplasia (CAH) arises when there is an enzymatic block in the complex biosynthetic pathways from cholesterol to cortisol and mineralocorticoid. Females usually present with the condition in the neonatal period showing an ambiguous genitalia. If left untreated, CAH is fatal. Clinical manifestations of classic CAH include one of two clinical syndromes:
- Salt-losing form.
- Simple virilizing form.

Therapy: glucocorticoid and mineralocorticoid replacement.

Adrenocortical hyperfunction

Cushing syndrome refers to a clinical condition characterized by manifestations of adrenocortical hyperfunction, with physical features of growth failure together with weight gain, 'moon facies', truncal obesity, formation of skin striae, hirsutism and poor wound healing. It is caused by a tumour in the pituitary gland secreting ACTH (Cushing disease) or in the adrenal gland, in which case treatment requires removal of the lesion surgically.

Neurology: seizures and epilepsy

Seizure: A transient occurrence of signs and/or symptoms because of abnormal excessive or synchronous neuronal activity in the brain.

Epilepsy: A disease of the brain defined by any of the following conditions:
- At least two unprovoked (or reflex) seizures occurring more than 24 hours apart.
- One unprovoked (or reflex) seizure and a probability of further seizures similar to the general recurrence risk (at least 60%) after two unprovoked seizures, occurring over the next 10 years.
- Diagnosis of an epilepsy syndrome.

Epilepsy syndrome: A cluster of features incorporating seizure types, electroencephalogram (EEG) findings and imaging features that tend to occur together.

TABLE 12.5 ■ **New terms used in the classification of seizures (International League Against Epilepsy, 2017)**

Old terms	New terms
Unconscious	Impaired awareness
Partial	Focal
Simple partial	Focal aware
Complex partial	Focal impaired awareness
Psychic	Cognitive
Secondarily generalized tonic–clonic	Focal to bilateral tonic–clonic
Arrest, freeze, pause, interruption	Behaviour arrest

Status epilepticus: A condition resulting either from the failure of mechanisms responsible for seizure termination or from the initiation of mechanisms, which leads to abnormally prolonged seizures (5 minutes after onset of seizure).

NEW CLASSIFICATION OF SEIZURES

A seizure has been redefined as a disease, not a disorder. A new classification and nomenclature of seizures and epilepsy was published in 2017 replacing some old terms with new descriptors (Table 12.5).

GENERAL CONSIDERATIONS

- The lifetime risk of developing epilepsy is 3.9%, with a slight preponderance of males.
- General recurrence risk after a single unprovoked seizure is about 60%.
- Up to 30% of patients have medically refractory epilepsy.
- Between 35% and 50% of children with epilepsy have psychiatric and behavioural disorders.
- One-third of patients who have seizures also have depression.

PAEDIATRIC SEIZURES AND EPILEPSY

Epilepsy in childhood is a relatively benign disease, often self-terminating, with good or excellent terminal remission after long-term follow-up. The outcome remains poor in 20% to 25% of patients, becoming intractable in 10% to 15% of children.

Febrile seizures are the most common neurologic disorder of childhood. They are defined as seizures occurring in children from 6 months to 5 years of age in association with a fever of 38° C (100.4° F) or higher without evidence of an intracranial cause (infection, head trauma, etc.), another definable cause of seizure or a history of an afebrile seizure.

- Some 30% to 40% of children will have a recurrence during early childhood.
- Benign, self-limiting, no intervention necessary.

DIAGNOSIS

Dependent on history, physical and neurological presentation, lab testing as indicated, EEG and neuroimaging findings.

MANAGEMENT

Most epilepsy treatment remains empirical without clear evidence as to how it works.
Antiepileptic drugs (AEDs):

- The occurrence of a single seizure does not always require initiation of AED.
- Reduce seizures by 30% to 40%, with this effect increasing over time.
- Diazepam rectal gel is used as a rescue medication for breakthrough seizures.

Responsive neurostimulation: In response to abnormal electrical activity, an implanted neurostimu-
lator (vagus nerve stimulator [VNS]) delivers electrical stimulation to the target-onset zone.

Status epilepticus (SE): IM midazolam or IV lorazepam are effective in early treatment.

Other treatments:

- Seizure surgery for intractable epilepsy (anterior temporal lobe resection.
- Ketogenic diets (high-fat, low-carbohydrate, low-protein diet).

LONG-TERM OUTCOMES OF SEIZURES AND EPILEPSY

- Two out of three patients with new-onset epilepsy will eventually enter a 5-year terminal
  remission.
- Mortality rate is higher for children than adults, particularly those with neurodeficits or
  severe epilepsy.
- Poor long-term outcome in relation to seizure control and cognition is seen in epilepsy
  syndromes.
- SE can have long-term sequelae, such as neuronal death, neuronal injury and alteration of
  neuronal networks. After 30 minutes of SE, there is increased risk of irreversible damage.

ORAL AND DENTAL CONSIDERATIONS

The major oro-dental concerns with epileptic children are gingival enlargement (Figure 12.18)
and the precipitation of a seizure in the dental surgery.

DENTAL MANAGEMENT

Management of gingival overgrowth is dependent on medication usage (phenytoin), oral hygiene
and the stage of dental development. In the permanent dentition, full mouth gingivectomy may
be required, but gingival overgrowth will recur if oral hygiene is not optimal and the medication
is not changed.

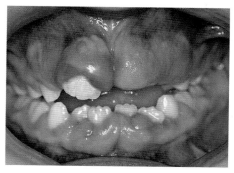

Figure 12.18   Gingival enlargement associated with phenytoin treatment. The initial enlargement is usually
seen in interdental papilla.

Maintenance of adequate oral hygiene may be especially difficult in children with additional intellectual disability and is highly dependent on the motivation and skill of caregivers. The use of chlorhexidine is effective in reducing the inflammatory component of the gingival overgrowth (i.e., biofilm). It is important to always keep the interests of the child in mind, particularly with regard to aggressive surgical treatment that may not benefit the child in the long term.

The general goal of dental management is the avoidance of a seizure. It is important to know the type of epilepsy and any precipitating factors, medications and dosage, compliance and degree of seizure control before commencing treatment. In addition to that, drug interactions with anticonvulsants are common, and their half-life and blood levels can be increased substantially. Consultation with the child's neurologist is essential before commencement of treatment.

The following management protocol is recommended for prevention and control of seizures in the dental surgery:

- Reduce stress to the child by behavioural management.
- Reduce direct overhead lighting, particularly for the photosensitive form of epilepsy.
- Avoid seizure-promoting medications, such as CNS stimulants.
- Emergency drugs such as oxygen, IV or rectal diazepam and IV phenobarbital sodium should be readily available.
- Call the emergency medical services after a seizure lasts more than 3 minutes.
- Prearranged transfer to a paediatric hospital, in case required.

GA is preferable in children with poor seizure control, as the abnormal neural activity is completely ablated during the procedure.

It is important to understand the patient's type of seizures and how well controlled they are.

- There is risk of aspiration of loose teeth, poorly retained appliances and crowns during a seizure.
- Electrocautery may damage the VNS generator; needs to be turned off during electrocautery use.
- Patients with epilepsy are prone to dental trauma during a seizure.
- Phenytoin causes gingival overgrowth, which can worsen with poor oral hygiene.
- Some AEDs may cause dry mouth and mood changes.
- Many patients with seizures may have a ventriculo-peritoneal shunt because of hydrocephalus. In these cases, careful manipulation of the head is necessary to avoid disconnection, breakage or migration of the shunt.
- There is no contraindication to the use of local anaesthetic with vasoconstrictors.
- Be prepared to handle a seizure emergency in office.

Respiratory disease

ASTHMA

General considerations

Asthma is a unique heterogeneous respiratory disease with a variable lifetime course. It is characterized by increased responsiveness of the airways to a wide variety of stimuli, leading to widespread narrowing of the airways resulting in symptoms of dyspnoea, wheezing and coughing. Precipitating factors include emotional stress, exercise, cold air, viral respiratory infections, air pollution and aspirin. The condition is reversible, either spontaneously or as a result of bronchodilator therapy. Currently, there is an emphasis on prophylactic medications to prevent episodes rather than simply treating acute attacks.

TABLE 12.6 ■ Risk factors for development of asthma

Genetic	Environmental	Natal and perinatal factors
Nonmodifiable	Maternal tobacco smoking in pregnancy	Neonatal jaundice
Allergic rhinitis		Preeclampsia
Obesity	Maternal diet in pregnancy	Caesarean section delivery
Boys are more likely to develop childhood asthma	High maternal sugar consumption	Chronic lung disease of prematurity
Risk is the same for both sexes in puberty	Passive tobacco smoking	Extreme preterm birth (23–27 weeks' gestation)
Girls have a higher risk after puberty	Outdoor and indoor air pollution, indoor dampness	Low birth weight
	Allergens such as house dust mites, pollens, pet allergens and fungal spores	
	Use of incense sticks/candles	
	Home cleaning chemicals	

Bronchodilators include β_2-adrenergic drugs such as salbutamol sulphate (Ventolin) and theophylline (Nuelin). Preventive agents include disodium cromoglycate (Intal), oral corticosteroids (prednisone) and inhaled corticosteroids, such as beclomethasone dipropionate (Beclovent) and salmeterol xinafoate (Seretide). Risk factors for the development of asthma are listed in Table 12.6.

- Childhood asthma has an overall high prevalence worldwide. Australia has one of the highest rates of childhood asthma in the world, with 1 in 5 children and 1 in 7 adolescents affected. Some 10% of children in the European Union and North America are affected. Almost 80% of asthma cases begin in the first 6 years of life, and there is a male predominance until puberty.
- Childhood asthma severity is associated with duration of symptoms, medication use, lung function, low socioeconomic status, racial/ethnic minorities and a neutrophilic phenotype.
- Childhood asthma leads to increased risk of chronic obstructive pulmonary disease in adulthood. These changes reflect airway size during different times of growth and development (smaller in boys during childhood, smaller in girls during puberty). Smaller airway size predisposes to worsened reactivity.
- Other factors include hormones, genetics, immunologic response and health-seeking behaviours.

Medical history:
- Presence of atopy: begins with atopic dermatitis (eczema) in infancy, followed by allergic rhinitis (hay fever) and then asthma later in childhood.
- Indoor allergen sensitization: dust mite, *Alternaria* (a fungus) mould, cockroach allergens.
- Recurrent croup.
- Rhinitis and food allergy may aggravate or mimic asthma.
- Medication exposure: exposure to antibiotics and antipyretics (acetaminophen, aspirin) both prenatally and during infancy increase risk of asthma.

Asthma presentation

Early childhood (≤6 years of age):
- Symptoms are varied and nonspecific: cough (dry and productive), wheeze, shortness of breath, work of breathing.
- Usually virally triggered rather than allergically triggered, particularly in the first 3 years.
- Therapy: based on recurrence of wheezing symptoms or in disease severity.

Late childhood (7–11 years):

- Symptoms transition from discrete episodes of wheezing attributed to viral infections to exacerbations because of allergies.
- Exercise-induced symptoms manifest more clearly in this age group.
- Severe attacks may occur in response to specific triggers, such as cold weather, cigarette smoke and seasonal allergies.

Adolescence (12–18 years):

- Predominant symptoms: shortness of breath with exertion, wheezing in response to triggers, chest pain, chest tightness, cough.
- Remission is common in adolescence.

Asthma therapy

The goal is to achieve and maintain clinical control, reduce future risks to the patient and enable the patient to lead a life without restrictions because of the disease. The majority of patients respond well to standard treatment:

- Inhaled corticosteroids (ICs) are general antiinflammatory agents that target airway inflammation (preventor/controller agents).
- Short- and long-acting beta agonists are bronchodilators that target bronchoconstriction of airway smooth muscle (relievers). Short-acting β-2-agonists provide quick symptom relief. Long-acting β-2-agonists are long-term control agents always used in conjunction with inhaled steroids.
- Immunomodulators (biologic therapies or monoclonal antibodies) are antiinflammatory agents (anti-IgE, mast cell stabilizers) and bronchodilators.

For patients with persistent asthma, daily use of preventer medication is the cornerstone of therapy. Well-controlled asthma means that the child has daytime symptoms twice a week or less, has no nocturnal or early awakening because of asthma, uses reliever medication twice a week or less and has no activity limitation because of asthma.

Severe asthma versus difficult-to-treat asthma:

In both situations, children seem not to respond to standard treatment, experiencing significant disease morbidity.

- These patients have severe anxiety and difficulty coping with the disease.
- Severe asthma: requires high-dose inhaled preventer and second controller medication and/or systemic corticosteroid to prevent it from becoming uncontrolled or remains uncontrolled despite this therapy.
- Child may have neutrophil-predominant asthma.
    Difficult-to-treat asthma: persistent symptoms and exacerbations caused by comorbidities, incorrect diagnosis, poor treatment adherence and/or incorrect inhaler technique.

Treatment comorbidities: allergic rhinitis, chronic exposure to allergens, obesity, GORD, obstructive sleep apnoea, vocal cord dysfunction, etc.

Oral and dental considerations

The major concern to the paediatric dentist is the exacerbation of an acute attack in the dental surgery.

- Avoid any known precipitating factors before dental treatment and ensure that the child has the appropriate medication (inhaler) for emergency use if an asthmatic attack occurs during dental treatment.
- Some bronchodilator and corticosteroid medications may cause extrinsic staining of the teeth because of changes in oral flora and may also predispose to oral candidiasis.

- Affected children are often mouth breathers, causing gingivitis and swelling of anterior gingival tissues.

Take a detailed asthma history:

- Number of exacerbations/attacks in the past year.
- Limitations on daily activity.
- Sleep disturbance.
- Medication use.
- Adherence to therapy.
- Comorbidities.
- Asthma doubles the risk of caries in both dentitions due to increased prevalence of mouth breathing because of nasal polyps, medication effects (xerostomia), dry powder inhalers that induce an oral pH under 5.5, enamel defects, long-term use of sucrose-rich medications, parental overindulgence.
- Increased consumption of carbonated drinks and juices because of xerostomia and following inhaler use to mask its bitter taste. Encourage patients to rinse mouth with water or fluoride mouthwashes following medication use and maintain optimal oral hygiene. Encourage patients to drink water instead of sweet drinks.
- The patient should bring the inhaler to dental appointments.
- Increased risk of dental erosion because of acidic medications and GORD.
- Long-term use of ICs and oral dryness facilitate the development of oral fungal infections.
- Fluoride varnishes that contain colophony, a natural resin that helps the varnish adhere to the tooth surface, should be avoided in severely asthmatic children as it may cause sensitivity reactions.
- Sedatives before dental visits may be used, but the patient's physician must be consulted first. Use of nitrous oxide inhalation and passive immobilization may be contraindicated in severely asthmatic children.
- Patients who have used ICs long term may be prone to adrenal crisis during dental appointments: check with the patient's physician if a supplemental dose of steroids is needed.
- The use of rubber dam isolation helps reduce the probability of an asthma attack because of aerosols, tooth dust and dental material residues.

CYSTIC FIBROSIS

General considerations

Cystic fibrosis (CF) is an autosomal recessive genetic multisystem disease caused by mutations in the gene encoding the CF transmembrane conductance regulator (CFTR) protein, which is found in the cell membrane of epithelial cells. CF affects all mucous-secreting exocrine glands, but clinically the most affected are the respiratory and GI systems. CFTR mutations cause aberrant chloride transport in epithelial tissues, leading to altered hydration and pH of the airway surface fluid, as well as viscous fluids.

- Organs that have functionally important cells expressing CFTR, such as respiratory tract, sweat gland, pancreas, hepatobiliary tract, salivary glands and vas deferens, are affected.
- CF is considered the most common lethal genetic disease in white populations: median predicted survival in the United States for patients with CF is 47.7 years.

Although the disease is currently incurable, aggressive symptomatic treatment has improved survival and quality of life in recent years. Long-term complications include sinusitis, pneumothorax, osteopenia, diabetes, and liver disease. The major cause of death is respiratory failure from recurrent chest infections. Patients need a high-fat, high-protein diet, larger and more frequent meals, increased salt, sweet foods and drinks, and dietary supplements.

Diagnosis

Newborn screening tests are available in many countries. The sweat test is the most readily available and clinically useful way of making the diagnosis of CF. In general, a diagnosis of CF can be made in a patient with clinical features of the disease if the concentration of chloride in sweat is 60 mmol/L (or more) or if it is in the intermediate range (30–59 mmol/L for infants <6 months of age, 40–59 mmol/L for older individuals) and two disease-causing mutations are identified.

Clinical manifestations of cystic fibrosis

Endocrine disorders:
- Pancreatic insufficiency is caused by the obstruction of intra-pancreatic ducts with thickened secretions and leads to fat-soluble vitamin deficiency and malnutrition caused by malabsorption.
- Patients must receive pancreatic enzyme replacement therapy.
  - Poor absorption of fat-soluble vitamins leads to acrodermatitis, neuropathy, night blindness, osteoporosis and prolonged bleeding.
  - CF-related diabetes develops when islet cells are no longer functional.
  - Focal biliary cirrhosis occurs because of obstruction of intrahepatic bile ducts.

Respiratory disease:
- Chronic airway infection is the hallmark of this disease. Deficient chloride and bicarbonate production cause thick secretions that lead to a vicious cycle of mucus obstruction, chronic infection and inflammation. Lung disease is a major cause of morbidity and 80% of mortality in patients with CF.
- Rapid colonization by *Haemophilus influenzae* and *S. aureus*, later by *Pseudomonas aeruginosa*.
- Acquiring *P. aeruginosa* is extremely dangerous; they synthesize an alginate coat and form biofilms that are difficult, if not impossible, to clear with standard antibiotic treatment.
- Approximately 15% to 20% of patients carry methicillin-resistant *S. aureus* (MRSA) in their airways.

Reproductive system:
- Vas deferens is very sensitive to CFTR dysfunction. All men with CF have azoospermia and are infertile because of congenital bilateral absence of vas deferens. Women with CF are fertile.

Liver disease:
- Cirrhosis caused by obstruction of intrahepatic bile duct.

Treatment: New drugs target the defective protein to enhance its function. Other treatment options being researched include targeted therapeutics, gene editing, stem cell therapy and alternative targets that can compensate for CFTR dysfunction.

Pulmonary disease:
- Daily inhaled Dornase alfa (recombinant human deoxyribonuclease) and inhaled tobramycin are standard of care. Macrolide antibiotics, oral antibiotics and high-dose oral ibuprofen are also used. IV antibiotics are used to treat flares of CF lung disease aggressively.
- Inhaled hypertonic saline draws water into the airways, improving mucociliary clearance.
- Airway clearance techniques that augment clearance of tenacious secretions.
- Physical exercise is important.
- Lung transplantation for individuals with end-stage lung disease.

Oral and dental considerations

- Always consult with a physician about the status of the lungs before providing dental procedures, including cleanings.

- Avoid scheduling more than one patient with CF at a time; they can cross-contaminate with *P. aeruginosa* and other dangerous bacteria.
- Verify the patient's respiratory system status; keep appointments short, especially for patients with severe lung disease.
- Special care for patients with lung transplantation because of immunosuppression issues.
- Risk of bleeding issues caused by vitamin K deficiency and liver disease.
- Consult with pulmonologist and anaesthesiologist when sedation and GA are considered for dental care.
- Nitrous oxide may be contraindicated in patients with poor lung function.
- Increased amount of calculus is possible because of altered amounts of calcium and phosphate in saliva.
- Use of inhaled meropenem, an antibiotic of the carbapenem family, may cause extrinsic black staining of teeth, and black 'hairy' tongue may appear because of increased use of antibiotics.
- Children with CF may be at lower risk for dental caries, but adolescents may not.

Antibiotic usage, good compliance with oral hygiene and use of pancreatic enzymes lead to salivary gland hypertrophy and reduction in plaque levels, higher salivary pH and buffering capacity because of CFTR defect in salivary gland. CFTR modulators may correct CFTR defect in salivary gland and lead to normal caries experience. There is a change in antibiotics in adolescence from penicillins to macrolides to protect against *P. aeruginosa*. Macrolides do not protect against cariogenic bacteria.

TUBERCULOSIS

General considerations

Tuberculosis is an infectious disease caused by *Mycobacterium tuberculosis* that involves granulomatous inflammation and caseating necrosis in the lung tissues. The most common presentation in children is malaise, anorexia and weight loss, fever and cough with signs of cervical lymphadenitis. Children are managed with long-term antibiotic treatment specific to the infectious organism. Chemoprophylaxis is given to other family members and contacts, to prevent spread of the disease. The bacille Calmette–Guérin (BCG) vaccine is used routinely in communities with a high prevalence of tuberculosis.

Genetics and dysmorphology

DIAGNOSIS

Although individually uncommon, many children with genetic disorders will present to the paediatric dentist with specific dental anomalies associated with their condition or medical problems that complicate their dental management. It is important not to assume that all conditions will have been diagnosed before they present, as many children are often diagnosed as having a significant genetic disorder late in childhood, either because the condition has late manifestations or because features have been missed. When taking a history, it is always useful to draw a simple three-generation family pedigree (Figure 12.19).

Many disorders do not follow mendelian inheritance patterns but are clearly of 'familial' or hereditary nature. Many important and common conditions fall into this group; they are often not single entities but causally heterogeneous and are seen as the end result of multiple gene effects against a variable environmental background (multifactorial or polygenic), for example, cleft lip and palate.

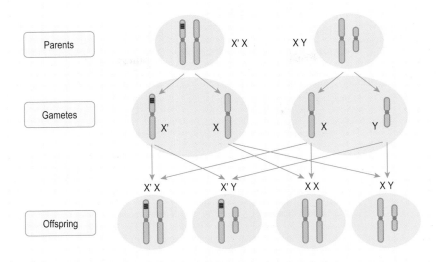

Figure 12.19   Calculation of risk in an X-linked recessive disorder. For a carrier mother (illustrated), there is a 50% chance that sons will be affected and a 50% chance that daughters will be carriers; for an affected father, no sons will be affected but all daughters will be carriers.

One in 170 live-born births has a major chromosomal abnormality. Chromosomal abnormalities, particularly those involving imbalance of the autosomes, usually result in developmental delay and dysmorphic features and often include multisystem anomalies. These include numerical abnormalities (trisomy 21 or Down syndrome) and structural abnormalities such as segmental deletions (Cri-du-chat syndrome), duplications and unbalanced translocations. Numerical abnormalities of the sex chromosomes are better tolerated than those of the autosomes and include conditions such as Turner syndrome (45, X) in females and Klinefelter syndrome (47, XXY) in males. Standard cytogenetic karyotyping is now being replaced by DNA-based chromosome micro-arrays (CMA) that can detect many more significant submicroscopic deletions and duplications (pathological copy number variations). Many other genetic disorders are caused by mutations within genes, which cannot be detected by karyotype or CMA analysis but may be able to be confirmed by targeted gene testing after a syndrome is recognized (Table 12.7).

The first step in making a diagnosis is the recognition that the child is dysmorphic or unusual looking. It is the pattern of dysmorphism and associated malformations rather than a single feature that aids diagnosis. Accurate diagnosis is the key to prognosis, management and sometimes the underlying genetic cause of the disorder. It also helps the parents because it removes the anxiety of uncertain aetiology and prognosis.

The diagnostic procedure involves history, clinical examination and laboratory investigations. Based on the previous information, children can be divided into three basic groups:
- Foetal environmental syndromes (teratogens, compression).
- Developmental anomalies.
- Genetic syndromes.

Referral to a genetic clinic is recommended for all children with multiple anomalies or dysmorphic features of unknown cause. Syndrome diagnosis aids (available by paid subscription),

TABLE 12.7 ■ Classification of genetic abnormalities

	Defect	Examples
Chromosomal structure	Aneuploidies (abnormal number of chromosomes)	Down syndrome, trisomy 21 Klinefelter syndrome (XXY)
		Turner syndrome (45,X)
	Chromosomal deletions, duplications and translocations	18q- (deletion of part of long arm of chromosome 18)
Single-gene defects	Autosomal dominant	Cleidocranial dysplasia
		Gorlin syndrome
		Osteogenesis imperfecta
	Autosomal recessive	Cystic fibrosis
	X-linked recessive	Haemophilia A, B
		Hypohidrotic ectodermal dysplasia
Polygenic disorders	Multiple minor gene abnormalities interacting with environmental influences	Cleft palate
		Diabetes mellitus
		Spina bifida
		Schizophrenia

(Modified from Jones, K.L., 1997. Smith's recognizable patterns of human malformation, 5th ed. WB Saunders, Philadelphia.)

such as POSSUM (www.possum.net.au) or the London Dysmorphology Databases (www.lmdatabases.com/), can assist. Laboratory investigations include radiographic survey, chromosomal or microarray analysis, biochemical screening of urine or blood, or cultured fibroblasts for specific enzymatic or protein deficiencies if a metabolic disorder is suspected. Referral to a genetics clinic is usually recommended to further elaborate a diagnosis and to assist with specialized genetic testing and genetic counselling.

It is not the intention of this section to detail those anomalies with a major craniofacial or orofacial manifestation, of which dental clinicians should be aware. The reader is directed to texts and online sources that more comprehensively cover these conditions (see References and further reading).

TERMS USED IN MORPHOGENESIS

Sequence

A pattern of multiple anomalies arising from a single structural defect or event; previously termed 'anomalad'. They usually originate early in development with single problems that create secondary anomalies and manifest with multiple defects at birth or later. These sequences may be divided into three basic groups.

Malformation sequence
- Poor formation of tissue.
- May be single or multiple but are primary structural abnormalities.

- Poor prognosis for normal growth in the areas affected.
- Recurrence rate of 1% to 5%.
- Example: cleft palate.

Malformations may present as:

- Accessory tissue (e.g., polydactyly, preauricular skin tags).
- Hamartomas (e.g., haemangioma/lymphangioma).
- Incomplete morphogenesis:
  - Agenesis (e.g., salivary gland agenesis).
  - Hypoplasia (e.g., enamel hypoplasia in amelogenesis imperfecta).
- Incomplete septation (e.g., ventral septal defect [VSD]).
- Incomplete migration of neuroectoderm cells (e.g., Di George association).
- Failure of cell death (apoptosis) (e.g., spina bifida, syndactyly).

Deformation sequence

- Unusual forces acting on normal tissues, usually from abnormal intrauterine pressures.
- Good prognosis for normal growth and a low risk of recurrence.
- Examples are:
  - (Some) isolated talipes.
  - Micrognathia.
  - Torticollis.

Disruption sequence

- Destruction or breakdown of normal tissue, which may result from vascular, infective or physical causes.
- Low risk of recurrence, poor prognosis for normal growth in affected areas.
- Examples:
  - Deafness from congenital rubella.
  - Facial clefting from amniotic bands.
  - Hemifacial microsomia (from stapedial artery haemorrhage).

Syndrome

- A recognizable pattern of malformation.
- Multiple defects of related pathogenesis, arising directly from a single cause (genetic or acquired).

Association

- Nonrandom occurrence of several morphologic defects not identified as a syndrome or sequence.
- Low risk of recurrence.
- Example: VATER association (V, vertebral anomalies; A, anal atresia; T-E, tracheo-esophageal fistula ± oesophageal atresia; R, radial and renal dysplasia).

RISK OF RECURRENCE IN GENETIC DISORDERS

Autosomal dominant

There is a 50% risk to each offspring of a single affected parent. Many dominant conditions have variable expression, and so the manifestations may be increased or reduced compared with the parent. New dominant genetic conditions can also occur.

Autosomal recessive

Carriers do not express the trait. If both parents are carriers, the risk of the child being affected (homozygous; the trait will be expressed) is 25%; the risk of being a carrier is 50% and the chance of neither being a carrier nor affected is 25%. If one parent is a carrier, there is a 50% chance of the child being a carrier.

X-linked (sex-linked)

- There is a 50% risk of transmission from female carriers to sons (who would then be affected) or daughters (who would then be a carrier).
- No male-to-male transmission from affected fathers to sons, but all daughters will be carriers.

The terms 'X-linked recessive' and 'X-linked dominant' are used to describe sex-linked conditions with an altered frequency of phenotypic expression. Males usually have only one X chromosome; males with an X-linked abnormality are described as hemizygous for the trait, and will be affected. Females usually have two X-chromosomes; female carriers of an X-linked trait are heterozygous. In X-linked recessive disorders, female carriers can be unaffected or affected (manifesting carrier), but the latter are usually much less severely affected than males. Rarely, females are homozygous for an X-linked trait, so will be affected as severely as a hemizygous male. 'X-linked dominant' traits manifest in females and males, but males are often more severely affected.

The degree of phenotypic expression in heterozygous females is determined by the pattern of X inactivation (Lyonization, see Chapter 11) in each tissue. For example, some female carriers of haemophilia A will show a measurable (but subclinical) reduction in factor VIII, and those that carry X-linked hypohidrotic ectodermal dysplasia may also show some phenotypic variation in the dentition such as microdontia and oligodontia, but not to the same extent as in hemizygous males. The markedly increased frequency of females seen with some 'X-linked dominant' conditions, such as incontinentia pigmenti or focal dermal hypoplasia (Goltz–Gorlin syndrome) is explained by male lethality for these mutations in most hemizygous males.

PRENATAL TESTS FOR GENETIC DISORDERS

Ultrasound

Ultrasound has become a routine investigation for most pregnancies. It is noninvasive to the mother and the foetus and there are many anomalies that may be diagnosed by this technique. Common ultrasound techniques include the first-trimester nuchal translucency measurement (a screening examination for Down syndrome risk) and the mid-trimester foetal morphology scan.

Amniocentesis

This is the sampling of cells from amniotic fluid at around 15 to 18 weeks. A number of tests can be performed including:
- Karyotyping.
- Sex determination.
- DNA diagnosis.
- Enzyme assays.

Chorionic villus sampling

This test is performed earlier than amniocentesis, at around 11 to 13 weeks. Similar tests are performed to those done with amniocentesis, although it has the advantage of earlier diagnosis.

Preimplantation genetic diagnosis

This is DNA testing of cells biopsied from IVF embryos. This is an option increasingly chosen by couples where genetic risk is high, abortion is not an acceptable option and targeted testing is possible (prior work-up is required).

Population screenings

- First-trimester combined maternal serum screening and nuchal translucency scan for Down syndrome risk.
- Mid-trimester maternal serum 'triple test' for Down syndrome risk.
- Mid-trimester maternal α-fetoprotein levels for neural tube defects.

Postnatal tests

Chromosome analysis (cytogenetic) or chromosomal microarrays (DNA-based). For any baby with dysmorphic features or multiple abnormalities.

DNA analysis. For specific disorders; direct mutation detection in selected gene(s).

Neonatal screening tests. A range of newborn screening tests is undertaken in each country, but the tests offered vary significantly between centres. Commonly performed tests include those for:
- Phenylketonuria.
- CF.
- Congenital hypothyroidism.
- Galactosaemia.
- Thalassaemia.
- SCD.
- Aminoacidopathies.
- Organic acidaemias.
- Fatty acid oxidation defects.

GENETIC COUNSELLING

Genetic counselling is the process of providing diagnostic assessment, information and support to families or individuals who have, or are at increased risk for, birth defects, chromosomal abnormalities or a variety of inherited conditions. Genetic counselling specialists include clinical geneticists and genetic counsellors. Clinical geneticists provide medical diagnostic assessment and investigation, interpretation of information about the disorder, analysis of inheritance patterns and risks of recurrence and review of available management options with the family. Genetic counsellors take a major role in providing information and supportive counselling to individuals and families, including facilitation of access to resources such as genetic support groups or other community or state support services.

DENTAL MANAGEMENT

- The aim of dental management should be a part of a team approach in the care of the child. The overall aim is to reduce the handicapping consequences of the condition. Restorative and surgical management of the specific dental disability (e.g., enamel hypoplasia or hypodontia) should be addressed with a long-term comprehensive management plan. This must involve several dental disciplines such as orthodontics, periodontics, oral surgery and restorative dentistry, working together to coordinate a treatment plan. Overall success in management is measured by the total rehabilitation of the child and family.

References and further reading

Asthma

Alavaikko, S., Jaakkola, M.S., Tjaderhane, L., et al., 2011. Asthma and caries: a systematic review and meta-analysis. American Journal of Epidemiology 174, 631–641.

Harrington, N., Pardo, N., Barry, S., 2016. Dental treatment in children with asthma – a review. British Dental Journal 220, 299–302.

Pijnenburg, M.W., Baraldi, E., Brand, P.L.P., et al., 2015. Monitoring asthma in children. European Respiratory Journal 45, 906–925.

Trivedi, M., Denton, E., 2019. Asthma in children and adults – what are the differences and what can they tell us about asthma? Frontiers in Pediatrics 7, 256.

Wechsler, M.E., 2009. Managing asthma in primary care: putting new guideline recommendations into context. Mayo Clinic Proceedings 84, 707–717.

Cardiology

Baltimore, R.S., Gewitz, M., Baddour, L.M., et al., 2015. Infective endocarditis in childhood: 2015 update. A scientific statement from the. American Heart Association. Circulation 132, 1487–1515.

Lantin-Hermoso, M.R., Berger, S., Bhatt, A.B., et al., 2017. The care of children with congenital heart disease in their primary medical home. Paediatrics 140, e20172607.

Pussinen, P.J., Paju, S., Koponen, J., et al., 2019. Association of childhood oral infections with cardiovascular risk factors and subclinical atherosclerosis in adulthood. JAMA Network Open 2, e192523.

Wahl, M.J., Miller, C.S., Rhodus, N.L., et al., 2018. Anticoagulants are dental friendly. Oral Surgery, Oral Medicine, Oral Pathology and Oral Radiology 125, 103–106.

Wilson, W.R., Gewitz, M., Lockhart, P.B., et al., 2021. Prevention of viridans group streptoccocal infective endocarditis. A scientific statement from the American Heart Association. Circulation 143, e963–e978.

Childhood cancer

da Fonseca, M.A., 1998. Paediatric bone marrow transplantation: oral complications and recommendations for care. Pediatric Dentistry 20, 386–394.

da Fonseca, M.A., 2000. Long-term oral and craniofacial complications following paediatric bone marrow transplantation. Pediatric Dentistry 22, 57–62.

da Fonseca, M.A., Hong, C., 2008. An overview of chronic oral graft-vs-host disease following paediatric hematopoietic stem cell transplantation. Pediatric Dentistry 30, 98–104.

Hong, C.H., da Fonseca, M., 2008. Considerations in the paediatric population with cancer. Dental Clinics of North America 52, 155–181.

Multinational Association of Supportive Care in Cancer. MASCC/ISOO clinical practice guidelines for the management of mucositis secondary to cancer therapy. Available: https://www.mascc.org/mucositis-guidelines.

Vesterbacka, M., Ringden, O., Remberger, M., et al., 2012. Disturbances in dental development and craniofacial growth in children treated with hematopoietic stem cell transplantation. Orthodontics & Craniofacial Research 15, 21–29.

Cystic fibrosis

American Diabetes Association, 2017. Classification and Diagnosis of Diabetes. Diabetes Care 40, S11.

Bornstein, S.R., Allolio, B., Arlt, W., et al., 2016. Diagnosis and treatment of primary adrenal insufficiency: an Endocrine Society Clinical Practice Guideline. Journal of Clinical Endocrinology and Metabolism 101, 364–389.

Chi, D.L., 2013. Dental caries prevalence in children and adolescents with cystic fibrosis: a qualitative systematic review and recommendations for future research. International Journal of Paediatric Dentistry 23, 376–386.

Farag, A.M., 2017. Head and neck manifestations of endocrine disorders. Atlas of the Oral and Maxillofacial Surgery Clinics of North America 25, 197–207.

Harrington, N., Barry, P.J., Barry, S.M., 2016. Dental treatment for people with cystic fibrosis. European Archives of Paediatric Dentistry 17, 195–203.

Padbury, A.D., Jr., Tözüm, T.F., Taba, M. Jr., et al., 2006. The impact of primary hyperparathyroidism on the oral cavity. Journal of Clinical Endocrinology and Metabolism 91, 3439–3445.

Pinto, A., Glick, M., 2002. Management of patients with thyroid disease: oral health considerations. Journal of the American Dental Association 133, 849–858.

Sutbeyaz, Y., Yoruk, O., Bilen, H., et al., 2009. Primary hyperparathyroidism presenting as a palatal and mandibular brown tumor. Journal of Craniofacial Surgery 20, 2101–2104.

Gastroenterology

Carvalho, F.K., Queiroz, A.M., Silva, R.A.B., et al., 2015. Oral aspects in celiac disease children: clinical and dental enamel chemical evaluation. Oral Surgery, Oral Medicine, Oral Pathology and Oral Radiology 119, 636–643.

Gupta, N., Bostrom, A.G., Kirschner, B.S., et al., 2008. Presentation and disease course in early- compared to later-onset paediatric Crohn's disease. American Journal of Gastroenterology 103, 2092–2098.

Khatib, M., Baker, R.D., Ly, E.K., et al., 2016. Presenting pattern of paediatric celiac disease. Journal of Pediatric Gastroenterology and Nutrition 62, 60–63.

Lourenço, S.V., Hussein, T.P., Bologna, S.B., et al., 2010. Oral manifestations of inflammatory bowel disease: a review based on the observation of six cases. Journal of the European Academy of Dermatology and Venereology 24, 204–207.

Radmand, R., Schilsky, M., Jakab, S., et al., 2013. Pre-liver transplant protocols in dentistry. Oral Surgery, Oral Medicine, Oral Pathology and Oral Radiology 115, 426–430.

Rowland, M., Fleming, P., Bourke, B., 2010. Looking in the mouth for Crohn's disease. Inflammatory Bowel Diseases 16, 332–337.

Smith, J.M., Hwong, C.S., Salamonik, E.B., et al., 2006. Sonic tooth brushing reduces gingival overgrowth in renal transplant recipients. Pediatric Nephrology 21, 1753–1759.

Haematology

da Fonseca, M., Oueis, H.S., Casamassimo, P.S., 2007. Sickle cell anemia: a review for the paediatric dentist. Pediatric Dentistry 29, 159–169.

Haghighi, A.G., Finder, R.G., 2016. Systemic disease and bleeding disorders for the oral and maxillofacial surgeon. Oral and Maxillofacial Surgery Clinics of the North America 28, 461–471.

Kotila, T.R., 2016. Sickle cell trait: a benign state? Acta Haematology 136, 147–151.

Laurence, B., Haywood Jr., C., Lanzkron, S., 2013. Dental infections increase the likelihood of hospital admissions among adult patients with sickle cell disease. Community Dental Health 30, 168–172.

Rotz, S.J., Ware, R.E., Kumar, A., 2018. Diagnosis and management of chronic and refractory immune cytopenias in children, adolescents, and young adults. Pediatric Blood & Cancer 65, e27260.

Immunodeficiencies

Deas, D.E., Mackey, S.A., McDonnell, H.T., 2000. Systemic disease and periodontitis: manifestations of neutrophil dysfunction. Periodontology 32, 82–104.

Dinauer, M.C., 2014. Disorders of neutrophil function: an overview. In: Quinn, M., DeLeo, F. (Eds.), Neutrophil methods and protocols. methods in molecular biology (methods and protocols). Humana Press, Totowa, NJ, pp. 501–515.

Hajishengallis, E., Hajishengallis, G., 2014. Neutrophil homeostasis and periodontal health in children and adults. Journal of Dental Research 93, 231–237.

McDonald-McGinn, D.M., Sullivan, K.E., Marino, B., et al., 2016. 22q11.2 deletion syndrome. Nature Reviews Disease Primers 1, 15071.

Seth, D., Ruehle, M., Kamat, D., 2019. Severe combined immunodeficiency: a guide for primary care givers. Clinical Pediatrics 58, 1124–1127.

Skokowa, J., Dale, D.C., Touw, I.P., et al., 2017. Severe congenital neutropenias. Nature Reviews Disease Primers 3, 17032.

Nephrology

Davidovich, E., Davidovits, M., Peretz, B., et al., 2009. The correlation between dental calculus and disturbed mineral metabolism in paediatric patients with chronic kidney disease. Nephrology, Dialysis, Transplantation 24, 2439–2445.

Gupta, M., Gupta, M., 2015. Oral conditions in renal disorders and treatment considerations – a review for paediatric dentist. Saudi Dental Journal 27, 113–119.

Proctor, R., Kumar, N., Stein, A., et al., 2005. Oral and dental aspects of chronic renal failure. Journal of Dental Research 84, 199–208.

Warady, B.A., Abraham, A.G., Schwartz, G.J., et al., 2015. Predictors of rapid progression of glomerular and nonglomerular kidney disease in children and adolescents: The Chronic Kidney Disease in Children (CKiD) Cohort. American Journal of Kidney Diseases 65, 878.

Seizures and epilepsy

Falco-Walter, J.J., Scheffer, I.E., Fisher, R.S., 2018. The new definition and classification of seizures and epilepsy. Epilepsy Research 139, 73–79.

Fisher, R.S., Cross, H.J., D'Souza, C., et al., 2017. Instruction manual for the ILAE 2017 operational classification of seizures. Epilepsia 58, 522–530.

Fisher, R.S., Cross, H.J., French, J.A., et al., 2017. Operational classification of seizure types by the International League Against Epilepsy: position paper of the ILAE Commission for Classification and Terminology. Epilepsia 58, 531–542.

Manford, M., 2017. Recent advances in epilepsy. Journal of Neurology 264, 1811–1124.

Tuberculosis

Cleveland, J.L., Robison, V.A., Panlilio, A.L., 2009. Tuberculosis epidemiology, diagnosis and infection control recommendations for dental settings. An update on the Centers for Disease Control and Prevention guidelines. JADA 140, 1092–1099.

Children with special needs

Neeta Prabhu ▪ Wendy J. Bellis ▪ Angus C. Cameron

...in order to treat some person equally, we must treat them differently.

Justice Blackmun 1985

Introduction

Although the oral health of people with special needs or 'disabilities' is similar to the rest of the population, it is generally accepted that many of these children have extensive treatment needs, which, for a variety of reasons, are not adequately met. Throughout the world, the standards of oral healthcare for this population have failed to achieve what would normally be expected for those without a disability.

WHAT IS SPECIAL CARE DENTISTRY?

It is a discipline targeted to meet the needs of individuals with a variety of limitations that require more than just routine dental care.

A disability may be:
- Intellectual.
- Physical.
- Developmental.
- Emotional (psychological or behavioural).
- Medical comorbidity (covered in the previous chapter).

BARRIERS TO CARE AND PHILOSOPHIES OF MANAGEMENT

Access to dentistry is often influenced by:
- The attitudes and willingness within the dental team to treat special needs children.
- A perception that the clinician may not have the skills or have the facilities to manage their care.
- Financial considerations.
- Physical access and transport barriers.
- Problems of self-image.
- Issues relating to consent for treatment.

The successful management of these children depends fundamentally on the dentist's ability to:
- Establish a rapport and form a partnership with the patient, the family and the carer.
- Clearly understand the condition of the child whom they are treating.
- Use appropriate behaviour management techniques based on the level of the patient's understanding.

CONSENT

Providing dental care for people with cognitive impairment who are unable to consent to treatment can raise ethical and legal problems for the practitioner. There is variation in the practice of consent, ranging from the ability of an individual to legally consent to their own treatment to the delegation of authority to their parents, caregivers or a guardianship board. Because these ethical predicaments are not obscure, healthcare professionals who routinely care for such patients must complement their clinical skills with their ability to recognize and clearly address these legal responsibilities.

WHERE ARE SPECIAL NEEDS CHILDREN TO BE MANAGED?

General dentists have often expressed concerns about a lack of adequate training in appropriately managing these patients in practice, leading to an increase in the number of referrals to tertiary hospitals. Although there has been an overall strategy of integration and normalization of these individuals into mainstream society, unfortunately, most have become reliant on the already stretched hospital-based healthcare system, leading to extended waiting times. It must be emphasized that children with special needs require dental appointments that are tailored to make best use of their abilities. The majority of children can be managed successfully in a general practice setting with appropriate training of the dental team. All of the required preventive and maintenance programmes and much of the restorative work can be performed under local anaesthesia and/or sedation. However, there will always be a cohort for whom dental treatment under general anaesthesia is the only alternative. This incurs high costs and has its own problems of access and additional risks and should be recommended only when all other forms of behaviour management have failed or are clearly inappropriate. Additionally, the patient's ability for oral health maintenance postoperatively must always be factored in the treatment planning process to avoid the misuse of these expensive facilities.

There is no doubt that the provision of care for many children with disabilities is challenging. Clinicians should be aware of their own limitations and should consider who and where the child is best managed.

PREVENTION

The best means of establishing good oral health is by a combination of early contact with dental services and increasing the awareness of regular dental check-ups. Many studies have demonstrated that certain groups of people with disabilities can be instructed in oral hygiene measures if sufficient encouragement and motivation were provided. It is important to introduce these measures from an early age, and clinicians should not be deterred from providing comprehensive preventive programmes.

Attention deficit hyperactivity disorder

Attention deficit hyperactivity disorder (ADHD) is a common developmental disorder affecting about 3% to 5% of the population. The term 'ADHD' is currently used to describe a range of children with varying functional difficulties who share the feature of poorly sustained attention. The exact causes remain unknown; however, most theories indicate abnormalities in the brain function that are mostly genetic in origin.

FEATURES OF ATTENTION DEFICIT HYPERACTIVITY DISORDER

- Boys are affected much more commonly than girls.
- They are characterized by developmentally inappropriate degrees of impulsivity, inattention and often hyperactivity.
- The symptoms arise in early childhood, usually well before school entry, and are present in all settings.
- Some children are extremely impulsive, some aggressive, others quiet and restless. Many have low self-esteem.
- Comorbidities include developmental language disorders, anxiety, oppositional-defiant behaviours, fine motor and coordination difficulties and specific learning disabilities.
- Virtually all children with ADHD have deficits in short-term auditory memory.

ASSESSMENT

The assessment of a child for the diagnosis of ADHD requires a number of essential components including:
- Detailed developmental history.
- Physical, neurological and neurodevelopmental examination.
- Detailed standardized behaviour rating scale data from at least two sources, usually school and home and psychometric testing.
  - Conners Parent and Teacher Rating Scale
  - ADD-H Comprehensive Teacher's Rating Scale
  - Child Behaviour Checklist

MANAGEMENT

Management of the child with ADHD involves three broad approaches:
- Behavioural.
- Educational.
- Pharmacological.

Many other approaches are commonly applied to these children, including dietary modification, 'natural' or complementary therapies of diverse types and behavioural optometry; however, there is little evidence to support the broad use of any of these interventions, although some individuals report benefits.

Pharmacological management

Psychostimulant medication is the principal pharmacological therapy for ADHD. The two stimulants most commonly prescribed are methylphenidate (Ritalin) and dexamphetamine.
- Onset of behavioural effect is usually noticeable within 30 to 60 minutes of ingestion.
- Significant clinical improvements in approximately 75% of correctly diagnosed children.
- Common oral side effects include dry mouth. Some of the medications can cause adverse interactions with drugs commonly used in dentistry – for example, local anaesthetics – and therefore monitoring vital signs during dental treatment is essential.
- Other medications sometimes used in ADHD include the antihypertensive drug clonidine, antidepressants (selective serotonin re-uptake inhibitors, reversible monoamine oxidase inhibitors and tricyclics) and occasionally neuroleptics.

DENTAL IMPLICATIONS

The visit to a dentist is likely to raise anxiety levels in any child and indeed their parents. In a child with ADHD, this anxiety may manifest in overexcited behaviour, and many parents worry about the effect of their child's behaviour on others. They have become accustomed to failure having taken their 'difficult' child to dentists only to be told that it is not possible to provide treatment/care. This may result in either an excessively protective/embarrassed parent with constant apologies on behalf of the child or else an overly firm parent exerting inappropriate, heavy-handed disciplinary actions throughout the encounter. In either situation, the child's behaviour is likely to be reactive towards the parent, thus precluding the establishment of a successful relationship with the dental practitioner.

Successful management of these children may be facilitated using similar strategies to those employed in other disabilities.
- It is important that the patient and the parent are managed positively and with confidence. By creating an atmosphere of confidence, the parental anxiety is often alleviated, allowing the child and the dentist to establish a relationship in a more relaxed environment. Similarly, a gentle but firm approach will convey to the child a confidence and structure to the situation within which it is easier for them to conform.
- It is useful for the practitioner to understand the current management strategies being employed by the family at home and in school and to adopt these techniques to maximize success in the dental clinic. For example, if a child is used to raising their hand before speaking, it is useful for the dentist to employ the same strategy. Clear instructions should be given to the child maintaining eye contact throughout and taking care not to overburden the short-term memory. Such instructions need to be given at a time when the child is not distracted by other activities in the dental surgery.
- The use of the tell–show–do method of behaviour direction has been shown to have value in the management of children with ADHD. Praise and encouragement have an important

role in the management of these children, and good behaviour should be reinforced and rewarded.

MANAGEMENT STRATEGIES

- The current medication scheme should be discussed with both the parents and the prescribing practitioner. It may be helpful to either change the dose or the timing of medication to optimize the action at the time of the dental visit. There is also some suggestion that morning appointments may be more successful; however, this may be related to the timing of medication rather than anything else.
- A preventive approach is essential. Toothbrushing and controlling diet both require concentration, motivation and understanding, all of which can be problematic for the child with ADHD. Toothbrushing charts for the child to take home and mark off daily are more likely to be successful than verbal instructions to brush daily.
- Repetition is important in building up self-confidence in the child.
- Multiple short visits have a higher chance of success than a few prolonged visits.
- Inhalation sedation can be a particularly useful adjunct to nonpharmacological behaviour management techniques.
- Finally, it is important to realize that oral health is only one of many priorities for the family of a child with ADHD, and the multiple demands made of the parents need to be weighed against the need for dental care. Again, it is important to realize that many of these children are already struggling to master other life skills.

Autism spectrum disorder

Autism is a lifelong developmental disability that affects how children perceive the world and interact with others. Children with autism have difficulties with everyday social communication, social interaction, repetitive behaviours and sensory issues. It has a wide range of presentations, and so is described as a 'spectrum'. Approximately 50% of people with autism have learning disabilities, although this may be difficult to assess accurately when the child is young. It is important to note that Asperger syndrome is a form of autism in which there may be average or above-average intelligence. Specific learning difficulties, such as dyslexia or difficulty understanding or processing language, may also be present.

AETIOLOGY

Although the exact cause of autism is still under investigation, there is overwhelming evidence of a combination of both a strong genetic and weaker environmental factors that alter brain structure and neurone function.

FREQUENCY

Approximately 1% of the population are thought to be affected, although this figure is likely to increase as our understanding of the condition develops and also as the definition of autism spectrum disorder (ASD) is revised in the future. There appears to be a male-to-female ratio of 4:1; however, girls are underdiagnosed because of their better language and social skills and ability to mask their difficulties to fit in with their peers. Because girls are not diagnosed early, they may display secondary difficulties, such as depression, severe anxiety and eating disorders, especially anorexia.

Because this is predominantly a genetic condition, siblings may also be affected as may be the parents themselves.

COMORBIDITIES

Some 10% of individuals may have other conditions such as Fragile X syndrome, tuberous sclerosis or syndromes including Down syndrome. These may compound the learning disability communication or behavioural problems. Epilepsy is a common association and, if not present in childhood, often manifests in adolescence. Injury to anterior teeth is not uncommon because of the association with epilepsy and dyspraxia.

ISSUES AFFECTING THE DENTAL TREATMENT OF A CHILD WITH AUTISM SPECTRUM DISORDER

The dental management of children with autism can be a great challenge for the paediatric dentist because of a combination of factors which can represent barriers to not only dental care but also oral health itself.

- Impaired communication

  Verbal communication is a major problem, and children may have limited speech and language. Children with autism may not fully understand colloquial speech, jokes and sarcasm.

  Many of these children never develop functional speech and are reliant on communication aids, and these are often visual aids. Clinicians need to be familiar with alternatives to facilitate communication. Pictorial communication aids such as Makaton or the Picture Exchange Communication System (PECS) may be used for some individuals. Makaton uses iconic symbols and line drawings to convey the meaning of words. The more user-friendly PECS system teaches nonspeaking children to exchange pictures of things that they want for the item, using their visual rather than verbal skills.

  Nonverbal communication is poorly understood by many children with autism, particularly facial expressions and tone of voice. Physical reinforcement such as patting or stroking may be ineffective and not be acceptable to the child.

- Behavioural differences

  The child's behaviour might appear disruptive, challenging, frightening and difficult to predict. This may include self-harming. Children with autism lack the 'theory of mind' (the ability to understand other peoples' thoughts and emotions) and are therefore not aware of how their behaviour is seen by those around them. The child may dislike, or be extremely frightened of, new situations and people.

- Sleep problems

  Sleep disruption is very common in children with autism and affects the whole family. As a result, the parent's and the child's resilience may be compromised because of chronic sleep deprivation.

- Sensory problems

  Sensory processing problems are extremely common in children with autism and may often trigger anxiety in a dental practice. Self-stimulatory behaviours are common. These repetitive habits ('stimming') can take many forms, including visual or tactile stimulation or movements such as rocking and hand flapping. Stimming is thought to provide reassurance in stressful situations and helps block out other unwanted sensory input. A child may be hyposensitive or hypersensitive to sights, sounds, smell, taste and touch, all of which are challenges in a dental office and waiting areas.

  It is important to identify elements of the dental surgery and waiting area that may present a sensory challenge to an autistic child. Some children are especially sensitive to light or noises.

  Some children may be very sensitive to an alteration in occlusion which occurs transiently following the placement of preformed metal crowns. Consequently, extra attention must be paid to ensuring that such crowns do not interfere with the occlusion. Oral care may be compromised, as the texture of the brush and the strong taste of the toothpaste may not be tolerated.

- Feeding and diet
  Children with autism have significantly more eating and feeding problems than nonautistic children. This is often linked to their sensory issues and is not necessarily associated with the severity of their autism.

  Dietary control and prevention may be made more difficult by rituals around eating or strong preference for food with particular packaging, colour or texture. There may be idiosyncratic behaviours such as food having to be arranged in a certain way on the plate. If the child receives too much sensory information, 'meltdown' can occur. This is an uncontrolled emotional or behavioural reaction to overwhelming stress or sensory overload that can trigger a 'fight or flight' reaction.

- Difficulty in expressing pain
  Pain perception can be a problem, and the child's response to pain may be different because of sensory integration issues. Localization of any pain can be difficult for the child. Parents are often worried that the child may have dental pain and be unable to inform the parent because of communication barriers. Therefore, dental professionals need to look out for alternative indicators of pain, such as sleep disruption, random emotional outbursts unusual for the child or problems eating.

  Many children with autism have mental health problems such as anxiety, obsessive compulsive disorder and depression. ADHD is frequently present, and patients may take methylphenidate (Ritalin) to help address this behaviour.

THERAPEUTIC INTERVENTIONS

A large number of suggested therapies relating to ASD are publicised on the internet, and although many of these approaches have a poor evidence base, they may be adopted by some families.

- Early intensive behavioural therapies
  These include a range of communication-based, behavioural and educational approaches used to support people with autism. These include approaches such as PECS, TEACCH (Treatment of Autistic and Communication Handicapped Children), ABA (Applied Behavioural Analysis), sensory integration, and speech and language therapy. These approaches can be adapted and used to help the child become familiar with the dental experience and oral care

- Diet modification
  Unusual diets are frequent because many parents exclude wheat, dairy products or yeast in an attempt to improve the symptoms associated with autism. In combination with the patient's own dietary demands, this may make dietary prevention advice very difficult. Confectionery may be being used for the reinforcement of good behaviour in addition to managing conflict with some children with autism.

  In addition to dietary restrictions, there may be imitations imposed on specific dental materials which a dentist might normally use, such as fluoride products.

- Medication
  Children with autism may be prescribed a number of medications aimed not only at addressing behavioural problems but also relating to any comorbidities present such as anxiety, ADHD, epilepsy and sleep problems.

  Because children with autism often have problems swallowing tablets (owing to sensory problems), they may be on liquid formulations for an extended period. These formulations may not be sugar free, and some can cause xerostomia.

CLINICAL MANAGEMENT

Late diagnosis

Unlike many other disabilities, the diagnosis of ASD is usually not possible around birth, and unfortunately, this delay often results in relatively late access to early preventive dental care.

Children with autism have a host of unique problems, resulting in a highly individualized approach being necessary, not only to preventive advice but also to their clinical management.

- Local anaesthesia and inhalation sedation usage is limited to those children who can understand and communicate; however, there are no contraindications.
- General anaesthesia and deep sedation are the most frequently used approaches, especially for those children who are young and present with extensive disease. Such treatment should obviously be definitive and comprehensive, including preventive as well as curative elements. If a general anaesthetic is indicated, space management should be considered proactively, as many may not be able to wear orthodontic appliances.

Important advice for management

Autism is associated with a strong need for routine. Individuals usually like events to be predictable, and new experiences may unbalance the whole day. These children dislike those things which are unfamiliar to them and definitely do not like surprises.

Both the child and the parents may be highly anxious about the dental visit, and therefore, the behaviour during the first few visits may be especially challenging. Some children may have a persistent occupation with certain objects, materials and electronic gadgets, which may initially appear unusual, and some will engage in repetitive body movements.

Because of the problems associated with communication and social interaction, traditional behaviour management approaches may need to be adapted. A lack of eye contact may make it difficult to gain and maintain attention (e.g., tell–show–do).

- Make contact with the families as soon as possible to encourage early access to services through the local child health networks and development teams.
- Send out a preappointment questionnaire-style letter and an information leaflet.
- Plan frequent short visits, making progress in small increments, until the child accepts dental examination sitting in the dental chair.
- Frequent visits to the dental setting will provide opportunities to learn about the child and give preventive support ('hello visits').
- Familiarize yourself with the different communication aids that the child may be using. Photographs or images can be put together in the form of a storyline/social story, so that the child is prepared for the dental visit. End the social story (book) with a 'reward picture'. This helps to reduce a build-up of anxiety by making events more predictable for the child.
- A 'social storyline' may help prepare the child for the next dental visit and reduce anxiety. This is a series of pictures or photographs telling the child what will happen and what is expected. Different children will respond to different styles and formats of social stories.
- Offer to have your photograph taken together with any images of the practice and staff involved.
- Establishing the behaviour of toothbrushing as early as possible is extremely important for these children, and not only for oral health and fluoride delivery; it is also the most successful way of initiating a dental examination.
- Use behavioural approaches such as ABA to establish patterns of behaviour around toothbrushing and also to teach the child to accept a dental examination.
- Where there are brushing problems, it is important to establish whether or not it is the brush or the toothpaste that the child dislikes. It may be the taste of the paste and the oral sensation, and you may need to explore acceptable flavours and low-foaming options.

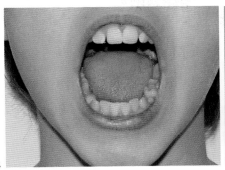
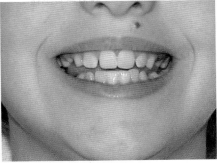

A   B

Figure 13.1 Encouraging echolalic children to copy expressions can aid in the examination and access to the oral cavity. (A) The 'AHHHH' sound helps open the mouth, whereas the sound 'EEEEEEE' (B) helps with access to the anterior teeth.

- Some echolalic children (automatic repetition of vocalizations) are able to copy words and expressions, and if this applies to the treating dentist, then the parents can be taught to encourage the child to say 'AHHHH'. This not only helps the parent to brush but also allows the dentist to examine the teeth visually and also facilitates examination of the pharynx by the child's medical practitioner. The sound 'EEEEEEE' can help display the upper anterior gingival margins, which are sometimes difficult to access (Figure 13.1).
- Actively look for evidence of trauma because of the association of ASD with epilepsy or self-injurious behaviours.
- Dietary advice must be specific to each individual child. If dietary reinforcers are being used, encourage the use of low-sugar safe snacks and consider the use of sugar-free confectionery.
- Establish time indicators. It is important to help the child realize that this experience does have a time limit. Visual or auditory timers (e.g., sand timers, buzzers, watch alarms) will help them to understand this and also to monitor the length of the experience.

Advise for improving communication

- Position yourself so that the child can see you.
- Get their attention by using the child's usual name at the beginning of the sentence.
- Use simple language without jokes, sarcasm or jargon.
- Use a minimum of social language (please and thank you) and avoid 'Childrenese'.
- Speak slowly to allow information to be processed.
- Limit any background noises in the surgery and use the same staff and a secluded dental surgery if possible.
- Positive reinforcement of desired behaviour should be 'celebrated' so that it is repeated. If the patient gets aggressive, maintain an unresponsive facial expression and use a calm tone.
- Try to engage the child. Knowing what he/she likes and dislikes is most important. Try to identify something in the surgery, perhaps moving the dental chair, playing with the light or a toy, that can be used to reinforce good behaviour.
- Humour has no effect and will not be understood.
- Be patient.

Paediatric dentists who care for a large number of these children need to have a full understanding of the nature of ASD and the specific issues and barriers to good oral health and dental care. As a paediatric dentist, it is important to remain flexible to meet the challenges which these children can present in the dental environment. Each child with autism is unique and requires a highly personalized management approach.

Developmental disabilities and intellectual disabilities

Developmental disabilities are described as differences in neurological-based functions that have their onset before birth, or during childhood, and are associated with long-term difficulties. People with intellectual disability have an IQ of less than 70 and deficits in adaptive functioning with an onset before 18 years of age. The term 'developmental disability' includes all people with an intellectual disability; however, not all people with a developmental disability have an intellectual disability. For example, children with cerebral palsy and autism have a developmental disability, but not all of them will be intellectually disabled.

TIPS FOR MANAGEMENT

- The first appointment is often one in which to familiarize both the dentist with the child's condition and the child with the dental environment.
- Consultation with the family and caregivers helps in finding out the patient's likes, dislikes and behaviour patterns.
- Determine each individual's level of communication; do not treat them as a 'homogenous group'. Be aware of your body language (nonverbal communication). Do not patronize but share the same social courtesies.
- Always allow extra time for your patients to familiarize; keep consistency with staff if possible. Short, early-morning appointments are preferable.
- Allow time for introduction of new concepts; prior explanation (announce each step) has better acceptance with patients as well as parents and caregivers.
- Repeat instructions when needed; offer praise and reinforce good behaviour. Be sensitive to your patient's gestures. Ask direct closed yes/no questions.
- 'Developmental delay' is a broad term covering children with a range of medical conditions and syndromes. It is essential that obscure syndromes be researched before performing treatment. Photocopy relevant information for the child's file.
- Support of the parent or caregivers is extremely important in reinforcing and administering preventive advice, oral hygiene practices and diet modification. Consultation with the school or institution may be required to modify diet.

PROBLEMS ASSOCIATED WITH INTELLECTUAL DISABILITIES

Management of poor plaque control

Patients with intellectual disabilities require assistance to maintain adequate oral hygiene to prevent gingivitis and periodontal disease. Carers should be trained in techniques to deliver oral care in a safe and effective manner. With some patients that may be tactile-defensive, referral to a speech pathologist for an oral desensitization programme before commencement of any oral hygiene programmes may be beneficial. These programmes include vibration and extraoral massage to treat tactile-defensive behaviour. The upper front teeth and gums are the most sensitive regions, so avoiding these areas until after complete desensitization of the oral cavity will assist in increasing compliance with tooth brushing.

Adjuncts to oral care

- When brushing, the parent or carer should stand behind and above the child whenever practicable to facilitate control of the head and the brush. This also allows better visual access. Other positions might include swaddling very young children, brushing while still in the wheelchair/feeding chair or sitting on the floor (Figure 13.2).

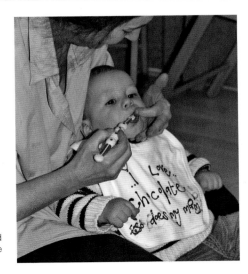

Figure 13.2 Sitting on the floor, supporting the child from behind, facilitates toothbrushing and oral hygiene for infants and young children with disabilities.

- A flexible 'three-headed toothbrush' simultaneously brushes the gums and teeth, making it easier for those with limited dexterity. It covers the entire tooth surface and is ideal for use in individuals with low tolerance or short attention span. Other toothbrushes with large handles assist patients with disabilities (Figure 13.3).
- Although electric toothbrushes have smaller heads and are easy to use, they run the risk of breaking or splitting inside the mouth and should be used with caution.
- Foam oral swabs (Figure 13.4) help to gently remove debris from the mouth in between brushing. They can be dipped into warm water, mouthwash or sodium bicarbonate (0.2%); however, they should not be substituted for regular tooth brushing.

MALOCCLUSION

There is a higher incidence of hypotonicity and hypertonicity of oral musculature in people with intellectual disabilities. These patients may also have unusual oral habits such as tongue thrusting, which creates malocclusions. Many patients with intellectual disabilities will be able to manage conventional orthodontics with an appropriate level of support, including with the use of relative

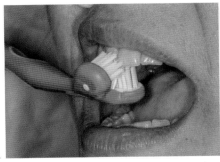
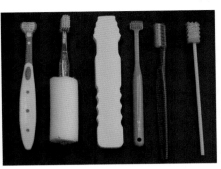

A   B

Figure 13.3 (A) Three-headed toothbrush. (B) A range of toothbrushes designed to facilitate improved brushing for patients with disabilities.

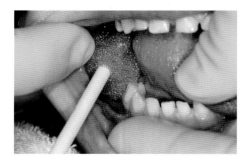

Figure 13.4 Foam tooth swabs are useful not only in children with disability but also in those children undergoing chemotherapy using sodium bicarbonate or chlorhexidine mouthwashes.

analgesia or sedation. However, for those patients with challenging behaviours, conventional orthodontics may not be possible. An orthodontist may consider interceptive orthodontic measures that might reduce the degree of malocclusion and the need for appliance wear. Early referral and consultation are beneficial for all children with a disability, who are developing a malocclusion in the mixed dentition stage.

MANAGEMENT OF TOOTH WEAR IN PATIENTS WITH AN INTELLECTUAL DISABILITY

Study models should be taken at the earliest signs of tooth wear to establish the rate of tooth wear over time. The causes of the tooth wear should be established and, if possible, eliminated. Gastro-oesophageal reflux is common in people with developmental disabilities and must be addressed by appropriate referral to gastroenterology. The incidence of tooth grinding is also higher in this population and should be addressed where possible by appropriate means.

Only treat the tooth wear restoratively if there is:
- Uncontrolled tooth wear over time.
- Loss of vitality or risk of loss of vitality.
- Aesthetic issues.
- Functional issues.

The restorative treatment of choice is overlaying of worn teeth using an indirect composite resin material with minimal tooth preparation. Two treatment sessions using sedation will be required for many patients with developmental disabilities to adequately take impressions and maintain isolation for cementation procedures.

Tooth grinding

Many parents and caregivers seek dental consultation because of tooth grinding and the worry or associated dental damage it can cause. It can be a social problem for families, teachers and caregivers, and consideration should be given to whether or not the behaviour has other implications, such as attention seeking in changed family circumstances. Tooth grinding is either physiological or pathological. It is quite commonly seen in individuals with neuromuscular and learning difficulties.

Physiological tooth grinding (Figure 13.5)

- Often occurs during times of concentration or at night during sleep, although it may occur at any time.
- Begins early during the development of the primary dentition, usually once the primary first molars erupt.
- Usually diminishes once the primary teeth have exfoliated.

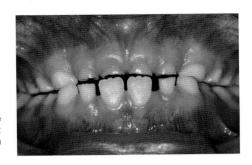

Figure 13.5 Physiological tooth wear can be quite extensive. Pulp exposure is uncommon; however, it is important to monitor the rate of tooth loss with serial photographs or, if possible, study models.

- No treatment is usually required other than parental reassurance.
- Use of soft or hard acrylic splints is indicated to protect the teeth; however, if the wear is excessive, threatening pulp exposure, then restorations using stainless steel crowns or extractions are indicated.
- Unusual to reflect any generalized systemic condition, and dental anthropologists regard this grinding as a phenomenon of 'tooth sharpening' termed 'thegosis'.

Pathological tooth grinding

- The amount of wear exceeds that which is felt to occur normally. Children may lose up to half the crown length in upper anterior teeth. Extensive enamel loss with wear facets and exposed dentine is unusual in posterior teeth.
- Often seen in children with underlying neurological disorders or medical problems such as Down syndrome, cerebral palsy or head injury. It has been hypothesized that tooth grinding in these patients stimulates endorphin production and is perceived to be a pleasurable activity.
- An increase in grinding intensity in these children may reflect other pathology such as otitis, salivary gland infection or generalized pain elsewhere in the body.

Management of tooth grinding

- If there has been extensive loss of tooth structure in the primary dentition, it will be essential to monitor any changes in the first permanent molars. Treatment may involve the placement of stainless steel crowns on the second primary molars. This will not only protect the permanent teeth but also preserve the vertical dimension of occlusion and tends to decrease grinding.
- Tooth grinding that is associated with self-mutilation of the soft tissues is extremely difficult to manage; some strategies have been discussed in Chapter 8.
- It must be noted that when, in the more severe cases, extractions of permanent teeth are contemplated, eventually all teeth will probably be lost. For those cases of intractable grinding and self-mutilation, the removal of only a few (anterior) teeth invariably leads to removal of all teeth in the arch.
- It is also important to identify other intrinsic or extrinsic factors such as reflux or an erosive diet that would contribute to further tooth surface loss.

Self-mutilation (self-injurious behaviours) (Figure 13.6)

A number of conditions exist which present with self-mutilation:
- Hereditary sensory neuropathies (congenital insensitivity to pain syndrome).
- Lesch–Nyhan syndrome (hypoxanthine guanine phosphoribosyltransferase deficiency).
- Hereditary neuropathies are rare inherited disorders affecting the number and distribution of small myelinated and unmyelinated nerve fibres. Most categories in classification systems

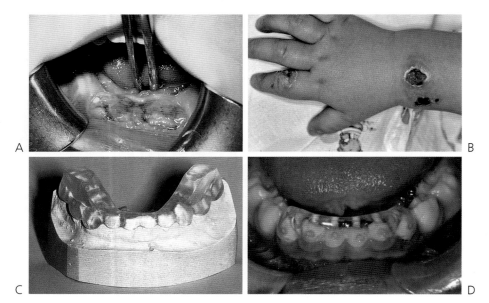

Figure 13.6 (A) Self-mutilation in a child with a peripheral sensory neuropathy. This child presented with exfoliation of the anterior teeth. She was investigated for many of the conditions described earlier until it was discovered that she herself was pulling out her teeth. Having no sensory nerve endings, she could feel no pain. (B) Finger-biting can also be a manifestation of neuropathies. (C) An appliance to prevent self-injury. All cases are different, and an appliance that is successful in one patient may not prove to be appropriate in another. (D) A lower acrylic splint to cover the teeth and prevent tongue biting. The holes on the labial aid in retention of the cement.

arise from the varied clinical presentations; terms used have included congenital indifference or insensitivity to pain, dysautonomia, sensory anaesthesia, painless whitlows of the fingers and recurrent plantar ulcers with osteomyelitis.

The term 'indifference to pain' in these cases is a misnomer in that indifference implies a cerebral inattention or cognitive dysfunction. Those patients with 'indifference' correctly receive painful stimuli but fail to react in the usual defensive manner by withdrawal. In those patients with 'insensitivity to pain', the deep tendon reflexes are preserved, as these are controlled by large-diameter myelinated fibres. The lack of pain perception is caused by a true peripheral neuropathy.

DIAGNOSIS

The diagnosis of these conditions is often made by exclusion and by careful observation of the child. It is not uncommon for many months to pass before a correct diagnosis is made and, in the absence of other pathologies, parents or caregivers may incorrectly be suspected of child abuse or Munchausen syndrome by proxy. Because of an inability to recognize or feel pain, these children may avulse teeth and inflict extensive trauma to the gingivae, tongue or mucosa with their fingers or by biting and chewing. Self-inflicted ulceration (factitious ulceration) may also occur as a habit (akin to nail biting) but may also be a manifestation of psychological disorders.

MANAGEMENT

- Selective grinding of tooth cusps or 'dome' build-ups of the occlusal table with composite resin to produce a smooth surface.

- Acrylic splints or cast silver splints to prevent gross laceration of the tongue or fingers.
- Extraction of teeth may be required as a last option in severe cases.

Initial management in young children often necessitates restraint to prevent these children from injuring themselves. Even for the most vigilant parents, constant supervision is impossible, and invariably these children will continue to sustain injuries despite the best care. The involvement of occupational therapists is invaluable to support parents and institute protective measures in the home such as the use of padded clothing, arm splints, helmets and other protective devices. Where lacerations to the tongue and other soft tissues occur, mouth guards and other appliances which prevent the teeth from occluding are required. Lower appliances are generally more suitable than those placed in the upper arch. In severe cases where the mutilation is intractable, botulinum toxin A (Botox) has been used to selectively paralyse the major mandibular elevator muscles (medial pterygoid and masseter).

PROGNOSIS

The prognosis for most children with peripheral sensory neuropathies is poor, and in one case managed by one of the authors, the child died of an undiagnosed pneumonia before 3 years of age. Children tend to have repeated hospital admissions, fractures of long bones, injuries to the extremities and recurrent chronic infections. This pattern of repeated traumatic injuries is characterized in one such patient managed by the authors:

- Premature loss of all lower anterior primary teeth.
- Chronic ulceration of the lower alveolus.
- Second-degree burn to right forearm from a radiator.
- Fracture of the left humerus (during hospital admission) with subsequent multifocal osteomyelitis.
- Fracture of left condyle and mandibular symphysis.
- Death from respiratory sepsis at 2 years of age.

Cerebral palsy

The cerebral palsies are a heterogeneous group of static encephalopathies that have in common a disorder of posture and movement. The motor disability is permanent, and the clinical manifestations are variable. Cerebral palsy can be simply classified into:

- Spastic (hemiplegia, paraplegia and quadriplegia).
- Dyskinetic (choreoathetoid and dystonic).
- Ataxia.
- Mixed.

Adverse prenatal and perinatal events that affect the brain account for the known causes of cerebral palsy, although most causes are unknown.

The cognitive ability of a child with cerebral palsy cannot be quickly determined. Time is required with these children to assess their physical and mental abilities. Many patients with cerebral palsy have no cognitive impairment at all and may use a form of verbal communication that requires an electronic aid and operator patience. It is often not necessary to change voice tone or level of language when addressing these children.

Maxillary protrusion and generalized anterior tooth spacing are common sequelae because of abnormal orofacial neuromuscular tone (Figure 13.7). Tongue thrust, dribbling, mouth breathing and perioral sensitivity are also common clinical presentations. Dental caries and periodontal disease may be severe because of neglect and following surgery to reposition the major saliva gland ducts to reduce drooling.

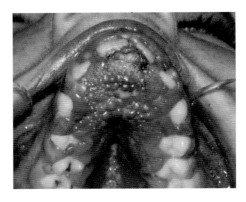

Figure 13.7 Severe phenytoin gingival enlargement, candidosis and papillary hyperplasia in the palate of a child with cerebral palsy. The hypertonicity of the oral musculature has caused the protrusion of the anterior teeth and an orthopaedic compression of the maxilla.

DENTAL MANAGEMENT

Reflex limb extension patterns may be triggered during dental visits if care is not taken. These contractions may occur during transfer of the patient from the wheelchair to the dental chair. Discuss the transfer with the parent or caregivers before offering assistance. Use the hoist option for a safe transfer when available. This reflex may also be stimulated if the child's head is loose or unsupported. Ensure that the child is stabilized in the chair with blankets and pillows or restrained with a belt or webbing. If a reflex pattern occurs where the limbs are in extension:

- Raise the chair.
- Stabilize the head in the midline.
- Bring the arms forwards.
- Reassure the child.

Some patients are best treated in their own motorized wheelchairs. Remember to lock the wheels, recline the chair and use adequate head support (Figure 13.8).

Gag, cough, bite and swallowing reflexes may be impaired or abnormal in children with cerebral palsy. If the gag reflex is more exaggerated, treat the patient in a more upright position with the neck in slight flexion and the knees bent upwards, if possible. Mouth props may be used; however, for those patients with impaired swallowing, there is an increased risk of aspiration. Hand-held props and a floss ligature help to reduce this possibility. Rubber dam is especially useful in these cases as well. If the patient's bite reflex to oral stimulation is still present, introduce instruments from the side rather than the front. To allow dental examination, apply gentle pressure with the forefinger on the anterior border of ascending ramus and in the retromolar triangle. This reduces the risk of a bitten finger. Alternatively, in some cases, foam mouth props are available to assist in providing a safe oral examination in those patients with unpredictable behaviour who

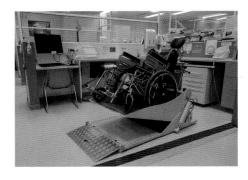

Figure 13.8 Motorized wheelchair lift, allowing the patient to remain in the chair during dental treatment.

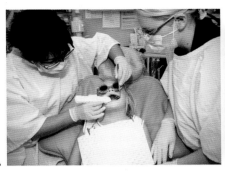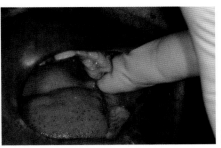

A   B

Figure 13.9 (A) A foam mouth-prop may also aid in oral examination or toothbrushing. (B) It is very important to protect your fingers from being bitten, not least to protect against the risk of infection but also potential damage. By placing the index finger in the buccal sulcus and behind the last molar, the mouth can be opened and the operator's fingers safe.

may unexpectedly bite down (Figure 13.9). Nitrous oxide sedation may help to reduce involuntary movements during dental treatment.

Hydrocephalus

Most cases of hydrocephalus result from obstruction to cerebrospinal fluid (CSF) flow, either within the cerebral ventricles or in the subarachnoid space. As the ventricles enlarge because of the accumulation of CSF, intracranial pressure increases, resulting in serious neurological impairment if not decompressed. The postnatal causes of hydrocephalus are varied, including bacterial infection, haemorrhage and neoplastic obstruction, but prenatal causes are often undiagnosable. Treatment by insertion of a shunt is usually appropriate in infants with severe hydrocephalus. Many children with hydrocephalus have other developmental deficits such as learning disabilities or paraplegia.

Children with hydrocephalus undergoing dental treatment may require antibiotic prophylaxis if they have shunts that directly empty into the major blood vessels (ventriculoatrial) to prevent septicaemia and shunt infection. It is generally considered that children with ventriculoperitoneal and spinoperitoneal shunts do not require prophylactic antibiotic cover, unless specified by the neurologist. In all instances it is wise to seek advice and manage the patient in consultation with their attending physician.

Spina bifida

In this condition, there is a herniation (meningomyelocele) of the spinal cord, nerve roots and meninges through a wide deficiency in the laminae and spinous process of one or more vertebrae, usually at the sacral or lumbosacral levels. The exposed cord is dysplastic and almost always nonfunctional, often resulting in paraplegia. Early operative closure is performed where possible to prevent infection, and subsequent orthopaedic and urological management is necessary. Rehabilitation is best provided by coordinated multidisciplinary clinics.

Children with spina bifida have a higher prevalence of latex allergy (gloves, rubber dam) compared with the general paediatric population. The use of vinyl gloves is recommended. Many children are confined to a wheelchair, and spinal comfort should be optimized in a similar way as for children with cerebral palsy. Otherwise, routine dental management can be undertaken in the clinic setting.

Muscular dystrophies

Muscular dystrophy is a progressive, genetically determined, primary degenerative myopathy. The clinical features include increasing muscle weakness, poor muscle tone, abnormal body movements, skin changes and progressive joint and skeletal deformity. Duchenne muscular dystrophy and myotonic dystrophy are the two most common forms and current treatment is to slow the effects of disuse atrophy. Ambulation is usually not possible after 12 years of age.

Oral manifestations include craniofacial deformity with protrusive spaced anterior teeth because of poor orofacial tone and associated mouth breathing, tongue thrust and open bite. Poor plaque control, gingivitis and anterior tooth trauma are common oral findings. Dental management strategies are similar to those used in children with cerebral palsy, using head and body supports and mouth props. Do not try and stop your patient's movements; instead, work around them. Use check retractors in patients with loose or rigid oral musculature.

Sedation and general anaesthesia are often necessary to manage children with muscular dystrophy because of their inability to tolerate routine procedures in the dental chair. Anaesthetic techniques must be modified to minimize intra- and postoperative respiratory and cardiovascular depression and invasive monitoring, and access to intensive care may be warranted. Depolarizing muscle relaxants like succinylcholine should be avoided because of the risk of hyperkalaemia. This may result in the release of large amounts of potassium ions from the muscle cell into the bloodstream, with a subsequent, rapid increase in potassium concentration in the blood, resulting in life-threatening cardiac rhythm disturbances. Malignant hyperthermia occurs relatively frequently in patients with muscular dystrophy in the presence of succinylcholine or inhalation anaesthetics. This is characterized by an extremely elevated metabolism within the muscle cell. As a result, the temperature of the entire body rises to life-threatening levels. It is of tremendous importance that this is promptly diagnosed and appropriate measures are implemented.

Vision impairment

In addition to the obvious barriers to care that present for a child with vision impairment, the inability to see the dentist, the environment and what treatment is being done are extremely threatening. Again, communication is the key to trust and success in treatment.

- The reception staff should introduce themselves and offer to lead the patient to the surgery and determine the level of assistance your patient needs. If the patient attends with a guide dog in harness, it indicates the dog is working.
- It is vital to assess the degree of visual impairment. Allow the child to make full use of their tactile sense and their sense of smell when familiarizing them with the dental environment and dental procedures.
- Always announce your entry and departure from the room. Offer verbal and physical reassurance to the child once a rapport has been established, as they cannot see nonverbal gestures.
- Paint a picture in the mind of your patients by describing the treatment and the environment throughout the procedure. A startle reflex may occur if patients are not warned before different instruments are introduced into the mouth.
- Many visually impaired people are photophobic. It is important to ask parents and children about light sensitivity. Safety glasses should preferably be tinted.
- All written information, including appointments and oral hygiene instructions, should be provided in large text or Braille.

Hearing impairment

Children with hearing impairment present a unique challenge for dentists because effective communication is the primary basis of successful child management. Hearing impairment may be sensorineural or conductive in origin, and range in degree of hearing loss from mild to profound. Recent advances, such as the development of the cochlear implant, new surgical procedures and future stem cell therapy, have improved hearing outcomes significantly for many, but not all, hearing-impaired children. It is useful to learn basic sign language or the appropriate manual finger-spelling alphabet (e.g., the two-handed alphabet in Britain, Australia and New Zealand or the one-handed alphabet in the USA and Canada and, with some variation, many other countries) (see Figure 13.10). It should be noted that even within the English-speaking world, there are

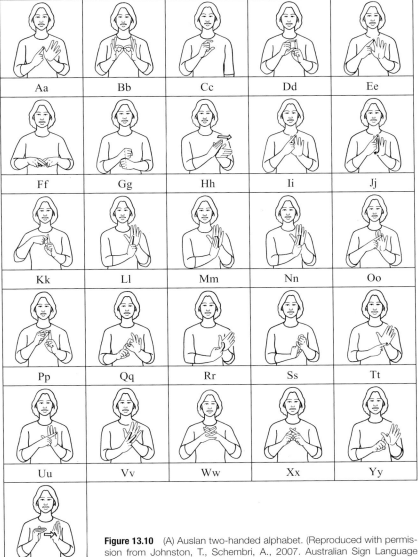

Figure 13.10 (A) Auslan two-handed alphabet. (Reproduced with permission from Johnston, T., Schembri, A., 2007. Australian Sign Language (Auslan): an introduction to sign language linguistics. Cambridge University Press, Cambridge.)

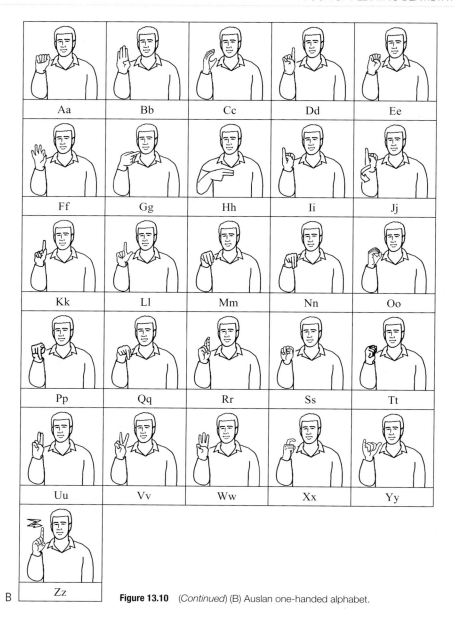

Figure 13.10 *(Continued)* (B) Auslan one-handed alphabet.

different sign languages which are mutually unintelligible (i.e., Auslan in Australia or American Sign Language in the USA and Canada). As with all behaviour management, it is essential to win the trust of the child, be cognizant of their special needs and understand the unique difficulties they have in communication.

- Investigate how the child communicates. If the child uses a sign language as their first or preferred language, use basic signs and finger-spelling if you have previously learned this or, preferably, use the services of a sign language interpreter.

- If the child is hearing impaired and can use their residual hearing with the help of hearing aids or a cochlear implant and lip-reading, use speech. A common fault is to talk loudly rather than slowly. Face the child and speak clearly and slowly. Remove your face mask and eliminate or reduce any background sounds (e.g., radio, etc.) before speaking with the child.
- Make it easy for patients to maintain visual contact, because these children may be startled if they are touched without visual contact.
- Children with hearing difficulties may be very sensitive to vibration, so introduce high-speed and low-speed drills carefully.
- If a hearing aid is worn, the volume may need adjustment. Try to avoid blocking the ears and the hearing aid with the forearms when operating, as this will create feedback.

Oro-motor dysfunction in patients with developmental disabilities

Children with cerebral palsy, trisomy 21 and global developmental delay often present with poor oral functions, including:

- Hypertonicity.
- Hypotonicity.
- Dysphagia (difficulty in swallowing).
- Dysphasia (difficulty in speaking).
- Sialorrhoea (difficulty in swallowing, resulting in drooling).

DROOLING

Parents will often present with their primary concern being excessive drooling. The paediatric dentist has a significant role in the management of sialorrhoea. Causes of drooling can range from poor competency of the lip and orofacial musculature, malocclusion, dysphagia, to oral habits.

The options for the management of drooling are:

Nonsurgical

- Eliminate aggravating factors (dental caries, habits, malocclusions).
- Referral to a multidisciplinary team for oro-motor function therapy.
- Biofeedback using mouth mirrors for lip posture and use of tongue suck and swallow reflex.

Surgical management

- Severance of the parasympathetic supply.
- Re-routing the submandibular duct to the posterior tonsillar pillar; 70% of cases are described as good to excellent.
- Salivary gland duct ligation.
- Salivary gland excision.

Risks and side effects

- Ranula formation.
- Loss of the gland.
- Increased caries risk.
- Aspiration of saliva because of dysphagia.

Pharmacological management

- Benztropine (*Cogentin*).
- Trihexyphenidyl hydrochloride (benzhexol hydrochloride; *Artane*).

- Scopolamine transdermal patches.
- Glycopyrrolate.
- Botulinum toxin A (*Botox*). It has a short duration of action (2–6 months) and necessitates the need for repeat general anaesthetics for some patients.

Side effects of medications include:

- Xerostomia.
- Dental caries.
- Urinary retention.
- Flushing.
- Drying of all mucous membranes.
- Trihexyphenidyl can cause behavioural changes.

ORO-MOTOR FUNCTION THERAPY

Oro-motor function therapy is carried out by multidisciplinary teams that may include speech pathologists, occupational therapists, physiotherapists and dentists. The focus of oro-motor function therapy is to develop the oral motor skills required to manage saliva control. This multifaceted approach may include a number of elements such as:

- Behaviour modification.
- Proprioceptive neuromuscular facilitation.
- Postural adaptations.
- Oral screens and dental appliances designed to stimulate oral musculature.

Dental appliances

These are individually designed to produce the desired movement of the tongue, lips or jaw (Figure 13.11). Common goals include:

- Establishment of correct tongue position.
- Stimulation of lip closure.
- Stimulation of tongue elevation, lateralization.
- Stimulation of jaw stabilization.
- Reduction in mouthing behaviour.

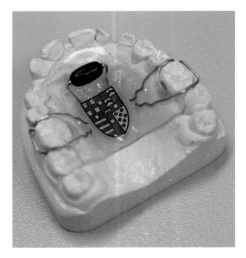

Figure 13.11 A dental appliance with a movable bead in palate for use in oro-motor function therapy.

TABLE 13.1 ■ Presentation of more common special-needs conditions

Condition	Common medical comorbidities	Dental associations
Williams syndrome	Mild to moderate intellectual disability, ADHD, distinctive facial features (elfin facies) like wide mouth, small upturned nose, hypertelorism, cardiovascular problems, hypercalcemia, short stature, speech delays, aversion to physical contact, sensitivity to loud noises	Malocclusion, aberration in tooth size and morphology, widely spaced teeth, agenesis of permanent teeth, taurodontism, enamel hypoplasia, increased prevalence of dental caries
Trisomy 21 (Down syndrome)	Congenital cardiac anomalies, intellectual disability, leukaemia, atlanto-axial instability, epilepsy, visual and conductive hearing impairment, hypotonia, early dementia	Over retained primary teeth, delayed tooth eruption, hypodontia, microdontia, taurodontism, hypoplasia, malocclusion Greater incidence of periodontal disease due to impaired host response Progressive loss of fine motor skills that compromise the ability to maintain oral hygiene
Fragile X syndrome	Congenital cardiac anomalies, epilepsy, intellectual disability, autism spectrum disorder, excessive laxity of joints	Root anomalies, malocclusion, drooling
Rett Syndrome	Rare genetic brain disorder causing repetitive hand movements, cardiac abnormalities, language and coordination difficulties, scoliosis/kyphosis, growth retardation, decreased or loss of use of fine motor skills	Bruxism, narrow and high arched palate, micrognathia, drooling, digit sucking, involuntary tongue
Muscular dystrophy	Progressive muscular wasting, poor body balance and waddling gait, scoliosis, progressive inability to walk becoming clinically evident when a child begins walking, respiratory difficulty, cardiomyopathy Duchenne muscular dystrophy (DMD) is the most common childhood form of muscular dystrophy, generally affecting only boys, some patients have a learning disability	Poor oral hygiene, increased dental decay, orofacial muscle weakness and drooling, disturbances in tooth number and form, anterior open bite, mouth breathing, xerostomia, reduced mouth opening
Foetal alcohol syndrome	Typical facial features, growth inhibition, learning and behaviour difficulties, hyperactivity, multiple organs can be affected	Extensive dental decay, xerostomia, cleft lip and palate, deep bite, developmental dental anomalies, impaired oro-motor functions causing speech difficulties
Tuberous sclerosis	It is usually linked to a triad of conditions comprising epilepsy, mental retardation, and angiofibromas, as well as to oral and skin manifestations. Multiple organs can be affected, patients also may have ASD and a speech impairment	Drooling, gingival hyperplasia, enamel pitting and hypoplasia, risk of bone cyst formation

Continued

TABLE 13.1 ■ *Continued*

Sotos syndrome	Typical facies with long, narrow head, high, protrusive forehead. Hypertelorism with downward slant of the eyes. Delayed oromotor developments and muscle weakness, sleep apnoea. Developmental delay, speech and learning difficulties	Hypodontia, high palate, excessive tooth wear, skeletal malocclusion, crossbite, ectopic tooth eruption
Cornelia de Lange	Low birth weight, excessive body hair, delayed growth, short arms and legs, deformities of the lower arms and hands. Congenital developmental, cardiac and gastrointestinal deformities. Facial dysmorphia with small head, low set ears, upturned nose, and synophrys (eyebrows meeting in the midline). Behavioural and speech impairments and some patients develop a hoarse voice	High arched palate, hypodontia, delayed tooth eruption, xerostomia, anterior open bite, Hutchinson-shaped maxillary central incisors, enamel hypomineralisation, drooling, erosion and bruxism
Mucopolysacc-aridoses	Metabolic disorder, multisystemic deterioration with cardiovascular and audiovisual impairments, sleep apnoea, impaired oro-motor function, dwarfism, hernias, coarse facial changes and progressive neurodegenerative disease	Enamel hypomineralisation, small jaws and malformed hypoplastic teeth, large tongue, drooling, high arched palate, delayed tooth eruption, gingival hyperplasia
Turner syndrome	Affects mainly women, short stature and infertility, congenital heart defects, hearing problems, behavioural and learning difficulties, webbing on the neck, soft upturned nails and low hairline	Early dental development and early tooth eruption, malocclusions, aberration in tooth morphology causing microdontia, short roots, enamel hypoplasia, widely spaced teeth, retrognathic mandible and large overjet
Noonan	Impaired growth hormone, short stature, cardiac defects, late-onset puberty in males, developmental and intellectual disability, poor muscle tone. Broad forehead, short and broad neck with webbing, low hairline at the nape of the neck, epicanthic fold in the inner corner of the eyes, ptosis, hypertelorism, low-set backward rotated ears	Micrognathia, high palate, delayed tooth eruption, missing teeth, giant cell lesions in the mandible
Angelman	Microcephaly, epilepsy, flat back of the head, poor muscle tone and ataxia, impaired psychosocial and intellectual disability, hyperactivity, delayed speech, hand flapping, happy social demeanour, epilepsy	Generalised spaced dentition, open bite, wide mouth, short upper lip, protruded tongue, drooling, features of mouth breathing
Tourette	Milder forms may closely resemble ADHD or OCD. Characterised by tics like blinking, facial grimace and one involuntary vocalisation like grunting, or barking, behavioural and learning and speech difficulties	Drooling, bruxism, self injurious behaviours

Further reading

Chew, L.C., King, N.M., O'Donnell, D., 2006. Autism: the aetiology, management and implications for treatment modalities from the dental perspective. Dental Update 33, 70–80.

Dougall, A., Fiske, J., 2008. Access to special care dentistry. Part 4: education. British Dental Journal 205, 119–130.

Estrella, M.R., Boynton, J.R., 2010. General dentistry's role in the care for children with special needs: a review. General Dentistry 58, 222–229.

Goyette, C.H., Conners, C.K., Ulrich, R.F., 1978. Normative data on revised Conners Parent and Teacher Rating Scales. Journal of Abnormal Child Psychology 6, 221–236.

Hussein, I., Kershaw, A.E., Tahmassebi, J.F., et al., 1998. The management of drooling in children and patients with mental and physical disabilities. International Journal of Pediatric Dentistry 8, 3–11.

Klein, U., Nowak, A.J., 1998. Autistic disorder: a review for the paediatric dentist. Pediatric Dentistry 20, 312–317.

Lawton, L., 2002. Providing dental care for special patients. Tips for the general dentist. Journal of the American Dental Association 133, 1666–1679.

Levine, M.D., Carey, W.B., 1983. Developmental–behavioral paediatrics. WB Saunders, Philadelphia.

Monroy, P.G., da Fonseca, M.A., 2006. The use of botulinum toxin-a in the treatment of severe bruxism in a patient with autism: a case report. Special Care in Dentistry 26, 37–39.

Moursi, A.M., Fernandez, J.B., Daronch, M., et al., 2010. Nutrition and oral health considerations in children with special health care needs: implications for oral health care providers. Pediatric Dentistry 32, 333–342.

Nunn, J., 2000. Disability and oral care. International Association for Disability and Oral Health and FDI. World Dental Press, London.

Pilebro, C., Bäckman, B., 2005. Teaching oral hygiene to children with autism. International Journal of Paediatric Dentistry 15, 1–9.

Websites

British Society for Disability and Oral Health. Available: www.bsdh.org.uk/guidelines.html.

Mn-H Center. Available: www.mun-h-center.se.

Management of cleft lip and palate

Julia Dando

Introduction

EPIDEMIOLOGY

Clefts of the lip and cleft palate are fusion disorders that affect the midfacial skeleton. They are one of the most common congenital anomalies, with a worldwide incidence of between 0.8 and 2.7 cases per 1000 live births. The incidence of clefting varies by region, gender, ethnicity and maternal characteristics. In general, it has been noted that incidence can be higher in first nation populations, followed by Asian, Caucasian and African Americans.

Aetiology

Despite being common, the aetiology of many clefts of the lip/palate remains obscure. In addition to chromosomal abnormalities and teratogenic effects, there are over 500 recognized Mendelian syndromes associated with a cleft of the lip/palate. In many instances, specific genetic mutations have been identified, for example, van de Woude syndrome (IRF6) and Treacher Collins (TCOF1). However, over 70% of clefts of the lip and palate and up to 50% of clefts of the palate only are apparently isolated anomalies. The aetiology of these nonsyndromic forms of cleft is multifactorial, and the relative genetic and environmental contributions remain unclear. Consequently, although it is understood that the offspring and siblings of individuals with a cleft have a higher risk of having a cleft themselves, this lack of clarity makes it difficult to give families accurate information regarding the recurrence risks or to offer informed genetic counselling.

Recent research has indicated that primary defects in regulators of epithelial cell adhesion are the most significant contributors to nonsyndromic cleft lip and palate that have been identified. These inherited single-gene variants explain a high proportion of the familial cases studied. This is in contrast to previously held views that many common genetic variants as well as environmental factors played a part in the risk of a child having cleft lip and palate. It is hoped that further research in this area may well lead to more specific counselling (Roscioli, 2018).

Embryology (Figure 14.1)

The structures of the lip and premaxilla develop between week 4 and week 6 in utero. The palate is formed slightly later, with the hard palate between weeks 6 and 8 and the soft palate at weeks 10 to 12.

Contributing to formation are
- The midline frontonasal prominence; from proliferation of neural crest cells ventral to the forebrain; and
- The bilateral maxillary processes and bilateral mandibular processes – from the first pharyngeal arch.

In week 5, nasal placodes appear in the frontonasal process and later form pits with medial and lateral nasal prominences on each side.

The medial nasal prominences are pushed into the midline by the expanding maxillary prominences, and at week 6, these structures fuse to form the lip, alveolus and premaxilla (primary palate). At this stage there is continuity between the oral and nasal cavities, and the maxillary prominences continue to expand vertically on either side of the tongue.

In the lower face, the mandibular processes fuse, and the resulting enlargement of the head and oral cavity allows the tongue to occupy a lower position.

In week 7, the palatal shelves can now elevate into a horizontal position, and in week 8, fusion occurs in the midline to form the hard palate. Palatal development then continues until completion of the soft palate in weeks 10 to 12.

Events that disrupt the fusion may result in clefting:
- Clefts of the primary palate (i.e., lip, alveolus and palate anterior to the incisive foramen) are caused by disruption of fusion of the medial nasal processes and maxillary prominences around week 6.
- Clefts of the secondary palate (i.e., hard and/or soft palate) are caused by disruption of the elevation and/or fusion of the palatal shelves around weeks 8 to 12.

The most severe anomalies will tend to occur early in embryonic development between weeks 4 and 8.

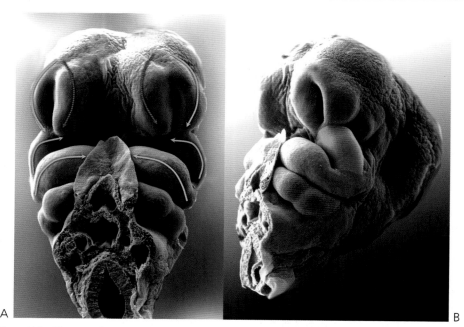

Figure 14.1 All mammalian embryos are similar in appearance in the early stages of development. Rat embryo at 35 days showing the development of the pharayngeal (branchial) arches that form the face and jaws. The cardiac sac has been sectioned and the neural tube is seen posteriorly and inferior. (A) The medial (*purple arrows*) and lateral nasal processes fuse early in development to join with the maxillary process (*green*). This explains the location of the majority of facial clefts being lateral to the premaxilla and not in the midline. (B) The maxillary process (*shaded green*) arises from the 1st branchial arch (mandibular arch – *shaded blue*) from which form the muscles of mastication. The 2nd arch (*shaded purple*) is the hyoid arch containing the facial nerve and the muscles of facial expression.

Anatomy

When describing a cleft, the anatomical structure, position and extent of the cleft should be noted:

- Lip, alveolus, palate or any combination.
- Right or left (unilateral).
- Both sides (bilateral).
- Partial thickness (incomplete).
- Full thickness (complete).

So, for example, a child with notching of the right side of the lip would be described as having a unilateral incomplete cleft lip. A cleft extending through the full thickness of the lip and into the palate, on both sides, would be described as having a bilateral complete cleft lip and palate.

Sometimes a child may have a complete cleft on one side with an incomplete cleft on the other or any combination of these.

CLEFTS OF THE LIP AND ALVEOLUS (PRIMARY PALATE) (Figures 14.5 and 14.3)

The clinical manifestation of a cleft in this region can vary from an incomplete cleft (*forme fruste*) to a minimal defect involving just the vermilion border, to a complete defect extending from the vermilion border to the floor of the nose with clefting of the alveolus. Even in the absence of a

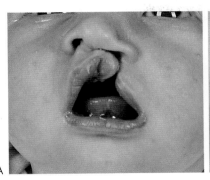 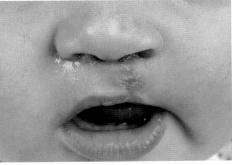

A   B

Figure 14.2 (A) Unilateral complete cleft lip and palate, showing the extent of the malformation with rotation of the alar base and the cleft extending into the nares. The columella and primary palate (lip and alveolus) are rotated superiorly and to the unaffected side. (B) Repair healing at 10 months of age, with equalization of the alar base and continuity of the vermilion border.

frank cleft of the bony alveolus there may be evidence of clefting in the form of a dental anomaly such as a missing or microdont lateral incisor (see Chapter 11).

CLEFT LIP AND PALATE

In a complete cleft of the lip and palate there is direct communication between the oral and nasal cavities on the cleft side (Figure 14.4A). There can be substantial variation in the degree of palatal shelf separation. Clinically this can result in either well-approximated segments or wide defects. In some cases oral function and tongue position can change the relative positions of the maxillary arch segments before surgery.

In the bilateral complete cleft lip and palate (Figure 14.4B), both nasal chambers are in direct communication with the oral cavity. The palatal processes are divided into two equal parts, and the turbinates are clearly visible within both nasal cavities. The nasal septum forms a midline structure that is firmly attached to the base of the skull but is fairly mobile anteriorly, where it supports the premaxilla and columella. In these clefts, the premaxilla protrudes considerably

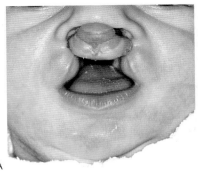 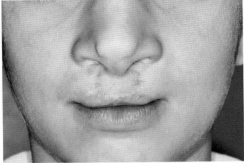

A   B

Figure 14.3 (A) Bilateral complete cleft lip and palate. The premaxillary segment is clearly visible as an extension of the nasal septum. The central incisors are contained within this process. The columella and philtrum are extremely short and there is a wide defect between the segments. (B) Repair at 8 years of age showing a relatively broad philtrum and short columella, but the alar base is symmetrical, although there is an accentuation of the cupid's bow and eversion of the vermilion border.

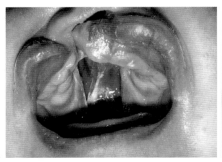 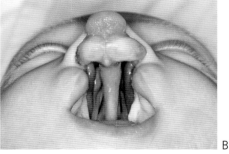

A   B

Figure 14.4   (A) Unilateral complete cleft of lip and palate showing the extent of the bony defect and deficiency of the palatal shelves. (B) Bilateral complete cleft of lip and palate. The upper anterior teeth are contained within the primary palate and are connected via the nasal septum and vomer.

forwards of the facial profile and is attached to a stalk-like vomer and the nasal septum. The 'lip' component of the medial segment contains only collagenous connective tissue. It is, therefore, grossly deficient in bulk and lacks the features normally produced by muscle.

CLEFT PALATE

A cleft of the palate may involve only the soft palate, both soft and hard palates or very occasionally the hard palate alone. Deficiencies of the mucosa and bone are the main features of clefts of the hard palate (Figure 14.4). The cleft may extend forward from the uvula to varying degrees, from a bifid uvula associated with a submucous cleft palate (see later and Figure 14.5) to a 'V'-shaped cleft extending through the hard palate to the incisive foramen. Some babies have a 'U'-shaped cleft of the palate that is described in 'Robin sequence' (Figure 14.6). Robin sequence is characterized by upper airway problems associated with extreme micrognathia and glossoptosis and is thought to be secondary to mandibular hypoplasia in the first trimester, which causes the tongue to sit high in the mouth and prevent fusion of the palatal shelves.

SUBMUCOUS CLEFT PALATE (Figure 14.5)

Clefting of the velum or soft palate can be 'submucous' where the mucous membrane remains intact, despite clefting of the underlying musculature. Submucous clefts of the palate occur in around 1 in 1200 live births, with only half of the cases having clinically significant symptoms.

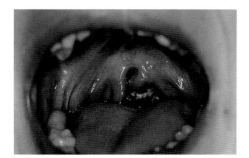

Figure 14.5   A bifid uvula associated with a submucous cleft palate. The fibres of tensor palati are not joined, although the epithelium is intact. These children may present with nasal air escape because of a shortened palate and velopharyngeal incompetence. There is often a notch felt at the posterior border of the hard palate and a bluish median line extends to the uvula.

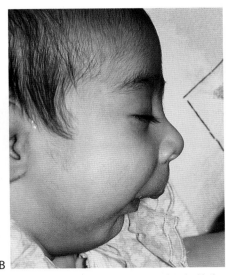

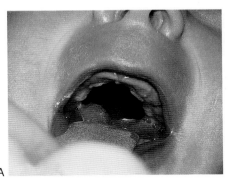

A   B

Figure 14.6 (A) Cleft of the palate with an intact lip and alveolus. This U-shaped cleft was associated with the Robin sequence and resulted from a failure of embryonic head rotation. This maintained the tongue in the oral cavity and the palatal shelves subsequently formed around the tongue, giving rise to the characteristic cleft shape. (B) Another manifestation of this condition is extreme micrognathia and glosoptosis.

OTHER FACIAL CLEFTS (Figure 14.7)

It is important to recognize that clefts are basically a failure of fusion of embryological processes and may occur in many other areas of the face and complex oro-facial or oro-ocular clefts form part of the spectrum of many craniofacial disorders.

Diagnosis

Clefting disorders are now increasingly diagnosed prenatally as part of routine ultrasound screening between 18 and 20 weeks in utero. The reported diagnostic accuracy of routine two-dimensional (2D) ultrasonography in a low-risk population varies between 9% and 100% for complete clefts of lip and palate but is much lower (0%–22%) for clefts of the palate only (Maarse et al., 2010). Much higher accuracy is achieved using 3D ultrasound, but again isolated clefts of the palate often remain undetected. Prenatal screening provides knowledge of the impending birth of a baby with a cleft, which allows both the family and appropriate clinicians to prepare for this event.

Management of individuals with clefts of the lip and/or palate

Although surgery can correct many of the structural defects, affected individuals can still face a lifetime of functional, social and aesthetic challenges. In addition, there is growing evidence that some individuals with cleft lip and palate may also have subtle neuropsychological and developmental deficits, which are associated with learning difficulties and other educational challenges. The care of these infants often starts antenatally and continues from birth through to adulthood

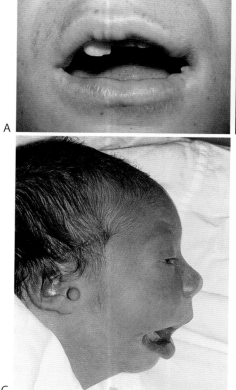

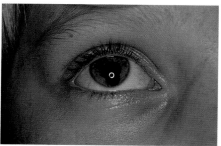

A

B

C

Figure 14.7 (A) Clefting may occur in many areas of the face (and body, e.g., spina bifida). This is a transverse cleft of the lateral commissure of the lip (Tessier Type 7) associated with segmental odonto-maxillary dysplasia. (B) An iris coloboma: a cleft of the iris that may feature in a number of craniofacial syndromes that include orofacial clefting. (C) This child has a cleft of the commissure (macrostomia) and a skin tag anterior to the ear, which is often seen in craniofacial microsomia.

and involves a large multidisciplinary team of clinicians. The specialties involved in this team vary greatly but usually include:

- Plastic surgery.
- Ear, nose and throat (otolaryngology) and/or maxillofacial surgery.
- Speech pathology and audiology.
- Orthodontics.
- Paediatric dentistry.
- Paediatrics.
- Psychology.
- Specialist nursing and social services.

In addition, genetics, ophthalmology, neurosurgery, periodontics, prosthodontics and implantology may be involved at different times. The range and length of treatment required place enormous burdens, both financial and psychosocial, on not just the individuals themselves but also their family.

Variation (and minimal high-level evidence) in the sequencing and timing of treatment and the clinical techniques and interventions used between cleft teams does exist. Overall, however, there are some commonly accepted aims and principles of treatment. Early support and advice for new parents are essential, especially if the birth is outside a centre used to caring for children with clefts. A specialist nurse and/or primary surgeon from a cleft team provides a rapid initial evaluation as soon as possible after the birth. Subsequent regular contact through either home visits or attendance at specialist cleft review clinics ensures that families are supported appropriately and social and psychological issues are identified and resolved early. Treatment plans should be formulated and implemented collaboratively by the multidisciplinary team in partnership with the families.

The goals of the treatment of a child with a cleft of the lip and/or palate are to restore both form (appearance) and function (especially speech and mastication) while optimizing general health and well-being.

Management in the neonatal period

FEEDING

Efficient feeding is important for growth and development in infancy. A baby with a cleft of any kind may experience feeding difficulties. However, babies with cleft palate or combined cleft lip and palate usually have more problems than those with cleft lip.

Feeding in babies is a reflex action that coordinates sucking, breathing and swallowing. A seal formed with the lips and negative pressure in the oral cavity are essential to draw milk from either the breast or the bottle. This is almost impossible for babies with a cleft, and they can become very fatigued when feeding. Much of the milk may be lost and lots of air swallowed, resulting in discomfort and the need to burp the child regularly.

The early involvement of specialist nurses with feeding expertise is essential. Special soft bottles that can be squeezed and teats that can direct milk to the back of the mouth are available. Although there is no doubt that breast-feeding is best for babies and should be encouraged, specialized bottle feeding (preferably using expressed breast milk) is often the most appropriate approach. Once a child is feeding well, and is progressively gaining weight, they will be able to cope with surgery.

PRESURGICAL ORTHOPAEDICS (Figure 14.8)

Presurgical orthopaedics (PSO) or nasoalveolar moulding (NAM) takes advantage of the plasticity of the nasal cartilage in the neonate by using orthodontic-like plates, with or without tapes and nasal stents, to reposition the maxillary segments and the nasal structures. PSO or NAM needs to

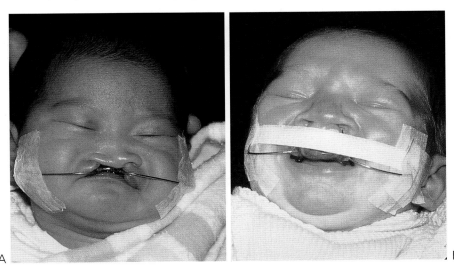

A　　　　　　　　　　　　　　　　　　　　　　　　　　　　　B

Figure 14.8 (A) Presurgical orthopaedic appliance. The plate is held by micropore tape to the cheeks. (B) Strapping aids in the positioning of the labial segments, especially in cases of bilateral complete clefts. Depending on the institution, these appliances are used in cases of bilateral cleft lip and those with very wide unilateral clefts as shown in (A).

be started as soon after birth as possible to maximize the chances of an infant tolerating the appliances. It is technically complex and demanding, not least because taking a maxillary impression in a neonate is particularly challenging with the associated risks to the airway. PSO or NAM should only be done by appropriately trained and experienced clinicians. Its use remains controversial, not least because of the associated financial burden coupled with the lack of strong long-term evidence of better outcomes.

COUNSELLING AND PARENT SUPPORT

Ongoing counselling by an appropriately informed cleft specialist is often needed by parents. In many cleft teams, this is provided by the specialist cleft nurses, who may schedule extra visits to provide additional support. Parents not only have many questions but are also often confused and anxious and may seek advice about the intermediate and long-term implications of the cleft defect and the necessary surgery. They also often appreciate, and benefit from, the assistance available from members of a parent support group such as CleftPALs (Australia), CLAPA (UK) and American Cleft Palate-Craniofacial Association.

PRIMARY SURGERY

Many surgical techniques have been described for the primary closure of cleft lip and palate. However, there is still controversy regarding the timing of surgery and which is the most reliable technique consistent with ensuring optimal growth of the face and development of speech.

- Lip repair is less controversial than palate repair and is generally undertaken around 10 to 12 weeks and almost certainly by 6 months of age, provided the infant is otherwise developing well. The aim of the lip repair is to restore the continuity of the orbicularis oris muscle of the lip and, with it, the appearance of the upper lip (Figures 14.2 and 14.3).
- Palate repair aims to reconstruct the abnormally inserted musculature of the soft palate to normalize movements of the soft palate and permit the development of normal speech. The extent and timing of palatal surgery are two of the major and continuing controversies in cleft management. This relates to the perceived balance between the benefits of good speech development (which is promoted by early closure) and the deleterious effects on midfacial growth through surgical trauma and associated scarring (which can be minimized by delaying the surgery).

To date, there is no strong evidence regarding the best approach to primary surgery. Attempts to address this gap in the evidence are being made through large multi-centre international clinical trials. Generally it will occur between the ages of 9 and 12 months of age. Eighteen months of age would be considered a late repair.

Management during childhood

SPEECH AND LANGUAGE AND EAR, NOSE AND THROAT PROBLEMS

Children with clefts and other craniofacial malformations are at an increased risk of speech and language difficulties. Regular assessments are required to monitor the speech and language acquisition process, to assist in making decisions about the need for either further surgery or speech therapy or both.

During childhood, care needs to be exercised to ensure hearing is optimal for speech and language development. Otitis media is common in infants and children with cleft palate, and some may also have sensorineural loss. Suboptimal hearing can affect speech and language development, so regular audiology assessments for all infants with clefts of the lip and palate is important.

VELOPHARYNGEAL INADEQUACY

Normal speech requires that the muscles that make up the velopharyngeal sphincter (predominantly the muscles of the soft palate and nasopharynx) work in a coordinated fashion. Defects in any aspect of the nasopharyngeal anatomy and/or physiology may lead to velopharyngeal inadequacy (VPI). It is uncommon for otherwise healthy individuals to have VPI. However, for individuals with anomalies of their velopharyngeal sphincter such as a cleft of the palate (hard and/or soft, repaired or unrepaired), VPI can, if severe, compromise speech production, rendering a child incomprehensible to others.

- The speech pathologist's assessment of speech production is critical in the identification and management of VPI, and they work closely with the primary cleft surgeons in deciding what, if any, intervention is required to optimize speech.
- If significant VPI is identified, then surgery is usually needed. There are a number of different approaches to the surgical management of VPI, including narrowing the velopharyngeal opening (pharyngoplasty), lengthening the soft palate (intravelar veloplasty) and bulking up the posterior pharyngeal wall (fat augmentation). Although surgery can be expected to improve structural obstacles which hinder the development of normal speech, postoperative speech therapy may still be needed (before and after surgery) to correct poor speech habits that have developed because of the structural malformation.
- Occasionally, surgical correction of VPI is not possible or does not bring resolution. In this case, a palatal obturator or a speech bulb may reduce the velopharyngeal space sufficiently for normal speech to develop.

ORTHODONTICS

Children with clefts of the lip and palate and those with cleft of the hard palate are at risk of compromised growth of the maxilla as a result of postsurgical scarring. If severe, the growth restriction of the maxilla which affects all three dimensions can lead to the development of a skeletal class III relationship and associated crossbites.

The first comprehensive orthodontic evaluation is generally at 7 to 8 years of age with an orthopantomogram to assess the developing dentition. Occasionally, there may be a need for earlier review.

In children with no alveolar involvement, the growth and dental development should be assessed as in any other child and interceptive treatment initiated if required. This may involve:

- Extractions for guided eruption of permanent teeth.
- Maxillary expansion to correct posterior crossbites.
- Correction of anterior crossbites with partial fixed appliances.
- Growth modification appliances.

ALVEOLAR DEFECTS (Figure 14.9)

When the cleft affects the alveolus (in some cases of cleft lip and all cases involving lip and palate), orthodontic intervention is usually required to facilitate alveolar bone grafting, to repair the bony defect.

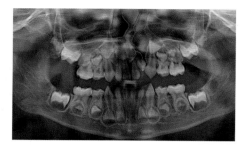

Figure 14.9 Orthopantomogram showing the extent of the bony defect in a child with a unilateral complete cleft of the lip and primary palate. The cleft (outlined in *red*) extends into the nasal cavity (outlined in *blue*). The upper left primary lateral incisor is partially erupted within the primary palate and the permanent tooth is absent. The primary and permanent canines are located in the lesser segment.

SECONDARY ALVEOLAR BONE GRAFTING (Figure 14.10)

Alveolar bone grafting should be timed to precede the eruption of the permanent canine tooth on the cleft side. The timing is indicated when this tooth shows between half and two-thirds of root development.

The aim of bone grafting is to:

- Restore the bony contour of the alveolus.
- Stabilize the maxillary expansion.
- Provide a bony matrix through which teeth (especially the canine) may erupt.
- Allow the teeth to have a healthy supporting periodontium.
- To support the alar base of the nose.

ORTHODONTIC PREPARATION FOR ALVEOLAR BONE GRAFTING

It is necessary to restore the arch dimension in preparation for surgery (Figure 14.11), and this is achieved by a maxillary expansion appliance and often a partial fixed appliance. This treatment also widens the defect and gives the surgeon much better access to place the bone graft.

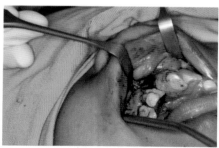

A

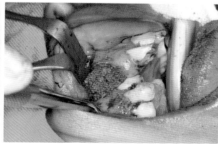

B

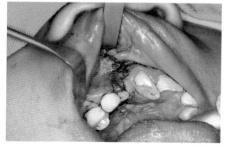

C

Figure 14.10 Bone grafting of a unilateral complete cleft palate. (A) The defect has been exposed and is then filled with cancellous bone harvested from the iliac crest. (B). The defect is closed on the nasal floor and orally (C). The aim of bone graft is not only to fill and stabilize the defect but also to allow the unerupted permanent canine to erupt through the bone.

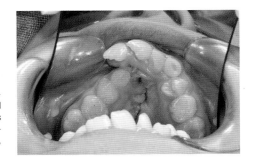

Figure 14.11 One of the major dental issues is collapse of the lesser segment. Rotation of the central incisor adjacent the cleft is often be seen. This is because of local crowding secondary to lack of alveolar bone. Palatal expansion corrects this collapse, and the arch is stabilized by the alveolar bone graft.

The type of appliance chosen is dependent on the movements required, and examples are seen in Figure 14.12.

Orthodontic preparation can take between 6 and 9 months, and the appliance is maintained up to 6 months postsurgery for bone healing and stability.

Occasionally there may be primary teeth or supernumerary teeth associated with the cleft (Figure 14.13). Ideally these should be removed and the mucosa given time to heal before the bone graft procedure. In reality, this is not always possible, and often they are removed by the surgeon at the same time.

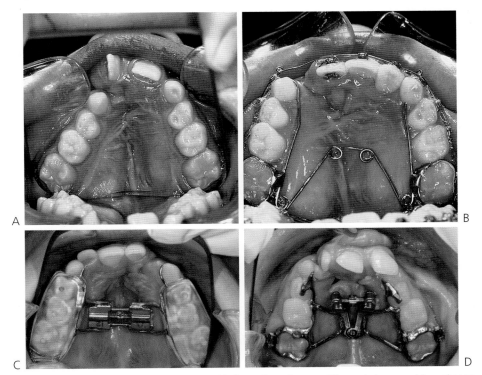

Figure 14.12 (A, B) Palatal expansion with a quad helix appliance to correct the posterior cross-bite and open space for the bone graft. A number of other appliances may be used depending on the requirements of each case. (C) A bonded rapid maxillary expansion device can be used if the occlusion is unfavourable or there is a vertical discrepancy. (D) A fan-type expander can be used if the intermolar width is adequate and more expansion is required anteriorly.

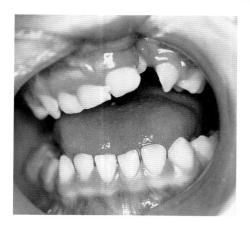

Figure 14.13 A tooth erupting in the cleft. Such teeth often become carious, but should be repaired and retained until bone grafting is performed. Where permanent teeth are congenitally absent, especially the lateral incisor, the supernumerary may be used if of adequate size.

Good oral hygiene is paramount in post-operative healing, and so the orthodontist should educate the child and parents on the importance of diet and cleaning and monitor for problems. Referral for treatment is essential if there are ongoing issues with this.

SURGICAL PROCEDURE FOR ALVEOLAR BONE GRAFTING

- Good exposure of the defect.
- Preparation of the donor site (usually iliac crest).
- Harvesting of cancellous bone.
- Repair of the nasal mucosa.
- Solid packing of the cancellous bone into the defect.
- Good soft tissue coverage of the graft to ensure 'water tight' closure.

Generally antibiotics are given and a post-surgical hygiene regime including mouthwash is prescribed.

POST BONE GRAFT MANAGEMENT

The child will be reviewed post surgery to monitor healing, and radiographic assessment of the bone graft is carried out no less than 6 months after the surgery.

The orthodontist will continue to monitor the dental development of the child and aim to correct any issues with alignment and eruption of the maxillary teeth.

Management in adolescence and early adulthood

ORTHODONTICS

The skeletal development of the child will determine the timing of definitive orthodontic treatment in the permanent dentition.

In cases where growth is favourable, orthodontic treatment can be initiated when the permanent dentition is established (excluding third molars) and completed before skeletal maturity.

The development of a skeletal class III discrepancy is common; however, this can delay definitive treatment until the cessation of growth.

The magnitude of the skeletal discrepancy and the facial appearance will determine the approach taken. In mild cases, orthodontic camouflage can still be considered, and the preference and concerns of the individual will guide this.

In more severe cases, it is necessary to have a combined orthodontic/surgical treatment approach to correct the discrepancy.

ORTHOGNATHIC SURGERY

Orthodontic preparation is vital to align and decompensate the teeth presurgery. This allows maximum movement of the jaws to achieve the most aesthetic and functional outcome.

The two most common procedures are Le Fort 1 advancement of the maxilla only and a bimaxillary procedure involving both jaws. In extremely severe cases, it is not physiologically possible to correct the discrepancy in a single operation. In these individuals, incremental surgeries, usually at least 12 months apart, can be required.

Another technique used for larger discrepancies is distraction osteogenesis. Osteotomy cuts are made in the maxilla, but there is no down fracture to complete mobilization. Instead, small distractors are placed on either side of the cuts, and the patient or carer is required to turn the screw mechanism daily. In this way the maxilla is advanced incrementally over a defined period, and much larger movements are made possible. The resulting defect is filled with new bone, as healing progresses.

POSTSURGICAL ORTHODONTICS AND RESTORATIVE CARE

Final detailing of the occlusion is carried out, with major settling in the first few weeks after surgery. Appliances are generally removed 3 to 6 months postsurgery and retainers provided.

For individuals with missing teeth, referral to a prosthodontist is required to complete oral rehabilitation with dental implants and associated crown and/or bridgework.

SOFT TISSUE CONSIDERATIONS

In some children, soft tissue procedures following primary surgery can be indicated. Functional lip and nose revisions can be combined with alveolar bone grafting to reduce the impact of the aesthetic deformity on the growing child. Final aesthetic procedures such as rhinoplasty are postponed until growth has ceased and any orthodontic or orthognathic surgery is completed.

Oral health in cleft care

Children born with a clefting condition require extensive interdisciplinary care throughout early life. Optimizing oral health is particularly important, as the presence of dental disease can severely compromise both surgical and orthodontic success. Both the orthodontist and paediatric dentist have an essential role in coordinating the oral healthcare for these individuals to ensure they reach adulthood with a healthy dentition and positive attitude to dental care. All aspects of dental treatment need to be coordinated with the rest of the cleft team, and as such it is important for them, or their representative, to regularly review the child with a cleft lip and palate.

THE FIRST APPOINTMENT

Babies born with a cleft of the lip and palate not uncommonly have a tooth present at, or erupting soon after, birth – a natal tooth. This can worry parents and may contribute to the existing anxiety around feeding. Such teeth often sit in the premaxillary region and may be very mobile. In most instances, they can be extracted simply using topical anaesthetic cream. Care should be taken to protect the airway while extracting the tooth.

In the absence of early eruption, babies should still be seen within the first 12 months, so that parents can be guided on the importance of oral health to the outcome of cleft care.

For parents, this initial consultation also provides a good opportunity to explain:

- The dental aspects of the clefting process.
- The likely course of dental management. The involvement of different specialties including restorative, radiological, orthodontic and possible later oral surgical care.
- The probability of the absence of the normal tooth in the region of the cleft and, conversely, the possibility of one or more supernumerary teeth in the cleft region should be mentioned (Figure 14.8).
- The likelihood of the presence of crown and/or root morphological abnormalities and enamel hypoplasia of the incisor and canine teeth adjacent to the cleft should be indicated, with the positive reassurance that these can be treated relatively simply soon after they appear.
- The absolute importance of sound preventive care and regular dental visits should be emphasized and the family encouraged to actively seek routine care with a dentist locally, either in primary care with a general dental practitioner (GDP) or a government dental clinic.

It will be necessary to reinforce this information and provide ongoing advice and support throughout the entire duration of the child's cleft care. Many cleft teams provide parents with handbooks containing, amongst other things, oral health information which is particularly useful.

PREVENTIVE DENTAL CARE

Children with clefts of the lip and/or palate may be at increased risk of developing dental caries for a number of reasons; however, the evidence is fairly weak. Reasons include:

- PSO (if carried out) may predispose infant oral cavity to colonization by mutans streptococci and, hence, to the early development of dental caries.
- Early infant feeding problems may lead to prolonged and more cariogenic feeding habits.
- Presence of developmental defects of enamel particularly around the cleft site.
- Presence of dental crowding, malocclusion and orthodontic appliances.
- Existence of other comorbidities, which may increase caries risk: for example, reduced salivary flow associated with velocardiofacial syndrome.
- Risk of being 'spoilt' with sugary treats to compensate for hospitalizations and other healthcare exposures.

Routine preventive dental care for children at increased risk of dental caries includes:

- Early and regular exposure to fluoridated toothpaste.
- Oral hygiene technique instruction – for parents and later for the individuals themselves.
- Home application of topical fluoride agents.
- Fissure sealing of both primary and permanent teeth.
- Dietary advice to child and parents.
- Appropriate use of bitewing radiographs (in line with national standards) to ensure early identification and treatment of carious lesions.

The prevention of dental caries and periodontal disease will help with cooperation for ultimate definitive orthodontic treatment, by reducing unnecessary visits for treatment in early childhood. Motivation is especially important for later orthodontic treatment in these patients. This should be assessed early and enhanced during preventive visits during childhood so as to ensure compliance.

In many countries, it is the role of the GDP to provide routine dental care to all children. Despite being at increased risk of dental disease, there is no reason why children with craniofacial anomalies cannot receive such care from their local GDP. In many cases, this will be geographically more convenient. However, it is important that the GDP establishes early contact with the cleft palate team or surgeon and maintains a frequent dialogue.

DENTAL EXTRACTIONS AND MINOR ORAL SURGERY

- Except in an emergency, dental extractions should not be performed for these children by the general dentist without reference to the orthodontist or paediatric dentist in the cleft team.
- Primary molars should be retained if at all possible (using standard techniques such as pulpotomies and preformed crowns) or the space maintained after extraction as advised by the orthodontist.
- Erupted supernumerary teeth should be retained until 6 to 7 years of age, unless impossible to clean, resulting in progressive dental caries or gingival or mucosal inflammation. Extraction of such teeth should then, in most cases, be carried out through the cleft team under either local or general anaesthetic. If a general anaesthetic is required for restorative treatment or other purpose, superficial or obstructing unerupted supernumerary teeth may be removed at the same time but only after discussion with the orthodontist.

DENTAL ANOMALIES (see also Chapter 11)

Dental anomalies are extremely common in children with orofacial clefting. The most commonly affected tooth is the maxillary lateral incisor on the cleft side. This is owing, in part, to disruption of the dental lamina. Anomalies may include:

- Agenesis of teeth.
- Supernumerary teeth.
- Concurrent agenesis and supernumerary teeth within or adjacent to the cleft.
- Disorders of morphogenesis (size and shape).
- Supernumerary teeth may occur in either the medial or distal segment and much less frequently in both segments (Figure 14.8).

COSMETIC RESTORATION OF MALFORMED ANTERIOR TEETH AND ALVEOLAR CLEFT

The appearance of the teeth can be improved at any time, depending on the child's perceptions and wishes.

- Composite resin restorations may be placed for hypoplastic or morphologically abnormal permanent incisor teeth adjacent to the cleft(s) soon after eruption; however, enamel-bonded crowns or veneers should be reserved until after passive eruption and establishment of the gingival margin at the cemento–enamel junction.
- As a temporary measure, and in suitable cases, an adhesive retained bridge may be placed to replace missing incisor teeth. This form of prosthesis is a superior alternative to a removable partial denture; however, an osseointegrated implant remains the ultimate treatment solution when space cannot be closed orthodontically.

Further reading

American Cleft Palate Association, 2009. Parameters for the evaluation and treatment of patients with cleft lip/palate and other craniofacial anomalies. Revised version. Online. Available: www.acpa-cpf.org.

Bergland, O., Semb, G., Abyholm, F.E., 1986. Elimination of the residual alveolar cleft by secondary bone grafting and subsequent orthodontic treatment. Cleft Palate Journal 23, 175–205.

Bessell, A., Hooper, L., Shaw, W.C., et al., 2011. Feeding interventions for growth and development in infants with cleft lip, cleft palate and cleft lip and palate (review). Cochrane Database of Systematic Reviews (2), CD003315.

Cheng, L.L., Moor, S.L., Ho, C.T.C., 2007. Predisposing factors to dental caries in children with cleft lip and palate: a review and strategies for early prevention. Cleft Palate-Craniofacial Journal 44, 67–72.

Cox, et al., 2018. The American Journal of Human Genetics 102, 1143–1157 (full article) and Roscioli. Available: https://www.neura.edu.au/news/breakthrough-in-cleft-lip-and-palate-research/.

Dixon, M., Marazita, M., Beaty, T., et al., 2011. Cleft lip and palate: understanding the genetic and environmental influences. Nature Reviews: Genetics 12, 167–178.

Eppley, B.L., van Aalst, J.A., Robey, A., et al., 2005. The spectrum of orofacial clefting. Plastic and Reconstructive Surgery 115, 101e–114e.

Guo, J., Li, C., Zhang, Q., et al., 2011. Secondary bone grafting for alveolar cleft in children with cleft lip or cleft lip and palate (review). Cochrane Database for Systematic Reviews (6), CD008050.

Hunt, O., Burden, D., Hepper, P., et al., 2005. The psychosocial effects of cleft lip and palate: a systematic review. European Journal of Orthodontics 27, 274–285 2005.

Levy-Bercowski, D., Abreu, A., DeLeon, E., et al., 2009. Complications and solutions in presurgical nasoalveolar moulding. Cleft Palate-Craniofacial Journal 46, 521–528.

Liao, Y.-F., Mars, M., 2006. Hard palate repair timing and facial growth in cleft lip and palate: a systematic review. Cleft Palate-Craniofacial Journal 43, 563–570.

Maarse, W., Berge, S.J., Pistorius, L., et al., 2010. Diagnostic accuracy of transabdominal ultrasound in detecting prenatal cleft lip and palate: a systematic review. Ultrasound in Obstetrics and Gynecology 35, 495–502.

Nelson, P., Glenny, A.M., Kirk, S., et al., 2012. Parents experience of caring for a child with a cleft lip and/or palate: a review of the literature. Child: Care, Health and Development 38, 6–20.

Tannure, P.N., Oliveira, C.A., Maia, L.C., et al., 2012. Prevalence of dental anomalies in nonsyndromic individuals with cleft lip and palate: a systematic review and meta-analysis. Cleft Palate-Craniofacial Journal 49, 194–200.

Speech, language and swallowing

Sarah Starr

Introduction

The ability to communicate effectively is vital to a person's functioning in society. Speech and language acquisition is a developmental process occurring most dramatically in the first years of life but one that proceeds throughout a person's lifetime. Difficulties may be encountered at any point during the language acquisition process. Children may experience problems acquiring the sounds of the language, learning how to combine words meaningfully or comprehending others' questions and instructions. In all cases, a speech and language pathologist is the primary healthcare professional responsible for the identification and treatment of individuals with communication problems. Paediatric dentists should be aware of the symptoms and problems associated with communication impairment, particularly when it relates to orofacial or dentofacial anomalies. They should know how to refer children and their families to a speech pathologist.

Communication begins at birth and continues throughout a child's life through adolescence and into adult life. A child's communication development is influenced by many variables, including neurological status and motor development, oromotor status (anatomical and physiological), cognition, hearing, birth order, environment, communication modelling and experiences, as well as their personality.

This chapter will briefly describe some of the main communication disorders that can present with particular focus for paediatric dentists.

Communication disorders

There are six main areas to be considered when assessing a child's communication:
- Oral motor and feeding problems.
- Articulation.
- Language.
- Voice.
- Fluency.
- Pragmatics.

ORAL MOTOR AND FEEDING PROBLEMS

Problems in this area constitute the earliest at which children are referred to a speech pathologist. Significant problems can result when an infant does not develop control of the oral mechanism sufficient for successful feeding. Early reflex development typically facilitates feeding behaviour, but neuromotor factors, prematurity, cleft lip and palate, tongue-tie, long-term nonoral feeding and other reasons may interfere with a child's development of the movement patterns essential for sucking, swallowing and feeding. Because these patterns form the scaffolding of movement for early speech sound development, children with a history of feeding difficulties may have subsequent difficulties in producing sounds for speech.

Reasons for referral

- Sucking, swallowing or chewing difficulties.
- Gagging, coughing or choking with feeds.
- Feeding refusal.
- Moist vocal quality during or after feeds.
- Poor cough or gag reflex.
- Persistent drooling (not coincident with teething).
- Recurrent chest infections.
- Presence of a craniofacial malformation.
- Parental report of feeding difficulty or refusal.
- Poor oral intake and associated poor weight gain in infants and young children.

ARTICULATION

Articulation refers to the production of speech sounds by modification of the breath stream using the various valves along the vocal tract: lips, tongue, teeth and palate. Problems in these areas can vary from a fairly mild distortion of sounds such as a lisp, where the child's speech is still easy to understand, through to a more severe speech production problem where all speech attempts are unintelligible or where the child makes very few speech attempts. Errors can be classified in the following ways:
- Speech sound omissions:
  - 'cu' for 'cup'.
  - 'te-y' for 'teddy'.
- Substitutions of sounds:
  - 'wed' for 'red'.
  - 'tun' for 'sun'.
- Distortions:
  - Lateral lisps – 's' that sounds slushy.

TABLE 15.1 ■ **Development of sounds with age**

Age (years)	Sounds correctly produced	Comments
2	m, n, h	Speech is sometimes difficult to understand, especially for unfamiliar people.
2½	p, b, ng, w, d, g All vowel sounds	
3	y, k, f, t	By 3 years of age, 80–90% of a child's speech should be easily understood.
3½	sh, ch, dge	
4	l, s,	Blends of sounds (i.e., st, cl, dr) are acquired later than the individual sounds but are usually mastered by 5 years.
5	z, zh (measure)	
	r	
5½	z	The ages quoted here are only a guideline as to when the average child acquires the sound, but by 8 years of age, all sounds should be mastered.
7½	th	
8	v	

Children learn to produce sounds in a developmental sequence, with adult-like sound systems expected by 8 years of age (Table 15.1). For example, it is quite acceptable for a 2-year-old to mispronounce an 's' sound, but it would be considered a problem if a similar error were made by a 7-year-old child.

LANGUAGE

In contrast to the fairly straightforward examples listed previously to illustrate speech sound learning, language development is much more complex. Skills emerge in two parallel levels.

Receptive language

This is the ability to understand language.

Expressive language

This refers to the ability to produce verbal and nonverbal communication in the form of gestures, body language, facial expression and words and sentences and may include speech and written language.

A child with a language disorder may present with difficulties in both comprehension and expression of language or in only one area of language learning. Language learning proceeds in a predictable order, but there is more variability in the emergence of these skills than the acquisition of speech sounds. Vocabulary grows as does a child's ability to progressively understand more complex language. Words are combined into phrases and eventually sentences, and comprehension becomes more adult-like over time. Eventually, language that is heard and said becomes the language of literacy, reading and writing. School success is highly correlated with language learning, especially in the early years.

Children may experience language learning problems at any stage of the acquisition process. There may be:

- Difficulties interpreting the meaning of words and gestures.
- Delays in the production of first words and phrases.

- A lack of understanding of questions and instructions.
- An inability to produce sentences that are grammatically correct.
- An inability to participate in conversations.

A delay at any single stage may not necessarily constitute a long-standing problem, although it should be investigated further. Problems with language acquisition are the most subtle indicators of difficulties with childhood development and therefore should never be ignored.

VOICE

Voice is produced when the vocal cords in the larynx are vibrated. Changes in air flow and the shape of the vocal folds can affect loudness, pitch and voice quality. Once voice is produced, its tone (resonance) and quality are modified by the throat, oral and nasal cavities. A child with a voice problem may present with the following:

Abnormal voice quality

Rough, breathy or hoarse voice in the absence of upper respiratory tract infection.

Abnormal resonance

Hypernasality (excessive nasal tone usually because of problems closing the velopharyngeal port during speech) or hyponasality (lack of nasal resonance usually caused by some type of nasopharyngeal obstruction).

Inappropriate loudness levels

Voice too soft to be heard or so loud that it is distracting from the message of the speaker.

Problems with pitch

Pitch too high or low for age or sex.

Voice problems may be caused by:
- Poor vocal use, for example, excessive yelling or screaming (in some cases producing vocal nodules).
- Neurological problems (e.g., cerebral palsy).
- Vocal pathology such as polyps or cysts.
- Muscular pathology.
- Vocal cord paralysis.
- Vocal irritants such as exposure to smoking, chemicals or aerosol sprays.
- Physical conditions including cleft palate, laryngectomy and hearing loss.

FLUENCY

Fluency refers to the smooth flow of speech. Where there are interruptions in the flow of speech, stuttering occurs. Many children experience brief periods of stuttering as they learn to speak in longer sentences, and this early form of dysfluency is not considered a disordered pattern, as it will usually pass. Early developmental dysfluency is best resolved by reacting to the message the child is attempting to convey rather than the dysfluency. When stuttering persists beyond the normal time period of approximately 3 to 6 months, and/or there is strong family history of stuttering or when it is becoming stressful for the child, referral to a speech pathologist is indicated.

A child or an adult with a stutter experiences involuntary repetition of sounds or words, prolongations of sounds in words and blocks where no sound is produced at all. Some speakers with a stutter will use words like 'um' to help them initiate speaking. Sometimes secondary features such as eye blinking and facial grimacing occur with the stutter.

Stutterers do not have more emotional or psychological problems when compared with the general population, nor is there evidence of decreased mental aptitude. Approximately 3% of the population stutter, with a predominance in males (3 : 1). The disorder usually has its onset in the early years of life, and treatment is most successful in the preschool years, hence the importance of prompt and early referral.

PRAGMATICS

Pragmatics refers to how we communicate with others through our verbal and nonverbal language as well as our tone of voice, stress, pausing, pitch and loudness. Pragmatics relates to our social use of language, including how we initiate, engage and maintain others in a communication dialogue through our eye contact, body language, physical space, choice and use of words, conversational turn taking and responses to others.

Pragmatic skills allow us to develop friendships and effectively communicate our messages in a social, educational and workplace setting. They are crucial to effective communication and develop from birth throughout our adult life. Pragmatic skills develop as part of normal cognitive development and are influenced by environmental and cultural modelling. Disorders in pragmatic skills can be isolated or part of a language, developmental, psychological or specific condition (e.g., autism).

Structural anomalies and their relationship to speech production and eating and drinking

The speech language pathologist is actively involved in the evaluation of orofacial, pharyngeal and laryngeal structures and functioning important for speech production and deglutition. Evaluation techniques may be perceptual or instrumental (e.g., video-fluoroscopic x-ray studies of swallowing) and are often a combination of both, with input from other members of a multidisciplinary team. Results of diagnostic structural and/or functional testing direct which management strategies are available to the patient.

Speech sounds may be acoustically or visually distorted because of abnormal structure and/or function of the articulators (most commonly the lips, tongue, teeth and palate). There are three main ways in which speech sound production is influenced, and these can co-exist, thus differential diagnosis is important in decision-making for management.

1. Speech sounds may be omitted, substituted or added during early childhood as mature speech patterns are mastered. For example, 3-year-old children often substitute alveolar sounds for velar sounds (cap → tap; go → do). Some children continue these substitutions for longer than expected and need speech therapy to learn mature speech patterns.

2. Speech sounds may be distorted because of underlying neurological impairment or oromotor planning/coordination problems. Speech may be termed 'dysarthric' (neurological) or 'dyspraxic' (motor planning), depending on the aetiology and characteristics noted.

3. Structural problems may affect speech (and swallowing) in a number of ways. These are outlined later.

DENTAL ANOMALIES

Malocclusion has the potential to greatly affect tongue position, jaw posturing and occlusion during eating and drinking and speech production. In some cases, patients may compensate for abnormal dental relationships.

HYPODONTIA/MISSING TEETH CAUSING INTERDENTAL SPACING

Biting and chewing difficulties may result, and a lateral or forward displacement of tongue during speech may occur, resulting in distortion of sounds. Missing middle incisors can impact biting, and this may in turn affect the way in which a child may compensate. For example, a child may demonstrate biting instead with more lateral incisors or molar teeth, others may avoid firm foods requiring biting, and still others may place large pieces of food in their mouth when unable to bite through a food. The presence or absence of teeth and the position of these teeth in the dental arch are thought to be more significant for speech production than the condition, size or texture of the teeth (Shprintzen & Bardach, 1995). In general, lingual-alveolar sounds (e.g., /s/, /z/) followed by lingual–palatal sounds ('j', 'sh', 'ch') are most affected by spaces in the dental arch. The tongue tends to move forwards into the interdental space, causing a central or lateral 'lisp'. The speech sounds most resistant to changes in the dental arch are the velar consonants /k/ and /g/ (Bloomer, 1971).

CLASS III MALOCCLUSION

A severe Class III malocclusion may be associated with distortion or interdentalization ('lisping') of sibilant and alveolar speech sounds (/s/, /z/, /t/, /d/, /n/, /l/) caused by difficulty elevating the tongue tip to the alveolar ridge. The sound most likely to be affected is /s/. This is probably because production relies on precise placement of the tongue tip and blade in addition to sufficient space being available anterior to the tip in the anterior portion of the palate (Bloomer, 1971). Forward tongue placement can also be associated with a tongue thrust swallow and more cumbersome oral preparation of food with poor lateral tongue transfers and imprecise tongue tip elevation during swallowing.

CLASS II MALOCCLUSION

A severe Class II malocclusion may interfere with lip closure during eating and drinking and may also affect biting of foods with middle incisors. Bilabial speech sounds (/p/, /b/, /m/) may be distorted or produced in a labiodental manner (with the upper incisors articulating with the lower lip). The speech sounds may be 'visually' distorted; that is, they may look different but be acoustically acceptable (sound near normal).

ANTERIOR OPEN BITE

An anterior open bite allows the tongue to move forwards into the interdental space, causing interdentalization ('lisping') or distortion of speech sounds, particularly those which involve the tongue tip contacting the alveolar ridge (/t/, /d/, /n/, /l/) and palate (/s/, /z/).

Swallowing may also be different for children with an anterior open bite, compared with those with a normal occlusion. For example, genioglossus muscle activity is significantly higher in patients with anterior open bite than those without (Alexander & Sudha, 1997). Difficulty biting with middle incisors is common when an anterior open bite is present with overfilling of the mouth, tearing of food or compensatory biting with more lateral teeth noted.

MAXILLARY COLLAPSE

This condition sometimes occurs after cleft palate surgery and leads to distortion of sounds requiring tongue and palatal contact ('s', 'z', 'sh', 'ch', 'j').

Speech and feeding problems are not always associated with these dental conditions. Each patient must be considered individually in light of their abilities to compensate for dental or occlusal anomaly. In cases where problems are identified, speech therapy is coordinated with dental and orthodontic management. Some children may not be able to improve their speech or feeding until their dental treatment is complete.

LIP ANOMALIES

Cleft lip

Breastfeeding and bottle-feeding issues may present because of poor lip seal closure during sucking, affecting the efficiency of milk intake and liquid loss from the mouth. Breast techniques and specific teats may be advised to facilitate lip seal and closure. Depending on the nature of the lip abnormality and range of lip movement, lip closure and protrusion during drinking (e.g., cup/straw drinking) or speech may be affected.

Sometimes, tissue deficiency and excessive tightness or scarring of tissue affect speech. The speech sounds most likely to be affected are the bilabials (/p/, /b/, /m/). Problems with the facial nerve affecting speech have been reported in syndromes such as hemifacial microsomia and Moebius syndrome (Shprintzen & Bardach, 1995).

Poor lip closure may relate to imprecise labial sounds (p, b, m) and poor lip protrusion associated with distortion of sounds such as 'w', 'oo', 'er'.

PALATAL ANOMALIES

The soft palate and pharyngeal walls work simultaneously to close the nasopharynx during speech production and swallowing (i.e., velopharyngeal closure). This action prevents excessive airflow into the nasal cavity during speech, maintains negative intraoral pressure during sucking and swallowing, and prevents nasal regurgitation of food or fluid during the swallow. If there is a palatal abnormality, velopharyngeal closure cannot take place efficiently, and there is often associated poor sucking, slow and inefficient feeding and possible escape of food and liquid into the nose. Speech is nasal and breathy, sounds are unclear and volume may be reduced.

Palatal anomalies may include:

- Cleft palate (with or without cleft lip).
- Submucous cleft palate, characterized by a bifid uvula, notching of the posterior margin of the hard palate, zona pellucida and abnormal insertion of the levator musculature into the free bony edge of the hard palate.
- Congenital palatal anomalies, including short palate, deep nasopharynx, poorly coordinated or inefficient velopharyngeal movement.
- Acquired palatal abnormalities resulting from neurological damage, surgery or neoplasms.
- Neurological abnormalities influencing palatal movement (e.g., cerebral palsy, cranial nerve IX and X abnormalities, muscular dystrophy).

Children with palatal anomalies are best referred to a specialist cleft palate clinic where they can receive coordinated multidisciplinary assessment and management (see Chapter 12).

LINGUAL ANOMALIES

Abnormalities of the tongue may affect the precision, range and speed of tongue movement, resulting in speech or feeding difficulties. The most common anatomical problem is ankyloglossia or tongue-tie. Tongue mobility, strength and coordination can directly affect sucking, swallowing and speech production.

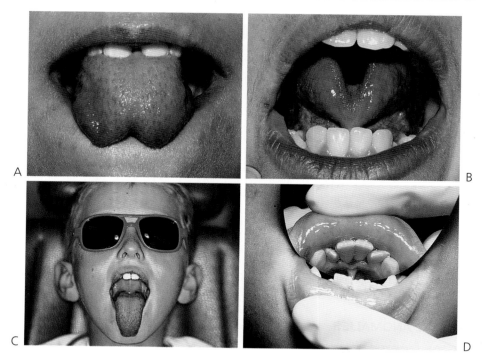

Figure 15.1   Ankyloglossia. (A, B) Notice the tethering of the frenum to the anterior tip of the tongue, restricting elevation and protrusion. It is important to assess the position of the frenum into the body of the tongue as well as any attachment into the gingival margin that may cause periodontal complications. (C) Extent of protrusion after lingual frenectomy. (D) Another indication for frenectomy is where the attachment inserts into the free gingival margin, causing potential periodontal problems.

Ankyloglossia (Figure 15.1)

Tongue-tie may occur with varying degrees of severity, which does not always correlate with the severity of functional impairment. Some children have no problems with eating/drinking or speech and others do. Some of the possible are:

- Feeding difficulties such as difficulty sucking in infancy, poor tongue movement and chewing because of restricted tongue movement laterally and persistent messy eating (attributed to the child being unable to clear food from the buccal cavities and the lips).
- Substitution and distortion of tongue tip (alveolar) sounds /l/, /t/, /d/, /n/, /s/, /z/ caused by restricted elevation of the tongue tip.
- Slower than normal speech rate or reduced speech intelligibility in conversational speech.
- Reduced speech precision during shouting. (Shouting requires the mouth to open more widely and thereby may result in the tongue-tie having a more negative effect on speech precision.)
- Difficulty breastfeeding in infancy and persistent messy eating, feeding refusal especially of food that requires chewing on the molar area in later childhood.

If a child's speech or feeding appears to be affected by tongue-tie, an assessment by a speech pathologist and a paediatric dentist is useful to determine whether lingual frenectomy is required.

Macroglossia

An abnormally large tongue may be associated with syndromes such as Beckwith–Wiedemann syndrome.

Infants with macroglossia may often have associated breathing, feeding and swallowing issues and require specific positioning and feeding techniques and equipment for successful oral feeding. Children with macroglossia may have difficulty correctly articulation dento–lingual sounds (e.g., 'th'), lingual–alveolar sounds /t/, /d/, /n/, /l/ and palatal–lingual sounds (e.g., 'ch', 'j', 'sh') because of forward tongue placement and difficulty configuring tongue placement within the oral cavity. In severe cases, the tongue will be protruded, affecting labial sounds and the blade of the tongue may contact the upper lip affecting vowels and glides (e.g., /r/ and /w/).

Microglossia

An abnormally small tongue may be associated with syndromes such as hypoglossia-hypodactyly. In these cases, the tongue tip may not contact the teeth, palate or alveolus sufficiently for precise consonant production. Compensatory articulation of sounds may need to be developed.

Maxillofacial surgery and its relation to speech production

When orthognathic surgery is being considered, a consultation with a speech pathologist should be made to determine the possible consequences of the procedure on speech production.

MAXILLARY ADVANCEMENT PROCEDURES

When the maxilla is advanced anteriorly, the hard palate and soft palate are also displaced forwards, increasing the distance that the soft palate must move to achieve velopharyngeal closure. Most patients seem able to compensate for this alteration in nasopharyngeal relationships, and their speech and swallowing are not affected. Some patients, however, are 'at risk' for deterioration in speech and swallowing characteristics (e.g., those with a repaired cleft palate). Forward displacement of the palatal structures may result in velopharyngeal insufficiency and hypernasal speech production. Forward placement of the maxilla also means that the tongue contact on the palate may be altered for some sounds. Therefore, tongue placement and sound production may be improved in cases with severe Class III malocclusion.

Given the potential impact of surgical interventions on velopharyngeal function, careful timing and selection of surgical techniques are recommended (Jacques et al., 1997). Postsurgical speech review and possible speech therapy may also be warranted.

Referral to a speech pathologist

When the presence of a communication or feeding problem is suspected, referral should be made as soon as possible.

Dentists should refer any child who experiences the difficulties outlined below.

FEEDING AND SWALLOWING

- Has difficulty sucking, swallowing, biting and chewing.
- Is coughing, gagging or choking during feeds.
- Is drooling excessively.
- Has reported breast, bottle, drinking or eating difficulties or refusal.

ARTICULATION

- Is not babbling a wide variety of sounds by 8 to 10 months.
- Is not easily understood by caregivers by 2 years.
- Is not easily understood by familiar adults by 3 years.
- Is having difficulty in producing sounds accurately by 5 years.

LANGUAGE

- Is not understanding simple instructions and questions by 18 months.
- Is not using single words by 18 months.
- Is not combining two words by 2 years (i.e., 'more drink').
- Has difficulty following instructions or answering questions.
- Gives inappropriate answers or frequently ignores language spoken to them.
- Is constructing sentences that are incorrect or immature by 3 to 4 years (i.e., 'me go to him house').
- Cannot maintain a topic of conversation by 4 years.

VOICE

- Has a hoarse or breathy voice or often loses their voice.
- Has a nasal voice.
- Often sounds as though they have a cold.
- Has a voice that seems too high or low for their sex or age.
- Continually speaks abnormally loudly or softly.
- Has a sudden onset of any of these problems.

FLUENCY

- Persistent stuttering at any age.

PRAGMATICS

- Does not initiate or engage others in communication at any age.
- Has poor eye contact.
- Constantly interrupts others.
- Displays inappropriate social use of language (e.g., inappropriate use of words for a situation).
- Talks excessively, does not take conversational turns or goes off on a tangent when speaking.

Referral procedures

It will be necessary to locate the most appropriate service to meet your patient's needs. Most often, access to a speech pathologist can be through a local community health centre or hospital. Some patients may require a more specialized service such as a developmental disability service, cleft palate clinic, feeding specialist or feeding clinic. Some patients may prefer the services of a private practitioner.

Referral is most efficient when the dentist provides a written referral outlining the areas of concern. Following an assessment, a treatment plan will be devised according to the individual needs of the patient. Treatment can be provided in individual or group sessions and it may extend over a period of time, depending on the nature and severity of the condition. Most speech, language and feeding problems are best treated with parental participation. Preschool or school-based programmes are important for older children.

Further reading

Alexander, S., Sudha, P., 1997. Genioglossus muscle electrical activity and associated arch dimensional changes in simple tongue thrust swallow pattern. Journal of Clinical Pediatric Dentistry 21, 213–222.

Bloomer, J.H., 1971. Speech defects associated with dental malocclusions and related abnormalities. In: Travis, L.E. (Ed.), Handbook of speech pathology and audiology. Prentice-Hall, Englewood Cliffs, NJ.

Jacques, B., Herzog, G., Muller, A., et al., 1997. Indications for combined orthodontic and surgical (orthognathic) treatments of dentofacial deformities in cleft lip and cleft palate patients and their impact on velopharyngeal function. Folia Phoniatrica et Logopaedica 49, 181–193.

Johnson, N.C., Sandy, J.R., 1999. Tooth position and speech – is there a relationship? Angle Orthodontist 69, 306–310.

Shprintzen, R.J., Bardach, J., 1995. Cleft palate speech management: a multidisciplinary approach. Mosby, St Louis.

Blood and serum testing and investigations

Angus C. Cameron ▤ Richard P. Widmer ▤ Benjamin Moran
▤ Mark Schifter

Laboratory examination may be divided into two general categories: screening and diagnostic. Screening studies are intended to identify individuals with disease in the early and asymptomatic stages. By definition, screening studies must be relatively simple and inexpensive, and are useful only when used to identify a disease which is relatively frequent (diabetes mellitus, anaemia, syphilis, blood disorders). Diagnostic examinations provide more specific information. The distinction between screening and diagnostic laboratory examination is not always rigid or absolute.

It must be remembered that laboratory examinations provide information that contributes to the diagnostic process. Seldom is this information of value by itself. The results must be interpreted in conjunction with other information that is available about the patient. It should also be noted that a laboratory value outside the normal range does not necessarily indicate disease. That value may represent normal for that specific patient. Usually, normal values are determined by testing supposedly healthy people, and these results are used to calculate the mean and normal range. Variables are not considered, and as a consequence, normal ranges are not always valid for all patients. Conversely, if a clinical diagnosis appears valid and is not substantiated by laboratory results, the tests should be repeated to rule out the possibility of laboratory error.

Haematology

FULL BLOOD COUNT

A full blood count (FBC) usually includes a white blood cell count (WBC), red cell blood count (RBC), haemoglobin (Hb), haematocrit (Hct) and red blood cell indices (mean corpuscular Hb, mean corpuscular volume, mean corpuscular Hb concentration and platelet count).

Platelet function tests are rarely ordered, usually only in consultation with a haematologist. If one asks for FBC and 'differential', one will also receive a breakdown of the RBC and WBC as listed on the form. If an FBC detects anaemia, then one should request serum ferritin, red cell folate and serum vitamin B_{12}. However, in interpretation of these results, one should seek counsel, as they are difficult.

COAGULATION AND BLEEDING TESTS

Problems relating to bleeding are relatively infrequent in dental practice. Most inherited defects will usually have been identified early in life, and so it is usually acquired bleeding problems about which the dentist must be aware. Screening studies will identify whether there is a bleeding problem, and in which of the three systems it is, namely, platelets, coagulation or vascular abnormalities.

TABLE A.1 ■ Normal blood values

	Children		Adults	
White blood cells	$4.0-15.0 \times 10^9$/L		$4.0-11.0 \times 10^9$/L	
Neutrophils	$1.5-7.5 \times 10^9$/L	50%	$2.0-8.0 \times 10^9$/L	60%
Lymphocytes	$1.0-8.6 \times 10^9$/L	42%	$0.5-4.0 \times 10^9$/L	33%
Monocytes	$0.5-1.5 \times 10^9$/L	5%	$0.2-1.0 \times 10^9$/L	4%
Eosinophils	$0.3-0.8 \times 10^9$/L		$0.04-0.5 \times 10^9$/L	
Basophils	$<0.1-0.2 \times 10^9$/L		$<0.01-0.2 \times 10^9$/L	
Red blood cells	$4.0-5.5 \times 10^{12}$/L	(3–12 years)	$4.5-6.5 \times 10^{12}$/L	Male
			$3.8-5.8 \times 10^{12}$/L	Female
Haemoglobin	115–145 g/L	(3–12 years)	130–180 g/L	Male
			115–165 g/L	Female
Mean corpuscular volume	70–90 fL		80–96 fL	
Mean corpuscular haemoglobin	23–31 pg		27–32 pg	
Platelets	$150-450 \times 10^9$/L			
Erythrocyte sedimentation rate	0–10 mm/h		0–5 mm/h	Male
			0–20 mm/h	Female
Reticulocytes	2.0–6.0% or mean 150×10^9/L	Infants	0.2%–2.0%	
	$10-100 \times 10^9$/L	Children		
Red cell folate	340–2500 nmol/L			
Serum folate	7–40 nmol/L			
Vitamin B_{12}	150–700 pmol/L			

TABLE A.2 ■ Tests for bleeding problems

Activated partial thromboplastin time (APTT)	24–38 sec
Prothrombin time	11–17 sec
Factor VIII assay	50%–200%
Mild haemophilia	20%–25%
Moderate	2%–5%
Severe	<1%
Skin bleeding time	<9 min

Clinical chemistry

It is not appropriate to simply request a multi-blood analysis in the hope of finding a diagnosis or abnormality. The following abbreviations are often used when ordering tests but will obviously differ from one institution or laboratory to another.

EUC	Electrolytes, urea, creatinine
LFTs	Liver profile, including serum proteins
CA	Calcium
PHOS	Inorganic phosphate, alkaline phosphatase

Blood chemistry

TABLE A.3 ■ **Normal blood chemistry**

Sodium		136–146 mmol/L
Potassium		3.4–5.5 mmol/L
Chloride		94–107 mmol/L
Total CO_2		24–31 mmol/L
Urea		2.5–6.5 mmol/L
Creatinine		60–125 mmol/L
Glucose	Fasting	3.9–6.1 mmol/L
	2 h postprandial	<7.8 mmol/L
Maintenance range for IDDM		4–10 mmol/L
Calcium		2.13–2.63 mmol/L
Phosphate		0.18–1.45 mmol/L
Osmolality		275–295 mmol/L
Lactate		0.63–2.44 mmol/L
Alkaline phosphatase		60–391 U/L

IDDM, insulin-dependent diabetes melitus.

LIVER FUNCTION TESTS

TABLE A.4 ■ **Liver function tests**

Total bilirubin	2–21 mmol/L
Total protein	63–79 g/L
Albumin	35–53 g/L
Alkaline phosphatase (ALP)	30–115 U/L
γ-Glutamyl-transpeptidase (γGT)	
Male	8–43 U/L
Female	5–30 U/L
Alanine aminotransferase (ALT)	7–47 U/L

IRON STUDIES

These tests are used when there is a suspicion of an underlying anaemia. The request for iron studies provides information regarding serum iron, total iron-binding capacity and percentage iron saturation.

TABLE A.5 ■ **Iron studies**

Ferritin	
Male	30–300 mg/L
Female: premenstrual	15–150 mg/L
Female: postmenstrual	25–200 mg/L
Iron	7.0–29.0 mmol/L
Transferrin	2.1–3.9 g/L
Saturation	0.09–0.52

Urine chemistry

TABLE A.6 ■ **Urine chemistry**

Sodium	40–220 mmol/L
Potassium	25–120 mmol/L
Creatinine	8.0–18.0 mmol/L
Total protein	<0.15 g/dL

ARTERIAL BLOOD GAS

TABLE A.7 ■ **Arterial blood gas**

pH	7.35–7.45
pCO_2	35–45 mmHg
pO_2	75–100 mmHg
HCO_3	22–26 mmol/L
Base excess	−3 to +3 mmol/L
SaO_2	0.95–0.98

Paediatric life support

Angus C. Cameron ■ Richard P. Widmer

apls
Advanced Paediatric
Life Support

Paediatric
basic life support

D → **Dangers?**

R → **Responsive?**

S → **Send** for help

A → Open **airway**

B → Normal **breathing?**
Give 2 breaths

C → **Check for signs of life**
+/- check pulse
Start CPR
15 compressions : 2 breaths

D → Attach **defibrillator** / monitor
Ensure help is coming

**Continue CPR until responsiveness or
normal breathing return**

Paediatric advanced life support

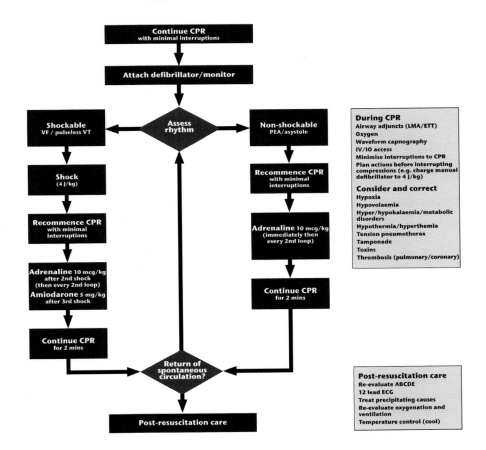

Continue CPR with minimal interruptions

Attach defibrillator/monitor

Assess rhythm

Shockable VF / pulseless VT

Non-shockable PEA/asystole

Shock (4 J/kg)

Recommence CPR with minimal interruptions

Recommence CPR with minimal interruptions

Adrenaline 10 mcg/kg after 2nd shock (then every 2nd loop)
Amiodarone 5 mg/kg after 3rd shock

Adrenaline 10 mcg/kg (immediately then every 2nd loop)

Continue CPR for 2 mins

Continue CPR for 2 mins

Return of spontaneous circulation?

Post-resuscitation care

During CPR
Airway adjuncts (LMA/ETT)
Oxygen
Waveform capnography
IV/IO access
Minimise interruptions to CPR
Plan actions before interrupting compressions (e.g. charge manual defibrillator to 4 J/kg)

Consider and correct
Hypoxia
Hypovolaemia
Hyper/hypokalaemia/metabolic disorders
Hypothermia/hyperthermia
Tension pneumothorax
Tamponade
Toxins
Thrombosis (pulmonary/coronary)

Post-resuscitation care
Re-evaluate ABCDE
12 lead ECG
Treat precipitating causes
Re-evaluate oxygenation and ventilation
Temperature control (cool)

Management of anaphylaxis

Angus C. Cameron ■ Richard P. Widmer ■ Benjamin Moran

Anaphylaxis

A symptom complex accompanying the acute reaction to a foreign substance to which the patient has been previously sensitized.

Anaphylaxis-like reactions (anaphylactoid)

Same symptoms but the reaction is nonimmunological or unknown.

Incidence

- Anaesthesia (paediatric): 1 : 40 000 (mortality is rare).
  Unlike adults who are usually paralyzed during anaesthesia, many children are maintained on volatile agents and are breathing spontaneously during anaesthesia, and consequently, few children receive muscle relaxants. Despite this, they are the most common trigger for paediatric anaphylaxis. The most common presentation of anaphylaxis is bronchospasm and hypotension.
- Radiographic contrast: 2%.
- Antibiotics: 1 : 5000.
- Latex allergy: 0.13%.
- Local anaesthetics: rare (usually to preservative).
- Foods, insects.

Latex sensitization in the general population is about 1%. Certain groups have a much higher incidence, such as the healthcare workforce, in which sensitization is estimated to be between 5% and 12%, and children with spina bifida, who are repeatedly exposed to latex from birth.

Timing

Some 98% occur within 5 min of drug administration, but may occur up to hours later, particularly if the trigger is an oral or topical medication.

Clinical presentation

PRODROME

- Metallic taste.
- Apprehension.
- Coughing.
- Choking sensation.
- Paraesthesia.
- Arthralgia.

CUTANEOUS

- Blushing.
- Urticaria.
- Angio-oedema.
- Pallor and cyanosis.

CARDIOVASCULAR

- Tachycardia.
- Hypotension.
- Shock.

RESPIRATORY

- Bronchospasm.
- Laryngeal obstruction.
- Pulmonary oedema.

GASTROINTESTINAL TRACT

- Nausea, vomiting, diarrhoea.
- Abdominal cramps.

OTHERS

- Disseminated intravascular coagulation.
- Fitting.

Treatment

Adrenaline and volume expansion are the mainstays of the treatment of anaphylaxis. Follow-up is essential. The patient must be transferred to an intensive care unit, as symptoms may return up to hours later. A letter must be sent with the patient describing the event and all the drugs used until skin testing can identify the offending drug. Skin testing of all drugs used is performed 3 months after the reaction. A *MedicAlert* bracelet should be worn by the child, identifying relevant drug reactions.

Notes on management (Figure C.1)

Adrenaline is the main drug used in the treatment of anaphylaxis and anaphylactoid reactions. Adrenaline must be used if anaphylaxis is suspected.

- The doses of adrenaline and colloid must be repeated if the patient's vital signs have not improved.

TABLE C.1 ■ **Treatment of anaphylaxis and anaphylactoid reactions with adrenaline**

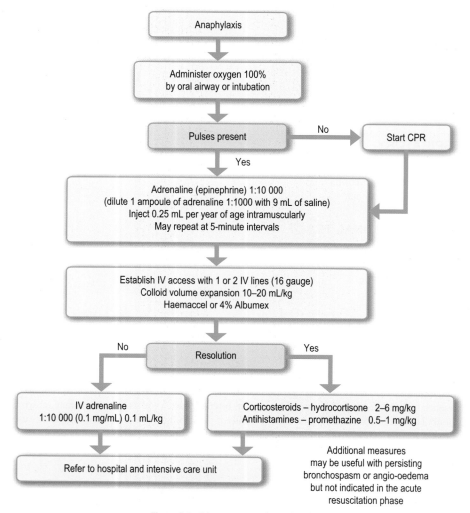

Figure C.1   Management of anaphylaxis.

Management of acute asthma

Angus C. Cameron ▦ Richard P. Widmer ▦ Benjamin Moran

Asthma is one of the most common childhood diseases and accounts for significant mortality and morbidity. The emphasis of treatment today is on prophylaxis rather than merely treating attacks. Most children with known asthma will have treatment plans prescribed by their doctor for use in acute episodes. However, there are children who have undiagnosed asthma who are at risk of acute attacks.

Essential equipment for an asthma kit

- Ventolin puffer (Figure D.1A).
- Bricanyl turbuhaler.
- Ventolin nebules (2.5 mg).
- Ventolin nebules (5 mg).
- Nebulizer unit and tubing for wall oxygen.
- Child mask for nebulizer.
- Small volume spacer with face mask.
- Volumatic spacer or small volume spacer with mouthpiece.

Bronchodilators (Figure D.1A)

VENTOLIN

- Inhaler (blue): 100 µg/puff.
- Dose: 4–12 puffs (weight dependent) via spacer.
- Nebules: 2.5 mg or 5 mg given via nebulizer.

BRICANYL

- Turbuhaler: 500 µg/inhalation.
- In acute situations: preferable to use puffer and a spacer.

Apparatus for administration of bronchodilators

SMALL VOLUME SPACER: CHILDREN 4 YEARS AND UNDER (Figure D.1B)

- Position AeroChamber with mask over child's face.
- Four puffs from Ventolin puffer; patient inhales four to six times for each puff.

VOLUMATIC SPACER: CHILDREN OVER 4 YEARS (Figure D.1C)

- Position spacer between lips.
- Four puffs from Ventolin puffer, patient inhales four to six times for each puff.
- Encourage child to breathe deeply for 6 to 10 seconds.

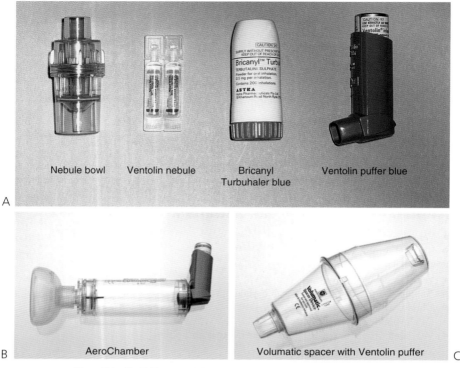

Figure D.1   (A–C) Drugs and devices used in the management of asthma.

NEBULIZER

- For very young children or in older children when the condition is not improved by puffer with spacer after 10 min.
- <5 years: 2.5 mg nebule.
- >5 years: 5 mg nebule.
- Place the contents of the nebule at the bottom of the nebule bowl, fix to face mask and apply oxygen or air to mask at 6 to 8 L/min flow rate. Add normal saline to Ventolin nebule solution to make up to 4 mL total.
- A fine mist will form, which the child breathes deeply for about 10 min.

Management

See Figure D.2.

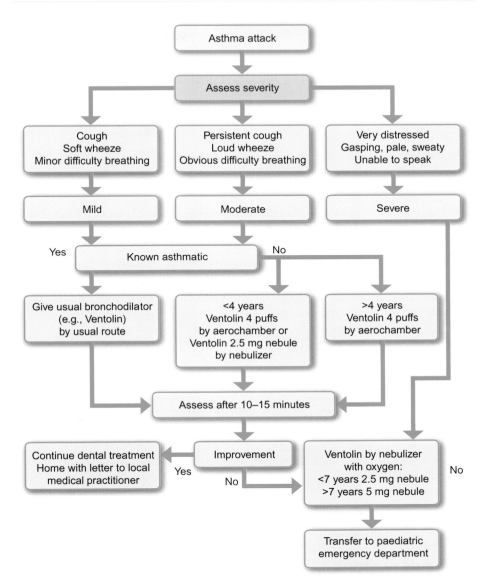

Figure D.2 Management of acute asthma.

Fluid and electrolyte balance

Angus C. Cameron ■ Richard P. Widmer ■ Benjamin Moran

Fluid and electrolyte replacement can be conveniently divided into:

- Maintenance replacement: The fluid and electrolyte losses occur during a normal day. These values are modified by other factors such as patient and environmental temperatures, age, weight and metabolic rate.
- Deficit replacement: To replace any existing or ongoing abnormal losses such as dehydration from vomiting or diarrhoea and blood loss.

Maintenance replacement

The need for water and electrolytes is a function of the metabolic rate, as they are substrates for metabolism. Thus, the younger the child, the higher the metabolic rate on a weight basis and the higher the turnover of water and electrolytes.

Water requirements

TABLE E.1 ■ Water requirements

Infants	Day 1	60 mL/kg/day
	Day 2	80 mL/kg/day
	Day 3	100 mL/kg/day
	Day 4 to 1 year	120 mL/kg/day
Children	<10 kg	4 mL/kg/h
	10–20 kg	2 mL/kg/h + 40 mL/h
	>20 kg	1 mL/kg/h + 60 mL/h

MODIFYING FACTORS

Increased maintenance requirement

- Fever: add 12% per degree above 37.5°C.
- Hyperventilation.
- Extreme activity.
- High environmental temperature.

Decreased maintenance requirement

- Cardiac failure.
- Inactivity (patient sedated in intensive care unit): decrease by 30%.
- Hypothermia: decrease 12% per degree <37.5°C.

- Head injury: decrease by 30%.
- Renal failure: decrease by 70% + urine output.

Electrolyte requirements

Normal electrolyte requirements are shown in Table E.2.

A total of 0.225% sodium chloride + 3.75% dextrose at normal maintenance rates will supply adequate sodium and chloride; potassium should only be added to intravenous fluids if replacement is to continue for more than 24 hours and adequate urine output is present. Although hypotonic solutions were recommended previously, the accepted routine replacement fluid in many centres is now an isotonic solution, such as Hartman or 0.9% saline. This is particularly important when managing children because of the risk of rapid osmotic shifts causing cerebral oedema or demyelination that might accompany the use of hypoptonic solutions.

TABLE E.2 ■ **Electrolyte requirements**

	0–10 kg	11–20 kg	>20 kg
Fluids (mL/kg/day)	100	50	20
Energy (cal/kg/day)	100	50	20
Na (mmol/kg/day)	3.0	1.5	0.6
K (mmol/kg/day)	2.0	1.0	0.4

Fluid deficit

Fluid deficit is usually expressed as a percentage of body weight. This allows for easy calculation of replacement fluids. Fluid imbalance may be as a result of any of the following:

WATER LOSS

- Decreased intake.
- Increased respiratory loss (especially seen in children with high respiratory rates).
- Renal concentration impairment.

WATER AND SALT LOSS

- Vomiting.
- Diarrhoea.
- Increased sweating.

BLOOD VOLUME LOSS

- Haemorrhage.
- Septic shock.
- Anaphylaxis.
- Burns.

Assessment of deficit

Deficit assessment is difficult even for experienced paediatricians. Some idea of the deficit can be gained from the history of the abnormal loss. For example:
- Has the vomiting persisted for more than 24 hours?
- Has the child passed urine in the past 12 hours?
- Is the child thirsty?

Dehydration is generally assessed by estimating weight loss.

MILD DEHYDRATION (2%–3% ACUTE WEIGHT LOSS)

- Thirst.
- Mild oliguria.
- No physical signs.

MODERATE DEHYDRATION (5% ACUTE WEIGHT LOSS)

- Slight decrease in skin tone.
- Sunken fontanelles in infants.
- Slight decrease in ocular tension.
- Tachycardia.

SEVERE DEHYDRATION (7%–8% ACUTE WEIGHT LOSS)

- Marked tachycardia.
- Loss of skin tone.
- Loss of ocular tension.
- Sunken eyes.
- Restlessness and apathy.

PROFOUND DEHYDRATION (>10% ACUTE WEIGHT LOSS)

- Circulatory collapse.
- Delirium and coma.
- Hyperpyrexia.
- Cyanosis.

Replacement of deficit

Usually, the deficit is replaced with the fluid that most closely approximates the fluid that has been lost. Replacement therapy is aimed at restoring the fluid compartments in the following order. If there is significant loss of blood volume, then this must be replaced as rapidly as is safely possible to preserve brain, heart and kidney perfusion.

BLOOD VOLUME LOSS

- Blood: packed red cells or whole blood.
- Colloid: 4% Albumin
- Hartmann solution or normal saline (minimize use because of risk of haemodilution or haemoglobin and coagulation factors)
- Inotropes if needed.

SALT AND WATER LOSS

■ Hartmann solution or normal saline.

It is important to note that treatment should be based on the aetiology of the deficit. Management of severe deficit should therefore occur in a monitored environment, such as an intensive care unit.

Calculation of deficit

Deficit (mL) = % dehydration × weight (kg) × 10.

Examples

MILD DEHYDRATION

Where there is no circulatory compromise, the loss will be water and electrolytes from all body compartments. This can be replaced with dextrose saline solution over many hours.

SEVERE DEHYDRATION

There is loss of intracellular, interstitial and, most importantly, blood volume. The priority is to rapidly restore blood volume and, with that, cardiac output with crystalloid solutions (20–40 mL/kg) to allow adequate vital organ perfusion.

SEVERE BLOOD LOSS

In cases of trauma or bleeding, there will initially be loss of blood volume. This is treated in the same way as earlier, that is, restoring circulating blood volume with blood and reassessment of losses. If the blood loss is unknown, then initial therapy is to start with 20 mL/kg over 10–20 min and then reassess. The measurement of blood pressure, which in adults is an important indicator of poor organ perfusion, is not indicative of such blood loss in children. Measurement of parameters such as heart rate and capillary return are more reliable indicators in the younger patient. The signs of adequate fluid replacement include urine output measurement and a return to normal values of heart rate and capillary return.

Notes on rehydration

The previous guidelines apply to previously healthy children. Those children with cardiac disease or significant systemic disease require intensive intravascular monitoring in a paediatric intensive care unit.

■ Constant reassessment of fluid therapy is essential throughout replacement.

■ Measurement of electrolytes is essential in the replacement of greater than moderate deficits and applies especially to potassium.

■ Measurement of acid–base status with arterial blood gases is often necessary, as fluid deficit causes organ hypoperfusion and subsequent metabolic acidosis. This will usually correct itself with correction of blood volume and cardiac output over many hours.

■ Fluid balance and acid–base disturbances are often very complex and life threatening; if there is any doubt as to management, then specialist paediatric intensivist or anaesthetic advice should be sought.

TRANSFUSION

$$\text{Volume (mL)} = \text{weight (kg)} \times \text{g\% Hb rise required} \times 3$$

TABLE E.3 ■ **Composition of intravenous crystalloid and colloid fluids**

	Na⁺ (mmol/L)	Cl– (mmol/L)	Lactate (mmol/L)	Ca²⁺ (mmol/L)	Dextrose (g/L)
Normal saline 0.9%	150	150			
Hartmann solution	130	110	5	3	
Albumin	140	128			

Antibiotic prophylaxis protocols for the prevention of infective endocarditis

Angus C. Cameron ■ Richard P. Widmer ■ Benjamin Moran

Infective endocarditis is a rare and potentially life-threatening disease with a reported annual incidence of 0.3 per 100 000 children in Western countries, which has remained unchanged in the past 40 years. Despite the advent of antibiotics, infective endocarditis still has a high rate of mortality, up to 25%, and is associated with significant morbidity.

Approved antibiotic prophylaxis regimens are still recommended for potentially at-risk patients receiving dental treatment, as there is evidence, predominantly based on animal models, that suggests infective endocarditis may follow dental treatment in susceptible patients. Recommendations differ from one institution to another and vary in different countries, and therefore it is the responsibility of clinicians to determine which guideline is the most suitable to their individual patient. However, no matter what recommendations are followed, the healthcare professional should offer patients at risk of infective endocarditis clear and consistent information about prevention, including:

- the importance of maintaining excellent dental hygiene and regular oral health checks.
- advice on the risk of body piercings and tattoos.
- seek medical advice in the event of prolonged unexplained febrile illness.
- benefits and risks of antibiotic prophylaxis and why AB prophylaxis is not routinely recommended for CHD patients during dental procedures.

Pathogenesis

- Characterized by inflammation of the inner surface of the heart (endocardium).
- Generally attributed to bacterial infection.
- Most commonly affecting the heart valves.
- May also involve nonvalvular areas.
- Implanted cardiac mechanical devices also affected, such as prosthetic heart valves.

Three conditions need to be met for infective endocarditis to occur:

- Pre-existing damage to the heart valve surface.
- Bacteraemia, that is, the introduction and circulation of bacteria in the bloodstream.
- Presence of bacteria of sufficient virulence to evade the body's innate defences, to attach, colonize, invade and so cause infection of the damaged heart valve surface.

Epidemiology

The at-risk population principally consists of those with:

- Rheumatic fever: Previously, the most common cause of heart valve damage was childhood rheumatic fever. Improved sanitation and living conditions and the availability of antibiotics have significantly reduced the incidence of rheumatic fever. In those areas with social and economic deprivation, rheumatic heart valve disease is still prevalent.
- Congenital heart disease.
- Prosthetic aortopulmonary shunts.

- Prosthetic heart valves.
- Patients with a previous history of endocarditis.
- Immunocompromised patients with long-term central venous lines.

Antibiotic prophylaxis

It has been long recognized that invasive dental procedures, typically extractions, cause an acute, substantive bacteraemia. However, there are increasing concerns regarding the cumulative bacteraemia associated with activities of daily living, such as chewing or toothbrushing, particularly in the presence of chronic dental disease. In spite of this, infective endocarditis is uncommon.

In an attempt to reduce the significant mortality and morbidity rates seen with infective endocarditis, numerous protocols recommending the prophylactic use of antibiotics have been published. Two of the most authoritative bodies, namely the American Heart Association (AHA) and the Working Party of the British Society for Antimicrobial Chemotherapy, have recently published significantly revised protocols for antibiotic prophylaxis for susceptible patients.

Cardiac conditions associated with the highest risk of adverse outcome from endocarditis for which prophylaxis with dental procedures is recommended:

- Previous history of infective endocarditis.
- Prosthetic cardiac valve replacement.
- Hypertrophic obstructive cardiomyopathy.
- Cardiac transplant recipients who develop valvulopathy.
- Post-percutaneous valve implantation (example: Melody valve).
- Specified congenital heart disease involving the presence or placement of shunts or conduits:
  - Unrepaired cyanotic shunts, including palliative shunts or conduits.
  - Completely repaired congenital heart defects with prosthetic material or device for at least 6 months after the procedure.
  - Repaired congenital heart disease with residual defects or adjacent to a site of prosthetic patch or material.

At-risk dental procedures

Antibiotic prophylaxis is now indicated for any and all dental procedures that involve manipulation of the gingival, mucosal or periapical tissues that is likely to cause bleeding (i.e., extractions, scaling, root canal instrumentation beyond the apex). The following procedures and events do not need prophylaxis:

- Routine anaesthetic injections through noninfected tissue.
- Taking dental radiographs.
- Placement of removable prosthodontic or orthodontic appliances.
- Adjustment of orthodontic appliances.
- Placement of orthodontic brackets
- Shedding of deciduous teeth.
- Bleeding from trauma to the lips or oral mucosa.

Guidelines for clinicians

PAST AND CURRENT MEDICAL HISTORY

It is essential that the patient's medical status and history be assessed with respect to their cardiac problem. Consultation with the patient's doctor or cardiologist is essential. Dentists should be prepared to discuss with the treating doctor any issues surrounding the dental care of their patient.

CONSIDERATIONS IN SELECTING APPROPRIATE ANTIBIOTICS

- Anaphylaxis must be considered a risk in all patients taking any antibiotic, but particularly with any of the penicillins.
- Does the patient have a convincing history of allergy to any of the recommended antibiotics?
- Is the patient on long-term antibiotics? Or have they recently been taking an antibiotic? Alternative agents should be used.
- Does the patient have impaired renal function that will necessitate dose modification?
- Is the patient able to accept oral medications? Is there a history of vomiting with oral antibiotics? If so, consider parenteral medication.

TREATMENT PLANNING

- 'Group' together a number of invasive dental procedures to be done in the minimal number of appointments to reduce the need for repeated courses of antibiotics.
- The same antibiotic should not be prescribed within 14 days.
- Is a general anaesthetic indicated? Consideration should be given to completing all possible treatment in one appointment.

RECOMMENDATIONS FOR USE OF PROTOCOLS FOR ANTIBIOTIC PROPHYLAXIS

The authors do not make a recommendation about the efficacy of one particular protocol over another. There are problems associated with prophylaxis regimens in that no two sets of guidelines are the same. Less than 10% of patients with endocarditis have had a recent invasive dental procedure and there is no direct evidence in humans that antibiotic prophylaxis is effective. Currently, there is disagreement over the efficacy of different protocols as to which patients and what dental procedures should be covered. Please note that the current Australian Guidelines make special reference for the need to provide antibiotic prophylaxis for indigenous Australians who have a history of rheumatic fever. The AHA Guidelines still recommend antibiotic prophylaxis for invasive dental procedures in select patients thought to be at higher risk of infective endocarditis. In contrast, the National Institute for Health and Clinical Excellence (NICE) published revised guidelines for the UK in 2008. The major recommendation of this group is that antibiotic prophylaxis is not recommended for patients at risk of infective endocarditis, undergoing any type of dental procedures, including invasive dental procedures. The NICE guidelines contend that the greatest risk of infective endocarditis is from the cumulative, incidental daily bacteremia. In light of this, the NICE guidelines place greater emphasis on the provision and maintenance of optimal oral hygiene and dental health. Of interest, since the introduction of the revised guidelines, there has not been an increase in the incidence of infective endocarditis in the United Kingdom.

PAEDIATRIC DOSING

- The dose for any child should be calculated up to, but not exceeding, the maximum adult dose.
- Dosage should always be prescribed according to weight (dose/kg).

OTHER CONSIDERATIONS

- It is expected that some cases of endocarditis will occur, despite the use of optimal prophylaxis protocols.
- In circumstances where appropriate prophylaxis has not been given, antibiotics prescribed up to 6 hours after a procedure may give effective cover.
- Good history-taking is essential.
- If in doubt, consult relevant medical authorities.

TABLE F.1 ■ Current protocols for susceptible patients

Situation	Agent	Regimen: single dose 30–60 minutes before procedure	
		Adults	Children[a]
Oral	Amoxicillin	2 g	50 mg/kg to adult dose
Unable to take oral medications	Ampicillin or Cefazolin or ceftriaxone	2 g IV or IM 1 g IV or IM	50 mg/kg IV or IM 50 mg/kg IV or IM
Oral but allergic to penicillins or ampicillin	Cefalexin[b,c] or Clindamycin or Azithromycin or clarithromycin	2 g 600 mg 500 mg	50 mg/kg 20 mg/kg 15 mg/kg
Allergic to penicillins or ampicillin and unable to take oral medications	Cefazolin or ceftriaxone or Clindamycin	1 g IV or IM 600 mg IM or IV	50 mg/kg IV or IM 50 mg/kg IV or IM

[a]Child dose must not exceed adult dose.
[b]Or other first- or second-generation cephalosporin in equivalent adult or paediatric dose.
[c]Cephalosporins should not be used in an individual with a history of anaphylaxis, angio-oedema or urticaria with penicillins or ampicillin.
IM, Intramuscular; *IV*, intravenous.
(From Wilson, W., Taubert, K.A., Gewitz, M., et al., 2007. Prevention of infective endocarditis. Guidelines from the American Heart Association. Prevention of infective endocarditis: A guideline from the American Heart Association Rheumatic Fever, Endocarditis and Kawasaki Disease Committee, Council on Cardiovascular Disease in the Young, and the Council on Clinical Cardiology, Council on Cardiovascular Surgery and Anesthesia, and the Quality of Care and Outcomes Research Interdisciplinary Working Group. Journal of the American Dental Association 138, 739–760.)

Further reading

Gould, F.K., Elliott, T.S., Foweraker, J., et al., 2006. Guidelines for the prevention of endocarditis: report of the Working Party of the British Society for Antimicrobial Chemotherapy. Journal of Antimicrobial Chemotherapy 57 (6), 1035–1042.

NICE, 2008. Clinical guideline 64. Prophylaxis against infective endocarditis: antimicrobial prophylaxis against infective endocarditis in adults and children undergoing interventional procedures. Online. Available: www.nice.org.uk/CG064. Updated September 2015–July 2016.

Sroussi, H.Y., Prabhu, A.R., Epstein, J.B., 2007. Which antibiotic prophylaxis guidelines for infective endocarditis should Canadian dentists follow? Journal of the Canadian Dental Association 73, 401–405.

Therapeutic Guidelines Ltd., 2007. Oral and dental, Version 1. Therapeutic Guidelines Limited, Melbourne. Online. Available at: www.tg.com.au.

Thornhill, M.H., Dayer, M.J., Forde, J.M., et al., 2011. Impact of the NICE guideline recommending cessation of antibiotic prophylaxis for prevention of infective endocarditis: before and after study. British Medical Journal 342, d2392.

Wilson, W., Taubert, K.A., Gewitz, M., et al., 2007. Prevention of infective endocarditis. Guidelines from the American Heart Association. Prevention of infective endocarditis: A guideline from the American Heart Association Rheumatic Fever, Endocarditis and Kawasaki Disease Committee, Council on Cardiovascular Disease in the Young, and the Council on Clinical Cardiology, Council on Cardiovascular Surgery and Anesthesia, and the Quality of Care and Outcomes Research Interdisciplinary Working Group. Journal of the American Dental Association 138, 739–760.

Glasgow Coma Scale

Angus C. Cameron ■ Richard P. Widmer ■ Benjamin Moran

The Glasgow Coma Scale (GCS) is a rating score for head injury, and the score gives an indication of degree of injury and level of consciousness. Table G.1 has been modified for children by the Adelaide Women's and Children's Hospital, as the response scores are usually lower in children. Children between 6 months and 2 years may localize pain but not obey commands, and before 6 months, the best score is withdrawal from pain or abnormal extension and flexion. There is no modification of the adult eye-opening scale. Verbal responses should be consistent with age.

Modified Glasgow Coma Scale

OUTCOMES

In children with GCS scores of 3 or 4, there are significant mortality rates (between 20% and 70%), whereas in those with scores over 5, there is low mortality and morbidity (<30%). If a child does not die within the first 24 hours, the risk of death falls to between 10% and 20%. Some 64% of children who do not open their eyes spontaneously within 24 hours will die or survive in a vegetative state. It is important to note that over 90% of children who are comatose initially with a GCS score greater than 3 will recover to an independent state, although 50% will have neurological impairment. If coma persists for longer than 3 months, there is almost always neurological and cognitive damage.

TABLE G.1 ■ **Modified Glasgow Coma Scale**

	Response	Response for infants	Score
Eye opening	Spontaneously	Spontaneously	4
	To speech	To speech	3
	To pain	To pain	2
	None	None	1
Verbal	Orientated	Coos and babbles	5
	Words	Irritable cries	4
	Vocal sounds	Cries to pain	3
	Cries	Moans to pain	2
	None	None	1
Motor	Obeys commands	Normal spontaneous movements	6
	Localizes	Withdraws to touch	5
	Withdraws from pain	Withdraws from pain	4
	Abnormal flexion to pain	Abnormal flexion	3
	Extension to pain	Abnormal extension	2
	None	None	1
Best possible score			15

(Modified for paediatric use by the Adelaide Women's and Children's Hospital.)

Common drug usage in paediatric dentistry

Angus C. Cameron ■ Richard P. Widmer ■ Benjamin Moran

TABLE H.1 ■ **Common drug usage in paediatric dentistry**

Drug	Route	Dose	Frequency	Max dose	Indications	Contraindications/notes
Antibiotics						
Amoxicillin	PO	15–25 mg/kg/dose	tds	4 g/day	Antibiotic of first choice, except in allergic patients	Syrup or chewable tablets for young children
	IV	25 mg/kg/dose	tds	8 g/day	Antibiotic of first choice, except in allergic patients	
	PO IV	50 mg/kg up to adult dose 2 g	60 min prior stat	2 g adult dose	Endocarditis prophylaxis	
Amoxicillin plus clavulanic acid	PO	22.5 mg/kg/dose	bd	1.5 g/day	Severe/persistent dental infections	For β-lactam resistant organisms only
Ampicillin	IV	25 mg/kg/dose	qid	12 g/day		
	IV	50 mg/kg up to adult dose 2 g	Stat	2 g adult dose	Endocarditis prophylaxis	
Benzylpenicillin	IV	30 mg/kg/dose	qid	1.2 g/dose	First IV drug of choice for odontogenic infections	
Phenoxymethylpenicillin potassium	PO	10–12.5 mg/kg/dose	qid	500 mg/dose		Must be given on an empty stomach

TABLE H.1 ◼ *Continued*

Drug	Route	Dose	Frequency	Max dose	Indications	Contraindications/notes
Cefalexin	PO	12.5–25 mg/kg/dose	qid	1 g/dose		
	PO	50 mg/kg up to adult dose 2 g	60 min prior	2 g adult dose	Endocarditis prophylaxis	Not for use in pregnancy
Cefalotin	IV	25 mg/kg/dose	qid	2 g/dose		
Cefazolin	IV	50 mg/kg up to adult dose 1 g	Stat	1 g adult dose	Endocarditis prophylaxis	
Metronidazole	IV	12.5 mg/kg/dose	b.d.	500 mg/dose	Supplement to penicillins in cases of severe or protracted infection	Not for use in pregnancy
	PO	10 mg/kg/dose	tds	400 mg/dose		
Clindamycin	PO IV	10 mg/kg/dose	tds	450 mg/dose	Antibiotic of first choice in penicillin-allergic patients	Low risk of pseudomembranous colitis with protracted use
	PO IV	20 mg/kg up to adult dose 600 mg	60 min prior stat	600 mg adult dose	Endocarditis prophylaxis	Oral 1 h or IV stat before procedure
Azithromycin Clarithromycin	PO	15 mg/kg up to adult dose 500 mg	60 min prior	500 mg adult dose	Alternative for endocarditis prophylaxis	Macrolide antibiotics: supersedes erythromycin
Antifungals						
Nystatin	PO	<2 years 50 000–100 000 U >2 years 100 000–500 000 U	qid		Topical antifungal	Drops: apply to affected area Tablets: chew slowly
Miconazole	PO	1/2 tbsp	bd–qid		Topical antifungal	Oral gel: apply to affected area

TABLE H.1 ■ *Continued*

Drug	Route	Dose	Frequency	Max dose	Indications	Contraindications/notes
Fluconazole	PO IV	3–6 mg/kg/day	Daily	400 mg/day	Systemic antifungal candidiasis prophylaxis and treatment in immunosuppressed patients	Warfarinized and renal patients. Change to oral as soon as possible. Multiple drug interactions
	PO	10 mg/dose (not kg)	6-hourly		Topical antifungal	Lozenge: patient to chew slowly
Amphotericin B	PO	100 mg/mL	6-hourly		Topical antifungal	Suspension: apply to affected area
	PO	3%	6-hourly		Topical antifungal	Ointment: apply to affected area
Antivirals						
Aciclovir	PO IV	20 mg/kg/dose 10 mg/kg/dose	5-hourly tds		Early primary herpetic gingivostomatitis	Immunosuppressed patients, should be prescribed within 72 hours of infection
Analgesics						
Xylocaine (viscous)	PO	2% 5 mL	3-hourly			Rinse mouth/gargle for 30 s. No food or drink for 1 hour after
Aspirin						Should not be used in children under 12 years of age because of the risk of Reye syndrome
Paracetamol	PO PR	15 mg/kg/dose	q4- to 6-hourly	60 mg/kg/day up to 4 g/day		Hepatotoxic if overdose. Be aware of different presentations of paracetamol
Ibuprofen	PO	5–10 mg/kg/dose	q6- to 8-hourly	40 mg/kg/day (2 g/day)		

TABLE H.1 ■ *Continued*

Drug	Route	Dose	Frequency	Max dose	Indications	Contraindications/notes
Naproxen	PO	10–20 mg/kg/day	q8- to 12-hourly	1 g/day		
Diclofenac	PO PR	1 mg/kg/dose	q8- to 12-hourly	3 mg/kg/day (150 mg/day)		Only in children >10 kg
Oxycodone	PO	0.1–0.25 mg/kg/dose	q4- to 6-hourly			
Morphine	PO IV IM	0.2–0.5 mg/kg/dose 100–200 µg/kg/dose	q4- to 6-hourly q2- to 4-hourly	15 mg/dose		Should only be used in admitted patients
Tramadol	PO	1–2 mg/kg/dose	q6-hourly	6 mg/kg/day (400 mg/day)		
Naloxone	IM IV	5–10 µg/kg	Single dose	10 mg total	Narcotic overdose	May be repeated at 2–3 min intervals if necessary
Midazolam	PO PN IV	0.3 mg/kg 0.2 mg/kg 0.1–0.2 mg/kg	Single dose	10 mg 5 mg	Sedation	
Flumazenil	IV	5 µg/kg repeated every minute up to 40 µg/kg	Every minute	Total 2 mg/dose	Benzodiazepine reversal	Complex to administer: refer to product information sheet. Requires IV access in emergency resuscitation.
Chloral hydrate	PO	10–20 mg/kg/dose 30–50 mg/kg	6-hourly Single dose	500 mg/dose 1 g	Sedation Hypnotic or premed	Avoid with renal or hepatic impairment
Temazepam	PO	0.3 mg/kg/dose	Single dose	20 mg/dose	Single dose for sedation	
Antiemetics						
Metoclopramide	PO IM IV	0.1–0.15 mg/kg	Single dose	0.5 mg/kg/day (30 mg/day)	Antinauseant/antiemetic	Single dose after narcotic if vomiting or nausea Dystonic extrapyramidal reactions may occur

TABLE H.1 ■ *Continued*

Drug	Route	Dose	Frequency	Max dose	Indications	Contraindications/notes
Ondansetron	IV	0.1–0.15 mg/kg	Single dose	4 mg/dose	Antinauseant/antiemetic Postoperative nausea and vomiting	Centrally acting Often used in chemotherapy recipients
Corticosteroids						
Kenalog in Orabase	PO	Triamcinolone 0.1%	4- to 6-hourly	–	Mild–moderate oral ulceration	Ointment: apply to ulcers but do not rub in
Betamethasone in Orabase	PO	0.1% compound 1:1 w/w with Orabase	4- to 6-hourly		Moderate to severe ulceration	Ointment severe ulceration Apply to ulcer but do not rub in
Dexamethasone	PO IV	0.1 mg/mL 0.1–0.2 mg/kg/dose	4- to 6-hourly Single dose		Moderate to severe ulceration Reduction in postsurgical inflammation	Mouthwash for very severe mucosal ulceration 5 mL rinse for 5 min and spit out well
Prednisolone	PO	'Pulse' dose of up to 2 mg/kg/day	6- to 12-hourly		Severe intractable immune-mediated oral ulceration	Weeklong course, rapid taper
Antifibrinolytics						
ε aminocaproic acid (EACA)	IV	30 mg/kg	Stat			Patients haemorrhagic diathesis loading dose of 100 mg/kg
Tranexamic acid	PO	15–20 mg/kg	qid			
Tranexamic acid	PO	10% compounded mouthwash	qid			Mouthwash – 5 mL rinse, then spit out well
Desmopressin	IV	0.3 mg/kg	Slowly infuse over 60 min	20 µg/dose	Give before surgery	Infused over 1 hour before surgery

Clinicians are warned to prescribe and administer any drug carefully. The dosages in this table are provided as a guide to the usage of medications in paediatric dental practice and clinicians should also consult their relevant pharmacopoeia. Take care when determining maximal dose and frequency of administration.

Radiography in children

Johan Aps

Radiographs are essential for accurate diagnosis. If, however, the information gained from such an investigation does not influence treatment decisions, both the timing and the need for the radiograph should be questioned.

Three basic principles are key:

- Justification — What diagnostic information is needed?
- Optimization — What imaging format is indicated?
- Limitation — ALARA – (as low as reasonably achievable)
  ALADA – (as low as diagnostically achievable)
  ALADAIP – (as low as diagnostically achievable being indication-oriented and patient specific)

This dovetails into the Image Gently in Dentistry® campaign (2014), which provided six practical steps to underline the principle that one size does not fit all:

- Select x-rays for a patient's individual needs, not as a routine.
- Use the fastest image receptor possible.
- Collimate the x-ray beam to expose only the area of interest.
- Use thyroid collars.
- Child-size the exposure.
- Use cone-beam computed tomography (CBCT) only when necessary.

The following radiographic techniques may be used in children:

Intraoral radiography

- Bitewing radiography.
- Periapical radiography.
- Occlusal radiography.

Extraoral radiography

- Panoramic radiography.
- Cephalometric radiography.
- Oblique lateral radiography.
- CBCT.

Medical imaging modalities

Medical imaging modalities can be valuable in cases where more specialized imaging of pathological conditions is required (e.g., parotitis, rhabdomyosarcoma, brain tumour). It is essential that paediatric dentists have knowledge of these techniques and their indications.

Positron emission tomography–computed tomography and single photon emission tomography are dual or hybrid imaging modalities because they allow for a combination of imaging of form (anatomy) and function. Radiopharmaceuticals are injected into the patient, which will be stored in specific target organs and tissues, which allows for accurate diagnosis of pathology (e.g., brain tumour). These are procedures which involve high patient radiation doses of up to 20000 μSv (compare with Table I.1).

Magnetic resonance imaging (MRI) does not involve ionizing radiation. This technique uses highly magnetic fields to influence the body's hydrogen nuclei. Several so-called sequences can be

TABLE I.1 ■ Typical effective radiation doses for a range of dental diagnostic exposures

Radiographic examination	Effective radiation dose µSv
Bitewing/periapical radiograph	3–22
Panoramic radiograph	2.7– 38
Upper standard occlusal radiograph	8
Lateral cephalometric radiograph	2.2–5.6
Posterior-anterior skull radiograph	20
CBCT–small field of view	10–670
CBCT–large field of view	30–1100
Radiation dose comparison for parents	
Chest x-ray	14

CBCT, Cone beam computed tomography.
(Modified from Whaites, E., N. Drage, 2013. Essentials of dental radiography and radiology. 5th ed. Churchill Livingstone Elsevier, London.)

applied to visualize soft tissue in particular (e.g., salivary glands, brain and tongue). Claustrophobia can be a serious issue in children when this imaging modality is used.

Questions are sometimes raised as to the use of stainless steel crowns (nickel chromium) and orthodontic appliances in children who require frequent MRIs. Stainless steel crowns are fabricated from Type 304 alloy and are considered to be no ferromagnetic. The latter have been studied extensively and are not considered to be a problem in regard to the safely in the magnet. However, they may result in the generation of considerable artefacts that may affect the diagnostic value of the scan. It is wise to consult with the child's neurologist and radiologist as to whether the use of other restorative materials might be more appropriate, especially in the maxilla. Further and updated information on dental materials can be found through this link: http://mrisafety.com/TMDL_list.php?qs=dental.

Ultrasonography is another technique that does not involve ionizing radiation. The different tissues' elastic impedance is used to acquire the image. This is a relatively easy and cheap technique which allows for quick and live imaging of soft tissues in the head and neck region (e.g., salivary glands, lymph nodes and arteries).

Guidelines for radiology in children

Different professional organisations such as the European Academy of Paediatric Dentistry, the American Academy of Pediatric Dentistry and the American Academy of Oral and Maxillofacial Radiology have formulated guidelines for the prescription of radiographs in children. Guidelines are recommendations only, and the clinical judgement of the dentist and the individual circumstance of the patient are essential in determining what is the most appropriate radiographic investigation that is required. In regard to the monitoring of caries progression, for example, a caries risk assessment is essential for each individual child, including fluoride history, current caries activity, diet analysis, and so on.

- The guidelines for prescribing radiographs in dental practice are shown in Figure I.1.
- Table I.2 summarizes what type of examination is indicated or recommended in different clinical circumstances.
- Figure I.2 shows the decision processes when CBCT is planned in a child or adolescent patient.

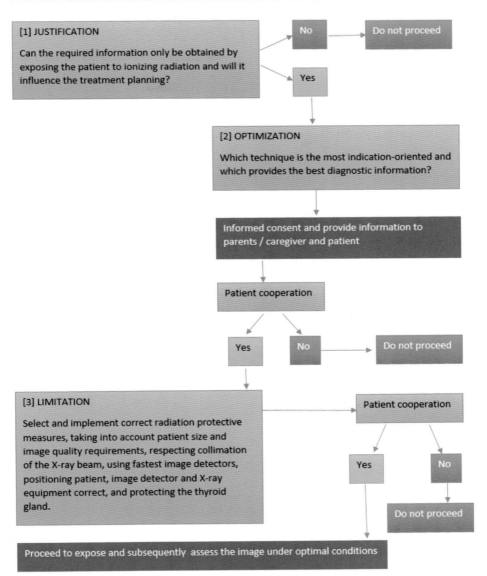

Figure I.1 Flow chart of the principle for prescription of radiographs (ionizing radiation exposure) in children and adolescents. (Modified from EAPD 2020 guidelines; Kühnisch, J., Anttonen, V., Duggal, M.S., et al., 2020. Best clinical practice guidance for prescribing dental radiographs in children and adolescents: an EAPD policy document. European Archives of Paediatric Dentistry 21, 375–386.)

Radiation dose (Table I.1)

Parents will always be concerned about the level of radiation to which their child might be exposed. It is important to be able to give parents good advice as to the need for radiographs and the relatively low doses that modern digital radiography can provide for appropriate diagnostic value. The doses are shown in Table I.1. The units of radiation measurement can be confusing

TABLE I.2 ■ Clinical-based and clinically judged indications of dental radiographs in children and adolescents

Type of appointment	Child		Adolescent
	Primary dentition 3–7 years	Mixed dentition 7–12 years	Permanent dentition >13 years
New patients	Bitewings if closed contacts between posterior teeth	Bitewings or extraoral bitewings from panoramic machine	
	Extra-oral bitewings from panoramic machine may have indication	Panoramic radiograph based on specific needs for assessment of growth and development or pathology	
	Children with no history of disease and where proximal contacts can be visualized may not require any radiographs	Selected periapical radiographs based on specific indications	
	Panoramic radiograph based on specific needs for the assessment of growth and development or pathology		
Recall patients			
No caries activity	Not recommended	Not recommended, however, at least one set of radiographs would be recommended in the mixed dentition in the absence of any other radiographic examination.	3–5 yearly
Enamel only	12–24 monthly	12–24 monthly	12–24 monthly
Caries beyond DEJ	12 monthly	12 monthly	6–12 monthly dependent on caries progression between examinations
Acute dental infection	Periapical or panoramic		
	If multiple carious teeth are present, then bitewings should also be taken.		

TABLE I.2 ■ *Continued*

Type of appointment	Child		Adolescent
	Primary dentition 3–7 years	Mixed dentition 7–12 years	Permanent dentition >13 years
Dental trauma			
Tooth fracture or luxation	Periapical radiographs Anterior maxillary occlusal are useful in the young child.		
Severe dentoalveolar trauma	Panoramic radiograph based on specific needs CBCT may be indicated in specific cases.		
Invasive cervical resorption	Periapical radiographs	Periapical radiographs Small field CBCT may be indicated to assess the extent of the resorptive lesion.	
Maxillofacial injuries	Panoramic radiographs and periapical radiographs as indicated/clinically judged CT scans as indicated. It is important to liaise with other treating clinicians, for example neurosurgeons. If a child required a CT scan to assess for head injuries, and maxillofacial injuries are suspected, the facial bones should be included in the scans		
Dental anomalies			
Hypodontia	A panoramic radiograph is useful when there is the suspicion of the absence of multiple teeth in the younger child	Periapical radiographs for localized hypodontia Panoramic radiographs when multiple teeth are absent	Panoramic or CBCT for orthodontic and surgical treatment planning Lateral cephalometric for orthodontics
Supernumerary teeth	Periapical or anterior maxillary/ mandibular occlusal	Periapical or panoramic radiographs as indicated A CBCT may be indicated to assist in the localization of deeply impacted supernumerary teeth when surgery is planned and for later orthodontic treatment planning for subsequent impacted teeth. Adjusted field of view CBCT to region of interest is recommended to keep radiation burden as low as possible. The exact proximity of the supernumerary to adjacent teeth is vitally important to prevent damage to these teeth	
Impacted teeth	Usually no radiographs indicated for this age group	Periapical or panoramic radiographs or CBCT as indicated, dependent on the number and the position of the affected teeth and the requirement for surgery or planning	
Molar-incisor hypomineralization	Bitewings for assessing hypoplastic second primary molars	Panoramic radiographs to assess for the development of second and third permanent molars for orthodontic treatment planning Bitewings for assessment of caries extent	

Continued

TABLE I.2 ■ *Continued*

Type of appointment	Child		Adolescent
	Primary dentition 3–7 years	Mixed dentition 7–12 years	Permanent dentition >13 years
Cleft lip and palate	Periapical radiographs or an anterior maxillary occlusal to assess the extent of the cleft and/or for the presence of supernumerary or missing teeth	Panoramic radiograph and CBCT if indicated for orthodontic and surgical treatment planning	Panoramic radiograph and CBCT if indicated for orthodontic and surgical treatment planning
Craniofacial syndromes	May not be required	Panoramic radiograph and CBCT if indicated for orthodontic and surgical treatment planning Lateral cephalometric radiograph for orthodontic treatment and/or surgery may be omitted if CBCT was taken and covered the required structures for cephalometric analysis	Panoramic radiograph and CBCT if indicated for orthodontic and surgical treatment Lateral cephalometric radiograph for cephalometric analysis
Amelogenesis / dentinogenesis imperfecta	May not be required Bitewings for caries assessment	Panoramic radiograph for restorative, orthodontic or surgical treatment planning	Panoramic radiograph and CBCT if indicated for restorative, orthodontic and surgical treatment planning Lateral cephalometric for orthodontics
Oral pathology			
Cysts and tumours	The choice of examination will be determined by the nature of the pathology. Simple bony lesions might be imaged with periapical radiographs whereas extensive lesions in the jaws require panoramic radiography. If CBCT is considered necessary, the child's cooperation should be assessed. If a CT is considered, sedation or general anaesthesia might be required if the child's cooperation is an issue for CT. If surgery is required, then it is recommended that the surgeon who is performing the procedure determines what imaging is required.		
Condylar morphology in patients with temporomandibular dysfunction	Panoramic radiography is usually not indicated for this age group unless other pathology is present (see previously)	Panoramic radiography is usually not indicated for this age group unless other pathology is present (see previously)	Panoramic and CBCT if indicated and judged clinically (caveat: temporomandibular disc is not visible on CBCT)
Periodontal disease	Young children with periodontal disease usually have systemic disease. In this age group, bitewing radiographs will give enough information concerning bone loss around primary molars.	Bitewing and periapical radiographs as clinically indicated Panoramic radiograph if considered clinically essential	

(Modified from recommendations of the EAPD, 2020, and AAPD, 2017.)

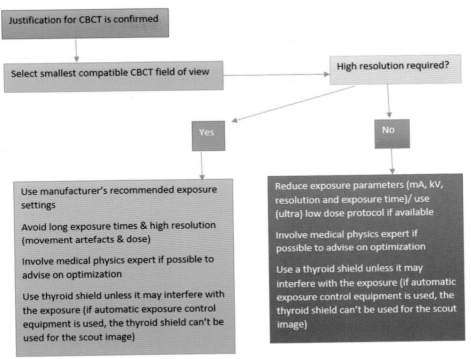

Figure I.2 Specific guidance when cone beam computed tomography is planned in a child or adolescent patient. *CBCT*, Cone beam computed tomography. (Modified from EAPD 2020 recommendations.)

and are complicated by usage or SI or Common units (roentgen, rads and rems) in different countries:

- Radiation absorbed dose (D)
  Takes into account the amount of energy absorbed from the radiation beam per unit mass of tissue (J/kg)
  Unit = Gray (Gy)
- Equivalent radiation dose (H)
  Takes into account the type of radiation
  Deals with radiobiological effectiveness of the radiation
  Weighting factor (W_R) for X-rays = 1
  $H = D \times W_R$ Unit = Sievert (Sv)
- Effective radiation dose (E)
  Takes into account the biological tissue
  Allows for investigations on different parts of the body to be compared as all doses are converted to an equivalent whole body dose
  Weighting factors (W_T) for different tissues (entire body $W_T = 1$)
  Unit = Sievert (Sv)
  $E = H \times W_T$ (or $E = D \times W_R \times W_T$)

Annual natural background radiation in Australia is around 1500 µSv, whereas in Europe it is 2500 µSv, and in the USA, 3500 µSv (1500 µSv is about 1500 single bitewing radiographs).

Further reading

American Academy of Paediatric Dentistry, 2019–2020. Prescribing dental radiographs for infants, children, adolescents, and individuals with special health care needs. In: The reference manual of pediatric dentistry. pp. 225–232.

Kühnisch, J., Anttonen, V., Duggal, M.S., et al., 2020. Best clinical practice guidance for prescribing dental radiographs in children and adolescents: an EAPD policy document. European Archives of Paediatric Dentistry 21, 375–386.

Van Acker, J.W.G., Pauwels, N.S., Cauwels, R.G.E.C., et al., 2020. Outcomes of different radioprotective precautions in children undergoing dental radiography: a systematic review. European Archives of Paediatric Dentistry 21, 463–508.

Whaites, E., Drage, N., 2013. Essentials of dental radiography and radiology, 5th ed. Churchill Livingstone Elsevier, London.

White, S.C., Scarfe, W.C., Schulze, R.K.W., et al., 2014. The Image Gently in Dentistry campaign: promotion of responsible use of maxillofacial radiology in dentistry for children. Oral Surgery, Oral Medicine, Oral Pathology, Oral Radiology 118, 1–5.

Ethics in paediatric dentistry

Richard Steffen

Ethics is a system of accepted beliefs that control our behaviour. This behaviour is determined by various moral codes, by our upbringing and origin, but also by the statutory environment and individual interpretation of these parameters. Our feeling to do the right thing is also controlled by our origin, our gender, our race and, last but not least, by any existing religion. Over the last hundred years, ethical values have shifted away from the perspective of the powerful to the common good. This applies in particular to attitude towards children, who used to be annoying, unfinished people of little value; but today, for many cultures, children are one of the most valuable assets in society. This is also reflected in the attitude of medicine and dentistry towards children. A development that was also urgently needed, it is still less than a hundred years ago when infants were still operated on without sufficient anaesthesia. The ethical goal in medicine and dentistry today is to keep our patients, children and young people, healthy.

'Health is a state of complete physical, mental and social well-being and not merely the absence of disease or infirmity'. This World Health Organization definition is still one of the best models to describe the term 'healthy'.

However, the concept of an ethical foundation for paediatric dentistry is far from being uniform or equally accepted everywhere. Although mainly Western, male-dominated concepts form the basis of many medical ethical treatises, there is now an almost uniform consensus as to which are the most important aspects in the treatment of children. These are:

Every child (every human being) should be treated equally and as optimally as possible, regardless of gender, race, age or religion.

But this is probably where our common ground ends. The combination of many different parameters creates a network of obligations, laws, taboos, externally determined constraints and individual decision criteria, which can lead to very different treatment concepts. Very quickly, the boundaries become blurred here when assessing what is right and what is wrong. To be able to make ethical decisions as well founded as possible anywhere in the world, it is therefore necessary to recognize and classify these many different parameters. The following scheme should help you to do this.

These principles ultimately lead to a partnership between practitioner and patient. This requires an acceptance of the professional skills of the practitioner on the patient's side, whereby the patient can also intervene in a controlling manner. On the side of dentistry, the aim should be to inform the patients as well as possible about the treatments and to involve the patients in therapy decisions within the bounds of possibility. A particular significance in the treatment of children is the lack of medical maturity. Depending on the age of the child, different levels of involvement of the legal guardians in the decision-making process regarding planned therapies are required. However, it is also difficult for therapeutic dentists to find the right path when making therapy decisions. This becomes more difficult the further such a therapy decision deviates from the everyday standard treatment. Research and teaching at universities and professional associations responsible for quality assurance face the same problem.

To be able to plan well-founded, secure treatment even in difficult situations, an ethically valid, comprehensively supported decision concept is required. It is **not enough** to base such decisions on evidence-based dentistry only.

Special ethical challenges in paediatric dentistry

Children represent a particularly vulnerable patient group. A special characteristic of children is their limited ability to consent and make decisions, which leads to a particularly pronounced social dependency relationship with a resulting increased need for protection. The vulnerability of children can be further increased by a precarious social constellation, physical or mental impairment or a particular medical emergency. Culture-specific aspects, in which practitioners and/or patients possess the repertoire of thought and action models, patterns of perception and moral values of cultures, can also play a role. Not least because of cultural backgrounds, there are big differences in the main problems of child treatment, the perception of fear and pain. One of the most controversial topics discussed in paediatric dentistry is the adequate handling of childhood fear and pain. It can be seen as ethically particularly problematic that anxious children under 14 years of age (not legally capable of will) can be treated by both parents and the dentist entirely opposite according to the child's will (= complete heteronomy). Research in developmental psychology has clearly pointed out the great damaging potential of unaccompanied coercive measures towards children. Purely coercive measures such as hand over mouth, active restraint or the holding of children by adults must therefore be firmly rejected. This is also in the knowledge that there are clear cultural differences between the perceptions of coercion. Nevertheless, forced treatment should never be applied to uncooperative children without accompanying consciousness-influencing measures, in particular sedation or anaesthesia. Children's dentistry encounters special problems not only in treatment but also in scientific research. Today, it is almost impossible to carry out a study, especially randomized clinical trials, on children that weighs therapeutic treatments against each other. Levine and co-authors have made this clear in their article, and just as clearly, the Helsinki Declaration advocates a safe ethical concept of clinical trials. Benefits factors (self-interest, group benefits, third-party benefits) are generally not recognized for clinical trials with children. The special need for protection has priority here. Good Clinical Practice includes exact and very strict conditions, such as an absolute noninvasivity of the trial, for approvals of studies in children.

At first glance, ethics in dentistry seems far less demanding than those of medicine, euthanasia for example. At any time, however, dentistry can also cause harm to patients or even death. This is particularly tragic for children and parents. We should not only be technically and medically prepared for incidents, but also emotionally, ethically and morally. Controversially discussed scientific topics such as stem cell research and organ donation are also an issue in paediatric dentistry.

We should be aware of what is a mistake and what is just a treatment failure. And without empathy for our children, patients and their caretakers, we cannot do our job anyway. Ethics is not moral philosophy. Ethical behaviour is the source of good paediatric dentistry.

Treatment error and treatment failure

Life without mistakes does not exist. The same things can be said about paediatric dentistry. Unwanted events, unintended damage, treatment errors and rule violations can quickly happen. There is a particular risk of error in the relationship between the patient and the dental professional, because the number of interventions is great, highly complex work processes exist and because, especially in paediatric dentistry, the treatment procedures are very often made considerably more difficult by a lack of cooperation. The desire for 'zero risk' dentistry is increasingly strengthening the pressure on dentists to provide patients with the least possible errors. Quality assurance systems, checklists and treatment standards are increasingly shaping everyday life in dentistry.

For this objective, it is necessary to define some key terms:

Adverse event: an event that may but does not necessarily result in harm to the patient. Example: An allergic reaction occurs during the administration of antibiotics.

- Preventable adverse event: an adverse event that could have been prevented by observing the due diligence rule. Example: If antibiotics are administered despite a known allergy, an allergic reaction occurs.
- Critical incident: an event with damaging potential that occurs if no suitable countermeasures are taken. Example: The patient is given an antibiotic but has not yet taken it. If there is no reaction, the patient is likely to be harmed when taking it.
- Error: an act or omission involving a deviation from a known treatment procedure. An injury need not be mandatory here. Example: Prescription of an antibiotic despite known allergy.
- Near miss: an incident that could lead to damage but which, because of timely intervention or lucky circumstances, did not occur. Example: A patient with a known allergy to antibiotics notices this himself before taking the antibiotics and draws the attention of the prescriber.

A wide variety of errors are possible in everyday practice (diagnostic errors, errors of medical treatment, nontreatment, errors in organization and information, cooperation errors and many others). For beginners, these are the most common mistakes when a difficult treatment is performed with limited professional experience. Overall, the most common medical errors are medication errors, and there is a wide range of possible errors, some of which have a high potential for damage.

Mistakes in dentistry are the same as moral misconduct, but mistakes carry the risk of causing such behaviour (denial, cover-up, shifting the blame). To avoid this and also because of the realization that mistakes will inevitably happen, it is ethically necessary to establish culture and strategies of error management in every dental institution.

Coping strategies for errors and medical mistreatment

The four main reasons which lead to an increased risk of error are:
- High time pressure to work and perform
- Physical mental and/or psychological stress
- Negligence
- Institutional deficits

The differences between the sources of error in small dental practices and large institutional clinics are huge. Although error management in small practices is usually in the hands of the practice owners, in large clinics, a real 'error infrastructure' must be built up. Such a corporate culture can consist of a responsible person, an internal weblog (e.g., Critical Incident Reporting System) and a periodic 'error conference' or this would be a paradoxical intervention, the published 'error of the month'. Essential in any size of business is an error reporting system to report incidents and critical situations. The easiest thing to do is to create a checklist for error reports. With the help of such a checklist, a solid error management can be built up, especially in a small, ambulant, clinical setting.

Checklist for management of errors and medical malpractice

A professional error happens quickly and is usually not an expression of personal failure. Ethical significance is attached to such a mistake by the way in which the mistake is dealt with and communicated.

Some important rules of communication are decisive:
- Errors should be reported as soon as possible.
- These communications/conversations should take place in a quiet, protected environment.

- A coworker who reports irregularities must not be deterred or otherwise hindered.
- Communication about errors is a 'chief matter' and should not be delegated.

Communication with patients should be handled in the following way:

- Presentation of the facts without whitewash.
- Expression of personal and sincere regret.
- Detailed information regarding consequences and possible remedies.
- Offer of a change of treatment provider.
- Indication that lessons and consequences are being learned from the error.
- Ensure that regular information and follow-up checks are carried out.
- Offer further assistance if necessary.

The points discussed here mainly concern error management in clinical operation. Special ethical and scientific requirements arise for scientific work. These are defined above all in the 'Good Scientific Practice' regulations. Scientific misconduct can be manifold but will not be further discussed here.

Further reading

Ashcroft, R., Baron, D., Benatar, S., et al., 1998. Teaching medical ethics and law within medical education: a model for the UK core curriculum. Journal of Medical Ethics 24, 188–192.

Beauchamp, T.L., Childress, J.F., 2009. Principles of biomedical ethics, sixth ed. Oxford University Press, New York.

FDI. FDI policy statement. Available: https://www.fdiworlddental.org/sites/default/files/media/documents/International-principles-of-ethics-for-the-dental-profession-1997.pdf. Accessed July 27, 2020.

Gross, D., 2012. Ethik in der Zahnmedizin. Quintessenz Publishing, Berlin, New York.

Holden, A.C.L., 2017. Blowing the whistle': the ethical, professional and legal implications of raising concerns and self-regulation within dentistry. Australian Dental Journal 63, 150–155.

Leroy, P., 2011. Medical errors: the importance of the bullet's blunt end. European Journal of Paediatrics 170, 251–252.

Levine, C., Faden, R., Grady, C., et al., 2010. Limitations of "vulnerability" as a projection for human research participants. American Journal of Bioethics 4, 44–49.

Schwartz, B., 2004. A call for ethics committees in dental organizations and in dental education. The Journal of the American College of Dentistry 71, 35–39.

World Health Organization, 2006. Constitution of the World Health Organization. Basic Documents, forty-fifth edition. World Health Organization, Geneva, Switzerland.

Somatic growth and maturity

Angus C. Cameron ■ Richard P. Widmer ■ Benjamin Moran

As soon as the child enters the surgery, assessment should begin. At the outset, the dentist should always look at a child's size, development, appearance and behaviour in relation to their chronological age. Dental examination will initially include an assessment of dental age (based on time of exfoliation, eruption status and root development) in relation to the chronological age. Any marked discrepancies should then be investigated further.

Basic indicators of somatic growth and development

HEIGHT AND WEIGHT

Height measurement

- Measure the child with shoes off, standing straight, with the Frankfort plane horizontal to the floor.
- Measurement is taken on deep inspiration of the patient.
- Sequential measurements are ideally taken at the same time of day.

Height abnormalities

- Short stature <3rd percentile, tall stature >97th percentile over a 6-month period.
- Rate of growth <3–5 cm/year; consider both for referral to specialist growth unit at a paediatric hospital.
- Measurements must be considered in relation to the height of the parents and skeletal age.
- Height prediction possible using methods of Tanner and Whitehouse (1983) or Bayley and Pinneau (1952).
- Prediction of adolescent growth spurt is achieved by serial measurements and may influence the subsequent timing of myofunctional orthodontic treatment.

Weight measurement

- Taken in light indoor clothing, with shoes off, ideally at the same time of day as height measurements.

Weight abnormalities

- Children with an endomorphic appearance tend to mature early, whereas those who are ectomorphic (especially boys) tend to mature late.
- Underweight: consider anorexia/bulimia.
- Overweight: may indicate nutritional problems.
- When children are markedly outside norms for age, early referral to a paediatrician or dietitian is essential.
- Gross obesity may significantly alter drug metabolism and will affect the calculation of drug dosages.

SKELETAL ASSESSMENT

- It has been consistently shown that bone age as determined from hand-wrist radiographs using the Greulich and Pyle or Tanner and Whitehouse systems has a high correlation with stature and general body development.
- Other rarely used methods of bone-age calculation include the FELS method (assess the skeletal maturity of the hand-wrist), use of knee joint or cervical vertebrae.
- Convention for anthropometric measurements uses the left hand.
- These methods assume that the bones of all patients consistently go through the same sequence of development, albeit at different rates. The Greulich and Pyle system is the most skeletally advanced for any age group, as it was derived in the USA from healthy children from a high socioeconomic group.

GREULICH AND PYLE METHOD

Each bone is matched with a similar-appearing bone in a series of standard radiographs of increasing age. Thus, each bone has a bone age assigned to it, and the modal (or most frequent) of these bone ages is taken as the bone age of the hand and wrist. Frequently, the step of assigning bone ages to each separate bone is omitted, and instead the patient's hand-wrist radiograph is matched to the nearest standard radiograph, thereby determining the patient's skeletal age. Radiographic standards are provided at 6- and 12-monthly intervals for both males and females.

TANNER AND WHITEHOUSE METHOD

This method scores specified bones according to their stage of development, using a written description and a radiographic standard of each stage of development. The total score for all bones is used to derive a skeletal age from tables provided. Generally, the TW-2 (13 bone score) is used in preference to the Tanner and Whitehouse 20-bone method, as it is about as accurate but is quicker to use. A computerized image analysis system for estimating TW-2 bone age has been shown to be more reliable than the manual rating system. The Tanner and Whitehouse TW-2 method is easier and more accurate than the Greulich and Pyle method for the occasional user.

SIGNIFICANCE

- Used to calculate potential for further increase in height.
- Used to predict adolescent growth spurt for timing of orthodontic treatment.
- Monitor growth abnormalities.

Dental development
ERUPTION TIMES

- The emergence of teeth in the primary and permanent dentitions is unreliable because of environmental influences (i.e., early extraction of primary teeth will delay eruption of the succedaneous tooth, whereas late extraction of a primary tooth will hasten the eruption of the permanent successor).
- Eruption is not a continuous event.
- Racial variations: published data on eruption times are generally of northern European populations. Earlier eruption times may be the norm in Asian peoples, and later eruption times are the norm in eastern and southern European groups.

ROOT DEVELOPMENT

- Use the scoring systems of Nolla, Moorees, Fanning, Demirijan and others. These quantify tooth development from initial calcification to final root closure, as seen on radiographs.

Sexual development: peak height velocity

- Hägg and Taranger (1980) observed that menarche occurred a mean 1.1 years after peak height velocity (PHV).
- Menarche is a highly reliable but not absolute indicator that PHV has been reached or passed.
- Menarche occurs at a bone age of 13.1 years.
- Boys attain a 'pubertal voice' (the pitch of the voice had changed noticeably but had not yet acquired adult characteristics) 0.2 years before PHV, and the 'male voice' (pitch of the voice had acquired adult characteristics), 0.9 years after PHV.
- Tanner (1978) found that in males, breaking of the voice happens relatively late in puberty and is caused by the increased length of the vocal cords, which follows the growth of the larynx. Voice breaking is often a gradual process and is not reliable as a criterion of puberty. Facial hair appears in boys usually somewhat later than the PHV.

Correlation between dental development and other maturity indicators

Evidence so far indicates that the skeletal system, as well as height and the onset of puberty, develops largely independently of the dental system. Teeth are partly of epithelial origin, whereas bone is derived from the mesoderm. Serious endocrinopathies, although severely retarding somatic growth and maturation, exert only a minor effect on the dentition. Demirjian (1978) found a very low correlation between dental age (root development) and skeletal age.

General observations on somatic growth

- Growth is nutrition dependent, and a well-fed infant gains length before it gains weight.
- The pubertal growth spurt is governed by growth hormone and anabolic steroids (testosterone and oestrogens).
- Girls enter the growth spurt about 2 years earlier than boys; however, they complete the growth spurt only about a year earlier than boys.
- The growth spurt is of greater magnitude and of shorter duration in boys than girls, as testosterone has a greater anabolic effect than oestrogen.
- Growth ceases from the feet upwards, so limb growth stops before spine growth.
- The pubertal growth spurt adds 25 to 30 cm to final height over the childhood growth curve. Boys on average end up 12 to 13 cm taller than girls, as their growth spurt occurs after an additional 2 years of childhood growth.

Further reading

Bayley, N., Pinneau, S., 1952. Tables for predicting adult height from skeletal age. Journal of Pediatrics 14, 432–441.

Demirjian, A., 1978. Dentition. In: Falkner, F., Tanner, J.M. (Eds.), Human growth. 2: Postnatal growth. Plenum Press, New York, pp. 413–444.

Fishman, L.S., 1988. Radiographic evaluation of skeletal maturation: a clinically oriented method based on hand wrist films. Angle Orthodontist 52, 88–112.

Hägg, U., Taranger, J., 1980. Skeletal stages of the hand and wrist as indicators of the pubertal growth spurt. Acta Odontologica Scandinavica 38, 187–200.

Hassel, B.A., Farman, A.G., 1995. Skeletal maturation evaluation using cervical vertebrae. American Journal of Orthodontics and Dentofacial Orthopedics 107, 58–66.

Tanner, J.M., 1978. Fetus into man. Harvard University Press, Cambridge, MA.

Tanner, J.M., Gibbons, R.D., 1994. A computerized image analysis system for estimating Tanner–Whitehouse 2 bone age. Hormone Research 42, 282–887.

Tanner, J.M., Whitehouse, R.H., Cameron, W.A., et al., 1983. Assessment of skeletal maturity and prediction of adult height (TW2 method), second ed. Academic Press, London.

Growth charts

Angus C. Cameron ■ Richard P. Widmer ■ Benjamin Moran

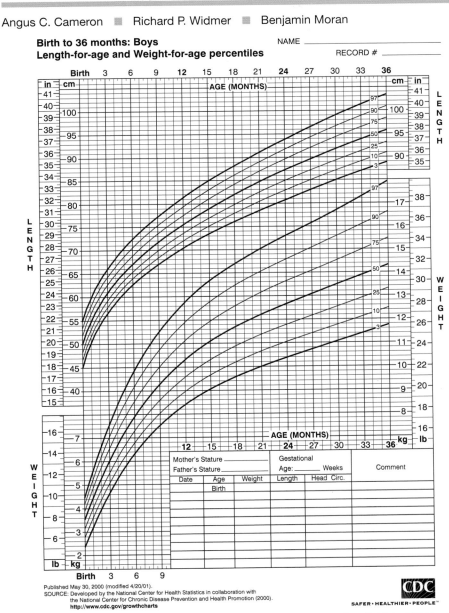

Figure L.1 Boys: Birth–36 months. Length-for-age and weight-for-age percentiles. (Published 30 May 2000; modified 20 April 2001. Developed by the National Center for Health Statistics in collaboration with the National Center for Chronic Disease Prevention and Health Promotion, 2000. Available: http://www.cdc.gov /growthcharts.)

531

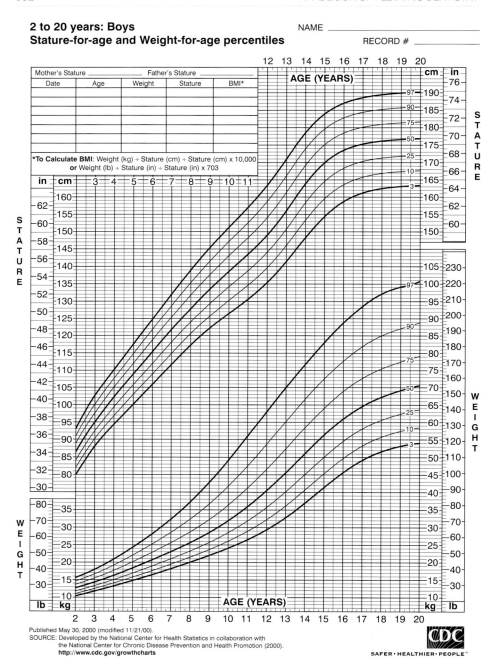

Figure L.2 Boys: Aged 2–20 years. Stature-for-age and weight-for-age percentiles. (Published 30 May 2000; modified 21 November 2000. Developed by the National Center for Health Statistics in collaboration with the National Center for Chronic Disease Prevention and Health Promotion, 2000. Available: http://www.cdc.gov /growthcharts.)

2 to 20 years: Boys
Body mass index-for-age percentiles

NAME _____

RECORD # _____

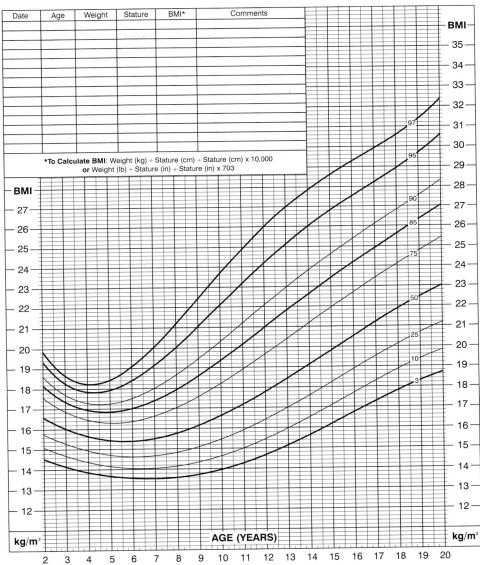

*To Calculate BMI: Weight (kg) ÷ Stature (cm) ÷ Stature (cm) x 10,000
or Weight (lb) ÷ Stature (in) ÷ Stature (in) x 703

AGE (YEARS)

Published May 30, 2000 (modified 10/16/00).
SOURCE: Developed by the National Center for Health Statistics in collaboration with
the National Center for Chronic Disease Prevention and Health Promotion (2000).
http://www.cdc.gov/growthcharts

SAFER · HEALTHIER · PEOPLE™

Figure L.3   Boys: Aged 2–20 years. Body mass index-for-age percentiles. (Published 30 May 2000; modified 16 October 2000. Developed by the National Center for Health Statistics in collaboration with the National Center for Chronic Disease Prevention and Health Promotion (2000), http://www.cdc.gov/growthcharts.)

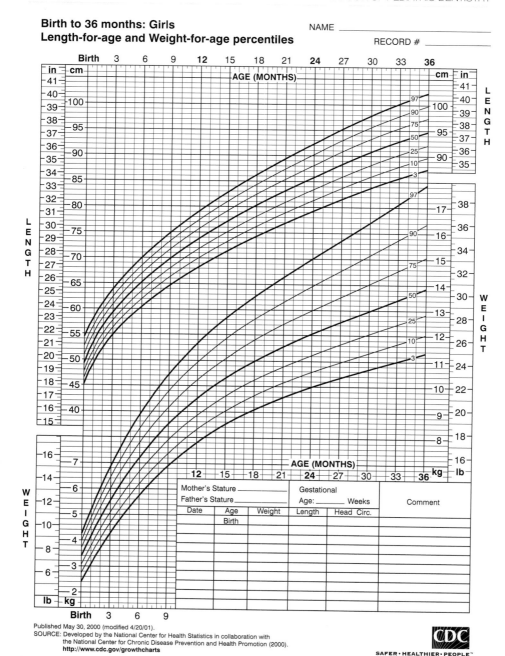

Birth to 36 months: Girls
Length-for-age and Weight-for-age percentiles

NAME _____

RECORD # _____

Published May 30, 2000 (modified 4/20/01).
SOURCE: Developed by the National Center for Health Statistics in collaboration with
the National Center for Chronic Disease Prevention and Health Promotion (2000).
http://www.cdc.gov/growthcharts

Figure L.4   Girls: Birth–36 months. Length-for-age and weight-for-age percentiles. (Published 30 May 2000; modified 20 April 2001. Developed by the National Center for Health Statistics in collaboration with the National Center for Chronic Disease Prevention and Health Promotion, 2000. Available: http://www.cdc.gov /growthcharts.)

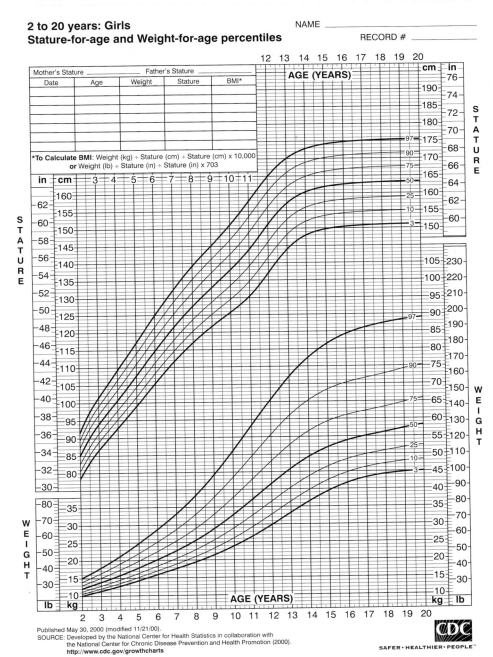

2 to 20 years: Girls
Stature-for-age and Weight-for-age percentiles

NAME _____

RECORD # _____

Published May 30, 2000 (modified 11/21/00).
SOURCE: Developed by the National Center for Health Statistics in collaboration with
the National Center for Chronic Disease Prevention and Health Promotion (2000).
http://www.cdc.gov/growthcharts

SAFER · HEALTHIER · PEOPLE™

Figure L.5 Girls: Aged 2–20 years. Stature-for-age and weight-for-age percentiles. (Published 30 May 2000; modified 21 November 2000. Developed by the National Center for Health Statistics in collaboration with the National Center for Chronic Disease Prevention and Health Promotion, 2000. Available: http://www.cdc.gov/growthcharts.)

2 to 20 years: Girls
Body mass index-for-age percentiles

NAME _____

RECORD # _____

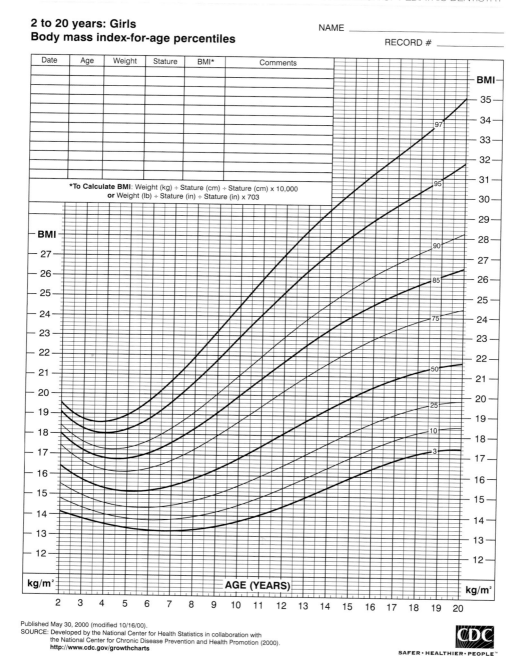

Published May 30, 2000 (modified 10/16/00).
SOURCE: Developed by the National Center for Health Statistics in collaboration with
the National Center for Chronic Disease Prevention and Health Promotion (2000).
http://www.cdc.gov/growthcharts

Figure L.6 Girls: Aged 2–20 years. Body mass index-for-age percentiles. (Published 30 May 2000; modified 16 October 2000. Developed by the National Center for Health Statistics in collaboration with the National Center for Chronic Disease Prevention and Health Promotion, 2000. Available: http://www.cdc.gov/growthcharts.)

Eruption dates of teeth

Angus C. Cameron ■ Richard P. Widmer ■ Benjamin Moran

Notes on eruption of teeth

All these values are based on work that was published over 50 years ago. At the time of this writing, there has been very little up-to-date work on the eruption of teeth. It should be noted that there is extreme variability within normal populations, and it is of more value to compare the eruption pattern of the whole dentition rather than one particular tooth. Eruption sequence is of particular importance and may be indicative of pathology (e.g., a supernumerary tooth blocking the eruption of a central incisor).

TABLE M.1 ■ Development of primary teeth

Tooth	Initiation (weeks in utero)	Calcification begins (weeks in utero)	Crown formation at birth (38–42 weeks)	Crown complete (months)	Eruption (months)
Central incisor	7	13–16	⅚ maxilla ⅗ mandible	1–3	6–9
Lateral incisor	7	14–16	⅔ maxilla ⅗ mandible	2–3	7–10
Canine	7.5	15–18	⅓	9	16–20
First molar	8	14.5–17	Cusps united Occlusal surface complete ½ to ¾ crown height	6	12–16
Second molar	10	16–23.5	Cusps united ¼ crown height	10–12	23–30

(From Logan, W.H., Kronfield, R., 1933. Development of the human jaw and surrounding structures from birth to the age of 15 years. Journal of the American Dental Association 20, 379–427; Shour, I., Massler, M., 1940. Studies in tooth development. The growth pattern of human teeth. Journal of the American Dental Association 27, 1918–1931.)

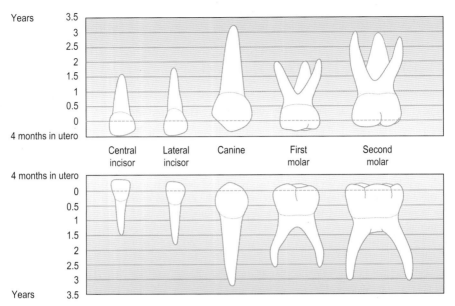

Figure M.1 Chronological development of primary dentition. (From Pindborg, J.J., 1970. Pathology of the dental hard tissues. WB Saunders, Philadelphia, with permission.)

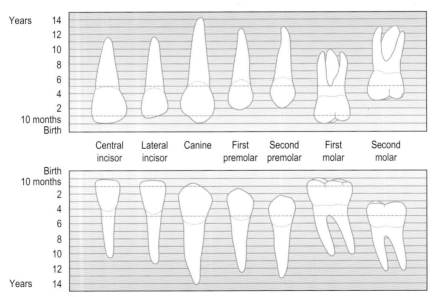

Figure M.2 Chronological development of permanent dentition. (From Pindborg, J.J., 1970. Pathology of the dental hard tissues. WB Saunders, Philadelphia, with permission.)

TABLE M.2 ■ **Development of permanent teeth**

Tooth	Initiation	Calcification begins	Crown complete (years)	Eruption (years)
Mandible				
Central incisor	5–5.25 miu	3–4 months	4–5	6–7
Lateral incisor	5–5.25 miu	3–4 months	4–5	7–8
Canine	5.5–6 miu	4–5 months	6–7	9–11
First premolar	Birth	1.75–2 years	5–6	10–12
Second premolar	7.5–8 months	2.25–2.5 years	6–7	11–12
First molar	3.5–4 miu	Birth	2.5–3	6–7
Second molar	8.5–9 months	2.5–3 years	7–8	11–13
Third molar	3.5–4 years	8–10	12–16	17–21
Maxilla				
Central incisor	5–5.25 miu	3–4 months	4–5	7–8
Lateral incisor	5–5.25 miu	11 months	4–5	8–9
Canine	5.5–6 miu	4–5 months	6–7	11–12
First premolar	Birth	1.25–1.75 years	5–6	10–11
Second	7.25–8 months	2–2.5 years	6–7	10–12
First molar	3.5–4 miu	Birth	2.5–3	6–7
Second molar	8.5–9 months	2.5–3 years	7–8	12–13
Third molar	3.5–4 years	7–9 years	12–16	17–25

miu, Months in utero.

Further reading

Logan, W.H., Kronfield, R., 1933. Development of the human jaw and surrounding structures from birth to the age of 15 years. Journal of the American Dental Association 20, 379–427.

Shour, I., Massler, M., 1940. Studies in tooth development. The growth pattern of human teeth. Journal of the American Dental Association 27, 1918–1931.

Construction of family pedigree

Angus C. Cameron ▦ Richard P. Widmer ▦ Benjamin Moran

Pedigree is a useful presentation of families in clinical notes. It displays information about past generations and the transmission of genetic traits through families. The symbols used in constructing pedigrees are shown in Figure N.1.

The affected individual at examination is termed the 'proband', and an arrow is placed indicating this patient. Generations are numbered with roman numerals, and arabic numbers are used to indicate individuals within each generation. An example of a family pedigree displaying a sex-linked transmission is shown in Figure N.2.

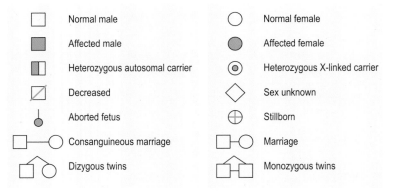

Figure N.1 Symbols used in the construction of pedigrees. (From Pindborg, J.J., 1970. Pathology of the dental hard tissues. WB Saunders, Philadelphia, with permission.)

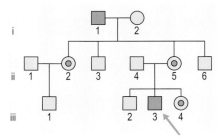

Figure N.2 A pedigree of a family with ectodermal dysplasia, demonstrating sex-linked inheritance. In the first generation, the grandfather (i1) of the proband (iii3) (*arrow*) had no hair, was hyperthermic and had only three permanent teeth. Of his offspring, all the females were heterozygotes (ii2 and ii5). The younger had sparse hair and eczema and was missing seven teeth, including the lower canines. It is important to note that there is no male-to-male transmission. The daughter then passed the mutation to one of her sons (iii3), who fully expresses the gene, and one of her daughters, who is a carrier. (From Pindborg, J.J., 1970. Pathology of the dental hard tissues. WB Saunders, Philadelphia, with permission.)

Calculating fluoride values for dental products

Angus C. Cameron ■ Richard P. Widmer ■ Benjamin Moran

The basic unit used for measuring and comparing fluoride products is parts per million (ppm). This is a water engineering term that has been adopted by the dental profession. One ppm is equal to 1 mg in 10^6 mg (or 1 kg). One ppm is 1 mg dissolved in 1 L of water; 1 L of water weighs 1 kg.

Some useful analogies for thinking about 1 ppm are as follows:

■ 1 inch in 16 miles.
■ 1 minute in 2 years.
■ 1 cent in $10 000.
■ 1 drop in 10 gallons
■ 1 mL in 1000 L.

The molecular weight ratio (MWR) is used to calculate the fluoride content of fluoride products. Most fluoride products are labelled with the concentration of the compound (e.g., 2% NaF), rather than the fluoride content. An exception to this labelling occurs with the 1.23% acidulated phosphate fluoride (APF) gels that are unusual in being labelled with the fluoride concentration (i.e., 1.23% F or 12 300 ppm F).

Sample calculations

SODIUM FLUORIDE

A NaF compound contains:

■ Na (atomic weight: 23) and F (atomic weight: 19)
■ NaF then contains $19 + 23 = 42$ (combined atomic weight for this compound).
■ F then represents $19/42 = 0.45$ (MWR for F).
■ Na represents $23/42 = 1.8$ (MWR for Na).

Consider a 2%NaF product:

To calculate the %F in this product, the numerical % concentration is multiplied by the MWR for F: $2 \times 0.45 = 0.91$%F.

To convert 0.91%F to ppm, multiply by 10^4 (because 1%F = 10 000 ppm F):

■ $0.91 \times 10^4 = 9100$ ppm F.

SODIUM MONOFLUOROPHOSPHATE

Na_2FPO_3:

■ 2Na (atomic weight: 46) and F (atomic weight: 19).
■ PO_3 (atomic weight .79).
■ For this compound the combined atomic weight is $46 + 19 + 79 = 144$.
■ F represents $19/144 = 0.132$% F.
■ A 0.76% sodium monofluorophosphate toothpaste contains: $0.76 \times 0.132 = 0.1$% F or 1000 ppm F.

COVID-19 and paediatric dentistry

Stephen Fayle

Commentary Stephen Fayle

The COVID-19 pandemic of 2020, caused by severe acute respiratory syndrome coronavirus 2 (SARS-CoV-2), has had a major impact across the full spectrum of healthcare in many parts of the globe. At the time of writing (September 2020), many countries are experiencing a 'second wave' of infection, and efforts are focussed on mitigating viral transmission, developing better treatments for the most severely ill and attempting to develop a suitable vaccine as rapidly as possible. In an effort to suppress viral transmission, social distancing and promotion of enhanced hand hygiene have been widely mandated. Many governments have also implemented extensive mitigation and suppression policies, often involving nationwide emergency stay-at-home/lockdown measures, to restrict unnecessary population movement and social interaction. This has been followed in many parts of the world by more targeted measures to control further outbreaks, the severity and extent of which have usually been informed by local and national incidence and prevalence data.

COVID-19 is a new disease, and many of the details of exactly how it spreads are still under investigation, but the main routes of infection seem to be via respiratory droplets and from contact with surfaces or objects previously contaminated by falling respiratory droplets of direct contact. As dentistry involves working in the respiratory tract, and some commonly used dental procedures generate aerosols, droplets and splatter (such as high-speed handpieces and ultrasonic scalers), the pandemic has produced major challenges to providers of oral healthcare and also those in the population in need of dental treatment. There has been major disruption to the provision of oral health care, both in severely limiting access and also because of the enhanced infection control processes required to mitigate the risk of infection during the delivery of dental treatment. This has been further complicated because in many individuals, the infection is either asymptomatic or very mild, and also some presymptomatic infected people can already be infectious. Hence, unless an individual has had a current positive coronavirus test, it is impossible to know with certainty whether or not an asymptomatic individual is infected.

Dental care for children is further complicated by a number of factors. Children suffering with active COVID-19 are often asymptomatic and are almost always brought to appointments by other family members. The significant reliance on aerosol-generating procedures (AGPs) and periods of restricted access to general anaesthesia during the worst phases of the pandemic have been important obstacles to care delivery. A significant proportion of children's dentistry clinics have open plan designs rather than individual surgeries.

Aerosol-generating procedures in dentistry

Dental clinicians operate close to a patient's respiratory tract and employ significant numbers of AGPs. Combinations of aerosol, droplets and splatter are generated by a range of operative dental procedures such as the use of high-speed air rotors. True aerosols comprise airborne particles under 5 µm (World Health Organization, 2014) and may carry virus particles (To et al., 2020);

however, the role of aerosols in the transmission of COVID-19 is currently unclear. Droplets and splatter potentially carry a greater viral load than aerosols and there is currently a greater consensus that these probably carry higher transmission risk.

Enhanced infection control measures

Whilst there is currently a paucity of scientific evidence addressing dental aerosols and associated viral transmission risk (Zemouri et al., 2017), the perceived risks associated with the provision of dental care have resulted in widespread adoption of additional measures to mitigate this risk. The exact measures employed vary considerably from one country/jurisdiction to another, but there are some common principles:

- Previsit planning and screening. Preoperative COVID-19 testing to screen children, and sometimes their parents, coupled with varying periods of self-isolation, has been widely used in some countries before admission to hospitals, but this is currently not in wide use in dentistry, often because of limited access to testing. Information about the dental appointment is often provided in advance, including advice not to attend if they have symptoms of COVID-19 or suspect they have come into contact with someone with COVID-19.
- Limiting accompanying adults with each child (usually to one).
- Temperature testing and COVID-19 screening questions on arrival.
- Hand cleansing, escorting of patients into and out of the clinic.
- Social distancing, measures to minimize waiting and contact with staff/fomites and hand disinfection. Mask/face coverings and pretreatment mouthrinses are advocated in some countries.
- Wider adoption of communication and consulting with parents/patients using telephone and internet-based video technologies.
- Enhanced personal protective equipment (PPE). Although there is wide consensus on the importance of strict observation of universal infection control precautions, and that enhanced PPE should be used when high-risk AGPs are planned, there is variation in exactly what procedures are deemed to constitute a 'high-risk AGP' and what 'enhanced' measures should be adopted in these circumstances. Use of a moisture-resistant IIR surgical mask, eye protection and single-use gloves during all patient contact is virtually universally mandated or endorsed. Other commonly endorsed/mandated measures for clinical staff where there is variation from one country to another include:
  - Wearing an FFP3, FFP2, N95 or similar respirators by clinical staff providing care during procedures perceived to carry high risk of transmission secondary to aerosol production.
  - Using full-face visors to protect from droplets and spatter.
  - Use of high-volume aspiration during perceived higher-risk AGPs.
  - Use of rubber dam where possible.
  - Wearing of moisture-resistant aprons or gowns.
  - 'Fallow time' between procedures to allow droplets to settle and enable effective cleaning of the environment. Fallow time can be reduced when air-changes are more frequent. Currently, in England, for example, a fallow time of 20 minutes is acceptable as long as surgery air-changes are greater than 10 to 12 per hour.
- Minimizing the delivery of traditional AGPs either by limiting these to special/urgent situations or by using other techniques less likely to cause aerosols/droplets. This has led to wider adoption of minimally invasive interventions, such as Hall crowns, intermediate glass ionomer cement restorations and silver diamine fluoride, and bonding techniques where the potential for aerosol generation during washing/drying is mitigated, or use of single-step bonding agents where washing is not necessary.

Social and economic impact

The prolonged reduction and, in some instances, interruption to dental services are likely to have had a significant detrimental effect on children's oral health, especially those with active disease or at high risk of developing disease. Evidence is emerging in some countries that waiting times for specialist paediatric dental care (already long in some parts of the world) have significantly increased, although the exact extent and impact of this on child oral health and well-being are as yet unknown. Paediatric dentists are facing considerable challenges balancing their desire to maintain a high standard of care for all their patients against the risks of viral transmission. In many countries, rapidly changing and evolving guidance/standards are making this even more of a challenge.

The pandemic has also brought with it serious economic pressures which have threatened the financial viability of practices and also limited some families' ability to pay for dental care.

Conclusion

At the time of writing this appendix, the exact timeline for this pandemic and the eventual impact, both in economic and health terms, are unknown. Such widespread and major disruption to modern healthcare systems is unprecedented, although dentistry has experienced a number of previous significant and disruptive infection control challenges including hepatitis B, new variant CJD and HIV/AIDS. Each of these previous challenges led to a revision of infection control standards in dentistry (often referred to as 'Universal Standards'), and this pandemic seems likely to lead to further revision. However, major upheaval has the potential to drive innovation and progress. The wider adoption of telephone and video to aid communication and oral health care, plus the use of alternative approaches to prevention and invasive dental treatment, may well continue as routine parts of the future paediatric dentistry oral health care armamentarium.

Although the future is currently even more uncertain than it normally is, paediatric dental teams will continue to focus on the well-being of their child patients and adapt to the challenges to delivering effective oral health care that the COVID-19 pandemic brings.

Stephen Fayle

Further reading

To, K.K., Tsang, O.T., Yip, C.C., et al., 2020. Consistent detection of 2019 novel coronavirus in saliva. Clinical Infectious Diseases 71 (15), 841–843.

World Health Organization, 2014. Infection prevention and control of epidemic and pandemic-prone acute respiratory infections in health care. WHO guidelines. Available https://www.who.int/csr/bioriskreduction/infection_control/publication/en/.

Zemouri, C., de Soet, H., Crielaard, W., et al., 2017. A scoping review on bioaerosols in healthcare and the dental environment. PLoS One 12, e0178007.

INDEX

Page numbers followed by 'f' indicate figures, 't' indicate tables, and 'b' indicate boxes.